Use this card to order extra copies of PDR® For Nonprescription Drugs

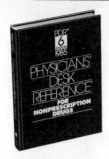

PDR For Nonprescription Drugs, 1985 is published in April, each year.

1 ☐ Send _____ copies of PDR For Nonprescription Drugs, 1985. My check is enclosed for $15.95 each.

2 ☐ Send _____ copies of PDR For Nonprescription Drugs, 1985. Bill me later for $17.95 each.

10% discount is granted for orders of 26 copies or more.

California and New Jersey residents add applicable sales tax.

Name _____

Institution _____

Street Address _____

City _____ State _____ Zip _____

Occupation _____

Signature _____

5N-AN-0

**MAIL THIS ORDER FORM,
IN AN ENVELOPE, TO:
PDR For Nonprescription Drugs
Box 2019
Mahopac, New York 10541**

DETACH ALONG DOTTED LINE

Use this card to order copies of PDR® For Ophthalmology

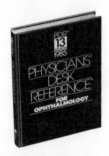

PDR For Ophthalmology 1985 was published in November, 1984.

1 ☐ Send _____ copies of PDR For Ophthalmology 1985. My check is enclosed for $21.95 each.

2 ☐ Send _____ copies of PDR For Ophthalmology 1985. Bill me later for $23.95 each.

10% discount is granted for orders of 26 copies or more.

California and New Jersey residents add applicable sales tax.

Name _____

Institution _____

Street Address _____

City _____ State _____ Zip _____

Occupation _____

Signature _____

5N-AN-0

**MAIL THIS ORDER FORM,
IN AN ENVELOPE, TO:
PDR For Ophthalmology
Box 2017
Mahopac, New York 10541**

DETACH ALONG DOTTED LINE

Use this card to order copies of Physicians' Desk Reference®

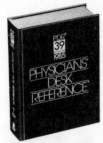

Physicians' Desk Reference is published in February, each year.

1 ☐ Send _____ copies of Physicians' Desk Reference, 1985. My check is enclosed for $25.95 each.

2 ☐ Send _____ copies of Physicians' Desk Reference, 1985. Bill me later for $27.95 each.

3 ☐ Send _____ copies of the 1985 PDR Supplements at $2.99 (Check must accompany order).

10% discount is granted for orders of 26 copies or more.

California and New Jersey residents add applicable sales tax.

Name _____

Institution _____

Street Address _____

City _____ State _____ Zip _____

Occupation _____

Signature _____

5N-AN-0

**MAIL THIS ORDER FORM,
IN AN ENVELOPE, TO:
Physicians' Desk Reference
Box 2017
Mahopac, New York 10541**

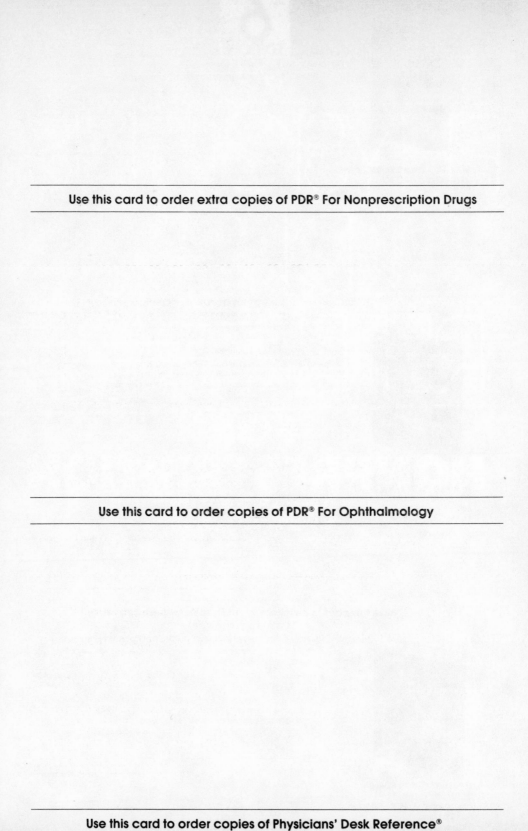

Use this card to order extra copies of PDR® For Nonprescription Drugs

Use this card to order copies of PDR® For Ophthalmology

Use this card to order copies of Physicians' Desk Reference®

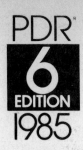

PDR®
6
EDITION
1985

PHYSICIANS' DESK REFERENCE

FOR NONPRESCRIPTION DRUGS

Publisher: EDWARD R. BARNHART

Director of Production: JEROME M. LEVINE

Managing Editor: BARBARA B. HUFF

Associate Editor: WILLIAM J. KNIPPING

Medical Consultant: IRVING M. LEVITAS, M.D.

Manager of Production Services: ELIZABETH H. CARUSO

Index Editor: ADELE L. DOWD

Editorial Assistants: F. EDYTHE PATERNITI
YVONNE HARLEY

Director of Printing: RALPH G. PELUSO

National Sales Manager: GARY J. GYSS

Account Managers: SALLY H. BERRIMAN
DAVID M. MJOLSNESS
PETER J. MURPHY
DEBRA E. REYNOLDS

Circulation Director: THOMAS S. KRAEMER

Assistant Circulation Director: LESLIE A. CLARK

Fulfillment Manager: JAMES SCIURBA

Research Director: CHARLOTTE SIBLEY

Officers of Medical Economics Company Inc.: Chairman and President, Charles P. Daly; Executive Vice President, Thomas J. McGill; Senior Vice Presidents: Theodore A. Maurer, Joseph M. Valenzano Jr.; Senior Vice President/Secretary, Stephen J. Sorkenn; Vice Presidents: Howard Clutterbuck, William J. Reynolds, Lewis A. Scaliti, Kathleen A. Starke.

ISBN 0-87489-880-3

Foreword to the Sixth Edition

Responsible self-medication is becoming ever more important in the health care of Americans. Self-medication continues to offer quick and inexpensive relief for minor health discomforts. Consumers of all socioeconomic levels have found the convenient availability and low cost of over-the-counter medicines (OTCs) an invaluable and welcome adjunct to the professional health care system.

In 1983, the final advisory panel report in the OTC Review (the government's exhaustive evaluation of the ingredients and labeling in OTC products) was published, completing the first phase of the Review. When the administrative phase of the Review is completed, the U.S. Food and Drug Administration (FDA) will have published some 75 "Final Monographs" defining which ingredients, dosages, and combinations, and labeling are "generally recognized" as safe and effective. At that time, OTC products not falling within the monograph criteria will need to obtain special approval from the FDA to continue to be considered "recognized" as safe and effective.

Of great interest to consumers and health professionals alike is a trend that began with the OTC Review, and is now continuing through several regulatory avenues: that of transferring some ingredients and dosages from prescription to OTC (nonprescription) status. This is broadening the range of effective products available to consumers for self-medication, while improved labeling helps ensure appropriate use.

The PHYSICIAN'S DESK REFERENCE® For NONPRESCRIPTION DRUGS is published annually by Medical Economics Company Inc., with the cooperation of the manufacturers whose products are described in the Product Identification, Product Information and Diagnostics, Devices and Medical Aids Sections. Its purpose is to make available essential information on nonprescription products.

The function of the Publisher is the compilation, organization, and distribution of this information. Each product description has been prepared by the manufacturer, and edited and approved by the manufacturer's medical department, medical director, and/or medical consultant. In organizing and presenting the material in PHYSICIANS' DESK REFERENCE® For NONPRESCRIPTION DRUGS, the Publisher is providing all the information made available to PHYSICIANS' DESK REFERENCE® For NONPRESCRIPTION DRUGS by manufacturers. Besides the information given here, additional information on any product may be obtained by the manufacturer. In making this material available it should be understood that the Publisher is not advocating the use of any product described herein.

EDWARD R. BARNHART
Publisher

HOW TO USE THIS EDITION

If you want to find . . .	And you already know . . .	Here's where to look . . .
the brand name of a product	the manufacturer's name	White Section: Manufacturers' Index
	its generic name	Yellow Section: Active Ingredients Index*
the manufacturer's name	the product's brand name	Pink Section: Product Name Index*
	the product's generic name	Yellow Section: Active Ingredients Index*
essential product information, such as: active ingredients indications actions warnings drug interaction precautions symptoms & treatment of oral overdosage dosage & administration how supplied	the product's brand name	Pink Section: Product Name Index*
	the product's generic name	Yellow Section: Active ingredients Index*
a product with a particular chemical action	the chemical action	Yellow Section: Active Ingredients Index*
a product with a particular active ingredient	the active ingredient	Yellow Section: Active Ingredients Index*
a similar acting product	the product classification	Blue Section: Product Category Index*
generic name of a brand name product	the product's brand name	Pink Section: Product Name Index. Generic name will be found under "Active Ingredients" in Product Information Section.

In the Pink, Blue and Yellow Sections, the page numbers following the product name refer to the pages in the Product Identification Section where the product is pictured and the Product Information Section where the drug is comprehensively described.

Contents

SECTION 1
Manufacturers' Index

The manufacturers whose names appear in this index have provided information concerning their products in either the Product Information Section, Product Identification Section, or the Diagnostics, Devices and Medical Aids Section.

Included in this index are the names and addresses of manufacturers, individuals or departments to whom you may address inquiries, a partial list of products as well as emergency telephone numbers wherever available.

The symbol ◆ indicates that the product is shown in the Product Identification Section.

PAGE

ABBOTT LABORATORIES—   **502**
ABBOTT PHARMACEUTICALS, INC.
North Chicago, IL 60064
    Address inquiries to:
Medical Director   (312) 937-7069
    Distribution Centers
ATLANTA
  Stone Mountain, GA 30302
  P.O. Box 5049   (404) 493-8330
CHICAGO
  Abbott Park
  North Chicago, IL 60064
  P.O. Box 68   (312) 937-5153
DALLAS
  Dallas, TX 75265
  P.O. Box 225295   (214) 387-1350
LOS ANGELES
  Los Angeles, CA 90060
  60162 Terminal Annex
       (213) 582-6341
PHILADELPHIA
  King of Prussia, PA 19406
  920 Eighth Ave., East
       (215) 265-9100
    OTC Products Available
Optilets-500
Optilets-M-500
Surbex-750 with Iron
Surbex-750 with Zinc
Surbex-T

ADRIA LABORATORIES   **403, 502**
Division of Erbamont Inc.
    Administrative Offices
5000 Post Road
Dublin, OH 43017

(◆ **Shown in Product Identification Section**)

PAGE

    Mailing Address
P.O. Box 16529
Columbus, OH 43216

    Address inquiries to:
Medical Dept.   (614) 764-8100
    OTC Products Available
efficin
Epsilan-M Capsules
Evac-Q-Kit
Evac-Q-Kwik
◆Modane
Modane Bulk Powder
◆Modane Plus Tablets
Modane Soft Capsules
◆Myoflex Creme
Pektamalt
Ratio Tablets
Taloin Ointment
W-T Lotion
Xylo-Pfan

ALBERTO-CULVER COMPANY   **506**
2525 Armitage
Melrose Park, IL 60160
    Address inquiries to:
Consumer Relations Dept.
       (312) 450-3163
    OTC Products Available
Mrs. Dash
SugarTwin

ALLERGAN   **403, 506**
PHARMACEUTICALS, INC.
2525 Dupont Drive
Irvine, CA 92713

PAGE

    Address Inquiries to:
Customer Service   (714) 752-4500
  For Medical Emergencies Contact:
Medical Research Dept.
       (714) 752-4500
    OTC Products Available
◆Lacri-Lube S.O.P.
Liquifilm Forte
◆Liquifilm Tears
◆Prefrin Liquifilm
◆Tears Plus

ALTANA INC.
See E. FOUGERA & CO. and
PHARMADERM
60 Baylis Road
Melville, NY 11747

AMERICAN HYGIENIC   **403, 507**
LABORATORIES INC.
555 Arthur Godfrey Road
Miami, FL 33140

    Address inquiries to:
Ben Grenald   (305) 538-7729
       (305) 673-8805
    OTC Products Available
◆Shuttle Blemish Discs
◆Shuttle First Aid Spray
◆Shuttle Lotion

AMES DIVISION,   **403, 734**
MILES LABORATORIES, INC.
P.O. Box 70
Elkhart, IN 46515

Address Inquiries to:
Customer Services   (219) 264-8901
For Medical Emergencies Contact:
Medical Department   (219) 264-8444
     After Hours   (219) 264-8111
OTC Products Available
◆Microstix-Nitrite Kit
Saltex
◆Visidex II Reagent Strips

ANABOLIC LABORATORIES, INC.   **507**
17802 Gillette Avenue
Irvine, CA 92714
Address inquiries to:
Georgiana Hennessy   (714) 546-8901
OTC Products Available
Ana-Pro (protein products)
Aqua-A
Aved-Eze
Aved-Gest
Aved-M
B6-Plus
B12-Plus
CPA
Cal-M
Calpadon
Cholagest
Chromease
Dermagen
Digestaid
Enhance (Vitamin E Topical)
Flexamide
Hy-C-3000
I-O-Plexadine
Immunase
K-Orotate
Lax Special
Lipall-Plus
Lysamin-C
Nutra-Cal
O-A-Crine
Osatate
Pro-Enz
Prostana
Sedaphan
Selenace
Sofn
Tercopan
Tri-88
Tri-Adrenopan
Tri-B3
Tri-B-Plex
Tri-C-500
Tryptophan-250
Vasotate
Vitamin C Wafer
Zinotate
Zymain

APOTHECARY PRODUCTS,   **403, 734**
INC.
11531 Rupp Drive
Burnsville, MN 55337
Address inquiries to:
Order Dept.   1 (800) 328-2742
        or (612) 890-1940
OTC Products Available
Custom-Imprinted Compliance Aids
Daily Pill Caddy
Drug Scanner (Controlled)
Eye Care Accessories
◆Ezy-Dose Compliance Products
◆Ezy-Dose Medicine Spoon
◆Ezy-Dose Nitro-Fresh Nitroglycerine Pill
   Holder
◆Ezy-Dose Oral Syringe with
   Dosage-Korc
◆Ezy-Dose 7-Day Pill Reminder
◆Ezy-Dose Spoon Dropper
Gallon-Spenser
Glass Medicine Dropper
Medication Twin Spoon
Medichron
Medicine Nursers
◆Medi-Set
Medispenser
◆Medtime-Minder
Normaline 250 mg Saline Solution
Oral Thermometer
Patient Advisory Leaflets
Patient Counseling System
Penaten Cream
Pill-Crusher

Pill-Pen
Pill Reminder (Electronic)
Pilltaker Cup
Reconstitube
Seaties Hygiene Products
Stat Count 30
Syringe Magnifier
Tablet Crusher
Warning Labels

ARCO PHARMACEUTICALS, INC.   **507**
105 Orville Drive
Bohemia, NY 11716
Address inquiries to:
Professional Service Dept.
                 (516) 567-9500
OTC Products Available
Arco-Cee Tablets
Arco-Lase Tablets
Arcoret Tablets
Arcoret w/Iron Tablets
Arcotinic Tablets
Co-Gel Tablets
Mega-B
Megadose

ARIZONA NATURAL PRODUCTS   **508**
7750 East Evans, #3
Scottsdale, AZ 85260
Address inquiries to:
      (800) 821-1989, Ext. 333
For Medical Emergencies Contact:
Mike Hanna   (602) 991-4414
OTC Products Available
Arizona Natural Odorless Garlic

B. F. ASCHER & COMPANY, INC.   **508**
15501 West 109th Street
Lenexa, KS 66219
Mailing Address: P.O. Box 827
Kansas City, MO 64141
Address inquiries to:
Joan F. Bowen   (913) 888-1880
For Medical Emergencies Contact:
Robert C. Mullins, R.Ph.
                 (913) 888-1880
OTC Products Available
Ayr Saline Nasal Drops
Ayr Saline Nasal Mist
Dalca Decongestant/Analgesic Tablets
Mobigesic Analgesic Tablets
Mobisyl Analgesic Creme
Soft 'N Soothe Anti-Itch Creme
Unilax Laxative Tablets

ASTRA PHARMACEUTICAL   **404, 508**
PRODUCTS, INC.
50 Otis Street
Westboro, MA 01581-4428
Address inquiries to:
Roy E. Hayward, Jr.   (617) 366-1100
For Medical Emergencies Contact:
Dr. Joseph C. Oakley   (617) 366-1100
OTC Products Available
◆Xylocaine Ointment 2.5%

AYERST LABORATORIES   **404, 509**
Division of American Home Products
Corp.
685 Third Ave.
New York, NY 10017
For Medical Information
Business hours only (9:00 A.M. to
5:00 P.M.), call   (212) 878-5900
For Medical Emergency Information
After hours or on weekends, call
             (212) 986-1000
             (212) 878-5000
             (212) 878-5900
Regional Sales Offices
South Plainfield, NJ 07080
4000 Hadley Rd.
          (201) 754-6220 (NJ)
          (212) 964-3903 (NY)
Rockville, MD 20852
6252 Montrose Rd.   (301) 984-9140
Chamblee, GA (Atlanta) 30341
3600 American Dr.   (404) 451-9578
          (404) 457-2510
Mobile, AL 36617
1110 Montlimar Dr., Suite 720
          (205) 344-1282
Mesquite, TX (Dallas) 75149
3601 Executive Blvd. (214) 285-6085
          (214) 285-8741

Ontario, CA 91764
2151 East D Street, Suite 121C
          (714) 984-2426
Foster City, CA 94404
1147 Chess Dr.   (415) 574-6065
Overland Park, KS 66214
10300 W. 103rd St.
Bldg. F, Suite 302 F, Suite 302
10300 W. 103rd St. (913) 492-0802
Chicago, IL 60648
7545 N. Natchez Ave.
          (312) 647-8948
          (312) 647-8840
Lakewood, OH (Cleveland) 44107
14701 Detroit Ave., Suite 440
          (216) 226-4128
          (216) 226-4274
Blue Ash, OH (Cincinnati) 45242
West Lake Center
4555 Lake Forest Dr., Suite 460
          (513) 563-0040
Springfield, MA 01115
Baybank Tower, Suite 1906
P.O. Box 15707
1500 Main Street   (413) 737-4594
Distribution Centers
Chamblee, GA 30341
3600 American Dr.   (404) 457-2518
Mesquite, TX 75149
3601 Executive Blvd. (214) 285-8741
Los Angeles, CA 90061
12833 S. Spring St.
          (213) 321-5550/1/2
Lenexa, KS 66210
10700 Pflumm Rd.   (913) 888-4310
Chicago, IL 60648
7545 N. Natchez Ave.
          (312) 763-0888 (Chicago)
          (312) 647-8840/1 (Niles)
Cleveland, OH 44135
15620 Industrial Pkwy.
          (216) 267-9090
OTC Products Available
Beminal-500
Beminal Forte w/Vitamin C
◆Beminal Stress Plus with Iron
◆Beminal Stress Plus with Zinc
Clusivol Capsules & Syrup
Clusivol 130 Tablets
◆Dermoplast
Enzactin Cream
◆Extra Strength Riopan Plus Suspension
◆Kerodex Cream 51 (for dry or oily
   work)
◆Kerodex Cream 71 (for wet work)
Larylgan Throat Spray
Riopan Antacid Chew Tablets
◆Riopan Antacid Suspension
Riopan Antacid Swallow Tablets
Riopan Rollpacks
Riopan Plus Chew Tablets
Riopan Plus Rollpacks
◆Riopan Plus Suspension
◆Riopan Plus Suspension - Extra
   Strength

BAKER/CUMMINS   **510**
Div. of Key Pharmaceuticals, Inc.
P.O. Box 693670
Miami, FL 33269-0670
          (305) 652-2276
Address inquiries to:
R. M. Scroggins
OTC Products Available
Complex 15 Moisturizing Cream &
   Lotion
P&S Liquid
P&S Plus
P&S Shampoo
Ultra Mide 25 Moisturizer Lotion
Xseb Shampoo
Xseb-T Shampoo

W. A. BAUM COMPANY, INC.   **735**
620 Oak Street
Copiague, NY 11726
Address inquiries to:
William A. Baum, Jr.   (516) 226-3940
OTC Products Available
Hi/Lo Baumanometer Blood Pressure
   Kit

BEACH PHARMACEUTICALS 404, 511
Division of Beach Products, Inc.
Executive Office
5220 S. Manhattan Ave.
Tampa, FL 33681   (813) 839-6565
Manufacturing and Distribution
Main St. at Perimeter Rd.
Conestee, SC 29605
           Toll Free 1-(800) 845-8210
Address inquiries to:
Victor De Oveo, R Ph, V.P., Sales
                       (803) 277-7282
Richard Stephen Jenkins, Exec. V.P.
                       (813) 839-6565
OTC Products Available
◆Beelith Tablets

**BECTON DICKINSON CONSUMER 511
PRODUCTS**
365 West Passaic Street
Rochelle Park, NJ 07662
Address inquiries to:
Consumer Service   (201) 368-7300
Toll Free Information Line
                       (800) 223-1134
OTC Products Available
B-D Glucose Tablets
Cankaid
Mercurochrome II

BEECHAM PRODUCTS   512, 735
P.O. Box 1467
Pittsburgh, PA 15230
Address inquiries to:
Professional Services Dept.
                     (800) BEECHAM
                     (412) 928-1050
OTC Products Available
Acu-Test In-Home Pregnancy Test
B.F.I. Antiseptic First-Aid Powder
Children's Hold
Cuprex
Deep-Down Pain Relief Rub
Eno Sparkling Antacid
FemIron Tablets
FemIron Multi-Vitamins and Iron
Geritol Complete Tablets
Geritol Liquid - High Potency Iron &
   Vitamin Tonic
Hold
Massengill Disposable Douche
Massengill Disposable Medicated
   Douche
Massengill Liquid Concentrate
Massengill Powder
N'ICE Medicated Sugarless Cough
   Lozenges
S.T.37
Scott's Emulsion
Serutan Concentrated Powder
Serutan Concentrated Powder - Fruit
   Flavored
Serutan Toasted Granules
Sominex Pain Relief Formula
Sominex 2
Sucrets (Regular and Mentholated)
Sucrets Children's Cherry Flavored
   Sore Throat Lozenges
Sucrets - Cold Decongestant Formula
Sucrets Cough Control Formula
Sucrets Maximum Strength
   Thermotabs
Vivarin Stimulant Tablets

BEIERSDORF, INC.   518
BDF Plaza
P.O. Box 5529
Norwalk, CT 06856-5529
Address Inquiries to:
Mr. Chauncey O. Johnstone
                     (203) 853-8008
Branch Offices
Bell, CA 90201
5651 Rickenbacker Rd.
                     (213) 264-7042
OTC Products Available
Aquaphor
Coverlet
Coverlet Eye Occlusor
Elastoplast
Eucerin Cleansing Bar
Eucerin Creme
Eucerin Lotion

Gelocast
Mediplast

BIGELOW-CLARK INC.   519
360 Meacham Avenue
Elmont, NY 11003
Address inquiries to:
                     (516) 775-5670
OTC Products Available
Work Out

BIO PRODUCTS, INC.   404, 519
55 Post Road West
Westport, CT 06880
Address Inquiries to:
J. H. Phelps   203-222-7645
For Medical Emergencies Contact:
J. H. Phelps   203-222-7645
Branch Offices
(Sales) Birmingham, AL 35216
2820 Columbiana Road
Suite 210   205-822-5970
(Distribution) Amityville, NY 11701
369 Bayview Avenue   516-789-1244
OTC Products Available
◆Q-vel Muscle Relaxant Pain Reliever

BLISTEX INC.   404, 519
1800 Swift Drive
Oak Brook, IL 60521
                     (312) 654-2870
                     (800) 323-7343
Address inquiries to:
Vice President, Technical Services
For Medical Emergencies Contact:
Manager, Quality Control
OTC Products Available
Blistex Lip Conditioner
◆Blistex Medicated Lip Ointment
Blistik Medicated Lip Balm
◆Foille First Aid Liquid, Ointment &
   Spray
◆Foille Plus First Aid Spray
Ivarest Medicated Cream & Lotion
◆Kank•A Medicated Formula

BLOCK DRUG COMPANY, INC.   521
257 Cornelison Avenue
Jersey City, NJ 07302
Address inquiries to:
Susan Stern   (201) 434-3000
For Medical Emergencies Contact:
James Gingold   (201) 434-3000
OTC Products Available
BC Powder
Nytol Tablets
Promise Toothpaste
Sensodyne Toothpaste
Sensodyne-F Toothpaste
Tegrin for Psoriasis Lotion & Cream
Tegrin Medicated Shampoo

**BOEHRINGER INGELHEIM   404, 522
PHARMACEUTICALS, INC.**
90 East Ridge
P.O. Box 368
Ridgefield, CT 06877
Address inquiries to:
Medical Services Dept.
                     (203) 438-0311
OTC Products Available
◆Dulcolax Suppositories
◆Dulcolax Tablets
◆Nōstril
◆Nōstrilla Long Acting Nasal
   Decongestant

**BOEHRINGER MANNHEIM   735
DIAGNOSTICS, INC.**
Bio-Dynamics Division
9115 Hague Road
Indianapolis, IN 46250
Address inquiries to:
                     (317) 845-2000
OTC Products Available
Accu-Chek bG Blood Glucose Monitor
Chemstrip bG Blood Glucose Test
Chemstrip bG Blood Glucose Test Kit
Chemstrip K Urine Ketones Test
Chemstrip uG Urine Glucose Test
Chemstrip uGK Urine Glucose &
   Ketones Test

**JOHN A. BORNEMAN AND   404, 524
SONS, INC.**
1208 Amosland Road
Norwood, PA 19074
Address inquiries to:
Jay P. Borneman, Vice President
                     (215) 532-2035
For Medical Emergencies Contact:
Technical Services Department
                     (215) 532-2035
OTC Products Available
◆Oscillococcinum

BRISTOL LABORATORIES   524
(Div. of Bristol-Myers Co.)
Thompson Rd. P.O. Box 4755
Syracuse, NY 13221-4755
                     (315) 432-2000
Address medical inquiries to:
Dept. of Medical Services
(315) 432-2838 or (315) 432-2000
*Orders may be placed by calling the
   following toll free numbers:*
Within New York State
                     1-(800) 962-7200
Continental U.S.   1-(800) 448-7700
Alaska - Hawaii   1-(800) 448-1100
*Mail orders and all inquiries should be
   sent to:*
Bristol Laboratories
Order Entry Department
P.O. Box 4755
Syracuse, NY 13221-4755
OTC Products Available
Naldecon-CX Suspension
Naldecon-DX Pediatric Syrup
Naldecon-EX Pediatric Drops

BRISTOL-MYERS PRODUCTS 405, 525
(Div. of Bristol-Myers Co.)
345 Park Avenue
New York, NY 10154
Address inquiries to:
Dr. Walter B. Elvers
In emergencies call:
Day   (212) 546-2752
Night   (212) 546-4700
OTC Products Available
Ammens Medicated Powder
◆Arthritis Strength Bufferin Analgesic
B.Q Cold Tablets
Ban Basic Antiperspirant
Ban Big Ball Antiperspirant
Ban Cream Antiperspirant
Ban Roll-on Antiperspirant
Body on Tap Shampoo and Conditioner
◆Bufferin Analgesic Tablets and
   Capsules
◆Comtrex Capsules
◆Comtrex Liquid
◆Comtrex Tablets
◆Congespirin Aspirin-Free Chewable Cold
   Tablets for Children
◆Congespirin Chewable Cold Tablets for
   Children
◆Congespirin Cough Syrup
◆Congespirin for Children Cough Syrup
◆Congespirin Liquid Cold Medicine
◆Excedrin Analgesic Capsules & Tablets
◆Excedrin P.M. Analgesic Sleeping Aid
◆Extra-Strength Bufferin Capsules &
   Tablets
◆Extra Strength Datril Capsules &
   Tablets
◆4-Way Cold Tablets
◆4-Way Long Acting Nasal Spray
4-Way Mentholated Nasal Spray
◆4-Way Nasal Spray
Minit-Rub Analgesic Balm
Mum Cream Deodorant
◆No Doz Keep Alert Tablets
◆Nuprin
Pazo Hemorrhoid Ointment/
   Suppositories
Score Hair Cream
Tickle Antiperspirant
Ultra Ban Aerosol
Ultra Ban Roll-on
Ultra Ban Solid Antiperspirant
Vitalis Dry Texture Hair Groom
Vitalis Hair Groom Liquid
Vitalis Hair Groom Tube

(◆ Shown in Product Identification Section)

Vitalis Regular Hold Hair Spray
Vitalis Super Hold Hair Spray

BURROUGHS WELLCOME CO. 406, 529
3030 Cornwallis Road
Research Triangle Park, NC 27709
Address Inquiries to:
Mr. C. A. Parish, Jr. (919) 248-3000
Branch Offices
Burlingame, CA 94010
1760 Rollins Rd. (415) 697-5630
OTC Products Available
Actidil Tablets & Syrup
◆Actifed Tablets & Syrup
Borofax Ointment
◆Empirin
Fedrazil Tablets
Marezine Tablets
◆Neosporin Ointment
Polysporin Ointment
◆Sudafed Cough Syrup
◆Sudafed Plus Tablets & Syrup
◆Sudafed S.A. Capsules
◆Sudafed Tablets and Syrup
◆Sudafed Tablets, Adult Strength
Wellcome Lanoline

CAMPBELL LABORATORIES INC. 532
300 East 51st Street
New York, NY 10022
Address Inquiries to:
Richard C. Zahn, President
P.O. Box 812, FDR Station
New York, NY 10150
(212) 688-7684
OTC Products Available
Herpecin-L Cold Sore Lip Balm

CARNATION COMPANY 533
5045 Wilshire Blvd.
Los Angeles, CA 90036
Address Inquiries to:
Ron Scott (213) 932-6535
OTC Products Available
Carnation Do-It-Yourself Diet Plan
Carnation Instant Breakfast
Carnation Nonfat Dry Milk
Slender Diet Food For Weight Control (Instant)
Slender Diet Meal Bars For Weight Control
Slender Diet Meal For Weight Control (Canned)

CARTER PRODUCTS 406, 534, 737
Division of Carter-Wallace, Inc.
767 Fifth Avenue
New York, NY 10153 (212) 758-4500
OTC Products Available
◆Answer At-Home Early Pregnancy Test Kit
◆Carter's Little Pills

CHATTEM CONSUMER PRODUCTS 407, 534
Division of Chattem, Inc.
1715 West 38th Street
Chattanooga, TN 37409
Address Inquiries to:
Joan Gutmann (615) 821-4571
OTC Products Available
Black-Draught Granulated
Black-Draught Lax-Senna Tablets
Black-Draught Syrup
Blis-To-Sol Liquid
Blis-To-Sol Powder
Pamprin Maximum Cramp Relief Formula Capsules & Tablets
Pamprin Tablets
◆PREMESYN PMS
Soltice Quick-Rub

CHURCH & DWIGHT CO., INC. 534
20 Kingsbridge Road
Piscataway, NJ 08854
Address inquiries to:
Mr. Stephen Lajoie (609) 683-5900
For Medical Emergencies Contact:
Mr. Stephen Lajoie (609) 683-5900
OTC Products Available
Arm & Hammer Pure Baking Soda

CIBA CONSUMER PHARMACEUTICALS 407, 535
Division of CIBA-GEIGY Corporation
Raritan Plaza III
Edison, NJ 08837
Address inquiries to:
(201) 225-6000
OTC Products Available
◆Acutrim Precision Release Tablets
Acutrim II
◆Slow Fe Tablets

CIBA PHARMACEUTICAL COMPANY 407, 536
Div. of CIBA-GEIGY Corporation
556 Morris Avenue
Summit, NJ 07901 (201) 277-5000
Shipping Branches
Eastern
14 Henderson Drive
West Caldwell, NJ 07006
(201) 575-6510
Central
7530 North Natchez Ave.
Niles, IL 60648 (312) 647-9332
Chicago, IL (312) 763-8700
Western
12850 Moore Street
Cerritos, CA 90701 (213) 404-2651
OTC Products Available
◆Nupercainal Cream & Ointment
◆Nupercainal Suppositories
◆Privine Nasal Solution
◆Privine Nasal Spray
Vioform Cream & Ointment

COLGATE-PALMOLIVE COMPANY 407, 537
A Delaware Corporation
300 Park Avenue
New York, NY 10022
Address inquiries to:
Consumers:
Consumer Affairs
300 Park Avenue
New York, NY 10022
(212) 310-2000
Physicians:
Medical Director
909 River Road
Piscataway, NJ 08854
(201) 878-7500
For Medical Emergencies Contact:
9 AM to 5 PM (201) 878-7500
5 PM to 9 AM (201) 547-2500
OTC Products Available
Colgate Dental Cream
◆Colgate MFP Fluoride Gel
◆Colgate MFP Fluoride Toothpaste
Colgate Toothbrushes
Curad Bandages
Dermassage Dish Liquid
◆Fluorigard Anti-Cavity Dental Rinse
Mersene Denture Cleanser
Ultra Brite Toothpaste

COMBE INCORPORATED 407, 538
1101 Westchester Avenue
White Plains, NY 10604
Address inquiries to:
Teresa C. Infantino (914) 694-5454
For Medical Emergencies Contact:
Mark K. Taylor (914) 694-5454
OTC Products Available
◆Gynecort Antipruritic 0.5% Hydrocortisone Acetate Creme
◆Lanabiotic First Aid Ointment
◆Lanacane Medicated Creme
◆Lanacort Anti-Itch Hydrocortisone Acetate 0.5% Creme and Ointment
◆Vagisil External Feminine Itching Medication

COMMERCE DRUG COMPANY 408, 539
Division of Del Laboratories, Inc.
565 Broad Hollow Road
Farmingdale, NJ 11735
Address inquiries to:
Peter Liman, V.P., Marketing
(516) 293-7070
OTC Products Available
Auro Ear Drops
◆Baby Orajel

Orajel, Maximum Strength
◆Orajel Mouth-Aid
◆Stye Ophthalmic Ointment

CONSOLIDATED CHEMICAL, INC 540
3224 S. Kingshighway Blvd.
St. Louis, MO 63139
Address Inquiries to:
John C. Brereton, Pres.
(314) 772-4610
For Medical Emergencies Contact:
Norman A. Van Rees (314) 772-4610
OTC Products Available
CC-500 Body Wash and Shampoo
Consept Skin and Hair Cleanser
Consol Concentrate Skin Cleanser
Formula Magic Lubricating Body Talc
GCP Shampoo, Geriatric Shampoo
Loving Lather Professional Hand Cleanser
New Consol "20" Skin Cleanser
Perineal/Ostomy Spray Cleaner
Satin Body Wash and Shampoo
Shower Team Body Wash and Shampoo
Skin Magic Lotion
Swirlsoft Whirlpool Moisturizer Additive

CREIGHTON PRODUCTS CORPORATION 409, 540
a Sandoz Company
(see also Ex-Lax Pharmaceutical Co., Inc.)
605 Third Avenue
New York NY 10158
Address inquiries to:
Karl Mohrmann (212) 370-0600
OTC Products Available
◆BiCozene Creme
◆Denclenz Denture Cleanser
◆Dietene Diet Shake Mix
◆Extra Strength Gas-X Tablets
◆Gas-X Tablets

DAYWELL LABORATORIES CORPORATION 541
78 Unquowa Place
Fairfield, CT 06430
Address inquiries to:
M. E. Norton (203) 255-3154
OTC Products Available
Vergo Cream

DERMIK LABORATORIES, INC. 542
500 Virginia Drive
Fort Washington, PA 19034
Distribution Centers
Oak Forest, IL 60452
4325 Frontage Road
(312) 687-7440
Langhorne, PA 19047
P.O. Box 247 (215) 752-1211
San Leandro, CA 94577
1550 Factor Avenue
P.O. Box 1569 (415) 357-9741
Tucker, GA 30084
4660 Hammermill Road
(404) 934-3091
OTC Products Available
Fomac Foam
Hytone Cream 1/2%
Loroxide Acne Lotion (Flesh Tinted)
Shepard's Formulations for Dry Skin Care
Shepard's Cream Lotion
Shepard's Skin Cream
Shepard's Soap
Vanoxide Acne Lotion
Vlemasque Acne Mask
Zetar Shampoo

DEWITT INTERNATIONAL CORPORATION 543
5 N. Watson Road
Taylors, SC 29687

Address inquiries to:
Bud Templeton   (803) 244-8521
For Medical Emergencies Contact:
Ron Romano   (803) 244-8521
OTC Products Available
Clinomint, the Smoker's Toothpaste
DeWitt's Absorbent Rub
DeWitt's Alertacaps
DeWitt's Antacid Powder
DeWitt's Aspirin
DeWitt's B Complex W/Vit. C Capsules
DeWitt's Baby Cough Syrup
DeWitt's Calamine Lotion
DeWitt's Camphor Spirits
DeWitt's Carbolized Witch Hazel Salve
DeWitt's Castor Oil
DeWitt's Children's Aspirin
DeWitt's Cold Capsules
DeWitt's Cold Sore Lotion
DeWitt's Creosant Cough Syrup
DeWitt's Feet Treat
DeWitt's Flowaway Tablets
DeWitt's Glycerin
DeWitt's Gumzor
DeWitt's Iodine
DeWitt's Joggers Lotion
DeWitt's Merthiolate
DeWitt's Multi Vitamins
DeWitt's Multi Vit./Iron
DeWitt's Oil for Ear Use
DeWitt's Oil of Cloves
DeWitt's Oil of Wintergreen
DeWitt's Olive Oil
DeWitt's Pills for Backache & Joint
  Pains
DeWitt's Pyrinyl
DeWitt's Spirit of Peppermint
DeWitt's Sweet Oil
DeWitt's Teething Lotion
DeWitt's Terpin Hydrate w/D.M.
DeWitt's Thera-M Vitamins
DeWitt's Toothache Drops
DeWitt's Turpentine
DeWitt's Vit. C 250 mg. Chewable
  Tablets
DeWitt's Vit. C 250 mg. Tablets
DeWitt's Vit. C 500 mg. Tablets
DeWitt's Vit. E 200 I.U. Capsules
DeWitt's Vit. E 400 I.U. Capsules
DeWitt's Vit. E 1000 I.U. Capsules
DeWitt's Zoo Chews Vitamins
DeWitt's Zoo Chews w/Iron Vitamins
HTO Stainless Manzan Hemorrhoidal
  Tissue Ointment

DORSEY LABORATORIES   408, 543
Division of Sandoz, Inc.
P.O. Box 83288
Lincoln, NE 68501
Address Medical Inquiries to:
Medical Department
Sandoz Pharmaceuticals
E. Hanover, N.J. 07936
                       (201) 386-7500
Other Inquiries to:
Dorsey Laboratories   (402) 464-6311
OTC Products Available
◆Acid Mantle Creme & Lotion
◆Cama Arthritis Pain Reliever
Chexit Tablets
◆Dorcol Children's Cough Syrup
◆Dorcol Children's Decongestant Liquid
◆Dorcol Children's Fever & Pain Reducer
◆Dorcol Children's Liquid Calcium
  Supplement
◆Dorcol Children's Liquid Cold Formula
Eclipse After Sun Moisturizer
Eclipse Sunscreen Gel & Moisturizing
  Lotion, Original
Eclipse Sunscreen Lip and Face
  Protectant
◆Eclipse Sunscreen Lotion, Total
  (Cooling Alcohol Base)
◆Eclipse Sunscreen Lotion, Total
  (Moisturizing Base)
Eclipse Suntan Lotion, Partial
Kanulase Tablets
Triaminic Allergy Tablets
Triaminic Chewables
◆Triaminic Cold Syrup
◆Triaminic Cold Tablets
◆Triaminic Expectorant
◆Triaminic-DM Cough Formula

◆Triaminic-12 Tablets
◆Triaminicin Tablets
◆Triaminicol Multi-Symptom Cold Syrup
◆Triaminicol Multi-Symptom Cold Tablets
Tussagesic Tablets & Suspension
Ursinus Inlay-Tabs

**EX-LAX PHARMACEUTICAL   409, 548
CO., INC.**
a Sandoz Company
(see also Creighton Products
  Corporation)
605 Third Avenue
New York, NY 10158
Address inquiries to:
Karl Mohrmann   (212) 370-0600
OTC Products Available
◆Ex-Lax Chocolated Laxative
◆Ex-Lax Pills, Unflavored
◆Extra Gentle Ex-Lax

FIBER-UP INC.   549
P.O. Box 288
Convent Station, NJ 07961
Address inquiries to:
Order Department   1-800-526-0169
For Medical Emergencies Contact
Customer Service   201-672-4255
OTC Products Available
Fiber-Up

FLEMING & COMPANY   549
1600 Fenpark Dr.
Fenton, MO 63026
Address inquiries to:
John J. Roth, M.D.   (314) 343-8200
OTC Products Available
Impregon Concentrate
Magonate Tablets
Marblen Suspension Peach/Apricot
Marblen Suspension Unflavored
Marblen Tablets
Nephrox Suspension
Nicotinex Elixir
Ocean Nasal Mist
Ocean-Plus
Purge Concentrate

**FOREST   419, 550
PHARMACEUTICALS, INC.**
Formerly O'Neal, Jones & Feldman
Pharmaceuticals
2510 Metro Boulevard
Maryland Heights, MO 63043
Address inquiries to:
Thomas Clark   (314) 569-3610
For Medical Emergencies Contact:
Jim Madison   (314) 569-3610
OTC Products Available
◆Banalg Hospital Strength Pain Reliever
◆Banalg Muscular Pain Reliever

FOTOMEDICS, INCORPORATED   738
5000 Cedar Plaza Parkway
St. Louis, MO 63128
Address inquiries to:
Mr. James Saitz   (314) 842-7135
For Medical Emergencies Contact:
Mr. James Saitz   (314) 842-7135
OTC Products Available
Cervicography

E. FOUGERA & COMPANY   550
Division of Altana Inc.
60 Baylis Road
Melville, NY 11747
Address inquiries to:
Customer Service   (800) 645-9833
For Medical Emergencies Contact:
E. Fougera & Co.   (800) 645-9833
OTC Products Available
Analgesic Balm
Antifungal Cream & Solution
Bacitracin Ointment, U.S.P.
Bacitracin-Neomycin-Polymyxin
  Ointment
Bacitracin-Polymyxin Ointment
Boric Acid Ointment
Cold Cream, U.S.P.
Dibucaine Ointment, U.S.P. 1%
Hydrocortisone Cream & Ointment,
  U.S.P. 0.5%
Lanolin, U.S.P.
Petrolatum White, U.S.P.

Swim Ear
Vitamin A + Vitamin D Ointment
Zinc Oxide Ointment, U.S.P.

FOX PHARMACAL, INC.   551
1750 W. McNab Road
Ft. Lauderdale, FL 33310
Address inquiries to:
Sandra Cook   (305) 971-4100
OTC Products Available
Odrinil
Quintrol
Super Odrinex

GEIGY PHARMACEUTICALS   409, 552
Div. of CIBA-GEIGY Corporation
Ardsley, NY 10502   (201) 277-5000
OTC Products Available
◆Otrivin Nasal Spray & Nasal Drops
◆Otrivin Pediatric Nasal Drops
◆PBZ Cream

GERBER PRODUCTS COMPANY
Fremont, MI 49412   (616) 928-2000
Address inquiries to:
Professional Communications Dept.
OTC Products Available
Gerber Biscuits
Gerber Cereals
     Barley Cereal
     Cereals with Fruit
     High Protein Cereal
     Mixed Cereal
     Oatmeal Cereal
     Rice Cereal
Gerber Chunky Foods
Gerber High Meat Dinners (Strained &
  Junior)
Gerber Junior Cookies
Gerber Junior Foods
Gerber Junior Meats
Gerber Strained Egg Yolks
Gerber Strained Food
Gerber Strained Juices
Gerber Strained Meats

**GLENBROOK   409, 552
LABORATORIES**
Division of Sterling Drug Inc.
90 Park Avenue
New York, NY 10016
Address inquiries to:
Medical Director   (212) 972-4141
OTC Products Available
◆Arthritis Bayer Timed-Release Aspirin
◆Bayer Aspirin
◆Bayer Children's Chewable Aspirin
Bayer Children's Cold Tablets
Bayer Cough Syrup for Children
◆Children's Panadol Chewable Tablets,
  Liquid, Drops
Cope
◆Cosprin 325
◆Cosprin 650
◆Cushies
◆Diaparene Baby Powder
◆Diaparene Baby Wash Cloths
◆Maximum Bayer Aspirin
◆Maximum Strength Panadol
◆Midol
◆Midol Maximum Strength for Cramps
◆Midol PMS
◆Phillips' Milk of Magnesia
Stri-Dex Maximum Strength Pads
Stri-Dex Regular Strength Pads
◆Vanquish

**GOODY'S MANUFACTURING   410, 556
CORPORATION**
P.O. Box 10518
Winston-Salem, NC 27108
Address inquiries to:
T.H. Chambers   (919) 723-1831
OTC Products Available
Goody's Extra Strength Tablets
◆Goody's Headache Powders
Isodettes DM Cough Relief Lozenges
Isodettes Sore Throat Spray
Sayman Soaps & Salves
Super Isodettes Sore Throat Lozenges

(◆ Shown in Product Identification Section)

HELENA LABORATORIES 410, 739
Home Health Care Division
1530 Lindbergh, P.O. Box 752
Beaumont, TX 77704
Address inquiries to:
Consumer Information(800) 231-4002
(800) 231-5663
In TX (800) 392-3126
OTC Products Available
◆ColoScreen Self-Test (CS-T)

HOECHST-ROUSSEL 410, 556
PHARMACEUTICALS INC.
Routes 202-206 North
Somerville, NJ 08876
Address medical inquiries to:
Scientific Services Dept.
(201) 231-2611
(8:30 AM-5:00 PM EST)
For medical emergency information
only, after hours and on weekends,
call: (201) 231-2000
OTC Products Available
◆Doxidan
◆Festal II
◆Surfak

HOLLAND-RANTOS COMPANY, 557
INC.
Post Office Box 385
865 Centennial Avenue
Piscataway, NJ 08854
See YOUNGS DRUGS PRODUCTS
CORPORATION

HYNSON, WESTCOTT 411, 557
& DUNNING
Division of Becton Dickinson and Co.
Charles & Chase Streets
Baltimore, MD 21201
(301) 837-0890
OTC Products Available
◆Lactinex Tablets & Granules
Thantis Lozenges

JEFFREY MARTIN, INC. 557
410 Clermont Terrace
Union, NJ 07083
Address inquiries to:
S.A. Geffken, Research Manager
During office hours (201) 687-4000
For Medical Emergencies Contact:
S.A. Geffken, Research Manager
During office hours (201) 687-4000
OTC Products Available
Ayds Appetite Suppressant Candy
Bantron Smoking Deterrent Tablets
Compoz Nighttime Sleep Aid
Cuticura Antibacterial Medicated Soap
Doan's Backache Spray
Doan's Pills
Porcelana Skin Bleaching Agent
Porcelana Skin Bleaching Agent with
Sunscreen
Pursettes Premenstrual Tablets

JOHNSON & JOHNSON 411, 558
BABY PRODUCTS
COMPANY
Grandview Road
Skillman, NJ 08558
For Medical Emergencies Contact:
Nancy C. Musso, RN (201) 874-1412
OTC Products Available
◆Johnson's Baby Cream
◆Sundown Sunblock Stick, Ultra
Protection
Sundown Sunscreen Lotions
Moderate Protection
Extra Protection
Maximal Protection
Ultra Protection
◆Sundown Sunscreen Stick, Maximal
Protection

JOHNSON & JOHNSON 411, 559
PRODUCTS,
INCORPORATED
501 George Street
New Brunswick, NJ 08903

Address inquiries to:
Room J526
Outside NJ (800) 526-2433
NJ (800) 352-4777
For Medical Emergencies Contact:
Outside NJ (800) 526-2433
NJ (800) 352-4777
OTC Products Available
AthletiCare Pretaping Underwrap
AthletiCare Sports Tape
◆Bioclusive Transparent Dressing
◆Johnson & Johnson Clinicydin
◆Johnson & Johnson First Aid Cream
◆K-Y Lubricating Jelly

THE KENDALL COMPANY 560
One Federal Street
Boston, MA 02101
Address inquiries to:
Peter Stratton (617) 423-2000
OTC Products Available
Dermassage Medicated Skin Lotion

KREMERS-URBAN COMPANY 560
See WILLIAM H. RORER, INC.

LACTAID INC. 411, 560
600 Fire Road
P.O. Box 111
Pleasantville, NJ 08232-0111
Address inquiries to:
Alan E. Kligerman (800) 257-8650
OTC Products Available
◆LactAid brand lactase enzyme

THE LANNETT COMPANY, INC. 561
9000 State Road
Philadelphia, PA 19136
Address inquiries to:
Medical Service Dept. (215) 333-9000
OTC Products Available
Acetaminophen Tablets & Elixir
Acnederm Lotion & Soap
Alphamul
Anulan Suppositories
Bellafedrol AH Tablets
Castaderm
Cebralan MT Tablets
Decavitamin Tablets
Disanthrol Capsules
Disodan Capsules
Disolan Capsules
Disonate Capsules
Disoplex Capsules
Lanamins
Lanatuss Expectorant
Lycolan Elixir
Magnatril Suspension & Tablets
Prelan Tablets
S-A-C Tablets
Salagen Tablets

LAVOPTIK COMPANY, INC. 561, 739
661 Western Avenue North
St. Paul, MN 55103
Address inquiries to:
661 Western Avenue North
St. Paul, MN 55103 (612) 489-1351
For Medical Emergencies Contact:
B. C. Brainard (612) 489-1351
OTC Products Available
Lavoptik Eye Cup
Lavoptik Eye Wash

LEDERLE LABORATORIES 411, 561
Division of American Cyanamid Co.
Wayne, NJ 07470 (201) 831-2000
Address inquiries on
medical matters to:
Professional Services Dept.
Lederle Laboratories
Pearl River, NY 10965
(914) 735-5000
Distribution Centers
ATLANTA
Bulk Address
Chamblee (Atlanta), GA 30341
5180 Peachtree Industrial Blvd.
Mail Address
Atlanta, GA 30302
P.O. Box 4272 (800) LEDERLE
(404) 455-0320

CHICAGO
Bulk Address
Rosemont, IL 60018
10401 W. Touhy Ave.
Mail Address
Chicago, IL 60666 (800) LEDERLE
P.O. Box 66189 (312) 827-8871
DALLAS
Bulk Address
Dallas, TX 75247
7611 Carpenter Freeway
Mail Address
Dallas, TX 75265 (800) LEDERLE
P.O. Box 225731 (214) 631-2130
LOS ANGELES
Bulk Address
Los Angeles, CA 90040
2300 S. Eastern Ave.
Mail Address
Los Angeles, CA 90051
T.A. Box 2202 (800) LEDERLE
(213) 726-1016
PHILADELPHIA
Fort Washington, PA 19034
185 Commerce Drive
(NY-NJ-MD-DE) (800) LEDERLE
(CT-VA-WV-DC) (800) LEDERLE
(Phila. Only) (215) 248-3900
(All Other) (215) 646-7000
OTC Products Available
Acetaminophen Capsules, Tablets, Elixir
Ascorbic Acid Tablets
Aureomycin Ointment 3%
◆Caltrate 600
◆Caltrate 600 + Vitamin D
◆Centrum
◆Centrum, Jr.
◆Centrum, Jr. + Extra C
◆Docusate Sodium (DSS) Capsules &
Syrup
Docusate Sodium w/Casanthranol
Capsules & Syrup
◆Ferro-Sequels
Ferrous Gluconate Iron Supplement
Ferrous Sulfate
Filibon Prenatal Vitamin Tablets
◆FootWork Athlete's Foot Cream 0.5 oz.
◆FootWork Athlete's Foot Cream 1.0 oz.
◆FootWork Athlete's Foot Powder
◆FootWork Athlete's Foot Solution
◆FootWork Athlete's Foot Spray Powder
Gevrabon Liquid
Gevral Protein Powder
Gevral Tablets
Gevral T Tablets
Guaifenesin Syrup
Guaifenesin w/D-Methorphan
Hydrobromide Syrup
Incremin w/Iron Syrup
Lederplex Capsules and Liquid
Neoloid Emulsified Castor Oil
Peritinic Tablets
Pseudoephedrine Syrup & Tablets
Pyridoxine HCl
Quinine Capsules
◆Spartus
◆Spartus + Iron
Stresscaps Capsules
◆Stresstabs 600 Tablets
◆Stresstabs 600 with Iron
◆Stresstabs 600 with Zinc
Thiamine HCl (Vitamin B-1) Tablets
Triprolidine with Pseudoephedrine
Syrup & Tablets
Vi-Magna Capsules
Vitamin A, Natural
Vitamin C Chewable
Vitamin E, Natural, USP
Vitamin E, USP
◆Zincon Dandruff Shampoo

LEEMING DIVISION 567
Pfizer Inc.
100 Jefferson Rd.
Parsippany, NJ 07054
Address inquiries to:
Research and Development Dept.
(201) 887-2100
OTC Products Available
Ben-Gay External Analgesic Products
Desitin Ointment
Rheaban Tablets
Unisom Nighttime Sleep Aid

(◆ Shown in Product Identification Section)

Visine A.C. Eye Drops
Visine Eye Drops

LEMAR LABORATORIES, 412, 569
INC.
Building B-200
10 Perimeter Way, N.W.
Atlanta, GA 30339
Address inquiries to:
Steve Barker (404) 952-3922
OTC Products Available
◆Healthbreak Smoking Deterrent Gum &
Lozenge

LOMA LINDA FOODS 569
Address inquiries to:
Marketing Office
11503 Pierce Street
Riverside, CA 92515 (714) 687-7800
800-932-5525
CA only 800-442-4917
OTC Products Available
Soyalac: Liquid Concentrate,
Ready-to-Serve and Powder
I-Soyalac: Liquid Concentrate and
Ready-to-Serve

LUYTIES PHARMACAL COMPANY 570
P. O. Box 8080
St. Louis, MO 63156
Address Inquiries to:
Customer Service (800) 325-8080
OTC Products Available
Yellolax

3M COMPANY 412, 570
Personal Care Products
3M Center
St. Paul, MN 55144
Address Inquiries to:
Sandy Lowe
3M Center (612) 736-0894
For Medical Emergencies Contact:
Riker Laboratories (213) 341-1300
Branch Offices
Atlanta, GA 30360
2860 Bankers Industrial Drive
(404) 447-7000
Independence, OH 44131
6100 Rockside Woods Blvd.
Suite 100 (216) 447-3050
LaMirada, CA 90638
14659 Alondra Boulevard
(213) 726-6351
Woodbury NY 11797
100 Crossways Park West
(516) 364-9400
OTC Products Available
Dorbane Tablets
Dorbantyl Capsules
Dorbantyl Forte Capsules
◆Titralac Liquid
◆Titralac Tablets

MACSIL, INC. 571
1326 Frankford Avenue
Philadelphia, PA 19125
(215) 423-5566
OTC Products Available
Balmex Baby Powder
Balmex Emollient Lotion
Balmex Ointment

A. G. MARIN PHARMACEUTICALS 571
P.O. Box 174
Miami, FL 33144

Address inquiries to:
Mr. Ricardo Mayo (305) 264-1241
OTC Products Available
MarEPA Marine Lipid Concentrate

MARION LABORATORIES, 412, 571
INC.
Marion Park Drive
Kansas City, MO 64137
For Medical Emergencies Contact:
Product Surveillance (816) 966-5000
OTC Products Available
◆Ambenyl-D Decongestant Cough
Formula
◆Debrox Drops
◆Gaviscon Antacid Tablets
◆Gaviscon Liquid Antacid

◆Gaviscon-2 Antacid Tablets
◆Gly-Oxide Liquid
◆Os-Cal 250 Tablets
◆Os-Cal 500 Tablets
Os-Cal Forte Tablets
Os-Cal-Gesic Tablets
Os-Cal Plus Tablets
◆Throat Discs Throat Lozenges

MARLYN COMPANY, INC. 413, 573
350 Pauma Place
Escondido, CA 92025
(714) 489-6115
OTC Products Available
Albumin 500 Tablets
C Speriden Tablets, Sustained Release
Daily Nutritional Packs
Care-4
◆ MARLYN PMS
Pro-Formance
Soft Stress
Hep-Forte Capsules
Marbec Tablets
Marlyn Formula 50 Capsules
Marlyn Prolonged Release Vitamins
Balanced B 125
Clock E, 400 I.U.
Iron-L
Niacin, 400 mg.
Super One Daily
Super Citro Cee
Ultimate One
Vitamin B$_{12}$, 1000 mcg.
Vitamin C, 1000 mg.

MAX FACTOR & CO. 413, 574
1655 N. McCadden Pl.
Hollywood, CA 90028
Address inquiries to:
Carol Walters (213) 856-6000
For Medical Emergencies Contact:
Joe DiSomma (805) 499-4560 (home)
(213) 856-6000 (work)
OTC Products Available
◆Erace Acne Control Cover-Up
◆For Your Eyes Only Mascara
◆Skin Principle Basic Clarifying Lotion
◆Skin Principle Daily Light Moisture
Lotion
◆Skin Principle Daily Rich Moisture
Lotion
◆Skin Principle Purifying Cleansing
Lotion
◆Skin Principle Serious Moisture
Supplement

MAYRAND INC. 575
P.O. Box 8869
Four Dundas Circle
Greensboro, NC 27419-0869
Address Inquiries to:
Vice-President, Sales (919) 292-5347
For Medical Emergencies Contact:
Technical Director (919) 292-5347
OTC Products Available
Eldertonic
EnTab-650 Tablets
Glytuss Tablets
Nu-Iron 150 Caps
Nu-Iron Elixir

McNEIL CONSUMER 413, 576
PRODUCTS CO.
McNeilab, Inc.
Fort Washington, PA 19034
Address inquiries to:
Professional Relations Department
Fort Washington, PA 19034
Manufacturing Divisions
Fort Washington, PA 19034
Southwest Manufacturing Plant
4001 N. I-35
Round Rock, TX 78664
Distribution Centers
Arlington, TX 76010
3129 Pinewood Drive
(817) 640-1167
Broadview, IL 60153
2122 Roberts Drive
(312) 343-1569

Doraville, GA 30360
2801 Bankers Industrial Drive
(404) 448-0200
Glendale, CA 91201
512 Paula Avenue (213) 245-1491
Montgomeryville, PA 18936
2 Progress Drive (215) 699-7081
OTC Products Available
◆Children's CoTYLENOL Chewable Cold
Tablets & Liquid Cold Formula
◆Children's TYLENOL Acetaminophen
Chewable Tablets, Elixir & Drops
◆CoTYLENOL Cold Medication Liquid
◆CoTYLENOL Cold Medication Tablets
and Capsules
◆Extra Strength SINE-AID Sinus
Headache Capsules
Extra-Strength TYLENOL
acetaminophen Adult Liquid Pain
Reliever
◆Extra-Strength TYLENOL
acetaminophen Tablets & Capsules
◆Infants' TYLENOL Drops
◆Junior Strength TYLENOL
acetaminophen Swallowable Tablets
◆Maximum Strength TYLENOL Sinus
Medication Capsules and Tablets
◆PEDIACARE 1 Children's Cough Relief
Liquid
◆PEDIACARE 2 Children's Cold Relief
Liquid
◆PEDIACARE 3 Children's Cold Relief
Liquid & Chewable Tablets
◆Regular Strength TYLENOL
acetaminophen Tablets & Capsules
◆SINE-AID Sinus Headache Tablets

MEAD JOHNSON 414, 583
NUTRITIONAL DIVISION
Mead Johnson & Company
2404 W. Pennsylvania St.
Evansville, IN 47721 (812) 426-6000
Address inquiries to:
Scientific Information Section
Medical Department
OTC Products Available
Casec
◆Ce-Vi-Sol
Criticare HN
◆Enfamil
Enfamil Nursette
◆Enfamil Ready-To-Use
◆Enfamil w/Iron
◆Enfamil w/Iron Ready-To-Use
Fer-In-Sol
◆Isocal
Isocal HCN
Isocal Tube Feeding Set
Lofenalac
Lonalac
Lytren
MCT Oil
◆Naturacil
Nutramigen
◆Poly-Vi-Sol Vitamins, Chewable Tablets
& Drops
◆Poly-Vi-Sol Vitamins, Circus Shapes,
Chewable with & without Iron & Zinc
◆Poly-Vi-Sol Vitamins w/Iron & Zinc,
Chewable Tablets
◆Poly-Vi-Sol Vitamins w/Iron, Drops
Portagen
Pregestimil
ProSobee
◆Smurf Chewable Vitamins
◆Smurf Chewable Vitamins with Iron and
Zinc
◆Sustacal Liquid
Sustacal Powder & Pudding
Sustacal HC
Sustagen
◆Tempra
TraumaCal
Trind
Trind-DM
◆Tri-Vi-Sol Vitamin Drops
◆Tri-Vi-Sol Vitamin Drops w/Iron

(◆ Shown in Product Identification Section)

MEAD JOHNSON   415, 594
PHARMACEUTICAL
DIVISION
Mead Johnson & Company
2404 W. Pennsylvania St.
Evansville, IN 47721 (812) 426-6000
    Address Inquiries to:
Scientific Information Section
  Medical Department
    OTC Products Available
◆Colace
 Natalins
◆Peri-Colace

MEDICONE COMPANY   595
225 Varick St.
New York, NY 10014
    Address inquiries to:
Professional Service Dept.
                    (212) 924-5166
    OTC Products Available
Derma Medicone
Medicone Dressing
Mediconet
Rectal Medicone Suppositories
Rectal Medicone Unguent

MEDTECH LABORATORIES, INC.   596
P.O. Box 2930
1501 Stampede Avenue
Cody, WY 82414-2930
    For Medical Emergencies Contact:
Carl J. Schmidlapp, III (307) 587-4973
                    (800) 443-4908
    Branch Offices
745 Fifth Avenue, Room 1106
New York, NY 10151 (212) 755-3200
    OTC Products Available
Iodex Regular
Iodex with Methyl Salicylate
New Skin Liquid Bandage
Nudit Depilatory Cream
ThexForte Capsules

MENLEY & JAMES   415, 596, 739
LABORATORIES
a SmithKline Beckman Company
One Franklin Plaza
P.O. Box 8082
Philadelphia, PA 19101
    Address inquiries to:
Medical Department (215) 751-5000
    OTC Products Available
◆A.R.M. Allergy Relief Medicine Tablets
◆Acnomel Cream
◆Benzedrex Inhaler
◆Congestac Tablets
◆Contac Capsules
◆Contac Cough Capsules
◆Contac Jr. Childrens' Cold Medicine
◆Contac Severe Cold Formula Capsules
◆Contac Severe Cold Formula Night
  Strength
◆Dietac Once-A-Day Maximum Strength
  Diet Aid Capsules
◆Ecotrin Maximum Strength Capsules
◆Ecotrin Regular Strength Capsules
◆Ecotrin Tablets
◆Ecotrin Maximum Strength Tablets
◆Feosol Capsules
◆Feosol Elixir
◆Feosol Plus Capsules
◆Feosol Tablets
◆Hemoccult Home Test
◆Ornacol Capsules
◆Ornex Capsules
◆Pragmatar Ointment
◆Sine-Off Extra Strength No Drowsiness
  Capsules
◆Sine-Off Extra Strength Sinus Medicine
  Aspirin-Free Capsules
◆Sine-Off Extra Strength Sinus Medicine
  Aspirin-Free Tablets
◆Sine-Off Sinus Medicine Tablets-Aspirin
  Formula
◆Teldrin Multi-Symptom Allergy Reliever
◆Teldrin Timed-Release Capsules
◆Troph-Iron Liquid
◆Trophite Liquid & Tablets

THE MENTHOLATUM COMPANY   604
1360 Niagara Street
Buffalo, NY 14213

    Address Inquiries to:
Sheila A. Eckert   (716) 882-7660
    OTC Products Available
Calmol 4 Suppositories
Fletcher's Castoria
Medi-Quik Aerosol Spray
Mentholatum Deep Heating Lotion
Mentholatum Deep Heating Rub
Mentholatum Lipbalm with Sunscreen
Mentholatum Ointment
Nytilax Tablets
Red Cross Toothache Medication
Resicort Cream

MERICON INDUSTRIES, INC.   606
8819 North Pioneer Rd.
Peoria, IL 61615
    Address inquiries to:
Thomas P. Morrissey (800) 242-6464
  In IL Collect (309) 693-2150
    OTC Products Available
Delacort
Orazinc Capsules
Orazinc Lozenges

MERRELL DOW   606
PHARMACEUTICALS INC.
Subsidiary of The Dow Chemical
Company
10123 Alliance Road
Cincinnati, OH 45242-9553
    Address inquiries to:
Professional Relations Manager
                    (513) 948-9111
    For Medical Emergencies Contact:
Merrell Dow Pharmaceuticals Inc.
                    (513) 948-9111
    OTC Products Available
Cēpacol Anesthetic Lozenges (Troches)
Cēpacol Mouthwash/Gargle
Cēpacol Throat Lozenges
CĒPASTAT Cherry Flavor Sore Throat
  Lozenges
CĒPASTAT Sore Throat Lozenges
Delcid
Kolantyl Gel
Kolantyl Wafers
Novahistine Cough & Cold Formula
Novahistine DMX
Novahistine Elixir
Simron Capsules
Simron Plus Capsules
Terpin Hydrate & Codeine Elixir

MERRICK MEDICINE   417, 611
COMPANY
501-503 South 8th (76706)
P.O. Box 1489 (76703)
Waco, TX
    Address inquiries to:
W.B. Clayton, President
                    (817) 753-3461
    OTC Products Available
◆Percy Medicine

MILES LABORATORIES, INC. 417, 611
1127 Myrtle Street
Elkhart, IN 46514
    Address inquiries to:
Manager, Consumer Affairs Dept.
                    (219) 264-8955
    For Medical Emergencies Contact:
Medical Department (219) 262-7886
    OTC Products Available
◆Alka-Mints Chewable Antacid
◆Alka-Seltzer Effervescent Antacid
◆Alka-Seltzer Effervescent Pain Reliever
  & Antacid
◆Alka-Seltzer Plus Cold Medicine
◆Bactine Antiseptic/Anesthetic First Aid
  Spray
◆Bactine Hydrocortisone Skin Care
  Cream
◆Biocal 250 mg Chewable Calcium
  Supplement
◆Biocal 500 mg Tablet Calcium
  Supplement
◆Bugs Bunny Children's Chewable
  Vitamins (Sugar Free)

 Bugs Bunny Children's Chewable
  Vitamins + Minerals with Iron &
  Calcium (Sugar Free)
◆Bugs Bunny Plus Iron Children's
  Chewable Vitamins (Sugar Free)
◆Bugs Bunny With Extra C Children's
  Chewable Vitamins (Sugar Free)
◆Flintstones Children's Chewable
  Vitamins
◆Flintstones Children's Chewable
  Vitamins Plus Iron
◆Flintstones Children's Chewable
  Vitamins With Extra C
◆Flintstones Complete With Iron, Calcium
  & Minerals Children's Chewable
  Vitamins
◆Miles Nervine Nighttime Sleep-Aid
◆One-A-Day Essential Vitamins
◆One-A-Day Maximum Formula Vitamins
  and Minerals
◆One-A-Day Plus Extra C Vitamins
◆Stressgard Stress Formula Vitamins
◆Within Multivitamin for Women with
  Calcium and Extra Iron

MILLER PHARMACAL GROUP   615
INC.
245 W. Roosevelt Road
West Chicago, IL 60185
    Address inquiries to:
Medical Service Dept. (312) 231-3632
    For Medical Emergencies Contact:
Medical Service Dept. (312) 231-3632
    OTC Products Available
A/G Pro Tablets
Amina-21 Capsules & Powder
B-60 Capsules
Ca/Mg Orotate
Ca-plus Protein Tablets
Calcium Ascorbate Powder
Calcium Aspartate Tablets
Calcium Orotate Tablets
Cardenz Tablets
Cemill 500 T.R. Tablets
Chenatal Tablets
Complere Tablets
D,L-Carnitine Capsules
Dequasine Tablets
Fe-plus Protein Tablets
Garlic with Lecithin Capsules
Glutamic Acid Tablets
Hyalex Tablets
Karbozyme Tablets
Mg-plus Protein Tablets
Magnesium Orotate Tablets
Miladregen Tablets
Milco Zyme Tablets
Ragus Tablets
Theramill Tablets
I-Tryptophan Capsules

MONOCLONAL ANTIBODIES, INC.   739
2319 Charleston Road
Mt. View, CA 94043
    Address inquiries to:
Customer Service   (800) 227-8855
                In CA (415) 960-1320
    For Medical Emergencies Contact:
OvuSTICK Hot Line (For patients)
                    (800) 332-1488
                In CA (800) 222-1488
    OTC Products Available
OvuSTICK Self-Test

MURO PHARMACEUTICAL, INC.   615
890 East Street
Tewksbury, MA 01876-9987
    Address inquiries to:
Professional Service Dept.
                1-(800) 225-0974
                    (617) 851-5981
    OTC Products Available
Duolube Ophthalmic Ointment
Murocel Ophthalmic Solution
Muro Tears
Salinex Nasal Mist & Drops

NATIONAL MAGNESIA CO., INC.   616
70-32 83rd Street
Glendale, NY 11385
    Address inquiries to:
Richard Neimeth   (718) 326-1500
    OTC Products Available
Citroma Oral Solution

(◆ Shown in Product Identification Section)

NATRA-BIO COMPANY 616
2615 Stanwell Drive
Concord, CA 94520

Address inquiries to:
Susan Lyon (415) 676-7201
(800) 533-1033
OTC Products Available
501 Indigestion
502 Cough
503 Nervousness
504 Injuries
505 Fever
506 Neuralgia
507 Sinus
508 Arthritis
509 Sore Throat
510 Menstrual
511 Nausea
512 Chest Cold
513 Head Cold
514 Earache
515 Headache
516 Prostate
517 Menopause
518 Bed Wetting
519 Hay Fever
520 Hemorrhoids
521 Laxative
522 Bladder Irritation
523 Insomnia
524 Diarrhea
525 Herpes
526 Acne
527 Flu
528 Exhaustion
529 Emotional
530 Eye Irritation
531 Teeth and Gums
532 Teething
533 Varicose Veins
534 Hair and Scalp
535 Insect Bites
536 Poison Oak/Poison Ivy
Natra-Bio Homeopathic-Style Glandulars
& Organs - Series 401-419
Natra-Bio Homeopathic Tissue Salts -
Series 301-315
Natra Med Homeopathic Ointments -
Series 600-606

THE NATREN COMPANY, 418, 616
INC.
10935 Camarillo Street
North Hollywood, CA 91602
Address inquiries to:
(818) 769-9300
OTC Products Available
Bifido Factor
◆Superdophilus

NATURE'S BOUNTY, INC. 617
105 Orville Drive
Bohemia, NY 11716
Address inquiries to:
Professional Service Dept.
(516) 567-9500
(800) 645-5412
OTC Products Available
Acerola C (100 mg)
Acidophilus Capsules
Alfalfa Tablets
I-Arginine
B-1 Tablets
B-2 Tablets
B-6 Tablets
B-12 & B-12 Sublingual Tablets
B-50 Tablets
B-100 Tablets
B-100 Time Release Tablets
B-125 Tablets
B-150 Tablets
B Complex & B-12 Tablets
B Complex & C (Time Release) Tablets
B & C Liquid
Bee Pollen Tablets
Beta-Carotene Capsules
Biotin Tablets
Bone Meal with Vitamin D Tablets
Brewer's Yeast Powder (Debittered)
Brewer's Yeast Tablets

C-250 with Rose Hips Tablets
C-300 with Rose Hips (Chewable)
Tablets
C-500 with Rose Hips Tablets
C-1000 with Rose Hips Tablets
C-Complex Tablets
C-Liquid
C-Time 500 Time Release Tablets
C-Time 750 Time Release Tablets
C-Time 1500 Time Release Tablets
Calciday-667
Calcium Ascorbate Tablets
Calcium Lactate Tablets
Calmtabs Tablets
Centrafree
Chelated Calcium Tablets
Chelated Chromium Tablets
Chelated Copper Tablets
Chelated Magnesium Tablets
Chelated Manganese Tablets
Chelated Multi-Mineral Tablets
Chelated Potassium Tablets
Chelated Zinc Tablets
Chew-Iron Tablets
Children's Chewable Vitamins
Children's Chewable Vitamins with Iron
Choline Tablets
Chromium, GTF Tablets
Citrus Bioflavonoids Tablets
Claws
Cocoa Butter Soap
I-Cysteine
Dolomite Tablets
E-200 Capsules
E-200 (Natural Complex) Capsules
E-400 Capsules
E-400 (Natural Complex) Capsules
E-600 (Natural Complex) Capsules
E-1000 (Natural Complex) Capsules
Emulsified E-200 Capsules
Evening Primrose Oil
Ferrous Sulfate Tablets
Folic Acid Tablets
Garlic Oil Capsules
Garlic & Parsley Capsules
Ginseng, Manchurian Capsules &
Tablets
Glucomannan Capsules
Glutamic Acid Tablets
I-Glutamine Tablets
Halibut Liver Oil Capsules
Herbal Laxative Tablets
I-Histidine (500 mg)
Inositol Tablets
Iron Tablets
Jojoba Shampoo
KLB6 Capsules
KLB6 Complete Tablets
KLB6 Diet Mix
Kelp Tablets
Lecithin Capsules
Lecithin Chewable Tablets
Lecithin Granules
Lecithin with Vitamin D Capsules
Liver W/B-12 Tablets
I-Lysine Tablets
Magnesium Tablets
Manganese Tablets
Mega V & M Tablets
Mega-B with C Tablets
Memory Booster
Multi-Mineral Tablets
Nature's Bounty Hair Booster Tablets
Nature's Bounty 1 Tablets
Nature's Bounty Slim
Niacin Tablets
Niacinamide Tablets
I-Ornithine
Oyster Calcium Tablets
Oystercal-D 250
Oystercal-500
PABA Tablets
Pantothenic Acid Tablets
Papaya Enzyme Tablets
I-Phenylalanine
Potassium Tablets
Potassium & B-6 Tablets
Protein For Body Building
Protein Tablets
RNA Tablets
RNA/DNA Tablets
Rutin Tablets

Selenium Tablets
Spirulina Tablets
Stress "1000" Tablets
Stress Formula "605" Tablets
Stress Formula "605" w/Iron Tablets
Stress Formula "605" w/Zinc Tablets
Superoxide Dismutase (SOD) Tablets
L-Tryptophan (200 mg)
L-Tryptophan (500 mg)
L-Tryptophan (667 mg)
Ultra "A" Capsules & Tablets
Ultra "A & D" Tablets
Ultra "D" Tablets
Ultra KLB6 Tablets
Ultra Vita-Time Tablets
Vitamin A Capsules & Tablets
Vitamin A & D Tablets
Vitamin C Crystals
Vitamin D Tablets
Vitamin K Tablets
Vita-Time Tablets
Water Pill with Iron (Natural Diuretic)
Water Pill with Potassium (Natural
Diuretic)
Wheat Germ Oil Capsules
Yeast Plus Tablets
Zacne Tablets
Zinc Tablets

NORCLIFF THAYER INC. 418, 621
303 South Broadway
Tarrytown, NY 10591
(914) 631-0033
OTC Products Available
◆A-200 Pyrinate Pediculicide Shampoo,
Liquid, Gel
AsthmaHaler Oral Inhalation for
Bronchial Asthma
AsthmaNefrin Solution Anti-Asthmatic
Inhalant
Esotérica Medicated Fade Cream
◆Liquiprin Acetaminophen
◆Nature's Remedy Laxative
◆NoSalt Salt Alternative, Regular
◆NoSalt Salt Alternative, Seasoned
◆Oxy Clean Lathering Facial Scrub
◆Oxy Clean Medicated Cleanser, Pads,
Soap
◆Oxy 10 Cover with Sorboxyl
◆Oxy 10 Wash Antibacterial Skin Wash
◆Oxy-5 Lotion with Sorboxyl
◆Oxy-10 Lotion with Sorboxyl
◆Tums Antacid Tablets, Regular and
Extra Strength

NOXELL CORPORATION 418, 624
11050 York Road
Hunt Valley MD 21030-2098
For Medical Emergencies Contact:
Edward M. Jackson, Ph.D.
(301) 628-4397
OTC Products Available
Noxzema Acne-12
Noxzema Antiseptic Skin Cleanser
Noxzema Cleansing Pads
◆Noxzema Medicated Skin Cream

NUAGE LABORATORIES, LTD. 624
4200 Laclede Avenue
St. Louis, MO 63108
Address inquiries to:
Customer Service (314) 533-9600
OTC Products Available
Biochemic Tissue Salts
Bioplasma
Calcium Fluoride
Calcium Phosphate
Calcium Sulfate
Ferrous Phosphate
Magnesium Phosphate
Potassium Chloride
Potassium Phosphate
Potassium Sulfate
Silica
Sodium Chloride
Sodium Phosphate
Sodium Sulfate
Tissue A
Tissue B
Ticcue C
Tissue D
Tissue E
Tissue G

(◆ Shown in Product Identification Section)

Tissue H
Tissue I
Tissue J
Tissue K
Tissue M
Tissue N
Tissue O
Tissue P

NUTRITIONAL FACTORS   **624**
2615 Stanwell Drive
Concord, CA 94520
Address inquiries to:
Susan Lyon   (415) 676-7201
(800) 533-1033
OTC Products Available
Acidaid
Amino Acid Tablets
Chelated Cal/Mag Tablets
Protesoy Protein Powder
Protesoy Protein Snacks

NUTRITIONAL SPECIALTY   **419, 624**
PRODUCTS
2210 Wilshire Blvd.
Suite 159
Santa Monica, CA 90403
Address inquiries to:
(213) 393-0827
Telex: 4996300 burx lsa (attn. nsp)
OTC Products Available
◆Geriavit Pharmaton

O'NEAL, JONES & FELDMAN   **419**
PHARMACEUTICALS
See FOREST PHARMACEUTICALS, INC.

OPTIMOX, INC.   **419, 625**
2720 Monterey Street
Suite 406
Torrance, CA 90503
Address Inquiries to:
Guy E. Abraham, M.D.(213) 618-9370
For Medical Emergencies Contact:
Guy E. Abraham, M.D.(213) 618-9370
OTC Products Available
◆Optivite for Women

ORANGE MEDICAL   **740**
INSTRUMENTS
3183-F Airway Avenue
Costa Mesa, CA 92626
Address inquiries to:
Customer Service   (714) 641-5836
For Medical Emergencies Contact
Customer Service   (714) 641-5836
OTC Products Available
BetaScan Reagent Strips, Blood
Glucose Test Strips
TrendStrips, Blood Glucose Test Strips

ORTHO   **419, 625, 741**
PHARMACEUTICAL
CORPORATION
Advanced Care Products Division
Route #202
Raritan, NJ 08869   (201) 524-0400
For Medical Emergencies Contact:
Dr. B. Malyk   (201) 524-5211
OTC Products Available
◆Advance Pregnancy Test
◆Conceptrol Birth Control Cream
◆Conceptrol Contraceptive Gel
◆Conceptrol Disposable Contraceptive
Gel
◆Daisy 2 Pregnancy Test
◆Delfen Contraceptive Foam
◆Dimensyn Maximum Strength Menstrual
Discomfort Relief
◆Fact Pregnancy Test
◆Gynol II Contraceptive Jelly
◆Intercept Contraceptive Inserts
◆Masse Breast Cream
◆Micatin Antifungal Cream
◆Micatin Antifungal Powder
Micatin Antifungal Spray Liquid
◆Micatin Antifungal Spray Powder
Micatin Jock Itch Cream
Micatin Jock Itch Spray Powder
◆Ortho Disposable Vaginal Applicators
◆Ortho Personal Lubricant
◆Ortho-Creme Contraceptive Cream
◆Ortho-Gynol Contraceptive Jelly

ORTHO PHARMACEUTICAL   **420, 629**
CORPORATION
Dermatological Division
Raritan, NJ 08869   (201) 524-0400
OTC Products Available
◆Purpose Dry Skin Cream
◆Purpose Shampoo
◆Purpose Soap

PADDOCK LABORATORIES, INC.   **629**
3101 Louisiana Ave. North
Minneapolis, MN 55427
Address inquiries to:
Robert E. Freye   (612) 546-4676
(800) 328-5113
For Medical Emergencies Contact:
Bruce G. Paddock   (800) 328-5113
OTC Products Available
Emulsoil
Glutose
Ipecac Syrup

PARKE-DAVIS   **420, 630**
Division of Warner-Lambert Company
201 Tabor Road
Morris Plains, New Jersey 07950
(201) 540-2000
For product information call:
1-(800) 223-0432
For medical information call:
(201) 540-3950
Regional Sales Offices
Atlanta, GA 30328
1140 Hammond Drive
(404) 396-4080
Baltimore (Hunt Valley), MD 21031
11350 McCormick Road
(301) 666-7810
Chicago (Schaumburg), IL 60195
1111 Plaza Drive   (312) 884-6990
Dallas (Grand Prairie), TX 75234
12200 Ford Road   (214) 484-5566
Detroit (Troy), MI 48084
500 Stephenson Highway
(313) 589-3292
Los Angeles (Tustin), CA 92680
17822 East 17th Street
(714) 731-3441
Memphis, TN 38119
1355 Lynnfield Road
(901) 767-1921
New York (East Hartford, CT) 06108
111 Founders Plaza
(203) 528-9601
Pittsburgh, PA 15220
1910 Cochran Road
(412) 343-9855
Seattle (Bellevue), WA 98004
301 116th Avenue, SE
(206) 451-1119
OTC Products Available
Abdec Baby Vitamin Drops
Acetaminophen (Tapar)
Agoral
Agoral, Marshmallow Flavor
Agoral, Raspberry Flavor
Alcohol, Rubbing (Lavacol)
Alophen Pills
◆Anusol Hemorrhoidal Suppositories
◆Anusol Ointment
Aspirin Tablets
◆Benadryl Antihistamine Cream
◆Benylin Cough Syrup
◆Benylin DM
◆Caladryl Cream, Lotion
Calcium Lactate Tablets
Cherry Syrup
Ferrous Sulfate Filmseals
◆Gelusil Liquid & Tablets
Gelusil-M Liquid & Tablets
Gelusil-II Liquid & Tablets
Geriplex-FS Kapseals
Geriplex-FS Liquid
Hydrogen Peroxide Solution
Lavacol
◆Myadec
Natabec Kapseals
Natabec-FA Kapseals
Peroxide, Hydrogen
Quinine Sulfate Capsules
Rubbing Alcohol (Lavacol)
Siblin Granules
Terpin Hydrate Elixir w/Codeine

Thera-Combex H-P Kapseals
Tucks Cream
Tucks Ointment
◆Tucks Premoistened Pads
Tucks Take-Alongs
Unibase
◆Ziradryl Lotion

THE PARTHENON COMPANY,   **634**
INC.
3311 West 2400 South
Salt Lake City, Utah 84119

Address inquiries to:
N. G. Mihalopoulos, Ph.D.
(801) 972-5184

For Medical Emergencies Contact:
N. G. Mihalopoulos   (801) 972-5184
(801) 266-3753
OTC Products Available
Devrom Chewable Tablets

PFIPHARMECS DIVISION   **420, 634**
Pfizer Inc.
235 E. 42nd Street
New York, NY 10017
Address inquiries to:
Pfizer Inc.   (212) 573-2323
Branch Offices
Clifton, NJ 07012
230 Brighton Rd.   (201) 546-7702
Doraville, GA 30340
4360 Northeast Expressway
(404) 448-6666
Hoffman Estates, IL 60712
2400 W. Central Road
(312) 381-9500
Grand Prairie, TX 75050
502 Fountain Parkway
(817) 261-9131
Irvine, CA 92705
16700 Red Hill Ave.
(714) 540-9180
OTC Products Available
◆Bonine
◆Coryban-D Capsules
◆Coryban-D Cough Syrup
◆Li-Ban Spray
◆RID
Terramycin Ointment
◆Wart-Off

PHARMACRAFT DIVISION   **421, 636**
Pennwalt Corporation
755 Jefferson Road
Rochester, NY 14623
Address inquiries to:
Professional Service Dept.
P.O. Box 1212
Rochester, NY 14603
(716) 475-9000
OTC Products Available
Allerest Eye Drops
Allerest Headache Strength Tablets
◆Allerest Sinus Pain Formula
◆Allerest Tablets, Children's Chewable
Tablets, & Timed-Release Capsules
Allerest 12 Hour Liquid
Allerest 12 Hour Nasal Spray
◆CaldeCORT Anti-Itch Hydrocortisone
Cream
◆CaldeCORT Anti-Itch Hydrocortisone
Spray
◆Caldesene Medicated Ointment
◆Caldesene Medicated Powder
◆Cold Factor 12 Liquid & Capsules
◆Cruex Antifungal Cream
◆Cruex Antifungal Powder
Cruex Antifungal Spray Powder
◆Desenex Antifungal Cream
◆Desenex Antifungal Foam
Desenex Antifungal Liquid
◆Desenex Antifungal Ointment
◆Desenex Antifungal Powder
◆Desenex Antifungal Spray Powder
Desenex Foot & Sneaker Spray
Desenex Soap
Fresh Antiperspirant Roll-on & Cream
Sinarest Nasal Spray
Sinarest Regular & Extra Strength
Tablets
Ting Antifungal Cream

Ting Antifungal Powder
Ting Antifungal Spray Powder

PHARMADERM   **421, 638**
a division of Altana, Inc.
60 Baylis Road
Melville, NY 11747
Address inquiries to:
Customer Service   (800) 645-9432
For Medical Emergencies Contact:
Pharmaderm   (800) 645-9432
OTC Products Available
Analgesic Balm
◆Athlete's Foot Cream & Solution
   (Tolnaftate 1%)
Bacitracin Ointment, USP
Bacitracin-Neomycin-Polymyxin
   Ointment
Bacitracin-Polymyxin Ointment
Boric Acid Ointment
Boric Acid Ophthalmic Ointment 5%
Cold Cream, USP
Dibucaine Ointment, USP 1%
Hydrocortisone Cream & Ointment,
   USP 0.5%
Hydrophilic Ointment
Ichthammol Ointment 10% & 20%
Lanolin, USP
Lanolin Anhydrous, USP
Petrolatum White, USP
Vitamin A + Vitamin D Ointment
Whitfield's Ointment, USP
Yellow Mercuric Oxide Ophthalmic
   Ointment 1% & 2%
Zinc Oxide Ointment, USP

PLOUGH, INC.   **421, 640**
3030 Jackson Avenue
Memphis, TN 38151
Address inquiries to:
Consumer Relations Dept.
         (901) 320-2386
For Medical Emergencies Contact:
Clinical Affairs Dept.   (901) 320-2011
OTC Products Available
◆Aftate for Athlete's Foot
◆Aftate for Jock Itch
◆Aspergum
◆Coppertone Sunscreen Lotion (SPF-6)
◆Coppertone Sunscreen Lotion (SPF-8)
◆Coppertone Sunscreen Lotion (SPF 15)
◆Correctol Laxative Liquid
◆Correctol Laxative Tablets
   Cushion Grip
◆Di-Gel
◆Duration Mild 4 Hour Nasal Spray
◆Duration 12 Hour Mentholated Nasal
   Spray
◆Duration 12 Hour Nasal Spray
◆Feen-A-Mint Gum
◆Feen-A-Mint Pills
◆Muskol Insect Repellent Aerosol Liquid
◆Muskol Insect Repellent Lotion
◆Regutol
◆St. Joseph Aspirin for Children
◆St. Joseph Aspirin-Free Chewable
   Tablets, Liquid & Infant Drops
◆St. Joseph Cold Tablets for Children
◆St. Joseph Cough Syrup for Children
◆Shade Sunscreen Lotion SPF 4
◆Shade Sunscreen Lotion SPF 6
◆Shade Sunscreen Lotion SPF 8
◆Shade Sunscreen Lotion SPF 15
◆Solarcaine

PROCTER & GAMBLE   **422, 643**
P.O. Box 171
Cincinnati, OH 45201
Address inquiries to:
Lawrence W. Farrell   (513) 530-2154
For Medical Emergencies Contact:
W.S. Lainhart, M.D.   (513) 627-7071
After hours, call Collect
         (513) 751-5525
OTC Products Available
◆Chloraseptic Preparations
◆   Children's Chloraseptic Lozenges
◆   Chloraseptic Liquid
◆   Chloraseptic Lozenges
◆Encaprin
◆Head & Chest Capsules
◆Head & Chest Liquid
◆Head & Chest Tablets

Head & Shoulders
◆Norwich Aspirin
◆Norwich Extra Strength Aspirin
◆Pepto-Bismol Liquid & Tablets
Scope

THE PURDUE FREDERICK   **647**
COMPANY
100 Connecticut Avenue
Norwalk, CT 06856   (203) 853-0123
Address inquiries to:
Medical Department
OTC Products Available
Arthropan Liquid
Betadine Aerosol Spray
Betadine Antiseptic Gauze Pad
Betadine Antiseptic Gel with Vaginal
   Applicator
Betadine Antiseptic Lubricating Gel
Betadine Disposable Medicated Douche
Betadine Douche
Betadine Douche Kit
Betadine Hēlafoam Solution
Betadine Mouthwash/Gargle
Betadine Ointment
Betadine Perineal Wash Concentrate
Betadine Shampoo
Betadine Skin Cleanser
Betadine Skin Cleanser Foam
Betadine Solution
Betadine Solution Swab Aid
Betadine Solution Swabsticks
Betadine Surgical Scrub
Betadine Surgi-Prep Sponge-Brush
Betadine Vaginal Suppositories
Betadine Viscous Formula Antiseptic
   Gauze Pad
Betadine Whirlpool Concentrate
Fibermed (Original & Fruit Flavors)
Fibermed High-Fiber Snacks
Senokap DSS Capsules
Senokot Suppositories
Senokot Syrup
Senokot Tablets/Granules
Senokot Tablets Unit Strip Pack
Senokot-S Tablets

REED & CARNRICK   **423, 649**
1 New England Avenue
Piscataway, NJ 08854
Address Inquiries to:
Professional Service Dept.
         (201) 981-0070
For Medical Emergencies Contact:
Medical Director   (201) 981-0070
OTC Products Available
Alphosyl Lotion, Cream
◆Phazyme Tablets
◆Phazyme-95 Tablets
◆Phazyme-125 Capsules Maximum
   Strength
◆proctoFoam/non-steroid
   Proxigel
◆R&C Lice Treatment Kit
◆R&C Shampoo
◆R&C Spray III
Trichotine Liquid, Vaginal Douche
Trichotine Powder, Vaginal Douche

REQUA MANUFACTURING   **651**
COMPANY, INC.
1 Seneca Place
Greenwich, CT 06830
Address inquiries to:
John L. Geils   (203) 869-2445
OTC Products Available
Charcoaid
Charcocaps

REXALL NUTRITIONAL   **651**
PRODUCTS, INC.
3901 N. Kingshighway Blvd.
St. Louis, MO 63115
Address inquiries to:
Director, Technical Affairs
         (314) 679-7100
For Medical Emergencies Contact:
Director, Technical Affairs
         (314) 679-7100
OTC Products Available
PMS Balance
Pac-Man Sugar Free Calcium for Kids
Pac-Man Sugar-Free Chewable
   Multivitamins plus Iron

RICHARDSON-VICKS INC.   **423, 651**
Personal Care Products Division
10 Westport Road
Wilton, CT 06897
Address inquiries to:
Vicks Research Center
         (203) 929-2500
For Medical Emergencies Contact
Medical Director
Vicks Research Center
         (203) 929-2500
OTC Products Available
Clearasil Acne Treatment Stick
◆Clearasil Adult Care - Medicated
   Blemish Cream
Clearasil Antibacterial Soap
Clearasil 10% Benzoyl Peroxide Lotion
   Acne Medication
◆Clearasil Pore Deep Cleanser
◆Clearasil Super Strength Acne
   Treatment Cream, Covering
◆Clearasil Super Strength Acne
   Treatment Cream, Vanishing
◆Topex 10% Benzoyl Peroxide Lotion
   Buffered Acne Medication

ORAL HEALTH PRODUCTS
Benzodent Analgesic Denture Ointment
Complete Denture Cleanser and
   Toothpaste in One
Denquel Sensitive Teeth Toothpaste
Fasteeth Denture Adhesive Powder
Fixodent Denture Adhesive Cream
Kleenite Denture Cleanser

RIKER LABORATORIES, INC.   **652**
255-1S-07 3M Center
St. Paul, MN 55144
Address Inquiries to:
Medical Services Dept.
For Medical Emergencies Contact:
         (612) 736-4930
Customer Service and other services:
         (612) 736-5747
Products Available
Cal•Sup Tablets
Medihaler-EPI

A. H. ROBINS COMPANY,   **423, 653**
INC.
CONSUMER PRODUCTS
DIVISION
3800 Cutshaw Avenue
Richmond, VA 23230
Address inquiries to:
The Medical Department
         (804) 257-2000
For Medical Emergencies Contact:
Medical Department   (804) 257-2000
(day or night)
If no answer, call answering service
         (804) 257-7788
OTC Products Available
◆Allbee C-800 Plus Iron Tablets
◆Allbee C-800 Tablets
◆Allbee with C Capsules
◆Chap Stick Lip Balm
◆Chap Stick Sunblock 15 Lip Balm
◆Dimacol Capsules
◆Dimetane Decongestant Elixir
◆Dimetane Decongestant Tablets
◆Dimetane Elixir
◆Dimetane Extentabs 8 mg
◆Dimetane Extentabs 12 mg
◆Dimetane Tablets
◆Extend-12 Liquid
◆Lip Soother Medicated Lip Cream
◆Robitussin
◆Robitussin-CF
◆Robitussin-DM
◆Robitussin-PE
◆Robitussin Night Relief
◆Z-Bec Tablets

ROCHE LABORATORIES   **425, 657**
Division of Hoffmann-La Roche Inc.
340 Kingsland Street
Nutley, NJ 07110
For Medical Information
Write: Professional Services Dept.

(◆ **Shown in Product Identification Section**)

Business hours only (8:30 a.m. to
5:00 p.m. EST), call
(201) 235-2355
For Medical Emergency Information
only after hours or on weekends,
call (201) 235-2355
Branch Warehouses
Belvidere, NJ 07823
Water Street (201) 475-5337
Des Plaines, IL 60018
105 E. Oakton St. (312) 299-0021
(Chicago) (312) 775-0733
OTC Products Available
◆Vi-Penta Infant Drops
◆Vi-Penta Multivitamin Drops

WILLIAM H. RORER, INC.   **425, 658**
500 Virginia Drive
Fort Washington, PA 19034
For Medical Emergencies Contact:
John F. A. Vance, M.D.
Medical Director (215) 628-6761
For Quality Matters Contact:
William E. Kinas, Vice President,
Quality Assurance (215) 628-6420
For Product Information Contact:
Ronald A. Amey, Marketing Services
Manager (215) 628-6492
Branch Offices
Langhorne, PA 19047
2201 Cabot Blvd. West
(215) 752-8555
Oak Forest, IL 60452
P.O. Box 280
4325 Frontage Rd. (312) 687-7440
San Leandro, CA 94577
P.O. Box 1569
1550 Factor Ave. (415) 357-9741
Tucker, GA 30084
4660 Hammermill Rd.
(404) 934-3091
OTC Products Available
◆Ascriptin Tablets
◆Ascriptin A/D Tablets
Calciferol Drops
Camalox Suspension & Tablets
◆Emetrol Solution
Fedahist Expectorant, Syrup & Tablets
Fermalox Tablets
Gemnisyn Tablets
Kudrox Suspension (Double Strength)
◆Lactrase
◆Maalox Suspension & Tablets
◆Maalox Plus Suspension & Tablets
◆Maalox TC Suspension & Tablets
Milkinol
◆Perdium Granules
◆Perdium Plain Granules

ROSS LABORATORIES   **426, 663**
Division of Abbott Laboratories USA
P.O. Box 1317
Columbus, OH 43216
Address Inquiries to:
Medical Director (614) 227-3333
OTC Products Available
Advance
◆Clear Eyes Eye Drops
◆Ear Drops by Murine
(See Murine Ear Wax Removal
System/Murine Ear Drops)
Isomil
Isomil SF
◆Murine Ear Wax Removal
System/Murine Ear Drops
◆Murine Eye Drops (Regular Formula)
◆Murine Plus Eye Drops
RCF-Ross Carbohydrate Free Soy
Protein Formula Base
◆Selsun Blue Dandruff Shampoo
(selenium sulfide lotion 1%)
Similac
Similac PM 60/40
Similac with Iron
Similac with Whey + Iron
◆Tronolane Cream
◆Tronolane Suppositories

ROWELL LABORATORIES, INC.   **671**
210 Main Street W.
Baudette, MN 56623

Address Inquiries to:
Professional Service Dept.
(218) 634-1866
For Medical Emergencies Contact:
V.P., Medical Affairs (218) 634-1866
OTC Products Available
Balneol
C-Ron
C-Ron Forte
C-Ron Freckles
Colrex Capsules
Colrex Expectorant
Colrex Syrup
Colrex Troches
Dermacort Lotion 0.5%
Hydrocil Instant
Quine 200
Quine 300

RYDELLE LABORATORIES,   **426, 671**
INC.
Subsidiary of S.C. Johnson & Son, Inc.
1525 Howe Street
Racine, WI 53403
Address inquiries to:
Carol Hansen
Consumer Affairs Director
(414) 631-4000
For Medical Emergencies Contact:
Richard D. Stewart (414) 631-3675
OTC Products Available
◆Fiberall, Natural Flavor
◆Fiberall, Orange Flavor

SCHERER LABORATORIES, INC.   **672**
14335 Gillis Road
Dallas, Texas 75244
Address Inquiries to:
F. R. Stravs (214) 233-2800
For Medical Emergencies Contact:
F. R. Stravs (214) 233-2800
OTC Products Available
HuMist Saline Nasal Mist
Xero-Lube - Saliva Substitute

SCHERING CORPORATION   **426, 672**
Galloping Hill Road
Kenilworth, NJ 07033
Address inquiries to:
Professional Services Department
(201) 558-4908
OTC Products Available
A and D Cream
◆A and D Ointment
◆Afrin Menthol Nasal Spray 0.05%
◆Afrin Nasal Spray 0.05%, Nose Drops
0.05%, Pediatric Nose Drops
0.025%
◆Afrinol Repetabs Tablets
◆Chlor-Trimeton Allergy Syrup, Tablets &
Long-Acting Repetabs Tablets
◆Chlor-Trimeton Decongestant Tablets
◆Chlor-Trimeton Long Acting
Decongestant Repetabs Tablets
◆Chlor-Trimeton Timed Release Allergy
Tablets
◆Cod Liver Oil Concentrate Tablets,
Capsules
◆Cod Liver Oil Concentrate Tablets
w/Vitamin C
Coricidin Cough Syrup
◆Coricidin 'D' Decongestant Tablets
Coricidin Decongestant Nasal Mist
◆Coricidin Demilets Tablets for Children
Coricidin Extra Strength Sinus
Headache Tablets
Coricidin Medilets Tablets for Children
◆Coricidin Tablets
◆Demazin Decongestant-Antihistamine
Repetabs Tablets & Syrup
◆Dermolate Anal-Itch Ointment
◆Dermolate Anti-Itch Cream & Spray
◆Dermolate Scalp-Itch Lotion
Disophrol Chronotab Sustained-Action
Tablets
Disophrol Tablets
◆Drixoral Sustained-Action Tablets
◆Emko Because Contraceptor Vaginal
Contraceptive Foam

◆Emko Pre-Fil Vaginal Contraceptive
Foam
◆Emko Vaginal Contraceptive Foam
◆Mol-Iron Tablets & Chronosule
Capsules
◆Mol-Iron Tablets w/Vitamin C
Sunril Premenstrual Capsules
◆Tinactin Aerosol Liquid 1%
◆Tinactin Aerosol Powder 1%
◆Tinactin Antifungal 1%, Cream,
Solution & Powder
◆Tinactin Jock Itch Cream 1%
◆Tinactin Jock Itch Spray Powder 1%

SEARLE CONSUMER   **428, 681**
PRODUCTS
Division of G. D. Searle & Co.
Box 5110
Chicago, IL 60680
Address inquiries to:
Medical Communications Department
G.D. Searle & Co.
4901 Searle Parkway
Skokie, IL 60077
For Medical Emergencies Contact:
Medical Department, G.D. Searle & Co.
Outside IL (business hours)
(800) 323-4204
Within IL (at other times)
(312) 982-7000
OTC Products Available
◆Dramamine Liquid
◆Dramamine Tablets
◆Equal Packets
◆Equal Sweet-tabs
◆Icy Hot Balm
◆Icy Hot Rub
◆Metamucil, Instant Mix, Orange Flavor
◆Metamucil, Instant Mix, Regular Flavor
◆Metamucil Powder, Orange Flavor
◆Metamucil Powder, Regular Flavor
◆Metamucil Powder, Strawberry Flavor
◆Metamucil Powder, Sugar Free, Regular
Flavor
◆Prompt

SOLGAR COMPANY, INC.   **428, 684**
410 Ocean Avenue
Lynbrook, NY 11563
Address inquiries to:
Rand Skolnick (516) 599-2442
OTC Products Available
Acidophilus Capsules
Alfalfa Tablets
Apple Pectin Powder
L-Arginine Capsules
B-Complex with C Stress Tablets
Beta Carotene Capsules
Biotin Tablets
Bone Meal Tablets
Bran Tablets, Miller's
Brewer's Yeast Tablets
Calcium 600
Calcium Ascorbate Tablets
Calcium Gluconate Tablets
Calcium Magnesium Tablets
Chews-Eze Tablets
Choline Tablets
Choline/Inositol Tablets
Citrus Bioflavonoid Complex
Cod Liver Oil Caps
L-Cysteine Capsules
Digestive Aid Tablets
Dolomite Tablets
Folic Acid Tablets
Formula B-50 Capsules
Formula B-100 Tablets
◆Formula VM-75 Tablets
Garlic Perles Capsules
Gelatin Capsules
L-Glutamic Acid Tablets
L-Glutamine Capsules
Glutathione Capsules
Hy-C Tablets
Inositol Tablets
Lecithin Capsules
Lecithin "95" Granules
Liver Tablets
L-Lysine Capsules
MaxEPA Capsules
Niacin Tablets
Niacinamide Tablets

(◆ Shown in Product Identification Section)

Octacosanol Capsules
L-Ornithine Capsules
Pantothenic Acid Tablets, 100 mg,
  200 mg & 500 mg
L-Phenylalanine Capsules
Potassium Gluconate Tablets
RNA/DNA Tablets
Rutin Tablets
Selenium Tablets
Spirulina Tablets
Taurine Capsules
L-Tryptophan Capsules
Vitamin A Capsules, 10,000 IU &
  25,000 IU
Vitamin B-1 Tablets
Vitamin B-2 Tablets
Vitamin B-6 Tablets
Vitamin B-12 Tablets
Vitamin C Tablets
Vitamin D Capsules 400 IU & 1000 IU
Vitamin E Capsules, 100 IU, 200 IU &
  400 IU D-Alpha Tocopherol plus
  Mixed Tocopherol
Vitamin E Capsules, 1000 IU D-Alpha
  Tocopherol plus Mixed Tocopherols
Vitamin K Tablets
Wheat Germ Oil Capsules
Zinc "50" Tablets

SPORTMED TECHNOLOGY LTD.   **741**
2180 Belgrave Avenue, Suite 495
Montreal, Quebec, Canada H4A 2L8
Address inquiries to:
Lawrence Klein, Vice President
    (514) 489-8251
    (800) 361-3651

For Medical Emergencies Contact:
Dr. H. K. Myers   (514) 731-9195
OTC Products Available
Sportmed Fitness Appraisal Kit

E. R. SQUIBB & SONS, INC.   **428, 685**
General Offices
P.O. Box 4000
Princeton, NJ 08540 (609) 921-4000
Address Inquiries to:
Squibb Professional Services Dept.
P.O. Box 4000
Princeton, NJ 08540 (609) 921-4006
Distribution Centers
ATLANTA, GEORGIA
  P.O. Box 16503
  Atlanta, GA 30321
State of GA Customers Call
    (800) 282-9103
Customers in States of AL, FL, MS, NC,
SC, and TN Call   (800) 241-1744
All Others Call   (800) 241-5364
CHICAGO, ILLINOIS
  P.O. Box 788
  Arlington Heights, IL 60006
State of IL Customers Call
    (800) 942-0674
All Others Call   (800) 323-0665
DALLAS, TEXAS
Mail or telephone orders and customer
service inquiries should be directed to
Atlanta, GA (see above)
State of MS Customers Call
    (800) 241-1744
All others call   (800) 241-5364
LOS ANGELES, CALIFORNIA
  P.O. Box 428
  La Mirada, CA 90638
State of CA Customers Call
    (800) 422-4254
State of HI Customers Call
    (714) 521-7050
All Others Call   (800) 854-3050
SEATTLE, WASHINGTON
Mail or telephone orders and customer
service inquiries should be directed to
Los Angeles, CA (see above)
States of AK and MT Customers Call
    (714) 521-7050
State of CA Customers Call
    (800) 422-4254
All Others Call   (800) 854-3050
NEW YORK AREA
  P.O. Box 2013
  New Brunswick, NJ 08903

State of NJ Customers Call
    (800) 352-4865
State of ME Customers Call
    (201) 469-5400
All Others Call   (800) 631-5244
OTC Products Available
E.T. The Extra-Terrestrial Children's
  Chewable Vitamins
E.T. The Extra-Terrestrial Children's
  Chewable Vitamins with Iron
Spec-T Sore Throat Anesthetic
  Lozenges
Spec-T Sore Throat/Cough Suppressant
  Lozenges
Spec-T Sore Throat/Decongestant
  Lozenges
Theragran Liquid
◆ Theragran Stress Formula
Theragran Tablets
◆ Theragran-M Tablets

STELLAR PHARMACAL   **428, 686**
CORP.
1990 N.W. 44th Street
R.R. 2, Box 904J
Pompano Beach, FL 33067
Address inquiries to:
Scott L. Davidson   (305) 972-6060
Customer Service & Order Department
    (800) 845-7827
OTC Products Available
◆ Star-Otic Ear Solution

STUART   **428, 686**
PHARMACEUTICALS
Div. of ICI Americas, Inc.
Wilmington, DE 19897
Address inquiries to:
Yvonne A. Graham, Manager
  Professional Services
    (302) 575-2231
For Medical Emergencies:
After hours & on weekends
    (302) 575-3000
OTC Products Available
◆ ALternaGEL Liquid
◆ Dialose Capsules
◆ Dialose Plus Capsules
◆ Effersyllium Instant Mix
  Ferancee Chewable Tablets
◆ Ferancee-HP Tablets
◆ Hibiclens
  Hibistat
◆ Kasof Capsules
◆ Mylanta Liquid
◆ Mylanta Tablets
◆ Mylanta-II Liquid
◆ Mylanta-II Tablets
◆ Mylicon (Tablets & Drops)
◆ Mylicon-80 Tablets
◆ Orexin Softab Tablets
◆ Probec-T Tablets
◆ The Stuart Formula Tablets
◆ Stuart Prenatal Tablets
◆ Stuartinic Tablets

SUNRISE & RAINBOW   **429, 691**
9526 West Pico Blvd.
Los Angeles, CA 90035
Address inquiries to:
    (213) 276-7237
OTC Products Available
Nursamil
◆ Nutrimil
Prenatamil

SYNTEX LABORATORIES, INC.   **691**
3401 Hillview Avenue
Palo Alto, CA 94304
Address medical inquiries to:
Medical Affairs   (415) 855-5545
Report adverse reactions to:
    (415) 852-1386
Address other inquiries to:
    (415) 855-5050
OTC Products Available
Carmol 10, 10% Urea Lotion
Carmol 20, 20% Urea Cream

THOMPSON MEDICAL   **430, 692**
COMPANY, INC.
919 Third Avenue
New York, NY 10022

Address inquiries to:
Dr. Edward L. Steinberg
    (212) 688-4420
OTC Products Available
◆ Appedrine, Maximum Strength Tablets
◆ Aqua-Ban Tablets
◆ Aqua-Ban, Maximum Strength Plus
  Tablets
◆ Aspercreme
◆ Control Capsules
◆ Cortizone-5 Creme & Ointment
◆ Dexatrim Capsules
◆ Dexatrim Extra Strength Capsules
◆ Dexatrim Extra Strength, Caffeine-Free
  Capsules
◆ Dexatrim Extra Strength Plus Vitamins
  Capsules
◆ Encare
◆ Prolamine Capsules, Maximum Strength
  Capsules
◆ Sleepinal, Maximum Strength Capsules
◆ Slim-Fast

THOUGHT TECHNOLOGY LTD.   **741**
2180 Belgrave Avenue, Suite 495
Montreal, Quebec, Canada H4A 2L8
Address inquiries to:
Lawrence Klein, Vice President
    (514) 489-8251
    (800) 361-3651
For Medical Emergencies Contact:
Dr. H.K. Myers   (514) 731-9195
OTC Products Available
Biofeedback 5
Calmset 3
EMG100T
GSR 2
GSR/Temp 2
HR/BVP 200T

ULMER PHARMACAL   **696**
A Krelitz Industries Company
2440 Fernbrook Lane
Minneapolis, MN 55441
Address Inquiries to:
Professional Services Dept.
  In MN (800) 292-7918
  In USA (800) 328-7157
OTC Products Available
Aerosan
Andoin Ointment
Bi-Amine
Chloral Methylol Ointment
Clinitar Cream
Clinitar Shampoo
Clinitar Stick
Gentle Shampoo
Kler-ro Liquid
Kler-ro Powder
Liquid Lather
Lobana Bath Oil
Lobana Body Lotion
Lobana Body Powder
Lobana Body Shampoo
Lobana Conditioning Shampoo
Lobana Derm-Ade Cream
Lobana Liquid Hand Soap
Lobana Peri-Gard
Lobana Perineal Cleanse
M.O.M. (Suspension of Magnesium
  Hydroxide)
Pheneen Solution
Reagent Alcohol
Surgel Liquid
Ta-Poff Aerosol
Ta-Poff Liquid
Versa-Quat
Verucid Gel
Vitamin A & D Ointment
Vleminckx' Solution

THE UPJOHN COMPANY   **430, 698**
7000 Portage Road
Kalamazoo, MI 49001
Address inquiries to:
Medical Information   (616) 323-6615
Pharmaceutical Sales Areas
and Distribution Centers
Atlanta (Chamblee)
  GA 30341   (404) 451-4822

(◆ Shown in Product Identification Section)

Boca Raton, FL 33432
    (305) 392-8500
Boston (Wellesley)
  MA 02181   (617) 431-7970
Buffalo (Cheektowaga)
  NY 14225   (716) 681-7160
Chicago (Oak Brook)
  IL 60521   (312) 654-3300
Cincinnati, OH 45237
    (513) 242-4574
Dallas, TX 75204   (214) 824-3028
Denver, CO 80216   (303) 399-3113
Hartford (Enfield)
  CT 06082   (203) 741-3421
Honolulu, HI 96813   (808) 538-1181
Kalamazoo, MI 49001
    (616) 323-7222
Kansas City, MO 64131
    (816) 361-2291
Los Angeles, CA 90038
    (213) 463-8101
Memphis, TN 38122 (901) 761-4170
Minneapolis, MN 55422
    (612) 588-2786
New York (Garden City)
  NY 11530   (516) 294-3530
Orlando, FL 32809   (305) 859-4591
Philadelphia (Wayne)
  PA 19087   (215) 265-2100
Pittsburgh (Bridgeville)
  PA 15017   (412) 257-0200
Portland, OR 97232 (503) 232-2133
St. Louis, MO 63146 (314) 872-8626
San Francisco (Palo Alto)
  CA 94306   (415) 493-8080
Washington, DC 20011
    (202) 882-6163

OTC Products Available
Alkets Tablets
Baciguent Antibiotic Ointment
Calcium Gluconate Tablets, USP
Calcium Lactate Tablets, USP
Cebenase Tablets
Cheracol Cough Syrup
◆Cheracol D Cough Formula
◆Cheracol Plus Head Cold/Cough
  Formula
Citrocarbonate Antacid
Clocream Skin Cream
◆Cortaid Cream
◆Cortaid Lotion
◆Cortaid Ointment
◆Cortaid Spray
Cortef Feminine Itch Cream
Diostate D Tablets
◆Kaopectate Anti-Diarrhea Medicine
◆Kaopectate Concentrate Anti-Diarrhea
  Medicine
◆Kaopectate Tablet Formula
Lipomul Oral Liquid
Myciguent Antibiotic Cream
Myciguent Antibiotic Ointment
◆Mycitracin Triple Antibiotic Ointment
Orthoxicol Cough Syrup
P-A-C Revised Formula Analgesic
  Tablets
Phenolax Wafers
◆Pyrroxate Capsules
Sigtab Tablets
Super D Perles
◆Unicap Capsules & Tablets
◆Unicap Jr Tablets
◆Unicap M Tablets
◆Unicap Plus Iron Tablets
◆Unicap Senior Tablets
◆Unicap T Tablets
Zymacap Capsules

UPSHER-SMITH   **431, 701**
LABORATORIES, INC.
14905 23rd Avenue North
Minneapolis, MN 55441
Address inquiries to:
Professional Service Department
    (612) 473-4412
For Medical Emergencies Contact:
Scientific Affairs Department
    (612) 473-4412
OTC Products Available
Acetaminophen Uniserts Suppositories
Aspirin Uniserts Suppositories
Bisacodyl Tablets
Bisacodyl Uniserts Suppositories

Daily-M Tablets
Docusate Sodium Capsules
Docusate Sodium with Casanthranol
  Capsules
Ferrous Gluconate Tablets
Ferrous Sulfate Tablets
Hemorrhoidal Uniserts Suppositories
Hemorrhoidal-HC Uniserts
  Suppositories
Hexavitamin Tablets
Kerasol Therapeutic Bath Oil
◆Lubrin Vaginal Lubricating Inserts
Sorbitol Solution
Stress-600 Tablets
Stress-600 with Zinc
Therapeutic B Complex with C
  Capsules
Therapeutic Multivitamin Tablets
Therapeutic Multivitamin & Mineral
  Tablets
Trofan Tablets (L-Tryptophan)

THE VALE CHEMICAL CO., INC   **701**
1201 Liberty St.
Allentown, PA 18102
Address inquiries to:
Elliot R. Davis   (215) 433-7579
OTC Products Available
Acedyne Tablets
Alkaline Aromatic Tablets
Ammonium Chloride Tablets
Antrin Tablets
Antussal Syrup
Aquabase (Beeler's) Hydrophylic
  Ointment Base
Ascorbic Acid Tablets
Aspir-10 Tablets
Aspirin Tablets, 5gr. & 10gr.
Belexal Tablets
Benzo-Menth Lozenges
Bismapec Tablets
Calfos-D Tablets
Dermaval Cream
Double-Sal Tablets
Duphrene Syrup & Tablets
Extract of Ox Bile Tablets
Ferate-C Tablets
Glucovite Tablets
Glycofed
Glycotuss Syrup & Tablets
Glycotuss-dM Syrup & Tablets
Hydra-Mag Tablets
Ironco-B Tablets
Magmalin Tablets & Suspension
Neofed
Neogesic Tablets
Neo-Tab Tablets
Niacin Tablets
Nyral Lozenges
Obeval
Oxynitral w/Veratrum Viride Tablets
Pedric Elixir & Tablets
Pedric Senior Tablets
Sodium Salicylate Tablets
Soothogel Cream
Synthetar Cream
Taystron Tablets
Terphan Elixir
Thiamine Hydrochloride Tablets
Tono-B Wafers
Trioval Tablets
Valax Tablets
Valcaine Ointment
Valcreme Lotion

VERA PRODUCTS, INC.   **431, 701**
601 West Jackson
Harlingen, TX 78550
Address inquiries to:
Todd Waller   (512) 428-6712
OTC Products Available
Lily of the Desert Aloe Vera Burn Aid
  (99.7%)
◆Lily of the Desert Aloe Vera Gelly
  (97%)
Lily of the Desert Aloe Vera Heat Rub
  (80%)
◆Lily of the Desert Aloe Vera Juice
  (99.8%)
Lily of the Desert Aloe Vera Lip Balm
  (20%)
Lily of the Desert Aloe Vera Ointment
  (75%)

Lily of the Desert Aloe Vera Shampoo
  (50%)
Lily of the Desert Aloe Vera Suntan
  Lotion (70%)

VICKS HEALTH CARE   **431, 701**
DIVISION
Richardson-Vicks Inc.
10 Westport Road
Wilton, CT 06897
Address inquiries to:
Director of Scientific & Regulatory
  Affairs
Vicks Research Center
    (203) 929-2500
For Medical Emergencies Contact
Medical Director
Vicks Research Center
    (203) 929-2500
OTC Products Available
◆Daycare Colds Capsules
◆Daycare Colds Liquid
Formula 44 Cough Control Discs
◆Formula 44 Cough Mixture
◆Formula 44D Decongestant Cough
  Mixture
◆Formula 44M Multisymptom Cough
  Mixture
◆Headway Capsules
◆Headway Tablets
◆Nyquil Nighttime Colds Medicine
Oracin Cherry Flavor Cooling Throat
  Lozenges
Oracin Cooling Throat Lozenges
◆Sinex Decongestant Nasal Spray
◆Sinex Long-Acting Decongestant Nasal
  Spray
◆Tempo Antacid with Antigas Action
◆Vaporub
Vaposteam
Vatronol Nose Drops
Vicks Blue Cough Drops
Vicks Childrens Cough Syrup
Vicks Cough Drops
  Regular Flavor
  Wild Cherry Flavor
  Lemon Flavor
  Blue Mint
Vicks Cough Silencers Cough Drops
Vicks Inhaler
Vicks Throat Lozenges
Victors Menthol-Eucalyptus Vapor
  Cough Drops
  Regular
  Cherry Flavor

VICKS PHARMACY   **432, 705**
PRODUCTS DIVISION
A subsidiary of Richardson-Vicks Inc.
10 Westport Road
Wilton, CT 06897
Address inquiries to:
Director of Scientific & Regulatory
  Affairs
Vicks Research Center
    (203) 929-2500
For Medical Emergencies Contact:
Medical Director
Vicks Research Center
    (203) 929-2500
OTC Products Available
Cremacoat 1
Cremacoat 2
Cremacoat 3
Cremacoat 4
◆Percogesic Analgesic Tablets

VIDAL SASSOON, INC.   **432, 707**
2049 Century Park East
Los Angeles, CA 90067
Address Inquiries to:
Vidal Sassoon Research Department
  Services   Toll free outside CA:
    (800) 421-4296
    California:
    (213) 998-2722
    (213) 873-7580

    (◆ Shown in Product Identification Section)

For Medical Emergencies Contact:
Vice President, Research and
Development   Toll free outside CA:
                              (800) 421-4296
                              California:
                              (213) 998-2722
                              (213) 873-7580
OTC Products Available
Sassoon D Hair and Scalp Conditioner
◆Sassoon D Shampoo

**WAKUNAGA OF AMERICA   432, 707
CO., LTD.**
Subsidiary of Wakunaga Pharmaceutical
Co., Ltd.
23510 Telo Avenue
Torrance, CA 90505
Address inquires to:
                              (213) 539-3381
OTC Products Available
◆Kyolic
◆   Kyolic-Aged Garlic Extract Flavor &
      Odor Modified Enriched with
      Vitamin B$_1$
      Kyolic-Aged Garlic Extract Flavor &
      Odor Modified Plain
      Kyolic-Formula 101 Capsules:
      Aged Garlic Extract (270 mg)
      Kyolic-Formula 101 Tablets: Aged
      Garlic Extract Powder (270 mg)
      Kyolic-Formula 103 Capsules:
      Aged Garlic Extract Powder
      (220 mg)
◆   Kyolic-Super Formula 100
      Capsules Aged Garlic Extract
      Powder (300 mg)
      Kyolic-Super Formula 100 Tablets:
      Aged Garlic Extract Powder (270
      mg)

WALKER, CORP & CO., INC.   707
20 E. Hampton Place
Syracuse, NY 13206
Address inquiries to:
P.O. Box 1320
Syracuse, NY 13201 (315) 463-4511
For Medical Emergencies Contact:
Robert G. Long   (315) 638-4763
OTC Products Available
Evac-U-Gen

WALKER PHARMACAL CO.   707
4200 Laclede
St. Louis, MO 63108
Address Inquiries to:
Customer Service   (314) 533-9600
OTC Products Available
HIKE Antiseptic Ointment
PRID Salve

WALLACE LABORATORIES   432, 708
Half Acre Road
Cranbury, NJ 08512
Address inquiries to:
Wallace Laboratories
Div. of Carter-Wallace, Inc.
P.O. Drawer #5
Cranbury, NJ 08512 (609) 655-6000
For Medical Emergencies:
                              (609) 799-1167
OTC Products Available
◆Maltsupex
◆Ryna
◆Ryna-C
◆Ryna-CX
◆Syllact

**WARNER-LAMBERT   432, 709
COMPANY**
201 Tabor Road
Morris Plains, NJ 07950
Address Inquiries to:
Robert Kirpitch   (201) 540-3204
For Medical Emergencies Contact:
Dr. Robert Gabrielson (201) 540-2301
OTC Products Available
◆e.p.t. Plus In-Home Early Pregnancy
  Test
◆Early Detector - In Home Test for
  Detection of Fecal Occult Blood
◆Efferdent Extra Strength
◆Halls Mentho-Lyptus Cough Tablets
◆Listerine Antiseptic
◆Listermint with Fluoride

Lubriderm Cream
◆Lubriderm Lotion
◆Lubriderm Lubath Bath-Shower Oil
  Maximum Strength Listerine Lozenges
◆Mediquell Chewy Cough Squares

**WARNER-LAMBERT   432, 709, 742
INC.**
Santurce, PR 00911
Address Inquiries to:
Robert Kirpitch   (201) 540-3204
For Medical Emergencies Contact:
Dr. Robert Gabrielson
                              (201) 540-2301
OTC Products Available
◆Rolaids
◆Sinutab Maximum Strength Capsules
◆Sinutab Maximum Strength Tablets
◆Sinutab Tablets
◆Sinutab II Maximum Strength No
  Drowsiness Formula Tablets &
  Capsules

**WESTWOOD   433, 712
PHARMACEUTICALS INC.**
100 Forest Avenue
Buffalo, NY 14213
Address inquiries to:
Consumer Affairs Department
                              (716) 887-3773
OTC Products Available
Alpha Keri Soap
◆Alpha Keri Therapeutic Shower & Bath
  Oil
Balnetar
Estar Gel
◆Fostex Medicated Cleansing Bar
  Fostex Medicated Cleansing Cream
◆Fostex 5% Benzoyl Peroxide Gel
◆Fostex 10% Benzoyl Peroxide
  Cleansing Bar
◆Fostex 10% Benzoyl Peroxide Gel
◆Fostex 10% Benzoyl Peroxide Tinted
  Cream
◆Fostex 10% Benzoyl Peroxide Wash
  Fostril
  Keri Creme
  Keri Facial Soap
◆Keri Lotion
  Lowila Cake
  Moisturel
  Pernox Lotion
  Pernox Medicated Lathering Scrub
  Pernox Shampoo
  PreSun 4 Creamy Sunscreen
  PreSun 8 Lotion, Creamy & Gel
◆PreSun 15 Creamy Sunscreen
◆PreSun 15 Sunscreen Lotion
  Sebucare
◆Sebulex & Sebulex Cream Shampoo
  Sebulex Shampoo with Conditioners
◆Sebulon Dandruff Shampoo
  Sebutone & Sebutone Cream Shampoo
  Transact
  Westcort Cream
  Westcort Ointment 0.2%

WHITEHALL LABORATORIES   434, 714
Division of American Home Products
  Corporation
685 Third Avenue
New York, NY 10017
Address inquiries to:
Medical Department   (212) 878-5508
OTC Products Available
◆Advil Ibuprofen Tablets
  Anacin Analgesic Capsules
◆Anacin Analgesic Tablets
  Anacin Maximum Strength Analgesic
  Capsules
  Anacin Maximum Strength Analgesic
  Tablets
◆Anacin-3 Children's Acetaminophen
  Chewable Tablets, Liquid, Drops
◆Anacin-3 Maximum Strength
  Acetaminophen Tablets & Capsules
  Anacin-3 Regular Strength
  Acetaminophen Tablets
◆Anbesol Baby Gel Antiseptic Anesthetic
◆Anbesol Gel Antiseptic Anesthetic

◆Anbesol Liquid Antiseptic Anesthetic
◆Arthritis Pain Formula by the Makers of
  Anacin Analgesic Tablets
  Arthritis Pain Formula Aspirin-Free by
  the Makers of Anacin Analgesic
  Tablets
◆Arthritis Pain Formula Safety Coated by
  the Makers of Anacin Analgesic
  Tablets
  Bisodol Antacid Powder
  Bisodol Antacid Tablets
  Bronitin Asthma Tablets
  Bronitin Mist
  Compound W Gel
  Compound W Liquid
  Denalan Denture Cleanser
◆Denorex Medicated Shampoo &
  Conditioner
◆Denorex Medicated Shampoo, Mountain
  Fresh Herbal
◆Denorex Medicated Shampoo, Regular
  Diet Gard 14 Day Diet Plan
◆Dristan Advanced Formula
  Decongestant/Antihistimine/
  Analgesic Capsules
◆Dristan Advanced Formula
  Decongestant/Antihistamine/
  Analgesic Tablets
  Dristan Cough Formula
  Dristan 12-Hour Nasal Decongestant
  Capsules
  Dristan Inhaler
◆Dristan Long Lasting Nasal Spray
◆Dristan Menthol Nasal Spray
  Dristan Nasal Spray
  Dristan Room Vaporizer
◆Dristan Ultra Colds Formula Nighttime
  Liquid
  Dristan Ultra Colds Formula Tablets &
  Capsules
  Dristan-AF Decongestant/
  Antihistamine/Analgesic Tablets
  Dry and Clear Acne Medicated Lotion &
  Double Strength Cream
  Dry and Clear Medicated Acne Cleanser
  Freezone Solution
  Heather Feminine Deodorant Spray
  Heet Analgesic Liniment
  Heet Analgesic Spray
  InfraRub Analgesic Cream
  Medicated Cleansing Pads by the
  Makers of Preparation H
  Hemorrhoidal Remedies
  Momentum Muscular Backache
  Formula
  Neet Aerosol Depilatory
  Neet Depilatory Cream
  Neet Depilatory Lotion
  Outgro Solution
  Oxipor VHC Lotion for Psoriasis
  Predictor In-Home Early Pregnancy
  Test
◆Preparation H Hemorrhoidal Ointment
◆Preparation H Hemorrhoidal
  Suppositories
  Prepcort Hydrocortisone Cream 0.5%
◆Primatene Mist
  Primatene Mist Suspension
◆Primatene Tablets - M Formula
◆Primatene Tablets - P Formula
  Quiet World Nighttime Pain Formula
◆Semicid Vaginal Contraceptive
  Suppositories
  Sleep-eze 3 Tablets
  Sudden Action Breath Freshener
  Sudden Beauty Country Air Mask
  Sudden Beauty Hair Spray
  Trendar Menstrual Relief Tablets
  Viro-Med Liquid
  Viro-Med Tablets
  Youth Garde Moisturizer Plus PABA

**WINTHROP-BREON   435, 721
LABORATORIES**
90 Park Ave.
New York, NY 10016
Address inquiries to:
Medical Department   (212) 907-2705
Main Office
90 Park Avenue
New York, NY 10016
                              (212) 907-2000

(◆ Shown in Product Identification Section)

OTC Products Available
◆Breonesin Capsules
Bronkolixir
◆Bronkotabs
◆Fergon Capsules
Fergon Elixir
◆Fergon Tablets
Measurin Tablets

**WINTHROP CONSUMER   722
PRODUCTS**
Division of Sterling Drug Inc.
90 Park Avenue
New York, NY 10016
Address inquiries to:
Winthrop Consumer Products
For Medical Emergencies Contact:
Medical Department   (212) 907-3027
                      (212) 907-3029
OTC Products Available
Bronkaid Mist
Bronkaid Mist Suspension
Bronkaid Tablets
Campho-Phenique Gel
Campho-Phenique Liquid
Haley's M-O, Regular & Flavored
NTZ Long Acting Spray & Drops
NāSal Saline Drops
NāSal Saline Spray
Neo-Synephrine Jelly
Neo-Synephrine Nasal Sprays
Neo-Synephrine Nasal Spray
  (Mentholated)
Neo-Synephrine Nose Drops
Neo-Synephrine II Long Acting Nasal
  Spray
Neo-Synephrine II Long Acting Nose
  Drops (Adult & Children's Strengths)
Neo-Synephrine II Long Acting Vapor
  Nasal Spray
Neo-Synephrine 12 Hour Nasal Spray
Neo-Synephrine 12 Hour Nose Drops
  (Adult & Children's Strengths)
Neo-Synephrine 12 Hour Vapor Nasal
  Spray
pHisoAc BP
pHisoDan
pHisoDerm
pHisoDerm-Fresh Scent
pHisoPUFF
Soapure
WinGel Liquid & Tablets

WYETH LABORATORIES   435, 726
Division of American Home Products
Corporation
P.O. Box 8299
Philadelphia, PA 19101

Address inquiries to:
Professional Service   (215) 341-2220
For EMERGENCY Medical Information
Day or night call   (215) 688-4400

Wyeth Distribution Centers
Andover, MA 01810
  P.O. Box 1776   (617) 475-9075
Atlanta, GA 30302
  P.O. Box 4365   (404) 873-1681
Baltimore, MD 21224
  101 Kane St.   (301) 633-4000
Boston Distribution Center
  see under Andover, MA
Buena Park, CA 90622-5000
  P.O. Box 5000   (714) 523-5500
  (Los Angeles) (213) 627-5374
Chicago Distribution Center
  see under Wheaton, IL
Cleveland, OH 44101
  P.O. Box 91549   (216) 238-9450
Dallas, TX 75238
  P.O. Box 38200   (214) 341-2299
Honolulu, HI 96814
  1013 Kawaiahao St.(808) 538-1988
Kansas City Distribution Center,
  see under North Kansas City, MO
Kent, WA 98064-5609
  P.O. Box 5609   (206) 872-8790
Los Angeles Distribution Center,
  see under Buena Park, CA
Memphis, TN 38101
  P.O. Box 1698   (901) 353-4680
North Kansas City, MO 64116
  P.O. Box 7588   (816) 842-0680
Philadelphia Distribution Center
  Paoli, PA 19301
  P.O. Box 61   (215) 644-8000
           (Phila.) (215) 878-9500
St. Paul, MN 55164
  P.O. Box 64034   (612) 454-6270
Seattle Distribution Center, see under
  Kent, WA
Wheaton, IL 60189-0140
  P.O. Box 140   (312) 462-7200

OTC Products Available
◆Aludrox Oral Suspension & Tablets
◆Amphojel Suspension & Suspension
  without Flavor
◆Amphojel Tablets
◆Basaljel Capsules
◆Basaljel Swallow Tablets
◆Basaljel Suspension & Extra Strength
  Suspension
◆Collyrium Eye Lotion
◆Collyrium 2 Eye Drops with
  Tetrahydrozoline
Nursoy Soy Protein Infant Formula
SMA Iron Fortified Infant Formula
SMA lo-iron
◆Simeco Suspension
◆Wyanoids Hemorrhoidal Suppositories

W. F. YOUNG, INC.   435, 729
111 Lyman Street
Springfield, MA 01103
Address Inquiries to:
Robert F. Ferrin   (413) 737-0201
For Medical Emergencies Contact:
Donald Smith   (413) 737-0201
OTC Products Available
Absorbine Arthritic Pain Lotion
Absorbine Athlete's Foot Powder
◆Absorbine Jr.

**YOUNGS DRUG PRODUCTS   729
CORPORATION**
P.O. Box 385
865 Centennial Avenue
Piscataway, NJ 08854
Sole Distributors for products
manufactured by HOLLAND-RANTOS
COMPANY, INC.

Address Inquiries to:
Mr. Phillip L. Frank or
Mr. Murray H. Glantz (201) 885-5777
OTC Products Available
Koromex Contraceptive Cream
Koromex Contraceptive Crystal Clear
  Gel
Koromex Contraceptive Foam
Koromex Contraceptive Jelly
Nylmerate II Solution Concentrate
Transi-Lube
Triple X - A Pediculicide

(◆ Shown in Product Identification Section)

SECTION 2
Product Name Index

In this section products are listed in alphabetical sequence by brand name or (if described) generic name. Only described products have page numbers to assist you in locating additional information. For additional information on other products, you may wish to contact the manufacturer directly. The symbol ◆ indicates the product is shown in the Product Identification Section.

(◆ Shown in Product Identification Section)   (Products without page numbers are not described)

(◆ Shown in Product Identification Section)   (Products without page numbers are not described)

◆K-Y Lubricating Jelly (Johnson & Johnson) p 411, 560
◆Kank.A Medicated Formula (Blistex) p 404, 520
Kanulase Tablets (Dorsey)
◆Kaopectate Anti-Diarrhea Medicine (Upjohn) p 430, 699
◆Kaopectate Concentrate Anti-Diarrhea Medicine (Upjohn) p 430, 699
◆Kaopectate Tablet Formula (Upjohn) p 431, 699
Karbozyme Tablets (Miller)
Kasof Capsules (Stuart) p 429, 688
Kelp Tablets (Nature's Bounty) p 619
Kerasol Therapeutic Bath Oil (Upsher-Smith)
Keri Creme (Westwood)
Keri Facial Soap (Westwood)
◆Keri Lotion (Westwood) p 433, 713
◆Kerodex Cream 51 (for dry or oily work) (Ayerst) p 404, 509
◆Kerodex Cream 71 (for wet work) (Ayerst) p 404, 509
Kleenite Denture Cleanser (Richardson-Vicks)
Kler-ro Liquid (Ulmer)
Kler-ro Powder (Ulmer)
Kolantyl (Merrell Dow) p 607
Koromex Contraceptive Cream (Youngs Drug Products) p 729
Koromex Contraceptive Crystal Clear Gel (Youngs Drug Products) p 729
Koromex Contraceptive Foam (Youngs Drug Products) p 729
Koromex Contraceptive Jelly (Youngs Drug Products) p 730
Kudrox Suspension (Double Strength) (Rorer) p 660
◆Kyolic (Wakunaga) p 432, 707
◆ Kyolic-Aged Garlic Extract Flavor & Odor Modified Enriched with Vitamin B₁ (Wakunaga) p 432
Kyolic-Aged Garlic Extract Flavor & Odor Modified Plain (Wakunaga)
Kyolic-Formula 101 Capsules: Aged Garlic Extract (270 mg) (Wakunaga)
Kyolic-Formula 101 Tablets: Aged Garlic Extract Powder (270 mg) (Wakunaga)
Kyolic-Formula 103 Capsules: Aged Garlic Extract Powder (220 mg) (Wakunaga)
◆ Kyolic-Super Formula 100 Capsules Aged Garlic Extract Powder (300 mg) (Wakunaga) p 432
Kyolic-Super Formula 100 Tablets: Aged Garlic Extract Powder (270 mg) (Wakunaga)

L

◆Lacri-Lube S.O.P. (Allergan) p 403, 506
◆LactAid (LactAid) p 411, 560
◆Lactinex Tablets & Granules (Hynson, Westcott & Dunning) p 411, 557
◆Lactrase (Rorer) p 425, 660
◆Lanabiotic First Aid Ointment (Combe) p 407, 538
◆Lanacane Medicated Creme (Combe) p 407, 538
◆Lanacort Anti-Itch Hydrocortisone Acetate 0.5% Creme and Ointment (Combe) p 407, 538
Lanamins (Lannett)
Lanatuss Expectorant (Lannett)
Lanolin, U.S.P. (Fougera) p 551
Lanolin, USP (Pharmaderm) p 639
Lanolin Anhydrous, USP (Pharmaderm) p 639
Larylgan Throat Spray (Ayerst)
Lavacol (Parke-Davis)
Lavoptik Eye Cup (Lavoptik) p 739
Lavoptik Eye Wash (Lavoptik) p 561
Lax Special (Anabolic)
Lecithin Capsules (Nature's Bounty) p 619
Lecithin Chewable Tablets (Nature's Bounty) p 619
Lecithin Granules (Nature's Bounty) p 619
Lecithin with Vitamin D Capsules (Nature's Bounty) p 619

Lederplex Capsules and Liquid (Lederle) p 565
◆Li-Ban Spray (Pfipharmecs) p 421, 635
Lily of the Desert Aloe Vera Burn Aid (99.7%) (Vera Products)
◆Lily of the Desert Aloe Vera Gelly (97%) (Vera Products) p 431, 701
Lily of the Desert Aloe Vera Heat Rub (80%) (Vera Products)
◆Lily of the Desert Aloe Vera Juice (99.8%) (Vera Products) p 431, 701
Lily of the Desert Aloe Vera Lip Balm (20%) (Vera Products)
Lily of the Desert Aloe Vera Ointment (75%) (Vera Products)
Lily of the Desert Aloe Vera Shampoo (50%) (Vera Products)
Lily of the Desert Aloe Vera Suntan Lotion (70%) (Vera Products)
◆Lip Soother Medicated Lip Cream (Robins) p 424, 655
Lipall-Plus (Anabolic)
Lipomul Oral Liquid (Upjohn)
Liquid Lather (Ulmer)
Liquifilm Forte (Allergan) p 506
◆Liquifilm Tears (Allergan) p 403, 506
◆Liquiprin Acetaminophen (Norcliff Thayer) p 418, 622
◆Listerine Antiseptic (Warner-Lambert Co.) p 433, 709
Listerine Maximum Strength Lozenges (Warner-Lambert Co.) p 709
◆Listermint with Fluoride (Warner-Lambert Co.) p 433, 710
Liver Tablets (Solgar) p 684
Liver W/B-12 Tablets (Nature's Bounty) p 619
Lobana Bath Oil (Ulmer) p 696
Lobana Body Lotion (Ulmer) p 696
Lobana Body Powder (Ulmer) p 697
Lobana Body Shampoo (Ulmer) p 697
Lobana Conditioning Shampoo (Ulmer) p 697
Lobana Derm-Ade Cream (Ulmer) p 697
Lobana Liquid Hand Soap (Ulmer) p 697
Lobana Peri-Gard (Ulmer) p 697
Lobana Perineal Cleanse (Ulmer) p 697
Lofenalac (Mead Johnson Nutritional) p 586
Lonalac (Mead Johnson Nutritional) p 587
Loroxide Acne Lotion (Flesh Tinted) (Dermik) p 542
Loving Lather Professional Hand Cleanser (Consolidated Chemical)
Lowila Cake (Westwood)
Lubriderm Cream (Warner-Lambert Co.) p 710
◆Lubriderm Lotion (Warner-Lambert Co.) p 433, 710
◆Lubriderm Lubath Bath-Shower Oil (Warner-Lambert Co.) p 433, 710
◆Lubrin Vaginal Lubricating Inserts (Upsher-Smith) p 431, 701
Lycolan Elixir (Lannett)
Lysamin-C (Anabolic)
l-Lysine Tablets (Nature's Bounty) p 619
Lytren (Mead Johnson Nutritional) p 587

M

MCT Oil (Mead Johnson Nutritional) p 588
Mg-plus Protein Tablets (Miller)
M.O.M. (Suspension of Magnesium Hydroxide) (Ulmer)
Mrs. Dash (Alberto-Culver) p 506
◆Maalox Suspension & Tablets (Rorer) p 425, 660
◆Maalox Plus Suspension & Tablets (Rorer) p 425, 661
◆Maalox TC Suspension & Tablets (Rorer) p 425, 661
Magmalin Tablets & Suspension (Vale)
Magnatril Suspension & Tablets (Lannett) p 561
Magnesium Orotate Tablets (Miller)
Magnesium Tablets (Nature's Bounty) p 619
Magonate Tablets (Fleming)
◆Maltsupex Powder, Liquid, Tablets (Wallace) p 432, 708

Manganese Tablets (Nature's Bounty) p 619
Marbec Tablets (Marlyn)
Marblen Suspensions & Tablets (Fleming) p 549
MarEPA Marine Lipid Concentrate (A. G. Marin) p 571
Marezine Tablets (Burroughs Wellcome) p 530
Marlyn Formula 50 Capsules (Marlyn)
◆Marlyn PMS (Marlyn) p 413, 573
Marlyn Prolonged Release Vitamins (Marlyn)
◆Masse Breast Cream (Ortho Pharmaceutical) p 419, 627
Massengill Disposable Douche (Beecham Products) p 514
Massengill Disposable Medicated Douche (Beecham Products) p 514
Massengill Liquid Concentrate (Beecham Products) p 514
Massengill Powder (Beecham Products) p 514
MaxEPA Capsules (Solgar)
◆Maximum Bayer Aspirin (Glenbrook) p 410, 554
Maximum Strength Orajel (See Orajel) (Commerce Drug)
◆Maximum Strength Panadol (Glenbrook) p 410, 555
Measurin Tablets (Winthrop-Breon) p 721
Medicated Cleansing Pads by the Makers of Preparation H Hemorrhoidal Remedies (Whitehall) p 718
Medication Twin Spoon (Apothecary Products)
Medichron (Apothecary Products)
Medicine Nursers (Apothecary Products)
Medicone Dressing Cream (Medicone) p 595
Mediconet (Medicone) p 595
Medihaler-EPI (Riker) p 653
Mediplast (Beiersdorf) p 518
◆Mediquell Chewy Cough Squares (Warner-Lambert Co.) p 433, 710
Medi-Quik Aerosol Spray (Mentholatum) p 604
◆Medi-Set (Apothecary Products) p 403, 735
Medispenser (Apothecary Products)
◆Medtime-Minder (Apothecary Products) p 403, 735
Mega V & M Tablets (Nature's Bounty) p 619
Mega-B (Arco) p 507
Mega-B with C Tablets (Nature's Bounty) p 619
Megadose (Arco) p 507
Memory Booster (Nature's Bounty) p 619
Mentholatum Deep Heating Lotion (Mentholatum) p 605
Mentholatum Deep Heating Rub (Mentholatum) p 605
Mentholatum Lipbalm with Sunscreen (Mentholatum) p 605
Mentholatum Ointment (Mentholatum) p 605
Mercurochrome II (Becton Dickinson Consumer) p 512
Mersene Denture Cleanser (Colgate-Palmolive)
◆Metamucil, Instant Mix, Orange Flavor (Searle Consumer Products) p 428, 683
◆Metamucil, Instant Mix, Regular Flavor (Searle Consumer Products) p 428, 683
◆Metamucil Powder, Orange Flavor (Searle Consumer Products) p 428, 683
◆Metamucil Powder, Regular Flavor (Searle Consumer Products) p 428, 682
◆Metamucil Powder, Strawberry Flavor (Searle Consumer Products) p 428, 683
◆Metamucil Powder, Sugar Free, Regular Flavor (Searle Consumer Products) p 428, 683
◆Micatin Antifungal Cream (Ortho Pharmaceutical) p 419, 627
◆Micatin Antifungal Powder (Ortho Pharmaceutical) p 419, 627
Micatin Antifungal Spray Liquid (Ortho Pharmaceutical) p 627
◆Micatin Antifungal Spray Powder (Ortho Pharmaceutical) p 419, 627

Micatin Jock Itch Cream (Ortho Pharmaceutical) p 627
Micatin Jock Itch Spray Powder (Ortho Pharmaceutical) p 627
◆Microstix-Nitrite Kit (Ames) p 403, 734
◆Midol (Glenbrook) p 410, 554
◆Midol Maximum Strength for Cramps (Glenbrook) p 410, 555
◆Midol PMS (Glenbrook) p 410, 554
Miladregen Tablets (Miller)
Milco Zyme Tablets (Miller)
◆Miles Nervine Nighttime Sleep-Aid (Miles Laboratories) p 418, 614
Milkinol (Rorer) p 662
Minit-Rub Analgesic Balm (Bristol-Myers)
Mobigesic Analgesic Tablets (Ascher)
Mobisyl Analgesic Creme (Ascher) p 508
◆Modane (Adria) p 403, 502
Modane Bulk Powder (Adria) p 503
◆Modane Plus Tablets (Adria) p 403, 503
◆Modane Soft Capsules (Adria) p 504
Moisturel (Westwood)
◆Mol-Iron Tablets & Chronosule Capsules (Schering) p 427, 680
◆Mol-Iron Tablets w/Vitamin C (Schering) p 427, 680
Momentum Muscular Backache Formula (Whitehall) p 718
Multi-Mineral Tablets (Nature's Bounty) p 619
Mum Cream Deodorant (Bristol-Myers)
◆Murine Ear Wax Removal System/Murine Ear Drops (Ross) p 426, 666
◆Murine Eye Drops (Regular Formula) (Ross) p 426, 666
◆Murine Plus Eye Drops (Ross) p 426, 666
Murocel Ophthalmic Solution (Muro) p 615
Muro Tears (Muro) p 615
◆Muskol Insect Repellent Aerosol Liquid (Plough) p 422, 641
◆Muskol Insect Repellent Lotion (Plough) p 422, 641
◆Myadec (Parke-Davis) p 420, 633
Myciguent Antibiotic Cream (Upjohn)
Myciguent Antibiotic Ointment (Upjohn) p 699
◆Mycitracin Triple Antibiotic Ointment (Upjohn) p 431, 699
◆Mylanta Liquid (Stuart) p 429, 689
◆Mylanta Tablets (Stuart) p 429, 689
◆Mylanta-II Liquid (Stuart) p 429, 689
◆Mylanta-II Tablets (Stuart) p 429, 689
◆Mylicon (Tablets & Drops) (Stuart) p 429, 689
◆Mylicon-80 Tablets (Stuart) p 429, 690
◆Myoflex Creme (Adria) p 403, 505

N

NTZ (Winthrop Consumer Products) p 724
Naldecon-CX Suspension (Bristol) p 524
Naldecon-DX Pediatric Syrup (Bristol) p 524
Naldecon-EX Pediatric Drops (Bristol) p 525
NāSal Saline Drops (Winthrop Consumer Products) p 723
NāSal Saline Spray (Winthrop Consumer Products) p 723
Natabec Kapseals (Parke-Davis) p 633
Natabec-FA Kapseals (Parke-Davis)
Natalins (Mead Johnson Pharmaceutical)
Natra-Bio Homeopathic-Style Glandulars & Organs - Series 401-419 (Natra-Bio)
Natra-Bio Homeopathic Tissue Salts - Series 301-315 (Natra-Bio)
Natra Med Homeopathic Ointments - Series 600-606 (Natra-Bio)
◆Naturacil (Mead Johnson Nutritional) p 414, 588
Nature's Bounty Hair Booster Tablets (Nature's Bounty) p 619
Nature's Bounty 1 Tablets (Nature's Bounty) p 619
Nature's Bounty Slim (Nature's Bounty) p 619
◆Nature's Remedy Laxative (Norcliff Thayer) p 418, 622
Neet Aerosol Depilatory (Whitehall)

Neet Depilatory Cream (Whitehall)
Neet Depilatory Lotion (Whitehall)
Neofed (Vale)
Neogesic Tablets (Vale)
Neoloid (Lederle) p 565
◆Neosporin Ointment (Burroughs Wellcome) p 406, 530
Neo-Synephrine (Winthrop Consumer Products) p 724
Neo-Synephrine Jelly (Winthrop Consumer Products)
Neo-Synephrine Nasal Sprays (Winthrop Consumer Products)
Neo-Synephrine Nasal Spray (Mentholated) (Winthrop Consumer Products)
Neo-Synephrine Nose Drops (Winthrop Consumer Products)
Neo-Synephrine II Long Acting Nasal Spray (Winthrop Consumer Products) p 723
Neo-Synephrine II Long Acting Nose Drops (Adult & Children's Strengths) (Winthrop Consumer Products) p 723
Neo-Synephrine II Long Acting Vapor Nasal Spray (Winthrop Consumer Products) p 723
Neo-Synephrine 12 Hour Nasal Spray, Nose Drops, & Vapor Nasal Spray (Winthrop Consumer Products) p 724
Neo-Tab Tablets (Vale)
Nephrox Suspension (Fleming) p 549
New Consol "20" Skin Cleanser (Consolidated Chemical)
New Skin Liquid Bandage (Medtech)
Niacin Tablets (Nature's Bounty) p 619
Niacinamide Tablets (Nature's Bounty) p 619
N'ICE Medicated Sugarless Cough Lozenges (Beecham Products) p 515
Nicotinex Elixir (Fleming) p 549
◆No Doz Tablets (Bristol-Myers) p 406, 529
Normaline 250 mg Saline Solution (Apothecary Products)
◆Norwich Aspirin (Procter & Gamble) p 423, 646
◆Norwich Extra Strength Aspirin (Procter & Gamble) p 423, 646
◆NoSalt Salt Alternative, Regular (Norcliff Thayer) p 418, 622
◆NoSalt Salt Alternative, Seasoned (Norcliff Thayer) p 418, 622
◆Nōstril (Boehringer Ingelheim) p 404, 523
◆Nōstrilla Long Acting Nasal Decongestant (Boehringer Ingelheim) p 404, 524
Novahistine Cough & Cold Formula (Merrell Dow) p 608
Novahistine DMX (Merrell Dow) p 608
Novahistine Elixir (Merrell Dow) p 609
Noxzema Acne-12 (Noxell)
Noxzema Antiseptic Skin Cleanser (Noxell)
Noxzema Cleansing Pads (Noxell)
◆Noxzema Medicated Skin Cream (Noxell) p 418, 624
Nudit Depilatory Cream (Medtech)
Nu-Iron 150 Caps (Mayrand) p 576
Nu-Iron Elixir (Mayrand) p 576
◆Nupercainal Cream & Ointment (Ciba Pharmaceutical) p 407, 536
◆Nupercainal Suppositories (Ciba Pharmaceutical) p 407, 536
◆Nuprin (Bristol-Myers)
Nursamil (Sunrise & Rainbow) p 691
Nursoy Soy Protein Infant Formula (Wyeth) p 727
Nutra-Cal (Anabolic)
Nutramigen (Mead Johnson Nutritional) p 588
◆Nutrimil (Sunrise & Rainbow) p 429, 691
Nylmerate II Solution Concentrate (Youngs Drug Products) p 730
◆Nyquil Nighttime Colds Medicine (Vicks Health Care) p 432, 703
Nyral (Sunrise & Rainbow) (Vale)
Nytilax Tablets (Mentholatum) p 605
Nytol Tablets (Block) p 521

O

O-A-Crine (Anabolic)
Obeval (Vale)

Ocean Mist (Fleming) p 549
Ocean-Plus (Fleming)
Octacosanol (Nature's Bounty) p 619
Odrinil (Fox) p 551
◆One-A-Day Essential Vitamins (Miles Laboratories) p 418, 614
◆One-A-Day Maximum Formula Vitamins and Minerals (Miles Laboratories) p 418, 614
◆One-A-Day Plus Extra C Vitamins (Miles Laboratories) p 418, 615
Optilets-500 (Abbott) p 502
Optilets-M-500 (Abbott) p 502
◆Optivite for Women (Optimox) p 419, 625
Oracin Cherry Flavor Cooling Throat Lozenges (Vicks Health Care)
Oracin Cooling Throat Lozenges (Vicks Health Care)
Orajel, Maximum Strength (Commerce Drug) p 539
◆Orajel Mouth-Aid (Commerce Drug) p 408, 539
Oral Thermometer (Apothecary Products)
Orazinc Capsules (Mericon) p 606
Orazinc Lozenges (Mericon) p 606
◆Orexin Softab Tablets (Stuart) p 429, 690
◆Ornacol Capsules (Menley & James) p 416, 601
◆Ornex Capsules (Menley & James) p 416, 601
l-Ornithine (Nature's Bounty) p 619
◆Ortho Disposable Vaginal Applicators (Ortho Pharmaceutical) p 420, 628
◆Ortho Personal Lubricant (Ortho Pharmaceutical) p 420, 628
◆Ortho-Creme Contraceptive Cream (Ortho Pharmaceutical) p 419, 628
◆Ortho-Gynol Contraceptive Jelly (Ortho Pharmaceutical) p 420, 628
Orthoxicol Cough Syrup (Upjohn)
Osatate (Anabolic)
◆Os-Cal 250 Tablets (Marion) p 413, 573
◆Os-Cal 500 Tablets (Marion) p 413, 573
Os-Cal Forte Tablets (Marion) p 573
Os-Cal-Gesic Tablets (Marion) p 573
Os-Cal Plus Tablets (Marion) p 573
◆Oscillococcinum (Borneman) p 404, 524
◆Otrivin (Geigy) p 409, 552
Outgro Solution (Whitehall) p 719
OvuSTICK Self-Test (Monoclonal Antibodies) p 739
Oxipor VHC Lotion for Psoriasis (Whitehall) p 719
◆Oxy Clean Lathering Facial Scrub (Norcliff Thayer) p 418, 623
◆Oxy Clean Medicated Cleanser, Pads, Soap (Norcliff Thayer) p 418, 622
◆Oxy 10 Cover with Sorboxyl (Norcliff Thayer) p 418, 623
◆Oxy 10 Wash Antibacterial Skin Wash (Norcliff Thayer) p 418, 623
◆Oxy-5 Lotion with Sorboxyl (Norcliff Thayer) p 418, 623
◆Oxy-10 Lotion with Sorboxyl (Norcliff Thayer) p 418, 623
Oxynitral w/Veratrum Viride Tablets (Vale)
Oyster Calcium Tablets (Nature's Bounty) p 619
Oystercal-D 250 (Nature's Bounty) p 619
Oystercal-500 (Nature's Bounty) p 619

P

PABA Tablets (Nature's Bounty) p 619
P-A-C Revised Formula Analgesic Tablets (Upjohn)
◆PBZ Cream (Geigy) p 409, 552
PMS Balance (Rexall) p 651
P&S Liquid (Baker/Cummins) p 510
P&S Plus (Baker/Cummins) p 510
P&S Shampoo (Baker/Cummins) p 511
Pac-Man Sugar Free Calcium for Kids (Rexall) p 651
Pac-Man Sugar-Free Chewable Multivitamins plus Iron (Rexall) p 651
Pamprin Maximum Cramp Relief Formula Capsules & Tablets (Chattem)
Pamprin Tablets (Chattem)
Pantothenic Acid Tablets (Nature's Bounty) p 620

(◆ Shown in Product Identification Section)   (Products without page numbers are not described)

(◆ Shown in Product Identification Section)   (Products without page numbers are not described)

(◆ Shown in Product Identification Section)　　　　　　　(Products without page numbers are not described)

Memorandum

Memorandum

SECTION 3
Product Category Index

Products described in the Product Information (White) Section are listed according to their classifications. The headings and subheadings have been determined by the OTC Review process of the U.S. Food and Drug Administration. Classification of products have been determined by the Publisher with the cooperation of individual manufacturers. In cases where there were differences of opinion or where the manufacturer had no opinion, the Publisher made the final decision.

A

ACNE PRODUCTS
(see under DERMATOLOGICALS)

AEROSOLS
CaldeCORT Anti-Itch Hydrocortisone Spray (Pharmacraft) p 421, 636
Cortaid Spray (Upjohn) p 430, 698
Cruex Antifungal Spray Powder (Pharmacraft) p 637
Desenex Antifungal Foam (Pharmacraft) p 637
Desenex Antifungal Spray Powder (Pharmacraft) p 421, 637
Desenex Foot & Sneaker Spray (Pharmacraft) p 637
Foille First Aid Liquid, Ointment & Spray (Blistex) p 404, 520
Foille Plus First Aid Spray (Blistex) p 404, 520
Medi-Quik Aerosol Spray (Mentholatum) p 604
R&C Spray III (Reed & Carnrick) p 423, 650
Tinactin Aerosol Liquid 1% (Schering) p 428, 680
Tinactin Aerosol Powder 1% (Schering) p 428, 680
Tinactin Jock Itch Spray Powder 1% (Schering) p 427, 680

ALLERGY RELIEF PRODUCTS
A.R.M. Allergy Relief Medicine Tablets (Menley & James) p 415, 596
Actidil Tablets & Syrup (Burroughs Wellcome) p 529
Actifed Tablets & Syrup (Burroughs Wellcome) p 406, 529
Afrin Menthol Nasal Spray (Schering) p 426, 672
Afrin Nasal Spray, Nose Drops, Pediatric Nose Drops (Schering) p 426, 672
Afrinol Repetabs Tablets (Schering) p 426, 673
Allerest Headache Strength Tablets (Pharmacraft) p 636

Allerest Sinus Pain Formula (Pharmacraft) p 421, 636
Allerest Tablets, Children's Chewable Tablets, & Timed-Release Capsules (Pharmacraft) p 421, 636
Ayr Saline Nasal Drops (Ascher) p 508
Ayr Saline Nasal Mist (Ascher) p 508
Caladryl Cream & Lotion (Parke-Davis) p 420, 631
Chlor-Trimeton Allergy Syrup, Tablets & Long-Acting Repetabs Tablets (Schering) p 426, 673
Chlor-Trimeton Decongestant Tablets (Schering) p 427, 674
Chlor-Trimeton Long Acting Decongestant Repetabs Tablets (Schering) p 427, 674
Cold Factor 12 Liquid & Capsules (Pharmacraft) p 421, 637
Congespirin Liquid Cold Medicine (Bristol-Myers) p 405, 527
Contac Capsules (Menley & James) p 415, 597
Coricidin Decongestant Nasal Mist (Schering) p 674
Coricidin Demilets Tablets for Children (Schering) p 427, 675
Coricidin Medilets Tablets for Children (Schering) p 675
Delacort (Mericon) p 606
Demazin Decongestant-Antihistamine Repetabs Tablets & Syrup (Schering) p 427, 676
Dimetane Decongestant Elixir (Robins) p 424, 655
Dimetane Decongestant Tablets (Robins) p 424, 655
Dimetane Elixir (Robins) p 424, 654
Dimetane Extentabs 8 mg (Robins) p 424, 654
Dimetane Extentabs 12 mg (Robins) p 424, 654
Dimetane Tablets (Robins) p 424, 654
Disophrol Chronotab Sustained-Action Tablets (Schering) p 677
Dorcol Children's Liquid Cold Formula (Dorsey) p 408, 544

Dristan Advanced Formula Decongestant/Antihistimine/Analgesic Capsules (Whitehall) p 434, 717
Dristan Advanced Formula Decongestant/Antihistamine/Analgesic Tablets (Whitehall) p 434, 717
Dristan Long Lasting Nasal Spray (Whitehall) p 434, 718
Dristan Nasal Spray (Whitehall) p 434, 718
Drixoral Sustained-Action Tablets (Schering) p 427, 678
4-Way Long Acting Nasal Spray (Bristol-Myers) p 406, 528
4-Way Nasal Spray (Bristol-Myers) p 406, 528
Fedrazil Tablets (Burroughs Wellcome) p 530
Headway Capsules (Vicks Health Care) p 431, 703
Headway Tablets (Vicks Health Care) p 431, 703
Nōstril (Boehringer Ingelheim) p 404, 523
Nōstrilla Long Acting Nasal Decongestant (Boehringer Ingelheim) p 404, 524
Novahistine Elixir (Merrell Dow) p 609
Pyrroxate Capsules (Upjohn) p 431, 699
Sinarest Regular & Extra Strength Tablets (Pharmacraft) p 638
Sinex Decongestant Nasal Spray (Vicks Health Care) p 432, 703
Sinex Long-Acting Decongestant Nasal Spray (Vicks Health Care) p 432, 703
Teldrin Multi-Symptom Allergy Reliever (Menley & James) p 417, 603
Teldrin Timed-Release Capsules, 8 mg., 12 mg. (Menley & James) p 417, 603
Triaminic Allergy Tablets (Dorsey) p 545
Triaminic Chewables (Dorsey) p 545

Triaminic Cold Syrup (Dorsey) p 408, 545

Triaminic Cold Tablets (Dorsey) p 408, 546

Triaminic-12 Tablets (Dorsey) p 408, 546

Triaminicin Tablets (Dorsey) p 409, 547

Ursinus Inlay-Tabs (Dorsey) p 548

Vatronol Nose Drops (Vicks Health Care) p 704

Visine A.C. Eye Drops (Leeming) p 568

ANALGESICS

Internal

Acetaminophen & Combinations

Allerest Headache Strength Tablets (Pharmacraft) p 636

Allerest Sinus Pain Formula (Pharmacraft) p 421, 636

Anacin-3 Children's Acetaminophen Chewable Tablets, Liquid, Drops (Whitehall) p 434, 715

Anacin-3 Maximum Strength Acetaminophen Tablets & Capsules (Whitehall) p 434, 715

Anacin-3 Regular Strength Acetaminophen Tablets (Whitehall) p 715

Children's Panadol Chewable Tablets, Liquid, Drops (Glenbrook) p 410, 555

Congespirin Aspirin-Free Chewable Cold Tablets for Children (Bristol-Myers) p 405, 526

Coricidin Demilets Tablets for Children (Schering) p 427, 675

Coricidin Extra Strength Sinus Headache Tablets (Schering) p 676

Daycare Multi-Symptom Colds Medicine Capsules (Vicks Health Care) p 431, 701

Daycare Multi-Symptom Colds Medicine Liquid (Vicks Health Care) p 431, 701

Dorcol Children's Fever & Pain Reducer (Dorsey) p 408, 544

Dristan Advanced Formula Decongestant/Antihistimine/Analgesic Capsules (Whitehall) p 434, 717

Dristan Advanced Formula Decongestant/Antihistamine/Analgesic Tablets (Whitehall) p 434, 717

Excedrin Capsules & Tablets (Bristol-Myers) p 405, 527

Excedrin P.M. Analgesic Sleeping Aid (Bristol-Myers) p 405, 528

Extra Strength Datril Capsules & Tablets (Bristol-Myers) p 405, 527

Formula 44M Multisymptom Cough Mixture (Vicks Health Care) p 431, 702

Gemnisyn Tablets (Rorer) p 659

Headway Capsules (Vicks Health Care) p 431, 703

Headway Tablets (Vicks Health Care) p 431, 703

Liquiprin Acetaminophen (Norcliff Thayer) p 418, 622

Maximum Strength Panadol (Glenbrook) p 410, 555

Nyquil Nighttime Colds Medicine (Vicks Health Care) p 432, 703

Ornex Capsules (Menley & James) p 416, 601

Percogesic Analgesic Tablets (Vicks Pharmacy Products) p 432, 706

Pyrroxate Capsules (Upjohn) p 431, 699

Robitussin Night Relief (Robins) p 425, 656

St. Joseph Aspirin-Free Chewable Tablets, Liquid & Infant Drops (Plough) p 422, 642

Sinarest Regular & Extra Strength Tablets (Pharmacraft) p 638

Sine-Aid, Extra Strength, Sinus Headache Capsules (McNeil Consumer Products) p 414, 579

Sine-Aid Sinus Headache Tablets (McNeil Consumer Products) p 414, 579

Sine-Off Extra Strength No Drowsiness Capsules (Menley & James) p 416, 602

Sine-Off Extra Strength Sinus Medicine Aspirin-Free Capsules (Menley & James) p 416, 601

Sinutab Maximum Strength Capsules (Warner-Lambert Co.) p 433, 711

Sinutab Maximum Strength Tablets (Warner-Lambert Co.) p 433, 711

Sinutab Tablets (Warner-Lambert Co.) p 433, 711

Sinutab II Maximum Strength No Drowsiness Formula Tablets & Capsules (Warner-Lambert Co.) p 433, 711

Sominex Pain Relief Formula (Beecham Products) p 515

Sunril Premenstrual Capsules (Schering) p 680

Tempra (Mead Johnson Nutritional) p 415, 592

Tussagesic Tablets & Suspension (Dorsey) p 548

Tylenol acetaminophen Children's Chewable Tablets, Elixir, Drops (McNeil Consumer Products) p 414, 580

Tylenol, Extra-Strength, acetaminophen Adult Liquid Pain Reliever (McNeil Consumer Products) p 582

Tylenol, Extra-Strength, acetaminophen Tablets, Capsules & Caplets (McNeil Consumer Products) p 413, 414, 582

Tylenol, Infants' Drops (McNeil Consumer Products) p 414, 580

Tylenol, Junior Strength, acetaminophen Swallowable Tablets (McNeil Consumer Products) p 414, 580

Tylenol, Maximum Strength, Sinus Medication Tablets & Capsules (McNeil Consumer Products) p 414, 582

Tylenol, Regular Strength, acetaminophen Capsules & Tablets (McNeil Consumer Products) p 413, 581

Aspirin & Combinations

Alka-Seltzer Effervescent Pain Reliever & Antacid (Miles Laboratories) p 417, 611

Anacin Analgesic Capsules (Whitehall) p 714

Anacin Analgesic Tablets (Whitehall) p 434, 714

Anacin Maximum Strength Analgesic Capsules (Whitehall) p 715

Anacin Maximum Strength Analgesic Tablets (Whitehall) p 715

Arthritis Bayer Timed-Release Aspirin (Glenbrook) p 410, 553

Arthritis Pain Formula by the Makers of Anacin Analgesic Tablets (Whitehall) p 434, 716

Arthritis Pain Formula Safety Coated by the Makers of Anacin Analgesic Tablets (Whitehall) p 434, 716

Arthritis Strength Bufferin (Bristol-Myers) p 405, 525

Ascriptin Tablets (Rorer) p 425, 658

Ascriptin A/D Tablets (Rorer) p 425, 658

Aspergum (Plough) p 421, 640

BC Powder (Block) p 521

Bayer Aspirin & Bayer Children's Chewable Aspirin (Glenbrook) p 409, 552

Bayer Children's Cold Tablets (Glenbrook) p 553

Bufferin Analgesic Tablets and Capsules (Bristol-Myers) p 405, 525

Cama Arthritis Pain Reliever (Dorsey) p 408, 543

Coricidin 'D' Decongestant Tablets (Schering) p 427, 674

Coricidin Tablets (Schering) p 427, 674

Cosprin 325 (Glenbrook) p 410, 554

Cosprin 650 (Glenbrook) p 410, 554

Ecotrin Maximum Strength Capsules (Menley & James) p 416, 599

Ecotrin Regular Strength Capsules (Menley & James) p 416, 600

Ecotrin Tablets (Menley & James) p 416, 599

Ecotrin Maximum Strength Tablets (Menley & James) p 416, 599

Empirin (Burroughs Wellcome) p 406, 530

Encaprin (Procter & Gamble) p 644

Excedrin Capsules & Tablets (Bristol-Myers) p 405, 527

Extra-Strength Bufferin Capsules & Tablets (Bristol-Myers) p 405, 526

4-Way Cold Tablets (Bristol-Myers) p 406, 528

Gemnisyn Tablets (Rorer) p 659

Goody's Headache Powders (Goody's) p 410, 556

Maximum Bayer Aspirin (Glenbrook) p 410, 554

Measurin Tablets (Winthrop-Breon) p 721

Midol (Glenbrook) p 410, 554

Midol Maximum Strength for Cramps (Glenbrook) p 410, 555

Momentum Muscular Backache Formula (Whitehall) p 718

Norwich Aspirin (Procter & Gamble) p 423, 646

Norwich Extra Strength Aspirin (Procter & Gamble) p 423, 646

St. Joseph Aspirin for Children (Plough) p 422, 642

St. Joseph Cold Tablets for Children (Plough) p 422, 642

Triaminicin Tablets (Dorsey) p 409, 547

Ursinus Inlay-Tabs (Dorsey) p 548

Vanquish (Glenbrook) p 410, 556

Ibuprofen

Advil Ibuprofen Tablets (Whitehall) p 434, 714

Others

Biochemic Tissue Salts (NuAGE Laboratories) p 624

DeWitt's Pills for Backache & Joint Pains (DeWitt) p 543

Doan's Pills (Jeffrey Martin) p 558

Momentum Muscular Backache Formula (Whitehall) p 718

Os-Cal-Gesic Tablets (Marion) p 573

Topical

Banalg Hospital Strength Pain Reliever (Forest) p 419, 550

Banalg Muscular Pain Reliever (Forest) p 419, 550

Lily of the Desert Aloe Vera Gelly (97%) (Vera Products) p 431, 701

Anesthetics

Anbesol Baby Gel Antiseptic Anesthetic (Whitehall) p 434, 716

Anbesol Gel Antiseptic Anesthetic (Whitehall) p 434, 716

Anbesol Liquid Antiseptic Anesthetic (Whitehall) p 434, 716

Baby Orajel (Commerce Drug) p 408, 539

Bactine Antiseptic/Anesthetic First Aid Spray (Miles Laboratories) p 417, 612

BiCozene Creme (Creighton Products) p 409, 540

Blistex Medicated Lip Ointment (Blistex) p 404, 520

Campho-Phenique Gel (Winthrop Consumer Products) p 722

Campho-Phenique Liquid (Winthrop Consumer Products) p 723

Cepacol Anesthetic Lozenges (Troches) (Merrell Dow) p 606

CEPASTAT Sore Throat Lozenges (Merrell Dow) p 607

Children's Chloraseptic Lozenges (Procter & Gamble) p 422, 644

Chloraseptic Liquid—Menthol or Cherry (Procter & Gamble) p 422, 644

Chloraseptic Liquid - Nitrogen Propelled Spray - Menthol or Cherry (Procter & Gamble) p 422, 644

Dermolate Scalp-Itch Lotion (Schering) p 427, 677
Dermoplast (Ayerst) p 404, 509
Gynecort Antipruritic 0.5% Hydrocortisone Acetate Creme (Combe) p 407, 538
Hytone Cream 1/2% (Dermik) p 542
Lanacane Medicated Creme (Combe) p 407, 538
Lanacort Anti-Itch Hydrocortisone Acetate 0.5% Creme and Ointment (Combe) p 407, 538
Noxzema Medicated Skin Cream (Noxell) p 418, 624
PBZ Cream (Geigy) p 409, 552
Resicort Cream (Mentholatum) p 605
Shepard's Cream Lotion (Dermik) p 542
Shepard's Skin Cream (Dermik) p 542
Shepard's Soap (Dermik) p 542
Tucks Cream & Ointment (Parke-Davis) p 634
Tucks Premoistened Pads (Parke-Davis) p 420, 633
Vagisil External Feminine Itching Medication (Combe) p 408, 539
Xylocaine 2.5% Ointment (Astra) p 404, 508
Zetar Shampoo (Dermik) p 543
Ziradryl Lotion (Parke-Davis) p 420, 634

Antipsoriasis Agents
Clinitar Cream (Ulmer) p 696
Clinitar Shampoo (Ulmer) p 696
Clinitar Stick (Ulmer) p 696
Denorex Medicated Shampoo & Conditioner (Whitehall) p 434, 717
Denorex Medicated Shampoo, Regular & Mountain Fresh Herbal (Whitehall) p 434, 717
Oxipor VHC Lotion for Psoriasis (Whitehall) p 719
P&S Liquid (Baker/Cummins) p 510
P&S Plus (Baker/Cummins) p 510
P&S Shampoo (Baker/Cummins) p 511
Tegrin for Psoriasis Lotion & Cream (Block) p 522
Tegrin Medicated Shampoo (Block) p 522
Xseb Shampoo (Baker/Cummins) p 511
Xseb-T Shampoo (Baker/Cummins) p 511
Zetar Shampoo (Dermik) p 543

Antiseborrhea
Clinitar Cream (Ulmer) p 696
Clinitar Shampoo (Ulmer) p 696
Clinitar Stick (Ulmer) p 696
Denorex Medicated Shampoo & Conditioner (Whitehall) p 434, 717
Denorex Medicated Shampoo, Regular & Mountain Fresh Herbal (Whitehall) p 434, 717
Fostex Medicated Cleansing Bar (Westwood) p 433, 712
Head & Shoulders (Procter & Gamble) p 645
P&S Liquid (Baker/Cummins) p 510
P&S Shampoo (Baker/Cummins) p 511
Pragmatar Ointment (Menley & James) p 416, 601
Sebulex & Sebulex Cream Shampoo (Westwood) p 433, 714
Sebulon Dandruff Shampoo (Westwood) p 433, 714
Tegrin Medicated Shampoo (Block) p 522
Xseb Shampoo (Baker/Cummins) p 511
Xseb-T Shampoo (Baker/Cummins) p 511
Zetar Shampoo (Dermik) p 543
Zincon Dandruff Shampoo (Lederle) p 412, 567

Astringents
Mediconet (Medicone) p 595
Tucks Premoistened Pads (Parke-Davis) p 420, 633

Bath Oils
Alpha Keri Therapeutic Shower & Bath Oil (Westwood) p 433, 712

Breast Creams
Masse Breast Cream (Ortho Pharmaceutical) p 419, 627

Coal Tar
Clinitar Cream (Ulmer) p 696
Clinitar Shampoo (Ulmer) p 696
Clinitar Stick (Ulmer) p 696
Denorex Medicated Shampoo & Conditioner (Whitehall) p 434, 717
Denorex Medicated Shampoo, Regular & Mountain Fresh Herbal (Whitehall) p 434, 717
Oxipor VHC Lotion for Psoriasis (Whitehall) p 719
P&S Plus (Baker/Cummins) p 510
Tegrin for Psoriasis Lotion & Cream (Block) p 522
Tegrin Medicated Shampoo (Block) p 522
Xseb-T Shampoo (Baker/Cummins) p 511
Zetar Shampoo (Dermik) p 543

Coal Tar & Sulfur
Pragmatar Ointment (Menley & James) p 416, 601

Conditioning Rinse
Denorex Medicated Shampoo & Conditioner (Whitehall) p 434, 717

Detergents
pHisoDerm (Winthrop Consumer Products) p 725
Selsun Blue Dandruff Shampoo (selenium sulfide lotion 1%) (Ross) p 426, 667
Zetar Shampoo (Dermik) p 543
Zincon Dandruff Shampoo (Lederle) p 412, 567

Emollients (softeners)
A and D Ointment (Schering) p 426, 672
Aquaphor (Beiersdorf) p 518
Balmex Baby Powder (Macsil) p 571
Balmex Emollient Lotion (Macsil) p 571
Balmex Ointment (Macsil) p 571
Balneol (Rowell) p 671
Blistex Lip Conditioner (Blistex) p 519
Blistex Medicated Lip Ointment (Blistex) p 404, 520
Blistik Medicated Lip Balm (Blistex) p 519
Borofax Ointment (Burroughs Wellcome) p 530
Carmol 10 Lotion (Syntex) p 691
Carmol 20 Cream (Syntex) p 692
Chap Stick Lip Balm (Robins) p 424, 654
Chap Stick Sunblock 15 Lip Balm (Robins) p 424, 654
Complex 15 Moisturizing Cream & Lotion (Baker/Cummins) p 510
Dermassage Medicated Skin Lotion (Kendall) p 560
Desitin Ointment (Leeming) p 567
Eucerin Creme (Beiersdorf) p 518
Eucerin Lotion (Beiersdorf) p 518
Herpecin-L Cold Sore Lip Balm (Campbell) p 532
Keri Lotion (Westwood) p 433, 713
Lanolin, U.S.P. (Fougera) p 551
Lily of the Desert Aloe Vera Gelly (97%) (Vera Products) p 431, 701
Lip Soother Medicated Lip Cream (Robins) p 424, 655
Lobana Bath Oil (Ulmer) p 696
Lobana Body Lotion (Ulmer) p 696
Lobana Peri-Gard (Ulmer) p 697
Lubriderm Cream (Warner-Lambert Co.) p 710
Lubriderm Lotion (Warner-Lambert Co.) p 433, 710
Lubriderm Lubath Bath-Shower Oil (Warner-Lambert Co.) p 433, 710
Noxzema Medicated Skin Cream (Noxell) p 418, 624
Petrolatum White, U.S.P. (Fougera) p 551
Purpose Dry Skin Cream (Ortho Dermatological) p 420, 629
Shepard's Cream Lotion (Dermik) p 542
Shepard's Skin Cream (Dermik) p 542
Shepard's Soap (Dermik) p 542

Skin Magic Lotion (Consolidated Chemical) p 540
Skin Principle Basic Clarifying Lotion (Max Factor) p 413, 575
Skin Principle Daily Light Moisture Lotion (Max Factor) p 413, 575
Skin Principle Daily Rich Moisture Lotion (Max Factor) p 413, 575
Skin Principle Serious Moisture Supplement (Max Factor) p 413, 575
Ultra Mide 25 Moisturizer Lotion (Baker/Cummins) p 511
Vitamin A + Vitamin D Ointment (Fougera) p 551
Wellcome Lanoline (Burroughs Wellcome) p 532

Foot Care
Desenex Foot & Sneaker Spray (Pharmacraft) p 637
FootWork Athlete's Foot Cream 0.5 oz. (Lederle) p 412, 563
FootWork Athlete's Foot Cream 1.0 oz. (Lederle) p 412, 563
FootWork Athlete's Foot Powder (Lederle) p 412, 563
FootWork Athlete's Foot Solution (Lederle) p 412, 563
FootWork Athlete's Foot Spray Powder (Lederle) p 412, 563
Freezone Solution (Whitehall) p 718
Outgro Solution (Whitehall) p 719
Wellcome Lanoline (Burroughs Wellcome) p 532

Fungicides
Athlete's Foot Cream & Solution (Tolnaftate 1%) (Pharmaderm) p 421, 638
Betadine Ointment (Purdue Frederick) p 648
Betadine Skin Cleanser (Purdue Frederick) p 647
Betadine Solution (Purdue Frederick) p 647
Caldesene Medicated Powder (Pharmacraft) p 421, 636
Cruex Antifungal Cream (Pharmacraft) p 421, 637
Cruex Antifungal Powder (Pharmacraft) p 421, 637
Cruex Antifungal Spray Powder (Pharmacraft) p 637
Desenex Antifungal Cream (Pharmacraft) p 421, 637
Desenex Antifungal Foam (Pharmacraft) p 637
Desenex Antifungal Liquid (Pharmacraft) p 637
Desenex Antifungal Ointment (Pharmacraft) p 421, 637
Desenex Antifungal Powder (Pharmacraft) p 421, 637
Desenex Antifungal Spray Powder (Pharmacraft) p 421, 637
FootWork Athlete's Foot Cream 0.5 oz. (Lederle) p 412, 563
FootWork Athlete's Foot Cream 1.0 oz. (Lederle) p 412, 563
FootWork Athlete's Foot Powder (Lederle) p 412, 563
FootWork Athlete's Foot Solution (Lederle) p 412, 563
FootWork Athlete's Foot Spray Powder (Lederle) p 412, 563
Tinactin Aerosol Liquid 1% (Schering) p 428, 680
Tinactin Aerosol Powder 1% (Schering) p 428, 680
Tinactin 1% Cream, Solution & Powder (Schering) p 427, 428, 680
Tinactin Jock Itch Cream 1% (Schering) p 427, 680
Tinactin Jock Itch Spray Powder 1% (Schering) p 427, 680

General
A and D Ointment (Schering) p 426, 672
Acid Mantle Creme & Lotion (Dorsey) p 408, 543
Acnederm Lotion (Lannett) p 561
Bactine Hydrocortisone Skin Care Cream (Miles Laboratories) p 417, 613

Balmex Ointment (Macsil) p 571
Caldesene Medicated Ointment
(Pharmacraft) p 421, 636
Cortaid Cream (Upjohn) p 430, 698
Cortaid Lotion (Upjohn) p 430, 698
Cortaid Ointment (Upjohn) p 430, 698
Cortaid Spray (Upjohn) p 430, 698
Desenex Soap (Pharmacraft) p 637
Desitin Ointment (Leeming) p 567
Hydrocortisine Cream & Ointment,
U.S.P. 0.5% (Fougera) p 551
Lobana Derm-Ade Cream (Ulmer)
p 697
Lubriderm Lotion (Warner-Lambert Co.)
p 433, 710
Purpose Dry Skin Cream (Ortho
Dermatological) p 420, 629
Shepard's Cream Lotion (Dermik)
p 542
Shepard's Skin Cream (Dermik) p 542
Shepard's Soap (Dermik) p 542

Keratolytics
Acnederm Lotion (Lannett) p 561
Carmol 10 Lotion (Syntex) p 691
Carmol 20 Cream (Syntex) p 692
Compound W Gel (Whitehall) p 717
Compound W Liquid (Whitehall) p 717
Fomac Foam (Dermik) p 542
Freezone Solution (Whitehall) p 718
Mediplast (Beiersdorf) p 518
Ultra Mide 25 Moisturizer Lotion
(Baker/Cummins) p 511

Powders
Aftate for Athlete's Foot (Plough)
p 421, 640
Aftate for Jock Itch (Plough) p 421,
640
Balmex Baby Powder (Macsil) p 571
Caldesene Medicated Powder
(Pharmacraft) p 421, 636
Cruex Antifungal Powder (Pharmacraft)
p 421, 637
Cruex Antifungal Spray Powder
(Pharmacraft) p 637
Desenex Antifungal Powder
(Pharmacraft) p 421, 637
Desenex Antifungal Spray Powder
(Pharmacraft) p 421, 637
Diaparene Baby Powder (Glenbrook)
p 410, 554
FootWork Athlete's Foot Powder
(Lederle) p 412, 563
FootWork Athlete's Foot Spray Powder
(Lederle) p 412, 563
Formula Magic Lubricating Body Talc
(Consolidated Chemical) p 540
Lobana Body Powder (Ulmer) p 697
Tinactin Aerosol Powder 1% (Schering)
p 428, 680
Tinactin Jock Itch Spray Powder 1%
(Schering) p 427, 680

Salicylic Acid
Stri-Dex Maximum Strength Pads
(Glenbrook) p 556
Stri-Dex Regular Strength Pads
(Glenbrook) p 556

Scabicides
Vleminckx' Solution (Ulmer) p 698

Shampoos
Clinitar Shampoo (Ulmer) p 696
Denorex Medicated Shampoo &
Conditioner (Whitehall) p 434, 717
Denorex Medicated Shampoo, Regular
& Mountain Fresh Herbal (Whitehall)
p 434, 717
Head & Shoulders (Procter & Gamble)
p 645
Lobana Body Shampoo (Ulmer) p 697
Lobana Conditioning Shampoo (Ulmer)
p 697
P&S Shampoo (Baker/Cummins) p 511
Purpose Shampoo (Ortho
Dermatological) p 420, 629
R&C Shampoo (Reed & Carnrick)
p 423, 650
Sassoon D Shampoo (Vidal Sassoon)
p 432, 707
Satin Body Wash and Shampoo
(Consolidated Chemical) p 540
Sebulex & Sebulex Cream Shampoo
(Westwood) p 433, 714

Sebulon Dandruff Shampoo (Westwood)
p 433, 714
Selsun Blue Dandruff Shampoo
(selenium sulfide lotion 1%) (Ross)
p 426, 667
Tegrin Medicated Shampoo (Block)
p 522
Xseb Shampoo (Baker/Cummins)
p 511
Xseb-T Shampoo (Baker/Cummins)
p 511
Zetar Shampoo (Dermik) p 543
Zincon Dandruff Shampoo (Lederle)
p 412, 567

Skin Bleaches
Esotérica Medicated Fade Cream
(Norcliff Thayer) p 621
Porcelana Skin Bleaching Agent (Jeffrey
Martin) p 558
Porcelana Skin Bleaching Agent with
Sunscreen (Jeffrey Martin) p 558

Skin Protectant
Ivarest Medicated Cream & Lotion
(Blistex) p 520
Johnson's Baby Cream (Johnson &
Johnson Baby Products) p 411, 558

Soaps & Cleansers
Betadine Skin Cleanser (Purdue
Frederick) p 647
Cuticura Antibacterial Medicated Soap
(Jeffrey Martin) p 558
Desenex Soap (Pharmacraft) p 637
Eucerin Cleansing Bar (Beiersdorf)
p 518
Fomac Foam (Dermik) p 542
Fostex Medicated Cleansing Bar
(Westwood) p 433, 712
Lobana Liquid Hand Soap (Ulmer)
p 697
Lobana Perineal Cleanse (Ulmer) p 697
Noxzema Medicated Skin Cream
(Noxell) p 418, 624
Oxy Clean Lathering Facial Scrub
(Norcliff Thayer) p 418, 623
Oxy Clean Medicated Cleanser, Pads,
Soap (Norcliff Thayer) p 418, 622
Oxy 10 Wash Antibacterial Skin Wash
(Norcliff Thayer) p 418, 623
Perineal/Ostomy Spray Cleaner
(Consolidated Chemical) p 540
pHisoDerm (Winthrop Consumer
Products) p 725
Purpose Soap (Ortho Dermatological)
p 420, 629
Satin Body Wash and Shampoo
(Consolidated Chemical) p 540
Shepard's Soap (Dermik) p 542
Skin Principle Purifying Cleansing
Lotion (Max Factor) p 413, 574

Sulfur & Salicylic Acid
Pragmatar Ointment (Menley & James)
p 416, 601

Sunburn Preparations
Bactine Antiseptic/Anesthetic First Aid
Spray (Miles Laboratories) p 417,
612
Balmex Ointment (Macsil) p 571
BiCozene Creme (Creighton Products)
p 409, 540
Blistex Medicated Lip Ointment
(Blistex) p 404, 520
Borofax Ointment (Burroughs
Wellcome) p 530
Dermoplast (Ayerst) p 404, 509
Dibucaine Ointment, U.S.P. 1%
(Fougera) p 551
Foille First Aid Liquid, Ointment &
Spray (Blistex) p 404, 520
Foille Plus First Aid Spray (Blistex)
p 404, 520
Lanacane Medicated Creme (Combe)
p 407, 538
Lobana Derm-Ade Cream (Ulmer)
p 697
Medi-Quik Aerosol Spray (Mentholatum)
p 604
Mercurochrome II (Becton Dickinson
Consumer) p 512
Shuttle First Aid Spray (American
Hygienic) p 403, 507
Shuttle Lotion (American Hygienic)
p 403, 507

Solarcaine (Plough) p 422, 643

Sunscreens
Blistex Lip Conditioner (Blistex) p 519
Blistex Medicated Lip Ointment
(Blistex) p 404, 520
Blistik Medicated Lip Balm (Blistex)
p 519
Chap Stick Lip Balm (Robins) p 424,
654
Chap Stick Sunblock 15 Lip Balm
(Robins) p 424, 654
Coppertone Sunscreen Lotion (SPF-6)
(Plough) p 422, 640
Coppertone Sunscreen Lotion (SPF-8)
(Plough) p 422, 640
Coppertone Sunscreen Lotion (SPF 15)
(Plough) p 422, 640
Eclipse Sunscreen Lotion, Total
(Cooling Alcohol Base) (Dorsey)
p 408, 545
Eclipse Sunscreen Lotion, Total
(Moisturizing Base) (Dorsey) p 408,
545
Herpecin-L Cold Sore Lip Balm
(Campbell) p 532
Mentholatum Lipbalm with Sunscreen
(Mentholatum) p 605
PreSun 15 Creamy Sunscreen
(Westwood) p 433, 713
PreSun 15 Sunscreen Lotion
(Westwood) p 433, 713
Shade Sunscreen Lotion SPF 4
(Plough) p 422, 643
Shade Sunscreen Lotion SPF 6
(Plough) p 422, 643
Shade Sunscreen Lotion SPF 8
(Plough) p 422, 643
Shade Sunscreen Lotion SPF 15
(Plough) p 422, 643
Sundown Sunblock Stick, Ultra
Protection (Johnson & Johnson Baby
Products) p 411, 558
Sundown Sunscreen, Extra Protection
(Johnson & Johnson Baby Products)
p 558
Sundown Sunscreen, Maximal
Protection (Johnson & Johnson Baby
Products) p 558
Sundown Sunscreen, Moderate
Protection (Johnson & Johnson Baby
Products) p 558
Sundown Sunscreen, Ultra Protection
(Johnson & Johnson Baby Products)
p 558
Sundown Sunscreen Stick, Maximal
Protection (Johnson & Johnson Baby
Products) p 411, 558

Wart Removers
Compound W Gel (Whitehall) p 717
Compound W Liquid (Whitehall) p 717
Vergo Cream (Daywell) p 541
Verucid Gel (Ulmer) p 697
Wart-Off (Pfipharmecs) p 421, 635

Wet Dressings
Tucks Premoistened Pads (Parke-Davis)
p 420, 633

Other
Bactine Hydrocortisone Skin Care
Cream (Miles Laboratories) p 417,
613
Bioclusive Transparent Dressing
(Johnson & Johnson) p 411, 559
Borofax Ointment (Burroughs
Wellcome) p 530
Cortaid Cream (Upjohn) p 430, 698
Cortaid Lotion (Upjohn) p 430, 698
Cortaid Ointment (Upjohn) p 430, 698
Cortaid Spray (Upjohn) p 430, 698
Cortef Feminine Itch Cream (Upjohn)
p 698
Derma Medicone Ointment (Medicone)
p 595
Diaparene Baby Wash Cloths
(Glenbrook) p 410, 554
Medicone Dressing Cream (Medicone)
p 595
pHisoPUFF (Winthrop Consumer
Products) p 725
PRID Salve (Walker Pharmacal) p 707
Resicort Cream (Mentholatum) p 605
Shepard's Cream Lotion (Dermik)
p 542

INFANT FORMULAS, SPECIAL PURPOSE

Carbohydrate-Free

Liquid Concentrate
RCF-Ross Carbohydrate Free Soy
 Protein Formula Base (Ross) p 666

Corn Free

Liquid Concentrate
Nursoy Soy Protein Infant Formula
 (Wyeth) p 727
I-Soyalac (Loma Linda) p 569

Liquid Ready-to-Feed
Nursoy Soy Protein Infant Formula
 (Wyeth) p 727
I-Soyalac (Loma Linda) p 569

Hypo-Allergenic

Liquid Concentrate
Isomil (Ross) p 664
Isomil SF (Ross) p 665
Nursoy Soy Protein Infant Formula
 (Wyeth) p 727
ProSobee (Mead Johnson Nutritional)
 p 590
Soyalac: Liquid Concentrate,
 Ready-to-Serve and Powder (Loma
 Linda) p 569
I-Soyalac (Loma Linda) p 569

Liquid Ready-to-Feed
Isomil (Ross) p 664
Isomil SF (Ross) p 665
Nursoy Soy Protein Infant Formula
 (Wyeth) p 727
ProSobee (Mead Johnson Nutritional)
 p 590
Soyalac: Liquid Concentrate,
 Ready-to-Serve and Powder (Loma
 Linda) p 569
I-Soyalac (Loma Linda) p 569

Powder
Isomil (Ross) p 664
Nutramigen (Mead Johnson Nutritional)
 p 588
Pregestimil (Mead Johnson Nutritional)
 p 589
ProSobee (Mead Johnson Nutritional)
 p 590
Soyalac: Liquid Concentrate,
 Ready-to-Serve and Powder (Loma
 Linda) p 569

Iron Supplement

Liquid Concentrate
Advance (Ross) p 663
Enfamil w/Iron Concentrated Liquid &
 Powder (Mead Johnson Nutritional)
 p 414, 584
SMA Iron Fortified Infant Formula
 (Wyeth) p 728
Similac with Iron (Ross) p 669
Similac with Whey + Iron (Ross) p 670

Liquid Ready-to-Feed
Advance (Ross) p 663
Enfamil w/Iron Ready-To-Use (Mead
 Johnson Nutritional) p 414, 585
SMA Iron Fortified Infant Formula
 (Wyeth) p 728
Similac with Iron (Ross) p 669
Similac with Whey + Iron (Ross) p 670

Powder
Enfamil w/Iron Concentrated Liquid &
 Powder (Mead Johnson Nutritional)
 p 414, 584
SMA Iron Fortified Infant Formula
 (Wyeth) p 728
Similac with Iron (Ross) p 669
Similac with Whey + Iron (Ross) p 670

Lactose Free

Liquid Concentrate
Nursoy Soy Protein Infant Formula
 (Wyeth) p 727
ProSobee (Mead Johnson Nutritional)
 p 590
Soyalac: Liquid Concentrate,
 Ready-to-Serve and Powder (Loma
 Linda) p 569
I-Soyalac (Loma Linda) p 569

Liquid Ready-to-Feed
Nursoy Soy Protein Infant Formula
 (Wyeth) p 727

ProSobee (Mead Johnson Nutritional)
 p 590
Soyalac: Liquid Concentrate,
 Ready-to-Serve and Powder (Loma
 Linda) p 569
I-Soyalac (Loma Linda) p 569

Powder
Portagen (Mead Johnson Nutritional)
 p 589
ProSobee (Mead Johnson Nutritional)
 p 590
Soyalac: Liquid Concentrate,
 Ready-to-Serve and Powder (Loma
 Linda) p 569

Low Phenylalanine

Powder
Lofenalac (Mead Johnson Nutritional)
 p 586

Medium Chain Triglycerides

Powder
Portagen (Mead Johnson Nutritional)
 p 589
Pregestimil (Mead Johnson Nutritional)
 p 589

Milk Free

Liquid Concentrate
Isomil (Ross) p 664
Isomil SF (Ross) p 665
Nursoy Soy Protein Infant Formula
 (Wyeth) p 727
ProSobee (Mead Johnson Nutritional)
 p 590
RCF-Ross Carbohydrate Free Soy
 Protein Formula Base (Ross) p 666
Soyalac: Liquid Concentrate,
 Ready-to-Serve and Powder (Loma
 Linda) p 569
I-Soyalac (Loma Linda) p 569

Liquid Ready-to-Feed
Isomil (Ross) p 664
Isomil SF (Ross) p 665
Nursoy Soy Protein Infant Formula
 (Wyeth) p 727
ProSobee (Mead Johnson Nutritional)
 p 590
Soyalac: Liquid Concentrate,
 Ready-to-Serve and Powder (Loma
 Linda) p 569

Powder
Isomil (Ross) p 664
ProSobee (Mead Johnson Nutritional)
 p 590
Soyalac: Liquid Concentrate,
 Ready-to-Serve and Powder (Loma
 Linda) p 569

Nutritional Beverage

Liquid Concentrate
Advance (Ross) p 663

Liquid Ready-to-Feed
Advance (Ross) p 663

Powder
Nutrimil (Sunrise & Rainbow) p 429,
 691

Protein Hydrolysate

Powder
Nutramigen (Mead Johnson Nutritional)
 p 588
Pregestimil (Mead Johnson Nutritional)
 p 589

Sucrose Free

Liquid Concentrate
Isomil SF (Ross) p 665
ProSobee (Mead Johnson Nutritional)
 p 590

Liquid Ready-to-Feed
Isomil SF (Ross) p 665
ProSobee (Mead Johnson Nutritional)
 p 590

Powder
ProSobee (Mead Johnson Nutritional)
 p 590

With Whey

Liquid Concentrate
Enfamil Concentrated Liquid & Powder
 (Mead Johnson Nutritional) p 414,
 584

Similac with Whey + Iron (Ross) p 670

Liquid Ready-to-Feed
Similac PM 60/40 (Ross) p 668
Similac with Whey + Iron (Ross) p 670

Powder
Enfamil Concentrated Liquid & Powder
 (Mead Johnson Nutritional) p 414,
 584
Similac PM 60/40 (Ross) p 668
Similac with Whey + Iron (Ross) p 670

INGROWN TOENAIL PREPARATIONS

Outgro Solution (Whitehall) p 719

INSECT BITE & STING PREPARATIONS

Anbesol Gel Antiseptic Anesthetic
 (Whitehall) p 434, 716
Anbesol Liquid Antiseptic Anesthetic
 (Whitehall) p 434, 716
B.F.I. (Beecham Products) p 512
Bactine Antiseptic/Anesthetic First Aid
 Spray (Miles Laboratories) p 417,
 612
Bactine Hydrocortisone Skin Care
 Cream (Miles Laboratories) p 417,
 613
BiCozene Creme (Creighton Products)
 p 409, 540
Borofax Ointment (Burroughs
 Wellcome) p 530
Dibucaine Ointment, U.S.P. 1%
 (Fougera) p 551
Foille First Aid Liquid, Ointment &
 Spray (Blistex) p 404, 520
Foille Plus First Aid Spray (Blistex)
 p 404, 520
Lanacane Medicated Creme (Combe)
 p 407, 538
Lanacort Anti-Itch Hydrocortisone
 Acetate 0.5% Creme and Ointment
 (Combe) p 407, 538
Medi-Quik Aerosol Spray (Mentholatum)
 p 604
Nupercainal Cream & Ointment (Ciba
 Pharmaceutical) p 407, 536
Shuttle First Aid Spray (American
 Hygienic) p 403, 507
Shuttle Lotion (American Hygienic)
 p 403, 507

INSECT REPELLENTS

Muskol Insect Repellent Aerosol Liquid
 (Plough) p 422, 641
Muskol Insect Repellent Lotion (Plough)
 p 422, 641

**INSULIN REACTION RELIEF
(see under BLOOD SUGAR
ELEVATING AGENTS)**

**IRON DEFICIENCY PREPARATIONS
(see under HEMATINICS)**

L

LAXATIVES

Bulk
Effersyllium Instant Mix (Stuart) p 428,
 687
Fiberall, Natural Flavor (Rydelle) p 426,
 671
Fiberall, Orange Flavor (Rydelle) p 426,
 671
Fibermed (Original & Fruit Flavors)
 (Purdue Frederick) p 648
Fiber-Up (Fiber-Up) p 549
Hydrocil Instant (Rowell) p 671
Maltsupex Powder, Liquid, Tablets
 (Wallace) p 432, 708
Metamucil, Instant Mix, Orange Flavor
 (Searle Consumer Products) p 428,
 683
Metamucil, Instant Mix, Regular Flavor
 (Searle Consumer Products) p 428,
 683
Metamucil Powder, Orange Flavor
 (Searle Consumer Products) p 428,
 683
Metamucil Powder, Regular Flavor
 (Searle Consumer Products) p 428,
 682

O

OBESITY AIDS
(see under APPETITE SUPPRESSANTS)

OPHTHALMICS

Devices
Lavoptik Eye Cup (Lavoptik) p 739

Medications
Clear Eyes Eye Drops (Ross) p 426, 664
Collyrium Eye Lotion (Wyeth) p 435, 727
Collyrium 2 Eye Drops with Tetrahydrozoline (Wyeth) p 435, 727
Lacri-Lube S.O.P. (Allergan) p 403, 506
Lavoptik Eye Wash (Lavoptik) p 561
Liquifilm Forte (Allergan) p 506
Liquifilm Tears (Allergan) p 403, 506
Murine Eye Drops (Regular Formula) (Ross) p 426, 666
Murine Plus Eye Drops (Ross) p 426, 666
Muro Tears (Muro) p 615
Prefrin Liquifilm (Allergan) p 403, 506
Stye Ophthalmic Ointment (Commerce Drug) p 408, 540
Tears Plus (Allergan) p 403, 506
Visine A.C. Eye Drops (Leeming) p 568
Visine Eye Drops (Leeming) p 568

ORAL HYGIENE AID
Colgate MFP Fluoride Gel (Colgate-Palmolive) p 407, 537
Colgate MFP Fluoride Toothpaste (Colgate-Palmolive) p 407, 537
Listerine Antiseptic (Warner-Lambert Co.) p 433, 709
S.T.37 (Beecham Products) p 516
Xero-Lube - Saliva Substitute (Scherer) p 672

P

PAIN RELIEVERS
(see under ANALGESICS)

PEDICULICIDES
A-200 Pyrinate Pediculicide Shampoo, Liquid, Gel (Norcliff Thayer) p 418, 621
Cuprex (Beecham Products) p 512
Li-Ban Spray (Pfipharmecs) p 421, 635
R&C Shampoo (Reed & Carnrick) p 423, 650
R&C Spray III (Reed & Carnrick) p 423, 650
RID (Pfipharmecs) p 421, 635
Triple X - A Pediculicide (Youngs Drug Products) p 730
Vleminckx' Solution (Ulmer) p 698

PINWORMS PREPARATIONS
(see under ANTHELMINTICS)

POISON IVY & OAK PREPARATIONS
Bactine Hydrocortisone Skin Care Cream (Miles Laboratories) p 417, 613
Caladryl Cream & Lotion (Parke-Davis) p 420, 631
CaldeCORT Anti-Itch Hydrocortisone Cream (Pharmacraft) p 421, 636
CaldeCORT Anti-Itch Hydrocortisone Spray (Pharmacraft) p 421, 636
Cortaid Cream (Upjohn) p 430, 698
Cortaid Lotion (Upjohn) p 430, 698
Cortaid Ointment (Upjohn) p 430, 698
Cortaid Spray (Upjohn) p 430, 698
Delacort (Mericon) p 606
Dermolate Anti-Itch Cream & Spray (Schering) p 427, 677
Hydrocortisine Cream & Ointment, U.S.P. 0.5% (Fougera) p 551
Hytone Cream 1/2% (Dermik) p 542
Ivarest Medicated Cream & Lotion (Blistex) p 520
Lanacane Medicated Creme (Combe) p 407, 538
Lanacort Anti-Itch Hydrocortisone Acetate 0.5% Creme and Ointment (Combe) p 407, 538
Resicort Cream (Mentholatum) p 605
Shuttle First Aid Spray (American Hygienic) p 403, 507
Ziradryl Lotion (Parke-Davis) p 420, 634

PREGNANCY TESTS
(see under DIAGNOSTICS, Pregnancy Tests)

PREMENSTRUAL THERAPEUTICS
(see under MENSTRUAL PREPARATIONS)

PRICKLY HEAT AIDS
(see under DERMATOLOGICALS, Antidermatitis & Powders)

S

SALIVA SUBSTITUTES
Xero-Lube - Saliva Substitute (Scherer) p 672

SALT SUBSTITUTES
Mrs. Dash (Alberto-Culver) p 506
NoSalt Salt Alternative, Regular (Norcliff Thayer) p 418, 622
NoSalt Salt Alternative, Seasoned (Norcliff Thayer) p 418, 622

SALT TABLETS
Thermotabs (Beecham Products) p 517

SCABICIDES
(see under DERMATOLOGICALS, Scabicides)

SHAMPOOS
(see under DERMATOLOGICALS, Shampoos)

SHINGLES RELIEF
(see under ANALGESICS)

SINUSITIS AIDS
(see under COLD PREPARATIONS)

SKIN BLEACHES
(see under DERMATOLOGICALS)

SKIN CARE PRODUCTS
(see under DERMATOLOGICALS)

SKIN DISEASE PREPARATIONS
(see under DERMATOLOGICALS)

SKIN PROTECTANTS
Caldesene Medicated Ointment (Pharmacraft) p 421, 636
Caldesene Medicated Powder (Pharmacraft) p 421, 636
Chap Stick Lip Balm (Robins) p 424, 654
Chap Stick Sunblock 15 Lip Balm (Robins) p 424, 654
Ivarest Medicated Cream & Lotion (Blistex) p 520
Johnson's Baby Cream (Johnson & Johnson Baby Products) p 411, 558
Kerodex Cream 51 (for dry or oily work) (Ayerst) p 404, 509
Kerodex Cream 71 (for wet work) (Ayerst) p 404, 509
Lobana Peri-Gard (Ulmer) p 697

SKIN REMEDIES
(see under DERMATOLOGICALS)

SKIN WOUND PREPARATIONS

Cleansers
Bactine Antiseptic/Anesthetic First Aid Spray (Miles Laboratories) p 417, 612
Betadine Solution (Purdue Frederick) p 647
Mercurochrome II (Becton Dickinson Consumer) p 512
S.T.37 (Beecham Products) p 516

Healing Agents
Johnson & Johnson Clinicydin (Johnson & Johnson) p 411, 559
Johnson & Johnson First Aid Cream (Johnson & Johnson) p 411, 560
Lanabiotic First Aid Ointment (Combe) p 407, 538
Medicone Dressing Cream (Medicone) p 595
Neosporin Ointment (Burroughs Wellcome) p 406, 530
Polysporin Ointment (Burroughs Wellcome) p 530
PRID Salve (Walker Pharmacal) p 707

Protectants
Boric Acid Ointment (Fougera) p 550
Medicone Dressing Cream (Medicone) p 595
S.T.37 (Beecham Products) p 516

SLEEP AIDS
Biochemic Tissue Salts (NuAGE Laboratories) p 624
Compoz Nighttime Sleep Aid (Jeffrey Martin) p 557
Miles Nervine Nighttime Sleep-Aid (Miles Laboratories) p 418, 614
Nytol Tablets (Block) p 521
Sleep-eze 3 Tablets (Whitehall) p 721
Sleepinal, Maximum Strength Capsules (Thompson Medical) p 430, 695
Sominex 2 (Beecham Products) p 516
Unisom Nighttime Sleep Aid (Leeming) p 568

SMOKING DETERRENTS
Bantron Smoking Deterrent Tablets (Jeffrey Martin) p 557
Healthbreak Smoking Deterrent Gum & Lozenge (Lemar) p 412, 569

SORE THROAT PREPARATIONS
(see under COLD PREPARATIONS, Lozenges)

SPORTS MEDICINE
AthletiCare Pretaping Underwrap (Johnson & Johnson) p 559
AthletiCare Sports Tape (Johnson & Johnson) p 559
Carnation Instant Breakfast (Carnation) p 533
Sportmed Fitness Appraisal Kit (Sportmed Technology) p 741
Work Out (Bigelow-Clark) p 519

STIFF NECK RELIEF
(see under ANALGESICS)

STIMULANTS
No Doz Tablets (Bristol-Myers) p 406, 529
Vivarin Stimulant Tablets (Beecham Products) p 517

SUGAR SUBSTITUTES
Equal (Searle Consumer Products) p 428, 682
SugarTwin (Alberto-Culver) p 506

SUN SCREENS
(see under DERMATOLOGICALS)

SUPPLEMENTS
(see under DIETARY SUPPLEMENTS)

T

TEETHING LOTIONS & GELS
Anbesol Baby Gel Antiseptic Anesthetic (Whitehall) p 434, 716
Anbesol Gel Antiseptic Anesthetic (Whitehall) p 434, 716
Anbesol Liquid Antiseptic Anesthetic (Whitehall) p 434, 716
Baby Orajel (Commerce Drug) p 408, 539

TENNIS ELBOW RELIEF
(see under ANALGESICS)

THROAT LOZENGES
Aspergum (Plough) p 421, 640
Cēpacol Anesthetic Lozenges (Troches) (Merrell Dow) p 606
Cēpacol Throat Lozenges (Merrell Dow) p 606

W

WART REMOVERS
(see under DERMATOLOGICALS)

WEIGHT CONTROL PREPARATIONS
(see under APPETITE SUPPRESSANTS or FOODS)

WET DRESSINGS
(see under DERMATOLOGICALS)

Memorandum

Memorandum

Memorandum

Memorandum

Memorandum

SECTION 4
Active Ingredients Index

In this section the products described in the Product Information (White) Section are listed under their chemical (generic) name according to their principal ingredient(s). Products have been included under specific headings by the Publisher with the cooperation of individual manufacturers.

A

Acerola
C-Complex Tablets (Nature's Bounty) p 617

Acetaminophen
Allerest Headache Strength Tablets (Pharmacraft) p 636
Allerest Sinus Pain Formula (Pharmacraft) p 421, 636
Anacin-3 Children's Acetaminophen Chewable Tablets, Liquid, Drops (Whitehall) p 434, 715
Anacin-3 Maximum Strength Acetaminophen Tablets & Capsules (Whitehall) p 434, 715
Anacin-3 Regular Strength Acetaminophen Tablets (Whitehall) p 715
Childrens CoTylenol Chewable Cold Tablets & Liquid Cold Formula (McNeil Consumer Products) p 414, 577
Children's Panadol Chewable Tablets, Liquid, Drops (Glenbrook) p 410, 555
Comtrex (Bristol-Myers) p 405, 526
Congespirin Aspirin-Free Chewable Cold Tablets for Children (Bristol-Myers) p 405, 526
Congespirin Liquid Cold Medicine (Bristol-Myers) p 405, 526
Contac Jr. Childrens' Cold Medicine (Menley & James) p 415, 599
Contac Severe Cold Formula Capsules (Menley & James) p 415, 598
Contac Severe Cold Formula Night Strength (Menley & James) p 415, 598
Coricidin Demilets Tablets for Children (Schering) p 427, 675
Coricidin Extra Strength Sinus Headache Tablets (Schering) p 676
Coryban-D Cough Syrup (Pfipharmecs) p 421, 635

CoTylenol Cold Medication Liquid (McNeil Consumer Products) p 414, 577
CoTylenol Cold Medication Tablets & Capsules (McNeil Consumer Products) p 414, 576
Daycare Multi-Symptom Colds Medicine Capsules (Vicks Health Care) p 431, 701
Daycare Multi-Symptom Colds Medicine Liquid (Vicks Health Care) p 431, 701
Dimensyn Maximum Strength Menstrual Discomfort Relief (Ortho Pharmaceutical) p 419, 626
Dorcol Children's Fever & Pain Reducer (Dorsey) p 408, 544
Dristan Advanced Formula Decongestant/Antihistimine/ Analgesic Capsules (Whitehall) p 434, 717
Dristan Advanced Formula Decongestant/Antihistamine/ Analgesic Tablets (Whitehall) p 434, 717
Excedrin Capsules & Tablets (Bristol-Myers) p 405, 527
Excedrin P.M. Analgesic Sleeping Aid (Bristol-Myers) p 405, 527
Extra Strength Datril Capsules & Tablets (Bristol-Myers) p 405, 527
Formula 44M Multisymptom Cough Mixture (Vicks Health Care) p 431, 702
Gemnisyn Tablets (Rorer) p 659
Goody's Headache Powders (Goody's) p 410, 556
Headway Capsules (Vicks Health Care) p 431, 703
Headway Tablets (Vicks Health Care) p 431, 703
Liquiprin Acetaminophen (Norcliff Thayer) p 418, 622
Maximum Strength Panadol (Glenbrook) p 410, 555
Midol PMS (Glenbrook) p 410, 554
Nyquil Nighttime Colds Medicine (Vicks Health Care) p 432, 703

Ornex Capsules (Menley & James) p 416, 601
Percogesic Analgesic Tablets (Vicks Pharmacy Products) p 432, 706
Prēmesyn PMS (Chattem) p 407, 534
Pursettes Premenstrual Tablets (Jeffrey Martin) p 558
Pyrroxate Capsules (Upjohn) p 431, 699
Robitussin Night Relief (Robins) p 425, 656
St. Joseph Aspirin-Free Chewable Tablets, Liquid & Infant Drops (Plough) p 422, 642
Sinarest Regular & Extra Strength Tablets (Pharmacraft) p 638
Sine-Aid, Extra Strength, Sinus Headache Capsules (McNeil Consumer Products) p 414, 579
Sine-Aid Sinus Headache Tablets (McNeil Consumer Products) p 414, 579
Sine-Off Extra Strength No Drowsiness Capsules (Menley & James) p 416, 602
Sine-Off Extra Strength Sinus Medicine Aspirin-Free Capsules (Menley & James) p 416, 601
Sine-Off Extra Strength Sinus Medicine Aspirin-Free Tablets (Menley & James) p 416, 602
Sinutab Maximum Strength Capsules (Warner-Lambert Co.) p 433, 711
Sinutab Maximum Strength Tablets (Warner-Lambert Co.) p 433, 711
Sinutab Tablets (Warner-Lambert Co.) p 433, 711
Sinutab II Maximum Strength No Drowsiness Formula Tablets & Capsules (Warner-Lambert Co.) p 433, 711
Sominex Pain Relief Formula (Beecham Products) p 515
Sunril Premenstrual Capsules (Schering) p 680
Teldrin Multi-Symptom Allergy Reliever (Menley & James) p 417, 603

Tempra (Mead Johnson Nutritional)
p 415, 592

Tussagesic Tablets & Suspension
(Dorsey) p 548

Tylenol acetaminophen Children's
Chewable Tablets, Elixir, Drops
(McNeil Consumer Products) p 414,
580

Tylenol, Extra-Strength, acetaminophen
Adult Liquid Pain Reliever (McNeil
Consumer Products) p 582

Tylenol, Extra-Strength, acetaminophen
Tablets, Capsules & Caplets (McNeil
Consumer Products) p 413, 414,
582

Tylenol, Infants' Drops (McNeil
Consumer Products) p 414, 580

Tylenol, Junior Strength,
acetaminophen Swallowable Tablets
(McNeil Consumer Products) p 414,
580

Tylenol, Maximum Strength, Sinus
Medication Tablets & Capsules
(McNeil Consumer Products) p 414,
582

Tylenol, Regular Strength,
acetaminophen Capsules & Tablets
(McNeil Consumer Products) p 413,
581

Vanquish (Glenbrook) p 410, 556

Acetic Acid

Star-Otic Ear Solution (Stellar) p 428,
686

Acetone Sodium Bisulfite

Dibucaine Ointment, U.S.P. 1%
(Fougera) p 551

Nupercainal Suppositories (Ciba
Pharmaceutical) p 407, 536

**Acetylsalicylic Acid
(see under Aspirin)**

Alcohol

Anbesol Gel Antiseptic Anesthetic
(Whitehall) p 434, 716

Anbesol Liquid Antiseptic Anesthetic
(Whitehall) p 434, 716

Coryban-D Cough Syrup (Pfipharmecs)
p 421, 635

Denorex Medicated Shampoo &
Conditioner (Whitehall) p 434, 717

Denorex Medicated Shampoo, Regular
& Mountain Fresh Herbal (Whitehall)
p 434, 717

Diaparene Baby Wash Cloths
(Glenbrook) p 410, 554

Freezone Solution (Whitehall) p 718

Oxipor VHC Lotion for Psoriasis
(Whitehall) p 719

Oxy Clean Medicated Cleanser, Pads,
Soap (Norcliff Thayer) p 418, 622

Stri-Dex Maximum Strength Pads
(Glenbrook) p 556

Stri-Dex Regular Strength Pads
(Glenbrook) p 556

Alfalfa

Alfalfa Tablets (Nature's Bounty) p 617

Allantoin

Blistik Medicated Lip Balm (Blistex)
p 519

Herpecin-L Cold Sore Lip Balm
(Campbell) p 532

Tegrin for Psoriasis Lotion & Cream
(Block) p 522

Allicin

Arizona Natural Odorless Garlic
(Arizone Natural) p 508

Aloe

Nature's Remedy Laxative (Norcliff
Thayer) p 418, 622

Shuttle First Aid Spray (American
Hygienic) p 403, 507

Aloe Vera

Lily of the Desert Aloe Vera Gelly
(97%) (Vera Products) p 431, 701

Lily of the Desert Aloe Vera Juice
(99.8%) (Vera Products) p 431, 701

d-Alpha Tocopherol

Vitamin E Capsules, 100 IU, 200 IU &
400 IU D-Alpha Tocopherol plus
Mixed Tocopherol (Solgar) p 685

Aluminum Acetate

Acid Mantle Creme & Lotion (Dorsey)
p 408, 543

Aluminum Carbonate

Basaljel Capsules (Wyeth) p 435, 726

Basaljel Swallow Tablets (Wyeth)
p 435, 726

Basaljel Suspension & Extra Strength
Suspension (Wyeth) p 435, 726

Aluminum Chlorohydrate

Desenex Foot & Sneaker Spray
(Pharmacraft) p 637

Aluminum Hydroxide

Camalox Suspension & Tablets (Rorer)
p 658

Delcid (Merrell Dow) p 607

Di-Gel (Plough) p 421, 641

Gaviscon Liquid Antacid (Marion)
p 412, 572

Gelusil-M (Parke-Davis) p 632

Gelusil-II Liquid & Tablets (Parke-Davis)
p 632

Maalox Suspension & Tablets (Rorer)
p 425, 660

Maalox Plus Suspension & Tablets
(Rorer) p 425, 661

Maalox TC Suspension & Tablets
(Rorer) p 425, 661

Nephrox Suspension (Fleming) p 549

Tempo Antacid with Antigas Action
(Vicks Health Care) p 432, 704

WinGel (Winthrop Consumer Products)
p 726

Aluminum Hydroxide Gel

ALternaGEL Liquid (Stuart) p 428, 686

Aludrox Oral Suspension & Tablets
(Wyeth) p 435, 726

Amphojel Suspension & Suspension
without Flavor (Wyeth) p 435, 726

Di-Gel (Plough) p 421, 641

Gelusil Liquid & Tablets (Parke-Davis)
p 420, 631

Kudrox Suspension (Double Strength)
(Rorer) p 660

Mylanta Liquid (Stuart) p 429, 689

Mylanta-II Liquid (Stuart) p 429, 689

Simeco Suspension (Wyeth) p 435,
728

Aluminum Hydroxide Gel, Dried

Aludrox Oral Suspension & Tablets
(Wyeth) p 435, 726

Amphojel Tablets (Wyeth) p 435, 726

Ascriptin Tablets (Rorer) p 425, 658

Ascriptin A/D Tablets (Rorer) p 425,
658

Gaviscon Antacid Tablets (Marion)
p 412, 572

Gaviscon-2 Antacid Tablets (Marion)
p 413, 572

Mylanta Tablets (Stuart) p 429, 689

Mylanta-II Tablets (Stuart) p 429, 689

Aluminum Hydroxide Preparations

Kolantyl (Merrell Dow) p 607

Magnatril Suspension & Tablets
(Lannett) p 561

Amino Acid Preparations

Amina-21 Capsules & Powder (Miller)
p 615

Yeast Plus Tablets (Nature's Bounty)
p 621

Aminobenzoic Acid

PreSun 15 Sunscreen Lotion
(Westwood) p 433, 713

Ammonium Alum

Massengill Powder (Beecham Products)
p 514

Ammonium Chloride

Aqua-Ban Tablets (Thompson Medical)
p 430, 692

Aqua-Ban, Maximum Strength Plus
Tablets (Thompson Medical) p 430,
692

Amylase

Festal II (Hoechst-Roussel) p 411, 556

Papaya Enzyme Tablets (Nature's
Bounty) p 620

Anethole

Vicks Cough Silencers Cough Drops
(Vicks Health Care) p 704

Antipyrine

Collyrium Eye Lotion (Wyeth) p 435,
727

Prefrin Liquifilm (Allergan) p 403, 506

l-Arginine

l-Arginine (Nature's Bounty) p 619

**Ascorbic Acid
(see under Vitamin C)**

Aspartame

Equal (Searle Consumer Products)
p 428, 682

Aspirin

Alka-Seltzer Effervescent Pain Reliever
& Antacid (Miles Laboratories)
p 417, 611

Alka-Seltzer Plus Cold Medicine (Miles
Laboratories) p 417, 612

Anacin Analgesic Capsules (Whitehall)
p 714

Anacin Analgesic Tablets (Whitehall)
p 434, 714

Anacin Maximum Strength Analgesic
Capsules (Whitehall) p 715

Anacin Maximum Strength Analgesic
Tablets (Whitehall) p 715

Arthritis Bayer Timed-Release Aspirin
(Glenbrook) p 410, 553

Arthritis Pain Formula by the Makers of
Anacin Analgesic Tablets (Whitehall)
p 434, 716

Arthritis Pain Formula Safety Coated by
the Makers of Anacin Analgesic
Tablets (Whitehall) p 434, 716

Arthritis Strength Bufferin
(Bristol-Myers) p 405, 525

Ascriptin Tablets (Rorer) p 425, 658

Ascriptin A/D Tablets (Rorer) p 425,
658

Aspergum (Plough) p 421, 640

BC Powder (Block) p 521

Bayer Aspirin & Bayer Children's
Chewable Aspirin (Glenbrook) p 409,
552

Bayer Children's Cold Tablets
(Glenbrook) p 553

Bufferin Analgesic Tablets and
Capsules (Bristol-Myers) p 405, 525

Cama Arthritis Pain Reliever (Dorsey)
p 408, 543

Congespirin Chewable Cold Tablets for
Children (Bristol-Myers) p 405, 527

Coricidin 'D' Decongestant Tablets
(Schering) p 427, 674

Coricidin Tablets (Schering) p 427,
674

Cosprin 325 (Glenbrook) p 410, 554

Cosprin 650 (Glenbrook) p 410, 554

Ecotrin Maximum Strength Capsules
(Menley & James) p 416, 599

Ecotrin Regular Strength Capsules
(Menley & James) p 416, 600

Ecotrin Tablets (Menley & James)
p 416, 599

Ecotrin Maximum Strength Tablets
(Menley & James) p 416, 599

Empirin (Burroughs Wellcome) p 406,
530

Encaprin (Procter & Gamble) p 644

Excedrin Capsules & Tablets
(Bristol-Myers) p 405, 527

Extra-Strength Bufferin Capsules &
Tablets (Bristol-Myers) p 405, 526

Oxipor VHC Lotion for Psoriasis (Whitehall) p 719
P&S Plus (Baker/Cummins) p 510
Pragmatar Ointment (Menley & James) p 416, 601
Tegrin for Psoriasis Lotion & Cream (Block) p 522
Tegrin Medicated Shampoo (Block) p 522
Xseb-T Shampoo (Baker/Cummins) p 511
Zetar Shampoo (Dermik) p 543

Cobalamin
B-12 & B-12 Sublingual Tablets (Nature's Bounty) p 617
B Complex & C (Time Release) Tablets (Nature's Bounty) p 617
B & C Liquid (Nature's Bounty) p 617
Chew-Iron Tablets (Nature's Bounty) p 618

Cocoa Butter
Calmol 4 Suppositories (Mentholatum) p 604
Nupercainal Suppositories (Ciba Pharmaceutical) p 407, 536

Cod Liver Oil
Calmol 4 Suppositories (Mentholatum) p 604
Desitin Ointment (Leeming) p 567
Medicone Dressing Cream (Medicone) p 595
Scott's Emulsion (Beecham Products) p 515

Cod Liver Oil Concentrate
Cod Liver Oil Concentrate Tablets, Capsules (Schering) p 427, 674
Cod Liver Oil Concentrate Tablets w/Vitamin C (Schering) p 427, 674

Codeine
Ryna-C Liquid (Wallace) p 432, 708
Ryna-CX Liquid (Wallace) p 432, 708

Codeine Phosphate
Naldecon-CX Suspension (Bristol) p 524

Copper
One-A-Day Maximum Formula Vitamins and Minerals (Miles Laboratories) p 418, 614
Stressgard Stress Formula Vitamins (Miles Laboratories) p 418, 615

Copper Amino Acid Chelate
Chelated Copper Tablets (Nature's Bounty) p 618

Copper Oleate
Cuprex (Beecham Products) p 512

Corn Silk Extract
Odrinil (Fox) p 551

Corn Starch
Diaparene Baby Powder (Glenbrook) p 410, 554
Lobana Body Powder (Ulmer) p 697

Cyanocobalamin
Bugs Bunny Children's Chewable Vitamins (Sugar Free) (Miles Laboratories) p 417, 613
Bugs Bunny Plus Iron Children's Chewable Vitamins (Sugar Free) (Miles Laboratories) p 417, 613
Bugs Bunny With Extra C Children's Chewable Vitamins (Sugar Free) (Miles Laboratories) p 417, 613
Flintstones Children's Chewable Vitamins (Miles Laboratories) p 417, 613
Flintstones Children's Chewable Vitamins Plus Iron (Miles Laboratories) p 417, 613
Flintstones Children's Chewable Vitamins With Extra C (Miles Laboratories) p 417, 613

Geritol Liquid - High Potency Iron & Vitamin Tonic (Beecham Products) p 513
One-A-Day Essential Vitamins (Miles Laboratories) p 418, 614
One-A-Day Maximum Formula Vitamins and Minerals (Miles Laboratories) p 418, 614
One-A-Day Plus Extra C Vitamins (Miles Laboratories) p 418, 615

Cyclizine Hydrochloride
Marezine Tablets (Burroughs Wellcome) p 530

D

DNA
RNA/DNA Tablets (Nature's Bounty) p 620

Danthron
Dorbane Tablets (3M Company) p 570
Dorbantyl Capsules (3M Company) p 570
Dorbantyl Forte Capsules (3M Company) p 570
Doxidan (Hoechst-Roussel) p 410, 556
Modane (Adria) p 403, 502
Modane Plus Tablets (Adria) p 403, 503

Desoxyephedrine-Levo
Vicks Inhaler (Vicks Health Care) p 705

Dexbrompheniramine Maleate
Disophrol Chronotab Sustained-Action Tablets (Schering) p 677
Drixoral Sustained-Action Tablets (Schering) p 427, 678

Dextromethorphan Hydrobromide
Ambenyl-D Decongestant Cough Formula (Marion) p 412, 571
Bayer Cough Syrup for Children (Glenbrook) p 553
Benylin DM (Parke-Davis) p 420, 631
Cheracol D Cough Formula (Upjohn) p 430, 698
Cheracol Plus Head Cold/Cough Formula (Upjohn) p 430, 698
Children's Hold (Beecham Products) p 514
Comtrex (Bristol-Myers) p 405, 526
Congespirin for Children Cough Syrup (Bristol-Myers) p 405, 526
Contac Cough Capsules (Menley & James) p 415, 597
Contac Jr. Childrens' Cold Medicine (Menley & James) p 415, 599
Contac Severe Cold Formula Capsules (Menley & James) p 415, 598
Contac Severe Cold Formula Night Strength (Menley & James) p 415, 598
Coricidin Cough Syrup (Schering) p 674
Coryban-D Cough Syrup (Pfipharmecs) p 421, 635
CoTylenol Cold Medication Liquid (McNeil Consumer Products) p 414, 577
CoTylenol Cold Medication Tablets & Capsules (McNeil Consumer Products) p 414, 576
Cremacoat 1 (Vicks Pharmacy Products) p 705
Cremacoat 3 (Vicks Pharmacy Products) p 706
Cremacoat 4 (Vicks Pharmacy Products) p 706
Daycare Multi-Symptom Colds Medicine Capsules (Vicks Health Care) p 431, 701
Daycare Multi-Symptom Colds Medicine Liquid (Vicks Health Care) p 431, 701
Dimacol Capsules (Robins) p 424, 654
Dorcol Children's Cough Syrup (Dorsey) p 408, 543
Formula 44 Cough Control Discs (Vicks Health Care) p 702

Formula 44 Cough Mixture (Vicks Health Care) p 431, 702
Formula 44D Decongestant Cough Mixture (Vicks Health Care) p 431, 702
Formula 44M Multisymptom Cough Mixture (Vicks Health Care) p 431, 702
Hold (Beecham Products) p 514
Mediquell Chewy Cough Squares (Warner-Lambert Co.) p 433, 710
Naldecon-DX Pediatric Syrup (Bristol) p 524
Novahistine Cough & Cold Formula (Merrell Dow) p 608
Novahistine DMX (Merrell Dow) p 608
Nyquil Nighttime Colds Medicine (Vicks Health Care) p 432, 703
Ornacol Capsules (Menley & James) p 416, 601
PediaCare 1 Children's Cough Relief Liquid (McNeil Consumer Products) p 413, 578
PediaCare 3 Children's Cold Relief Liquid & Chewable Tablets (McNeil Consumer Products) p 413, 578
Robitussin-CF (Robins) p 424, 656
Robitussin-DM (Robins) p 424, 656
Robitussin Night Relief (Robins) p 425, 656
St. Joseph Cough Syrup for Children (Plough) p 422, 643
Sucrets Cough Control Formula (Beecham Products) p 517
Sudafed Cough Syrup (Burroughs Wellcome) p 406, 531
Triaminic-DM Cough Formula (Dorsey) p 409, 546
Triaminicol Multi-Symptom Cold Syrup (Dorsey) p 409, 547
Triaminicol Multi-Symptom Cold Tablets (Dorsey) p 409, 547
Trind-DM (Mead Johnson Nutritional) p 594
Tussagesic Tablets & Suspension (Dorsey) p 548
Vicks Childrens Cough Syrup (Vicks Health Care) p 704
Vicks Cough Silencers Cough Drops (Vicks Health Care) p 704

Dextromethorphan Polystirex
Extend-12 Liquid (Robins) p 424, 655

Dextrose
B-D Glucose Tablets (Becton Dickinson Consumer) p 511
Glutose (Paddock) p 629
Thermotabs (Beecham Products) p 517

Dibucaine
Dibucaine Ointment, U.S.P. 1% (Fougera) p 551
Dibucaine Ointment, USP 1% (Pharmaderm) p 639
Nupercainal Cream & Ointment (Ciba Pharmaceutical) p 407, 536

Diethyl-m-Toluamide
Muskol Insect Repellent Aerosol Liquid (Plough) p 422, 641
Muskol Insect Repellent Lotion (Plough) p 422, 641

Dihydroxyalumin Sodium Carbonate
Rolaids (Warner-Lambert Co.) p 433, 710

p-Diisobutylphenoxypolyethoxyethanol
Ortho-Gynol Contraceptive Jelly (Ortho Pharmaceutical) p 420, 628

Dimenhydrinate
Dramamine Liquid (Searle Consumer Products) p 428, 681
Dramamine Tablets (Searle Consumer Products) p 428, 681

Dimethicone
Complex 15 Moisturizing Cream & Lotion (Baker/Cummins) p 510
Johnson's Baby Cream (Johnson & Johnson Baby Products) p 411, 558

One-A-Day Essential Vitamins (Miles Laboratories) p 418, 614
One-A-Day Maximum Formula Vitamins and Minerals (Miles Laboratories) p 418, 614
One-A-Day Plus Extra C Vitamins (Miles Laboratories) p 418, 615
Simron Plus (Merrell Dow) p 610
Stressgard Stress Formula Vitamins (Miles Laboratories) p 418, 615
The Stuart Formula Tablets (Stuart) p 429, 690
Stuart Prenatal Tablets (Stuart) p 429, 690
Tri-B-Plex (Anabolic) p 507

Frangula
Herbal Laxative Tablets (Nature's Bounty) p 619

G

Garlic Extract
Arizona Natural Odorless Garlic (Arizone Natural) p 508
Kyolic (Wakunaga) p 432, 707

Garlic Oil
Garlic Oil Capsules (Nature's Bounty) p 618
Garlic & Parsley Capsules (Nature's Bounty) p 619

Gelatin
Gelocast (Beiersdorf) p 518

Gingseng
Geriavit Pharmaton (Nutritional Specialty) p 419, 624
Ginseng, Manchurian Capsules & Tablets (Nature's Bounty) p 619

Glucose Oxidase
BetaScan Reagent Strips, Blood Glucose Test Strips (Orange Medical) p 740
TrendStrips, Blood Glucose Test Strips (Orange Medical) p 740

Glutamic Acid
Glutamic Acid Tablets (Nature's Bounty) p 619

l-Glutamine
l-Glutamine Tablets (Nature's Bounty) p 619
Memory Booster (Nature's Bounty) p 619

Glycerin
Complex 15 Moisturizing Cream & Lotion (Baker/Cummins) p 510
Debrox Drops (Marion) p 412, 571
Gly-Oxide Liquid (Marion) p 413, 572
Mediconet (Medicone) p 595
S.T.37 (Beecham Products) p 516
Shuttle Lotion (American Hygienic) p 403, 507
Ultra Mide 25 Moisturizer Lotion (Baker/Cummins) p 511

Glyceryl Guaiacolate
(see under Guaifenesin)

Glyceryl PABA
Eclipse Sunscreen Lotion, Total (Cooling Alcohol Base) (Dorsey) p 408, 545

Glyceryl Stearate
Johnson & Johnson First Aid Cream (Johnson & Johnson) p 411, 560
Shepard's Skin Cream (Dermik) p 542

Gotu-Kola
Memory Booster (Nature's Bounty) p 619

Guaifenesin
Ambenyl-D Decongestant Cough Formula (Marion) p 412, 571
Breonesin Capsules (Winthrop-Breon) p 435, 721

Bronkaid Tablets (Winthrop Consumer Products) p 722
Bronkolixir (Winthrop-Breon) p 721
Bronkotabs (Winthrop-Breon) p 435, 721
Cheracol D Cough Formula (Upjohn) p 430, 698
Congestac Tablets (Menley & James) p 415, 597
Coricidin Cough Syrup (Schering) p 674
Coryban-D Cough Syrup (Pfipharmecs) p 421, 635
Cremacoat 2 (Vicks Pharmacy Products) p 705
Cremacoat 3 (Vicks Pharmacy Products) p 706
Dimacol Capsules (Robins) p 424, 654
Dorcol Children's Cough Syrup (Dorsey) p 408, 543
Formula 44D Decongestant Cough Mixture (Vicks Health Care) p 431, 702
Formula 44M Multisymptom Cough Mixture (Vicks Health Care) p 431, 702
Glycotuss Syrup & Tablets (Vale) p 701
Glytuss Tablets (Mayrand) p 575
Head & Chest (Procter & Gamble) p 423, 645
Naldecon-CX Suspension (Bristol) p 524
Naldecon-DX Pediatric Syrup (Bristol) p 524
Naldecon-EX Pediatric Drops (Bristol) p 525
Novahistine DMX (Merrell Dow) p 608
Robitussin (Robins) p 424, 656
Robitussin-CF (Robins) p 424, 656
Robitussin-DM (Robins) p 424, 656
Robitussin-PE (Robins) p 425, 656
Ryna-CX Liquid (Wallace) p 432, 708
Sudafed Cough Syrup (Burroughs Wellcome) p 406, 531
Triaminic Expectorant (Dorsey) p 408, 546
Vicks Childrens Cough Syrup (Vicks Health Care) p 704

H

HCG Antibodies
Daisy 2 Pregnancy Test (Ortho Pharmaceutical) p 419, 741

HCG Antiserum (rabbit)
Acu-Test In-Home Pregnancy Test (Beecham Products) p 735
Answer At-Home Early Pregnancy Test Kit (Carter Products) p 406, 737
Fact Pregnancy Test (Ortho Pharmaceutical) p 419, 741

HCG Monoclonal Antibody
Advance Pregnancy Test (Ortho Pharmaceutical) p 419, 741
e.p.t. Plus In-Home Early Pregnancy Test (Warner-Lambert Co.) p 432, 742

Halibut Liver Oil
Halibut Liver Oil Capsules (Nature's Bounty) p 619

Hemicellulose
Serutan Concentrated Powder (Beecham Products) p 515
Serutan Concentrated Powder - Fruit Flavored (Beecham Products) p 515
Serutan Toasted Granules (Beecham Products) p 515

Hesperidin Complex
C-Complex Tablets (Nature's Bounty) p 617
Hy-C Tablets (Solgar) p 684

Hexylresorcinol
Listerine Maximum Strength Lozenges (Warner-Lambert Co.) p 709
S.T.37 (Beecham Products) p 516

Sucrets (Regular and Mentholated) (Beecham Products) p 516

l-Histidine
l-Histidine (500 mg) (Nature's Bounty) p 619

Homeopathic Medications
Biochemic Tissue Salts (NuAGE Laboratories) p 624
501 Indigestion (Natra-Bio) p 616
502 Cough (Natra-Bio) p 616
503 Nervousness (Natra-Bio) p 616
504 Injuries (Natra-Bio) p 616
505 Fever (Natra-Bio) p 616
506 Neuralgia (Natra-Bio) p 616
507 Sinus (Natra-Bio) p 616
508 Arthritis (Natra-Bio) p 616
509 Sore Throat (Natra-Bio) p 616
510 Menstrual (Natra-Bio) p 616
511 Nausea (Natra-Bio) p 616
512 Chest Cold (Natra-Bio) p 616
513 Head Cold (Natra-Bio) p 616
514 Earache (Natra-Bio) p 616
515 Headache (Natra-Bio) p 616
516 Prostate (Natra-Bio) p 616
517 Menopause (Natra-Bio) p 616
518 Bed Wetting (Natra-Bio) p 616
519 Hay Fever (Natra-Bio) p 616
520 Hemorrhoids (Natra-Bio) p 616
521 Laxative (Natra-Bio) p 616
522 Bladder Irritation (Natra-Bio) p 616
523 Insomnia (Natra-Bio) p 616
524 Diarrhea (Natra-Bio) p 616
525 Herpes (Natra-Bio) p 616
526 Acne (Natra-Bio) p 616
527 Flu (Natra-Bio) p 616
528 Exhaustion (Natra-Bio) p 616
529 Emotional (Natra-Bio) p 616
530 Eye Irritation (Natra-Bio) p 616
531 Teeth and Gums (Natra-Bio) p 616
532 Teething (Natra-Bio) p 616
533 Varicose Veins (Natra-Bio) p 616
534 Hair and Scalp (Natra-Bio) p 616
535 Insect Bites (Natra-Bio) p 616
536 Poison Oak/Poison Ivy (Natra-Bio) p 616
Oscillococcinum (Borneman) p 404, 524
Yellolax (Luyties) p 570

Human Chorionic Gonadotropin (HCG)
Advance Pregnancy Test (Ortho Pharmaceutical) p 419, 741
Answer At-Home Early Pregnancy Test Kit (Carter Products) p 406, 737
Daisy 2 Pregnancy Test (Ortho Pharmaceutical) p 419, 741
Fact Pregnancy Test (Ortho Pharmaceutical) p 419, 741

Hydrocortisone
Bactine Hydrocortisone Skin Care Cream (Miles Laboratories) p 417, 613
CaldeCORT Anti-Itch Hydrocortisone Spray (Pharmacraft) p 421, 636
Cortaid Spray (Upjohn) p 430, 698
Cortizone-5 Creme & Ointment (Thompson Medical) p 430, 693
Delacort (Mericon) p 606
Dermolate Anal-Itch Ointment (Schering) p 427, 677
Dermolate Anti-Itch Cream & Spray (Schering) p 427, 677
Dermolate Scalp-Itch Lotion (Schering) p 427, 677
Hydrocortisine Cream & Ointment, U.S.P. 0.5% (Fougera) p 551
Hydrocortisone Cream & Ointment, USP 0.5% (Pharmaderm) p 639
Hytone Cream 1/2% (Dermik) p 542
Resicort Cream (Mentholatum) p 605

Hydrocortisone Acetate
CaldeCORT Anti-Itch Hydrocortisone Cream (Pharmacraft) p 421, 636
Cortaid Cream (Upjohn) p 430, 698
Cortaid Lotion (Upjohn) p 430, 698
Cortaid Ointment (Upjohn) p 430, 698

Mentholatum Deep Heating Rub (Mentholatum) p 605
Sinex Decongestant Nasal Spray (Vicks Health Care) p 432, 703
Vatronol Nose Drops (Vicks Health Care) p 704
Vicks Inhaler (Vicks Health Care) p 705
Work Out (Bigelow-Clark) p 519

Methylbenzethonium Chloride

Diaparene Baby Powder (Glenbrook) p 410, 554
Lobana Body Powder (Ulmer) p 697

Methylcellulose

Murocel Ophthalmic Solution (Muro) p 615

Methylparaben

Shuttle Blemish Discs (American Hygienic) p 403, 507
Shuttle First Aid Spray (American Hygienic) p 403, 507
Transi-Lube (Youngs Drug Products) p 730

Miconazole Nitrate

Micatin Antifungal Cream (Ortho Pharmaceutical) p 419, 627
Micatin Antifungal Powder (Ortho Pharmaceutical) p 419, 627
Micatin Antifungal Spray Liquid (Ortho Pharmaceutical) p 627
Micatin Antifungal Spray Powder (Ortho Pharmaceutical) p 419, 627
Micatin Jock Itch Cream (Ortho Pharmaceutical) p 627
Micatin Jock Itch Spray Powder (Ortho Pharmaceutical) p 627

Milk Of Magnesia

Haley's M-O (Winthrop Consumer Products) p 723
Shuttle Lotion (American Hygienic) p 403, 507

Mineral Oil

Agoral, Plain (Parke-Davis) p 630
Agoral Raspberry & Marshmallow Flavors (Parke-Davis) p 630
Alpha Keri Therapeutic Shower & Bath Oil (Westwood) p 433, 712
Balneol (Rowell) p 671
Complex 15 Moisturizing Cream & Lotion (Baker/Cummins) p 510
Haley's M-O (Winthrop Consumer Products) p 723
Keri Lotion (Westwood) p 433, 713
Lacri-Lube S.O.P. (Allergan) p 403, 506
Lobana Bath Oil (Ulmer) p 696
Lobana Body Lotion (Ulmer) p 696
Milkinol (Rorer) p 662
Nephrox Suspension (Fleming) p 549
Ultra Mide 25 Moisturizer Lotion (Baker/Cummins) p 511

Multiminerals

Chelated Multi-Mineral Tablets (Nature's Bounty) p 618

Multivitamins

KLB6 Complete Tablets (Nature's Bounty) p 619
KLB6 Diet Mix (Nature's Bounty) p 619
Stress "1000" Tablets (Nature's Bounty) p 620
Stress Formula "605" Tablets (Nature's Bounty) p 620

Multivitamins with Minerals

Carnation Do-It-Yourself Diet Plan (Carnation) p 533
Carnation Instant Breakfast (Carnation) p 533
Centrum, Jr. + Extra C (Lederle) p 412, 562
Children's Chewable Vitamins with Iron (Nature's Bounty) p 618
Dietene Diet Shake Mix (Creighton Products) p 409, 541
Mega V & M Tablets (Nature's Bounty) p 619

Multi-Mineral Tablets (Nature's Bounty) p 619
Nature's Bounty 1 Tablets (Nature's Bounty) p 619
Nursamil (Sunrise & Rainbow) p 691
Nutrimil (Sunrise & Rainbow) p 429, 691
Optilets-500 (Abbott) p 502
Optilets-M-500 (Abbott) p 502
Slender Diet Food For Weight Control (Instant) (Carnation) p 533
Slender Diet Meal Bars For Weight Control (Carnation) p 534
Slender Diet Meal For Weight Control (Canned) (Carnation) p 533
Spartus (Lederle) p 412, 565
Spartus + Iron (Lederle) p 412, 566
Stress Formula "605" w/Iron Tablets (Nature's Bounty) p 620
Stress Formula "605" w/Zinc Tablets (Nature's Bounty) p 620
Surbex-750 with Iron (Abbott) p 502
Surbex-750 with Zinc (Abbott) p 502
Ultra Vita-Time Tablets (Nature's Bounty) p 620
Vita-Time Tablets (Nature's Bounty) p 621

N

Naphazoline Hydrochloride

Clear Eyes Eye Drops (Ross) p 426, 664
4-Way Nasal Spray (Bristol-Myers) p 406, 528
Privine Nasal Spray & Solution 0.05% (Ciba Pharmaceutical) p 407, 536

Neomycin Sulfate

Bacitracin-Neomycin-Polymyxin Ointment (Fougera) p 550
Bacitracin-Neomycin-Polymyxin Ointment (Pharmaderm) p 639
Johnson & Johnson Clinicydin (Johnson & Johnson) p 411, 559
Lanabiotic First Aid Ointment (Combe) p 407, 538
Myciguent Antibiotic Ointment (Upjohn) p 699
Mycitracin Triple Antibiotic Ointment (Upjohn) p 431, 699
Neosporin Ointment (Burroughs Wellcome) p 406, 530

Niacin

Allbee C-800 Plus Iron Tablets (Robins) p 424, 653
Allbee C-800 Tablets (Robins) p 423, 653
Allbee with C Capsules (Robins) p 424, 653
B Complex & B-12 Tablets (Nature's Bounty) p 617
Bugs Bunny Children's Chewable Vitamins (Sugar Free) (Miles Laboratories) p 417, 613
Bugs Bunny Plus Iron Children's Chewable Vitamins (Sugar Free) (Miles Laboratories) p 417, 613
Bugs Bunny With Extra C Children's Chewable Vitamins (Sugar Free) (Miles Laboratories) p 417, 613
Flintstones Children's Chewable Vitamins (Miles Laboratories) p 417, 613
Flintstones Children's Chewable Vitamins Plus Iron (Miles Laboratories) p 417, 613
Flintstones Children's Chewable Vitamins With Extra C (Miles Laboratories) p 417, 613
Niacin Tablets (Nature's Bounty) p 619
One-A-Day Essential Vitamins (Miles Laboratories) p 418, 614
One-A-Day Maximum Formula Vitamins and Minerals (Miles Laboratories) p 418, 614
One-A-Day Plus Extra C Vitamins (Miles Laboratories) p 418, 615
Stressgard Stress Formula Vitamins (Miles Laboratories) p 418, 615
Z-Bec Tablets (Robins) p 425, 657

Niacinamide

B-100 Tablets (Nature's Bounty) p 617
B Complex & C (Time Release) Tablets (Nature's Bounty) p 617
B & C Liquid (Nature's Bounty) p 617
Geritol Liquid - High Potency Iron & Vitamin Tonic (Beecham Products) p 513
Mega-B (Arco) p 507
Megadose (Arco) p 507
Niacinamide Tablets (Nature's Bounty) p 619
Tri-B-Plex (Anabolic) p 507

Nicotinic Acid
(see also under Niacin)

Nicotinex Elixir (Fleming) p 549

Nonfat Dry Milk

Carnation Do-It-Yourself Diet Plan (Carnation) p 533
Carnation Instant Breakfast (Carnation) p 533
Carnation Nonfat Dry Milk (Carnation) p 533
Slender Diet Food For Weight Control (Instant) (Carnation) p 533

Nonoxynol-9

Conceptrol Birth Control Cream (Ortho Pharmaceutical) p 419, 625
Conceptrol Contraceptive Gel (Ortho Pharmaceutical) p 419, 626
Conceptrol Disposable Contraceptive Gel (Ortho Pharmaceutical) p 419, 626
Delfen Contraceptive Foam (Ortho Pharmaceutical) p 419, 626
Emko Because Contraceptor Vaginal Contraceptive Foam (Schering) p 427, 678
Emko Pre-Fil Vaginal Contraceptive Foam (Schering) p 427, 679
Emko Vaginal Contraceptive Foam (Schering) p 427, 679
Encare (Thompson Medical) p 430, 694
Gynol II Contraceptive Jelly (Ortho Pharmaceutical) p 419, 626
Intercept Contraceptive Inserts (Ortho Pharmaceutical) p 419, 627
Koromex Contraceptive Crystal Clear Gel (Youngs Drug Products) p 729
Koromex Contraceptive Foam (Youngs Drug Products) p 729
Koromex Contraceptive Jelly (Youngs Drug Products) p 730
Ortho-Creme Contraceptive Cream (Ortho Pharmaceutical) p 419, 628
Semicid Vaginal Contraceptive Suppositories (Whitehall) p 434, 720

O

Octacosanol

Octacosanol (Nature's Bounty) p 619

Octoxynol

Koromex Contraceptive Cream (Youngs Drug Products) p 729

Octoxynol 9

Massengill Liquid Concentrate (Beecham Products) p 514

Octyl Dimethyl PABA

Blistex Lip Conditioner (Blistex) p 519
Blistik Medicated Lip Balm (Blistex) p 519
Eclipse Sunscreen Lotion, Total (Cooling Alcohol Base) (Dorsey) p 408, 545
Eclipse Sunscreen Lotion, Total (Moisturizing Base) (Dorsey) p 408, 545
Mentholatum Lipbalm with Sunscreen (Mentholatum) p 605
Porcelana Skin Bleaching Agent with Sunscreen (Jeffrey Martin) p 558
Sundown Sunblock Stick, Ultra Protection (Johnson & Johnson Baby Products) p 411, 558

Neo-Synephrine II Long Acting Nose Drops (Adult & Children's Strengths) (Winthrop Consumer Products) p 723

Neo-Synephrine II Long Acting Vapor Nasal Spray (Winthrop Consumer Products) p 723

Otrivin (Geigy) p 409, 552

Y

Yeast

Brewer's Yeast Powder (Debittered) (Nature's Bounty) p 617

Brewer's Yeast Tablets (Nature's Bounty) p 617

Chromease (Anabolic) p 507

Yellow Mercuric Oxide

Stye Ophthalmic Ointment (Commerce Drug) p 408, 540

Yellow Mercuric Oxide Ophthalmic Ointment 1% & 2% (Pharmaderm) p 640

Z

Zinc

Beminal Stress Plus with Zinc (Ayerst) p 404, 509

Megadose (Arco) p 507

One-A-Day Maximum Formula Vitamins and Minerals (Miles Laboratories) p 418, 614

Poly-Vi-Sol Chewable Vitamins with Iron and Zinc (Mead Johnson Nutritional) p 414, 589

Smurf Chewable Vitamins with Iron and Zinc (Mead Johnson Nutritional) p 415, 591

Stressgard Stress Formula Vitamins (Miles Laboratories) p 418, 615

Z-Bec Tablets (Robins) p 425, 657

Zinc Amino Acid Chelate

Chelated Zinc Tablets (Nature's Bounty) p 618

Zinc Chloride

Orajel Mouth-Aid (Commerce Drug) p 408, 539

Zinc Gluconate

Chromease (Anabolic) p 507

Megadose (Arco) p 507

Orazinc Lozenges (Mericon) p 606

Zacne Tablets (Nature's Bounty) p 621

Zinc Tablets (Nature's Bounty) p 621

Zinc "50" Tablets (Solgar) p 685

Zinc Oxide

Anusol Ointment (Parke-Davis) p 420, 630

Anusol Suppositories (Parke-Davis) p 420, 630

Balmex Baby Powder (Macsil) p 571

Balmex Ointment (Macsil) p 571

Caldesene Medicated Ointment (Pharmacraft) p 421, 636

Calmol 4 Suppositories (Mentholatum) p 604

Derma Medicone Ointment (Medicone) p 595

Desitin Ointment (Leeming) p 567

Gelocast (Beiersdorf) p 518

Medicone Dressing Cream (Medicone) p 595

Nupercainal Suppositories (Ciba Pharmaceutical) p 407, 536

Pazo Hemorrhoid Ointment/ Suppositories (Bristol-Myers) p 529

Rectal Medicone Suppositories (Medicone) p 595

Rectal Medicone Unguent (Medicone) p 596

Shuttle Lotion (American Hygienic) p 403, 507

Wyanoids Hemorrhoidal Suppositories (Wyeth) p 435, 729

Zinc Oxide Ointment, U.S.P. (Fougera) p 551

Zinc Oxide Ointment, USP (Pharmaderm) p 640

Ziradryl Lotion (Parke-Davis) p 420, 634

Zinc Pyrithione

Sebulon Dandruff Shampoo (Westwood) p 433, 714

Zincon Dandruff Shampoo (Lederle) p 412, 567

Zinc Sulfate

Orazinc Capsules (Mericon) p 606

Surbex-750 with Zinc (Abbott) p 502

Visine A.C. Eye Drops (Leeming) p 568

Zinc Undecylenate

Cruex Antifungal Cream (Pharmacraft) p 421, 637

Cruex Antifungal Spray Powder (Pharmacraft) p 637

Desenex Antifungal Cream (Pharmacraft) p 421, 637

Desenex Antifungal Ointment (Pharmacraft) p 421, 637

Desenex Antifungal Powder (Pharmacraft) p 421, 637

Desenex Antifungal Spray Powder (Pharmacraft) p 421, 637

Memorandum

Memorandum

SECTION 5

Product
Identification
Section

This section is designed to help you identify products and their packaging.

Participating manufacturers have included selected products in full color. Where capsules and tablets are included they are shown in actual size. Packages generally are reduced in size.

For more information on products included, refer to the description in the PRODUCT INFORMATION SECTION or check directly with the manufacturer.

While every effort has been made to reproduce products faithfully, this section should be considered only as a quick-reference identification aid.

INDEX BY MANUFACTURER

ADRIA

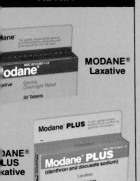

MODANE®
Laxative

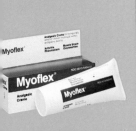

MODANE®
PLUS
Laxative

Allergan

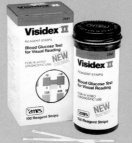

0.7 fl oz

0.7 fl oz Sterile

PREFRIN™ LIQUIFILM®
Ocular Decongestant
(phenylephrine HCl 0.12%)

Ames Division

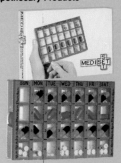

VISIDEX™ II
Reagent Strips

Blood Glucose Test
for Visual Reading

Apothecary Products

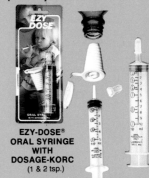

MEDI-SET™
Patient Compliance Device for
Multi-Medication Therapy

Allergan

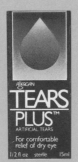

½ fl oz

Also available: 1 fl oz
TEARS PLUS™
Artificial Tears

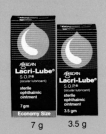

MYOFLEX®
Analgesic Creme

APOTHECARY PRODUCTS

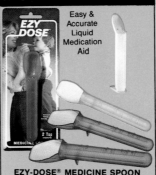

Easy &
Accurate
Liquid
Medication
Aid

EZY-DOSE® MEDICINE SPOON
(1 2 & 3 Tsp.)

Apothecary Products

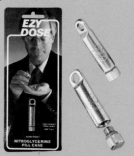

EZY-DOSE®
ORAL SYRINGE
WITH
DOSAGE-KORC
(1 & 2 tsp.)

Efficient, Non-Spill Liquid
Medication Administration

ALLERGAN

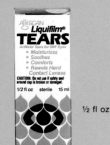

7 g   3.5 g

Also available: .7 g unit dose (24 pack)

LACRI-LUBE® S.O.P.®
Sterile Ophthalmic Ointment

AMERICAN HYGIENIC

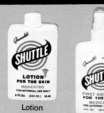

Lotion

First Aid Spray

SHUTTLE®
Medicated Lotion
First Aid Spray
and
Blemish Discs

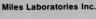

Blemish
Discs

Apothecary Products

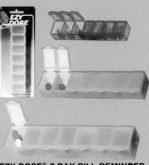

EZY-DOSE® 7-DAY PILL REMINDER
(Small, Medium, Large)

Apothecary Products

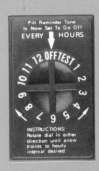

EZY-DOSE®
NITRO-FRESH® PILL HOLDER
Air-Tight, Waterproof, Light-Resistant
Nitroglycerine Pill Holder

Allergan

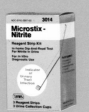

½ fl oz

Also available: 1 fl oz

LIQUIFILM® TEARS
Artificial Tears

AMES DIVISION

Miles Laboratories Inc.

3014

Microstix-
Nitrite

MICROSTIX®-NITRITE

Reagent Strip Kit

An Indicator of Urinary
Tract Infection

Apothecary Products

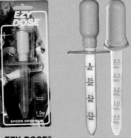

EZY-DOSE®
SPOON DROPPER
(½ & 1 tsp.)
Allows Controlled Placement of
Oral Liquid Medication

Apothecary Products

Pill Reminder Tone
Is Now Set To Go Off
EVERY   HOURS

OFFTEST

INSTRUCTIONS:
Rotate dial in either
direcion until arrow
Points to hourly
interval desired.

MEDTIME MINDER™
Automatic Medication Reminder

ASTRA

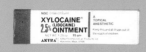

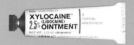

Available in 35g Tube

XYLOCAINE® 2.5% OINTMENT
(lidocaine)

Ayerst

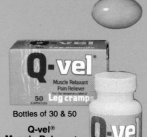

Available in 12 fl oz Suspension, Chew and Swallow Tablets (60s and 100s), and Rollpacks

RIOPAN®
(magaldrate)
Antacid

BIO PRODUCTS

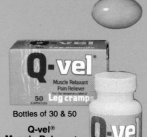

Bottles of 30 & 50

Q-vel®
Muscle Relaxant Pain Reliever

For the temporary relief of night leg cramps

Boehringer Ingelhei

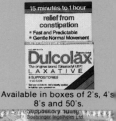

Available in boxes of 2's, 4's 8's and 50's.

10 mg.

Dulcolax® Suppositories
(bisacodyl USP)

AYERST

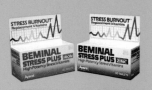

BEMINAL STRESS PLUS™ with Iron **BEMINAL STRESS PLUS™ with Zinc**

Stress Burnout™ replacement vitamins

Bottles of 60

Ayerst

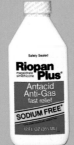

Available in 12 fl oz Suspension, Chew Tablets (60s and 100s), and Rollpacks

RIOPAN PLUS®
(magaldrate and simethicone)
Antacid/Anti-Gas

BLISTEX INC.

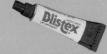

Blistex Lip Ointment For Cold Sores

Also available: .5 oz. tube

BLISTEX® LIP OINTMENT
(camphor and phenol)

Boehringer Ingelheim

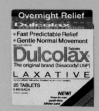

Available in boxes of 25's, 50's, 100's, bottles of 1,000

12   5 mg.

Dulcolax® Tablets
(bisacodyl USP)

Ayerst

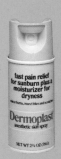

DERMOPLAST®
Topical Anesthetic First Aid Spray
(20% benzocaine and 0.5% menthol)

Ayerst

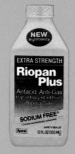

Available in 12 fl oz Suspension

EXTRA STRENGTH RIOPAN PLUS®
(magaldrate and simethicone)

High-Potency Antacid/Anti-Gas

Blistex Inc.

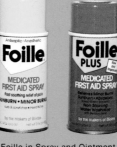

Foille in Spray and Ointment

FOILLE® and FOILLE® PLUS
(benzocaine and chloroxylenol)

Boehringer Ingelheim

Metered One-Way Pump Spra for Nasal Decongestion

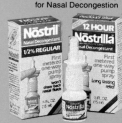

Nostril®
(phenylephrine HCl)

12 Hour Nostrill
(0.05% oxymetazo HCl)

Nostril® available in 0.25% (¼% Mild) and 0.5% (½% Regul Phenylephrine HCl

---

Ayerst

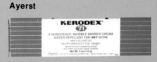

KERODEX® 71 for Wet Work

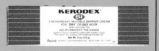

KERODEX® 51 for Dry Work

Barrier Skin Cream
Available in 4 oz tubes and 1 lb jars

BEACH

Front

Back

BEELITH
(magnesium oxide 600 mg; pyridoxine HCl 25 mg)

Blistex Inc.

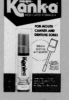

Kank-A For Canker Sores

KANK-A®
(benzocaine, cetylpyridinium chloride, tincture of benzoin)

BORNEMAN

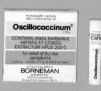

3 tubes per box

OSCILLOCOCCINUM®
Homeopathic remedy for relief flu-like symptoms

BRISTOL-MYERS

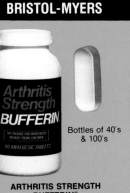
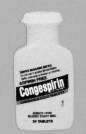
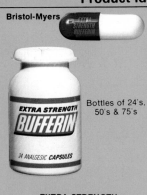
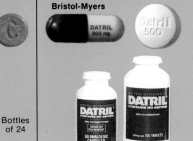

Bottles of 40's & 100's

ARTHRITIS STRENGTH BUFFERIN®
(aspirin)

Bottles of 24's, 50's & 75's

EXTRA STRENGTH BUFFERIN® CAPSULES
(aspirin)

Bottles of 24

ASPIRIN FREE CONGESPIRIN®
(acetaminophen 81 mg., phenylephrine 1.25 mg.)

Bottles of 24 & 50 Capsules   Bottles of 30, 60 & 100 Tablets

EXTRA STRENGTH DATRIL® CAPSULES and TABLETS
(acetaminophen)

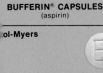
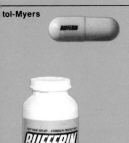
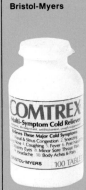
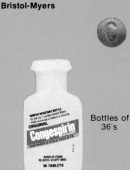
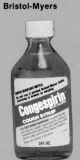
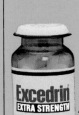

Bottles of 30, 50 & 75

BUFFERIN® CAPSULES
(aspirin)

Bottles of 6 & 10 oz.

COMTREX® LIQUID

Bottles of 36's

CONGESPIRIN® COLD TABLETS

Bottles of 24's, 40's & 60's

EXCEDRIN® CAPSULES
Aspirin/Acetaminophen/Caffeine

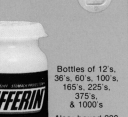

Bottles of 12's, 36's, 60's, 100's, 165's, 225's, 375's, & 1000's

Also: boxed 200 x 2 tablets foil packets

BUFFERIN®
(aspirin)

Bottles of 24's & 50's

COMTREX® TABLETS

3 oz. Bottles

5 mg. per 5 ml teaspoon

CONGESPRIN® COUGH SYRUP
(dextromethorphan, hydrobromide)

Bottles of 12's, 36's, 60's, 100's, 165's, 225's & 375's

EXCEDRIN® TABLETS
Aspirin/Acetaminophen/Caffeine

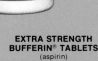
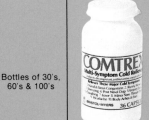
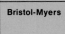
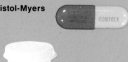
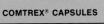
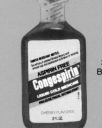
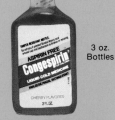
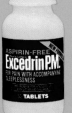

Bottles of 30's, 60's & 100's

EXTRA STRENGTH BUFFERIN® TABLETS
(aspirin)

Bottles of 16's & 36's

COMTREX® CAPSULES

3 oz. Bottles

CONGESPRIN® LIQUID COLD MEDICINE

Bottles of 10's, 30's, 50's & 80's

EXCEDRIN P.M.®

Bristol-Myers

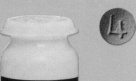

Bottles of 15's, 36's & 60's

4-WAY® COLD TABLETS

Bristol-Myers

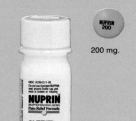

200 mg.

Bottles of 50 and 100

NUPRIN™
(ibuprofen)

Burroughs Wellcome

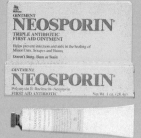

Available in ½ and 1 oz. tubes

NEOSPORIN®
TRIPLE ANTIBIOTIC
FIRST AID OINTMENT

Burroughs Wellcome

10

SUDAFED®
60 mg TABLETS

Bristol-Myers

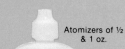

Atomizers of ½ & 1 oz.

4-WAY® NASAL SPRAY

BURROUGHS WELLCOME

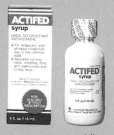

4 fl. oz.

ACTIFED® SYRUP

Burroughs Wellcome

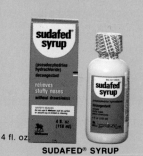

8 fl. oz.   4 fl. oz.

SUDAFED® COUGH SYRUP

Burroughs Wellcome

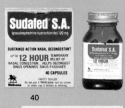

4 fl. oz.   24

48

SUDAFED® PLUS
SYRUP & TABLETS

Bristol-Myers

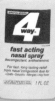

½ oz.
Atomizers

4-WAY® LONG ACTING NASAL
SPRAY
(oxymetazoline hydrochloride 0.05%)

Burroughs Wellcome

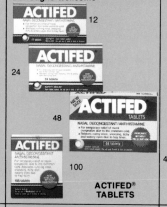

12

24

48

100

ACTIFED®
TABLETS

Burroughs Wellcome

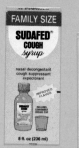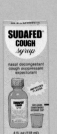

4 fl. oz.

SUDAFED® SYRUP
Decongestant

Also available in pints

Burroughs Wellcome

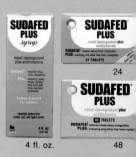

40

1

Sudafed® S.A.

Also available in 100s
SUDAFED® S.A. CAPSULES

Bristol-Myers

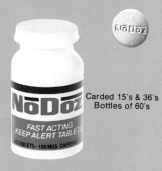

Carded 15's & 36's
Bottles of 60's

NO-DOZ® TABLETS
(caffeine)

Burroughs Wellcome

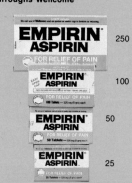

250

100

50

25

EMPIRIN® ASPIRIN TABLETS

Burroughs Wellcome

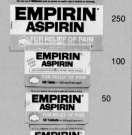

100

48

24

SUDAFED® TABLETS
Decongestant

CARTER PRODUCTS

Division of Carter-Wallace In

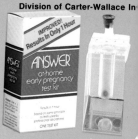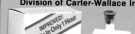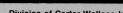

ANSWER®
At-home early pregnancy test k

er Products

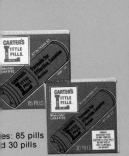

CARTER'S LITTLE PILLS
(5 mg. bisacodyl)

es: 85 pills
d 30 pills

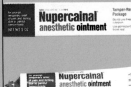

Available in 2 oz and 1 oz tubes

NUPERCAINAL®
Anesthetic Ointment

CIBA

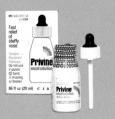

.66 fl oz

PRIVINE®
Nasal Solution

COMBE

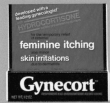

½ oz.

GYNECORT®
Antipruritic 0.5% Hydrocortisone
Acetate Creme

---

ttem Consumer Products

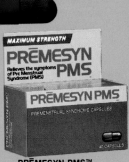

PREMESYN PMS™
menstrual Syndrome Capsules

CIBA

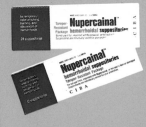

Available in boxes of
12 and 24 suppositories

NUPERCAINAL®
Hemorrhoidal Suppositories

For more detailed information on products illustrated in this section, consult the Product Information Section or manufacturers may be contacted directly.

Combe

Please note: recent packaging
no longer carries word NEW.

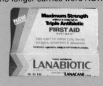

1 oz.

Also available in ½ oz.
LANABIOTIC®
Triple Antibiotic First Aid
Ointment

CIBA CONSUMER

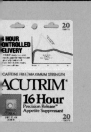

able in packages of 20 & 40 tablets

ACUTRIM™
16 Hour Precision Release™
Appetite Suppressant

CIBA

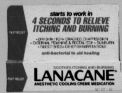
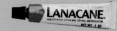

1½ oz

NUPERCAINAL®
Pain-Relief Cream

COLGATE-PALMOLIVE

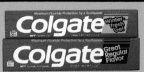

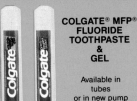

COLGATE® MFP®
FLUORIDE
TOOTHPASTE
&
GEL

Available in
tubes
or in new pump
dispensers

Combe

1 oz.
Also available in 2.0 oz. tube

LANACANE®
Anesthetic Cooling Creme Medication

---

a Consumer

SLOW FE™
Slow Release Iron

Available in packages of
30 & 100 tablets

CIBA

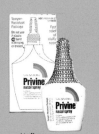

½ fl oz

PRIVINE®
Nasal Spray

Colgate-Palmolive

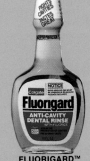

FLUORIGARD™
Anti-Cavity Dental Rinse
With Fluoride

Combe

½ oz. and
1 oz.

LANACORT® CREME

½ oz.

LANACORT® OINTMENT
Anti-Itch Hydrocortisone
Acetate 0.5%

Combe

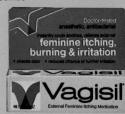

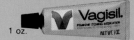

1 oz.

Also available in 2 oz. tube

VAGISIL®
External Feminine Itching Medication

DORSEY

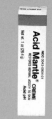

Creme
1 oz, 4 oz, 1 lb

Lotion
4 oz

ACID MANTLE®
CREME AND LOTION
(aluminum acetate)

Dorsey

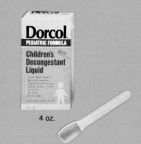

4 oz.

DORCOL™
CHILDRÉN'S DECONGESTANT
LIQUID

Dorsey

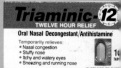

10's, 20's

TRIAMINIC-12® TABLETS
(Sustained Release)

COMMERCE DRUG

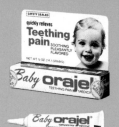

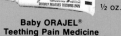

½ oz.

Baby ORAJEL®
Teething Pain Medicine

Benzocaine 7.5% in a
special base

Dorsey

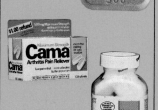

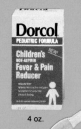

100's and 250's

CAMA®
ARTHRITIS PAIN RELIEVER

Dorsey

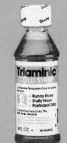

4 oz.

DORCOL™
CHILDREN'S FEVER & PAIN
REDUCER

Dorsey

4 oz, 8 oz

TRIAMINIC®
COLD SYRUP

Commerce Drug

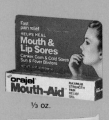

⅓ oz.

⅓ oz.

ORAJEL® Mouth-Aid
Benzocaine 20%, benzalkonium chloride
0.12%, zinc chloride 0.1% in a special
emollient base

Dorsey

4 oz., 8 oz.

DORCOL™
CHILDREN'S COUGH
SYRUP

Dorsey

4 oz.

DORCOL™
CHILDREN'S LIQUID
CALCIUM SUPPLEMENT

Dorsey

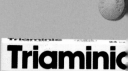

24's and 48's

TRIAMINIC®
COLD TABLETS

Commerce Drug

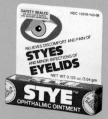

0.125 oz.

STYE™
Ophthalmic Ointment

Yellow mercuric oxide, cod liver oil,
boric acid and zinc sulfate in a
special ophthalmic base

Dorsey

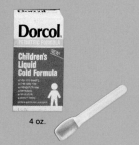

4 oz.

DORCOL™
CHILDREN'S LIQUID
COLD FORMULA

Dorsey

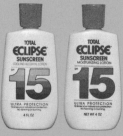

Cooling Alcohol
Lotion
4 oz.

Moisturizing
Lotion
4 oz., 6 oz.

ECLIPSE® SUNCARE PRODUCTS

Dorsey

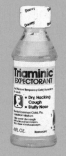

4 oz, 8 oz

TRIAMINIC®
EXPECTORANT

orsey

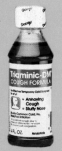

4 oz, 8 oz

**TRIAMINIC-DM®
COUGH FORMULA**

EX-LAX PHARMACEUTICAL

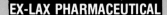
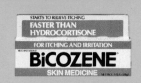
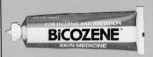

1 oz. (28 g.)

BICOZENE® CREME

Ex-Lax Pharmaceutical

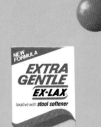

EXTRA GENTLE
EX-LAX
laxative with *stool softener*

For gentle,
more comfortable relief
24 PILLS

EXTRA GENTLE EX-LAX®

Geigy

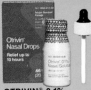

OTRIVIN® 0.1%
Nasal Drops

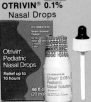

OTRIVIN® 0.05%
Pediatric Nasal Drops

---

orsey

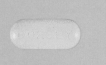

Triaminicin® Tablets

DECONGESTANT
ANALGESIC ANTIHISTAMINIC
For relief of
*Nasal Congestion
and Headache due to
Common Cold/Hay Fever*

24 TABLETS

12's, 24's, 48's, 100's

**TRIAMINICIN®
TABLETS**

Ex-Lax Pharmaceutical

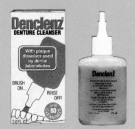

Denclenz®
DENTURE CLEANSER

2 fl. oz. and 3.5 fl. oz.

**DENCLENZ®
Denture Cleanser**

Ex-Lax Pharmaceutical

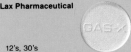

12's, 30's

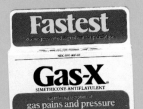

Fastest

Gas-X®
SIMETHICONE ANTIFLATULENT

gas pains and pressure

GAS-X®
(80 mg. simethicone)

Geigy

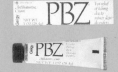

PBZ

PBZ

Cream

PBZ®
(tripelennamine hydrochloride)

---

orsey

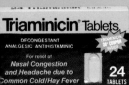

Triaminicol®
MULTI-SYMPTOM COLD SYRUP

4 oz, 8 oz

**TRIAMINICOL®
MULTI-SYMPTOM COLD SYRUP**

Ex-Lax Pharmaceutical

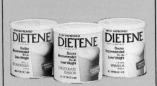

DIETENE **DIETENE** **DIETENE**

16 oz. (1 lb.)
Strawberry, Chocolate and Vanilla

**DIETENE®
Diet Shake Mix**

Ex-Lax Pharmaceutical

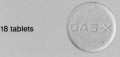

18 tablets

**EXTRA STRENGTH
Gas-X®**
SIMETHICONE-ANTIFLATULENT
STRONGEST, FASTEST
gas pains and pressure

EXTRA-STRENGTH GAS-X®
(125 mg. simethicone)

GLENBROOK

**Division of
Sterling
Drug Inc.**

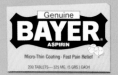

**Genuine
BAYER**
ASPIRIN
Micro-Thin Coating · Fast Pain Relief

Available in packs of 12 tablets
and bottles of 24's, 50's,
100's, 200's and 300's

BAYER® ASPIRIN

---

orsey

Triaminicol®
MULTI-SYMPTOM COLD TABLETS
with Cough Suppressant

For Effective Temporary Cold Symptom Relief of:
• Nasal Congestion • Runny Nose
• Frequent Cough
Due to common cold, flu, bronchial irritation

24 Tablets

24's and 48's

**TRIAMINICOL®
ULTI-SYMPTOM COLD TABLETS**

Ex-Lax Pharmaceutical

Gentle,
dependable
overnight relief
FOR RELIEF OF CONSTIPATION

EX-LAX®
PILLS
30 PILLS · UNFLAVORED

Pill

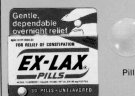

EX-LAX
THE CHOCOLATED LAXATIVE
18 TABLETS

Chocolated
Tablet

EX-LAX®

GEIGY

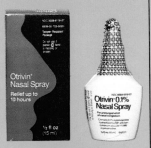

Otrivin®
Nasal Spray
Relief up to
10 hours

½ fl oz
(15 ml)

Otrivin® 0.1%
Nasal Spray

OTRIVIN® 0.1%
Nasal Spray

Glenbrook

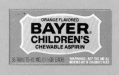

ORANGE FLAVORED
**BAYER®
CHILDREN'S**
CHEWABLE ASPIRIN

Available in bottle
of 36 tablets

**BAYER® CHILDREN'S
CHEWABLE ASPIRIN**

Glenbrook

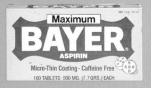

500 mg.
**MAXIMUM
BAYER® ASPIRIN**
Micro-Thin Coating—Caffeine Free

Glenbrook

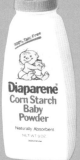

Available in 4 oz., 9 oz.. and
14 oz. containers
DIAPARENE® BABY POWDER

Glenbrook

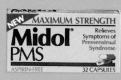

Available in packages of 8, 16, 32 capsules

**MIDOL® PMS
MAXIMUM STRENGTH**

Glenbrook

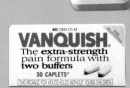

Available in packages
of 30, 60 and 100
**VANQUISH®
Extra-strength pain formula
with two buffers**

Glenbrook

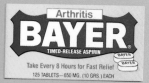

Available in bottles of
30, 72, and 125 tablets
**ARTHRITIS BAYER®
TIMED-RELEASE ASPIRIN**

Glenbrook

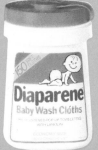

Available in 70
and 150 cloth canisters
**DIAPARENE®
BABY WASH CLOTHS**

Glenbrook

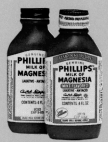

Available in regular and mint
flavor 4 oz., 12 oz. and 26 oz.
PHILLIPS'® MILK OF MAGNESIA

6 Powders

HEADACHE POWDERS

Glenbrook

325   650

COSPRIN
325
COSPRIN
650

**COSPRIN®
Enteric Release Aspirin**

Glenbrook

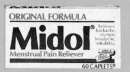

Available in packages of 12, 30
and 60 Caplets®

MIDOL®

Glenbrook

Liquid

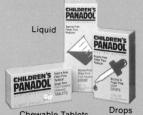

Chewable Tablets   Drops

**CHILDREN'S PANADOL®
Chewable Tablets, Liquid
and Drops**
Acetaminophen

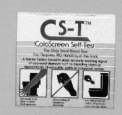

**CS-T™
ColoScreen Self-Test**
Stool Blood Test

Glenbrook

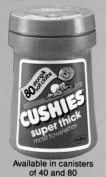

Available in canisters
of 40 and 80
**CUSHIES®
Moist Towelettes**

Glenbrook

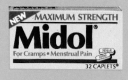

Available in packages of 8, 16, 32 caplets

**MIDOL®
MAXIMUM STRENGTH**

Glenbrook

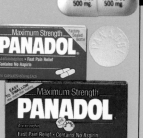

**MAXIMUM STRENGTH
PANADOL**
Capsules and Coated Tablets
Acetaminophen

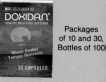

Packages
of 10 and 30,
Bottles of 100

Laxative and Stool Softener

DOXIDAN®
(docusate calcium USP and
danthron USP)

chst-Roussel

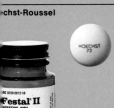

Bottles
of 100
Tablets

Digestive Aid

FESTAL® II
(digestive enzymes)

JOHNSON & JOHNSON

Baby Products Company

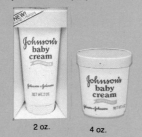

2 oz.   4 oz.

**JOHNSON'S
BABY CREAM**

Johnson & Johnson

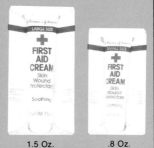

1.5 Oz.   .8 Oz.

**FIRST AID CREAM
Skin Wound Protectant**

Lederle

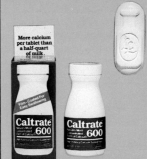

**CALTRATE™ 600
High Potency Calcium
Supplement**

---

chst-Roussel

50 mg
Packages of
30 and 100

240 mg.
Packages of
7 and 30,
Bottles of 100

Stool Softener

Surfak®
(docusate calcium USP)

Baby Products Company

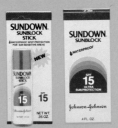

Also available: Also available:
SPF 8   SPF 4, 6 and 8

**SUNDOWN® SUNBLOCK
Lotion and Stick**

Johnson & Johnson

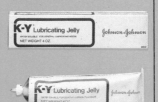

K-Y™ LUBRICATING JELLY
Water Soluble, for General
Lubricating Needs

Lederle

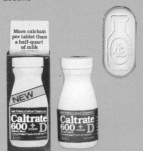

**CALTRATE™ 600+D
High Potency Calcium
Supplement**

---

son, Westcott & Dunning

duct must be refrigerated

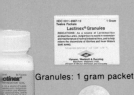

Granules: 1 gram packet

ets: bottles of 50

**LACTINEX®
Tablets & Granules**
(Lactobacillus acidophilus and
Lactobacillus bulgaricus)

JOHNSON & JOHNSON

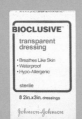

2 in. × 3 in. dressings
**BIOCLUSIVE™
TRANSPARENT DRESSING**
• Breathes Like Skin • Waterproof
• Hypo-Allergenic

LACTAID

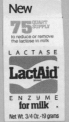

4 qt. size, 12 qt. size,
30 qt. size, 75 qt. size
LactAid®
(lactase enzyme)

Lederle

C1

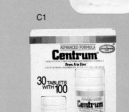

**Advanced Formula
CENTRUM®
High Potency Multivitamin/
Multimineral Formula**

For more detailed in-
formation on products
illustrated in this sec-
tion, consult the Prod-
uct Information Sec-
tion or manufacturers
may be contacted di-
rectly.

Johnson & Johnson

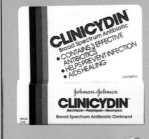

**CLINICYDIN™
Broad Spectrum Antibiotic Ointment**

LEDERLE

**LEDERMARK™
Product Identification
Code**

Many Lederle tablets and capsules
bear an identification code, and
these codes are listed with each
product pictured. A current listing
appears in the Product Information
Section of the 1985 Physicians' Desk
Reference.

Lederle

60 tablets

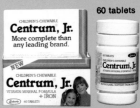

**CENTRUM®, JR.
Children's Chewable
Vitamin/Mineral Formula + Iron
More Essential Nutrients**

Lederle

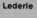

60 tablets

CENTRUM, JR.®
Children's Chewable
Vitamin/Mineral Formula+Extra C

Lederle

S22

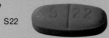

Bottles of 60

SPARTUS®
High Potency Vitamins
& Minerals plus
Electrolytes

Lederle

S3

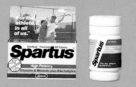

Bottles of 30 & 60

**Advanced Formula
STRESSTABS® 600
with ZINC**
High Potency Stress Formula
Vitamins

MARION

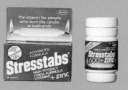
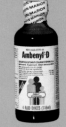

4 fl. oz.

AMBENYL®-D
Decongestant Cough Formula

Lederle

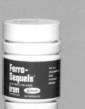

Bottles of 30, 100 and 1000

FERRO-SEQUELS®
Sustained Release Iron Capsules

Lederle

S23

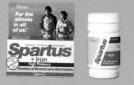

Bottles of 60

SPARTUS®
High Potency Vitamins
& Minerals plus
Electrolytes + Iron
Tablets

Lederle

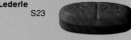
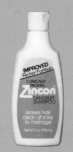

4 fl oz (118 ml)

ZINCON® Dandruff Shampoo

Marion

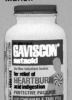
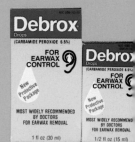

1 fl. oz.   ½ fl. oz.

DEBROX®
Drops

Lederle

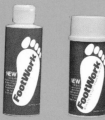

Powder   Spray Powder

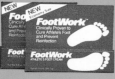
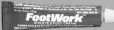

Cream: 0.5 oz. and 1.0 oz.

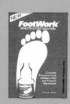

Solution
FOOTWORK™
Athlete's Foot Remedy

Lederle

S1

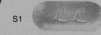
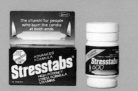

Bottles of 30, 60
& 500

**Advanced Formula
STRESSTABS® 600**
High Potency Stress Formula
Vitamins

LEMAR

Medicated
Chewing
Gum

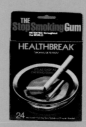

HEALTHBREAK™
Smoking Deterrent

Marion

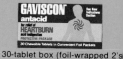

100-tablet
bottle

30-tablet box (foil-wrapped 2's)
GAVISCON®
Antacid Tablets

Lederle

S2

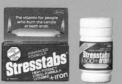

Bottles of 30 & 60

**Advanced Formula
STRESSTABS® 600
with IRON**
High Potency Stress Formula
Vitamins

3M/PERSONAL CARE

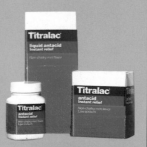

**TITRALAC®
ANTACID
TABLETS and LIQUID**

Marion

Available
6- and 12-
oz. bottle

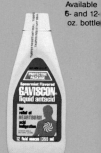

12 fl. oz.

GAVISCON®
Liquid Antacid

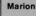
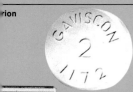

Box of 48
foil-wrapped
tablets

**GAVISCON®-2
Antacid Tablets**

Marion

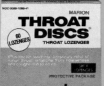

Box of 60 lozenges

**THROAT DISCS®
Throat Lozenges**

½ fl. oz.

Available in 2- and ½-fl.-oz. bottles

GLY-OXIDE® Liquid

MARLYN

Boxes of
60 Paks,
135 Paks

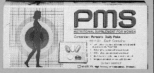

**MARLYN PMS™
Nutritional Supplement For
Women**

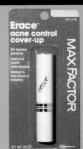

Bottles
of 100
and 240
tablets

**OS-CAL® 250
Tablets**
(calcium with vitamin D)

MAX FACTOR & CO.

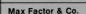

Erace® Acne
Control in 4
skin tones:
- Soft Natural
- Medium Tone
- Fair Tone
- Truly Tan

Dries and
clears acne
pimples

ERACE® ACNE CONTROL COVER-UP
5% Benzoyl Peroxide
Shaded to help blend in naturally

Marion

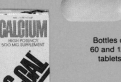

Bottles of
60 and 120
tablets

**OS-CAL® 500
Tablets**

Max Factor & Co.

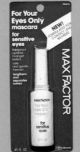

Shades:
Velvet Black
Black
Black/Brown

Formulated
for contact
lens wearers.

.45 fl. oz.

FOR YOUR EYES ONLY™ Mascara
For sensitive eyes, flakeproof,
ophthalmologist tested, safe and
gentle formula

Max Factor & Co.

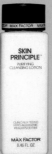

Purifying
Cleansing
Lotion

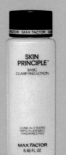

Basic Clarifying Lotion

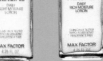

Daily Light
Moisture Lotion

Daily Rich
Moisture Lotion

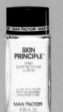

Serious
Moisture
Supplement

SKIN PRINCIPLE™ PRODUCTS
Hypo-Allergenic Fragrance Free
Collagen Enriched

McNEIL CONSUMER

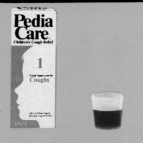

Available in 4 fl. oz. bottle with
child-resistant safety cap and convenient
dosage cup.
**PEDIACARE™ 1
Children's Cough Relief**

McNeil Consumer

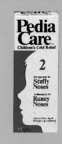

Available in 4 fl. oz. bottle with
child-resistant safety cap and convenient
dosage cup.
**PEDIACARE™ 2
Children's Cold Relief**

McNeil Consumer

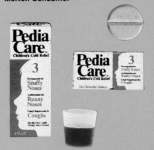

Available in 4 fl. oz. bottle with convenient
dosage cup and in bottles of 24 tablets,
both with child-resistant safety cap.
**PEDIACARE™ 3
Children's Cold Relief**

McNeil Consumer

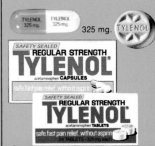

325 mg.

Capsules available in tamper-resistant
bottles of 24, 50 and 100. Tablets available in tamper-resistant tins and vials
of 12 and bottles of 24, 50, 100 and 200.
REGULAR STRENGTH TYLENOL®
acetaminophen Capsules & Tablets

McNeil Consumer

500 mg.

Capsules: tamper-resistant vials of 8 and
bottles of 24, 50, 100 and 165. Tablets
available in tamper-resistant vials
of 10 and bottles of 30, 60, 100 and 200.
Liquid: 8 fl. oz.
EXTRA-STRENGTH TYLENOL®
acetaminophen
Capsules, Tablets & Liquid

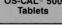
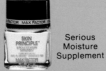

McNeil Consumer

500 mg.

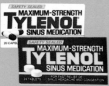

Caplets: tamper-resistant bottles of
24, 50 and 100.

EXTRA-STRENGTH TYLENOL®
acetaminophen Caplets

McNeil Consumer

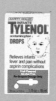

Available in ½ fl. oz. bottle with
child-resistant safety cap and
calibrated dropper.

INFANTS' TYLENOL®
acetaminophen
Alcohol Free Drops

McNeil Consumer

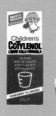

Available in bottles of 24 tablets
with child-resistant safety cap.

CHILDREN'S COTYLENOL®
Chewable Cold Tablets

Mead Johnson Nutritional Division

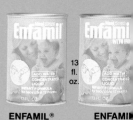

ENFAMIL®   **ENFAMIL®**
               With Iron

Infant Formula for
Baby's First Twelve Months

McNeil Consumer

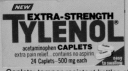

**MAXIMUM-STRENGTH
TYLENOL®
SINUS MEDICATION**

Capsules: bottles of 20 & 40
Tablets: bottles of 24 & 50

McNeil Consumer

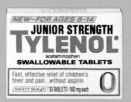

Available in
child-resistant blister-pack of 30
JUNIOR STRENGTH TYLENOL®
acetaminophen
Swallowable Tablets

McNeil Consumer

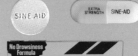

Available in 5 fl. oz. bottle with
child-resistant safety cap and convenient
dosage cup enclosed.

CHILDREN'S COTYLENOL®
Liquid Cold Formula

Mead Johnson Nutritional Division

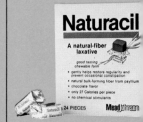

NATURACIL®
A natural-fiber laxative

McNeil Consumer

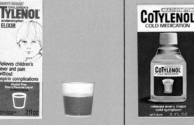

Available in bottles of 30 with
child-resistant safety cap.

CHILDREN'S TYLENOL®
acetaminophen
Chewable Tablets

McNeil Consumer

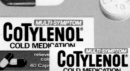

Capsules available in blister-pack of
20 and bottle of 40.
Tablets available in blister-
pack of 24 and bottles of 50 and 100.

**COTYLENOL®
COLD MEDICATION**
Tablets and Capsules

McNeil Consumer

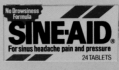

SINE-AID®

**EXTRA STRENGTH
SINE-AID®**
For sinus headache pain and pressure

Mead Johnson Nutritional Division

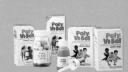

**POLY-VI-SOL®
CHEWABLE VITAMINS**
with and without iron and zinc

**POL-VI-SOL®
VITAMIN DROPS**
with and without iron

McNeil Consumer

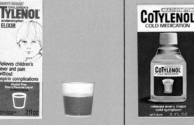

Available in 2 & 4 fl. oz. bottles
with child-resistant safety cap and
convenient dosage cup.

CHILDREN'S TYLENOL®
acetaminophen
Alcohol Free Elixir

McNeil Consumer

Available in 5 fl. oz. bottle with
child-resistant safety cap and convenient
dosage cup enclosed.

**COTYLENOL®
LIQUID COLD MEDICATION**

MEAD JOHNSON NUTRIT.

CE-VI-SOL® VITAMIN C DROPS

Mead Johnson Nutritional Division

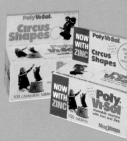

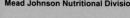

**POLY-VI-SOL® CIRCUS SHAPES
CHEWABLE VITAMINS**
with and without iron and zinc

...ad Johnson Nutritional Division

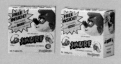

**SMURF™
CHEWABLE VITAMINS**
with and without iron and zinc

MEAD JOHNSON PHARM.

NDC 0087-0713-02
CAPSULES
COLACE®
DOCUSATE SODIUM
STOOL SOFTENER
Store below 86°F/30°C.
Protect from freezing.
60 CAPSULES
Mead Johnson

50 mg

100 mg

Bottles of 30, 60, 250 and 1000
Stool Softener
COLACE®
(docusate sodium)

Menley & James

**BENZEDREX®
INHALER**
for stuffed-up noses

BENZEDREX®
INHALER
nasal decongestant

BENZEDREX® INHALER
(propylhexedrine, SK&F)

Menley & James

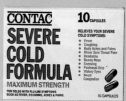

CONTAC SEVERE COLD FORMULA
MAXIMUM STRENGTH
10 CAPSULES
RELIEVES YOUR SEVERE COLD SYMPTOMS:
• Fever
• Coughing
• Body Aches and Pains
• Minor Sore Throat Pain
• Headache
• Runny Nose
• Sneezing
• Postnasal Drip
• Watery Eyes
• Nasal Congestion
FOR COLDS WITH FLU-LIKE SYMPTOMS
SUCH AS FEVER, COUGHING, ACHES & PAINS.

Packages of 10 and 20 capsules
**CONTAC®
SEVERE COLD FORMULA**

...ad Johnson Nutritional Division

ISOCAL®
COMPLETE LIQUID DIET
READY TO USE

SUSTACAL®
READY TO USE

ISOCAL®   **SUSTACAL®**
Ready To Use

Nutritionally Complete Food

**Mead Johnson
Pharmaceutical Division**

NDC 0087-0715-02
CAPSULES
PERI-COLACE®
CASANTHRANOL and DOCUSATE SODIUM
**LAXATIVE PLUS
STOOL SOFTENER**
A GENTLE, PREDICTABLE LAXATIVE
60 CAPSULES
Mead Johnson

Bottles of 30, 60, 250 and 1000
Laxative and Stool Softener
PERI-COLACE®
(casanthranol and docusate sodium)

Menley & James

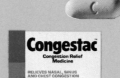

Congestac
Congestion Relief Medicine
RELIEVES NASAL, SINUS AND CHEST CONGESTION
HELPS YOU BREATHE EASIER
NO ANTIHISTAMINE DROWSINESS
12 TABLETS

Packages of 12 and 24 tablets
Bottles of 50 tablets
CONGESTAC™
Congestion Relief Medicine
Decongestant/Expectorant

Menley & James

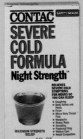

**CONTAC SEVERE COLD FORMULA
Night Strength™**
RELIEVES SEVERE COLD SYMPTOMS FOR HOURS SO YOU CAN SLEEP
• Coughing
• Body Aches and Pain
• Fever
• Headache
• Runny Nose
• Sneezing
• Postnasal Drip
• Watery Eyes
• Nasal Congestion
MAXIMUM STRENGTH RELIEF
5 FL. OZ.

Measured dose cup

**CONTAC®
SEVERE COLD FORMULA
NIGHT STRENGTH**

...ad Johnson Nutritional Division

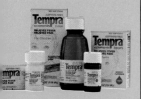

Tempra
RELIEVES FEVER RELIEVES PAIN

**Aspirin-free
TEMPRA®**
Acetaminophen for children

MENLEY & JAMES

ACNOMEL®
acne cream
NET WT. 1 OZ. (28 GRAMS)

ACNOMEL® ACNE CREAM
(resorcinol, sulfate, alcohol)

Menley & James

Packages of 10, 20, 30 and 40 capsules

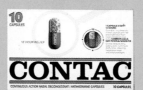

10 CAPSULES
12 HOUR RELIEF
CONTAC
CONTINUOUS ACTION NASAL DECONGESTANT / ANTIHISTAMINE CAPSULES   10 CAPSULES

**CONTAC®
CONTINUOUS ACTION
DECONGESTANT CAPSULES**

Menley & James

Complete Cold Medicine for Children
CONTAC Jr.
• Gentle decongestant
• Safe cough quieter
• Pain and fever reducer
• Non-narcotic
ASPIRIN-FREE
4 FL. OZ.

Includes dose-by-weight cup

**CONTAC JR.®
COLD MEDICINE FOR CHILDREN**

...ad Johnson Nutritional Division

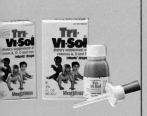

Tri-Vi-Sol
dietary supplement of vitamins A, D, C and iron
infants' drops
Mead Johnson

**TRI-VI-SOL®
VITAMIN DROPS**
with and without iron

Menley & James

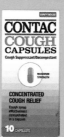

NEW FORMULA
**A.R.M.
ALLERGY RELIEF MEDICINE**
MAXIMUM STRENGTH
HAY FEVER / ALLERGY / SINUS CONGESTION
20 TABLETS

Packages of 20 and 40 tablets
A.R.M.® ALLERGY RELIEF MEDICINE
(chlorpheniramine maleate, phenylpropanolamine HCl)

Menley & James

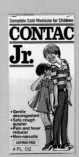

**CONTAC
COUGH CAPSULES**
Cough Suppressant/Decongestant
MAXIMUM STRENGTH
CONCENTRATED COUGH RELIEF
Cough syrup effectiveness concentrated in a capsule
10 CAPSULES

Packages of 10 and 20 capsules
**CONTAC®
COUGH CAPSULES**

Menley & James

Packages of 20 and 40 capsules

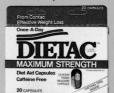

From Contac
Effective Weight Loss
Once-A-Day
DIETAC
MAXIMUM STRENGTH
Diet Aid Capsules
Caffeine Free
12 HOUR TIMED RELEASE CAPSULE
20 CAPSULES

**Once-A-Day
DIETAC™ MAXIMUM STRENGTH**
Diet Aid Capsules

Menley & James

- RELIEVES PAIN AND INFLAMMATION
- PROTECTS AGAINST STOMACH UPSET
- EASY TO SWALLOW

Ecotrin
SAFETY-COATED ASPIRIN
for arthritis pain
100 TABLETS 325 MG (5 GR.) EACH

In 36, 100, 250 and 1000
tablet bottles

ECOTRIN® TABLETS
Duentric® coated 5 gr. aspirin

Menley & James

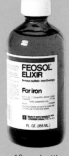

**FEOSOL
ELIXIR**
ferrous sulfate—iron therapy

For iron

FL. OZ. (355 ML.)

16 oz. bottle
FEOSOL® ELIXIR
(ferrous sulfate USP)

Menley & James

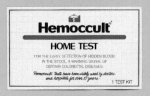

Hemoccult®
HOME TEST
FOR THE EARLY DETECTION OF HIDDEN BLOOD
IN THE STOOL, A WARNING SIGNAL OF
CERTAIN COLORECTAL DISEASES.

Hemoccult Tests have been widely used by doctors
and hospitals for over 10 years.

1 TEST KIT

HEMOCCULT® HOME TEST
For the early detection of hidden blood
in the stool, a warning signal of certain
colorectal diseases.

Menley & James

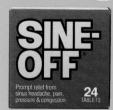

SINE-OFF
Prompt relief from
sinus headache, pain,
pressure & congestion
24
TABLETS

Packages of 24,
48, and 100 tablets

SINE-OFF® REGULAR STRENG
ASPIRIN FORMULA

Menley & James

**MAXIMUM
STRENGTH
Ecotrin**
SAFETY-COATED ASPIRIN
60 TABLETS 500 MG EACH
for arthritis pain

In 24, 60 and 150
tablet bottles

**MAXIMUM STRENGTH
ECOTRIN® TABLETS**
Duentric® coated 7.69 gr. aspirin

Menley & James

Feosol
SPANSULE® CAPSULES
ferrous sulfate—iron therapy

For iron
Controlled-release formula for simple
iron deficiency and iron deficiency anemia
30 CAPSULES

In 30 capsule package and
100 and 500 capsule bottles

FEOSOL® CAPSULES
(ferrous sulfate USP)

Menley & James

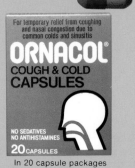

For temporary relief from coughing
and nasal congestion due to
common colds and sinusitis

ORNACOL®
COUGH & COLD
CAPSULES

NO SEDATIVES
NO ANTIHISTAMINES
20 CAPSULES

In 20 capsule packages

**ORNACOL® COUGH & COLD
CAPSULES**

Menley & James

20 tablet
package

SINE-OFF

EXTRA STRENGTH
ASPIRIN-FREE PAIN RELIEVER
Prompt relief from
sinus headache, pain,
pressure & congestion
20
TABLETS

**SINE-OFF®
EXTRA STRENGTH
NON-ASPIRIN TABLETS**

Menley & James

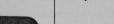

**REGULAR
STRENGTH
Ecotrin** NEW!
SAFETY-COATED ASPIRIN
70 CAPSULES 325 MG
for arthritis pain

In 70 and 140 capsule bottles

ECOTRIN® CAPSULES
Safety-coated aspirin encapsulated
Duentric® 5 gr. aspirin

Menley & James

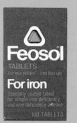

In 100 and 1,000 tablet bottles

Feosol
TABLETS
ferrous sulfate—iron therapy

For iron
Specially coated tablet
for simple iron deficiency
and iron-deficiency anemia
100 TABLETS

FEOSOL® CAPSULES
(ferrous sulfate USP)

Menley & James

ORNEX®
DECONGESTANT/ANALGESIC
For temporary relief of nasal
congestion, headache, aches,
pains and fever due to
**COLDS ·
SINUSITIS
& FLU**
NO
ANTIHISTAMINE
DROWSINESS
24 CAPSULES

In 24, 48 and 100
capsule packages

ORNEX® CAPSULES
Decongestant/Analgesic

Menley & James

20 capsule
package

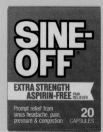

SINE-OFF

EXTRA STRENGTH
ASPIRIN-FREE PAIN RELIEVER
Prompt relief from
sinus headache, pain,
pressure & congestion
20
CAPSULES

**SINE-OFF®
EXTRA STRENGTH
NON-ASPIRIN CAPSULES**

Menley & James

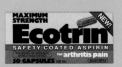

**MAXIMUM
STRENGTH
Ecotrin** NEW!
SAFETY-COATED ASPIRIN
50 CAPSULES 500 MG
for arthritis pain

In 50 and 100 capsule bottles

**MAXIMUM STRENGTH
ECOTRIN® CAPSULES**
Safety-coated aspirin encapsulated
Duentric® 7.7 gr. aspirin

Menley & James

Feosol Plus
iron plus vitamins
For simple iron and iron-
deficiency
anemia
100 CAPSULES

FEOSOL PLUS®
Iron Plus Vitamins

Menley & James

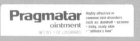

Pragmatar®
ointment
slightly effective in
common skin disorders
such as: dandruff • eczema
• itchy, scaly skin
• "athlete's foot"
NET WT 1 OZ (28 GRAMS)

Dermatologic Ointment

1 oz. tube
PRAGMATAR® OINTMENT

Menley & James

20 capsule
package

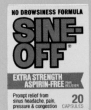

NO DROWSINESS FORMULA
SINE-OFF

EXTRA STRENGTH
ASPIRIN-FREE PAIN RELIEVER
Prompt relief from
sinus headache, pain,
pressure & congestion
20
CAPSULES

**SINE-OFF®
EXTRA STRENGTH NO DROWS**
CAPSULES

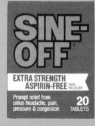

Menley & James

In packages of 12;
bottles of 50

8 mg.

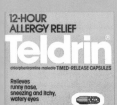

12-HOUR ALLERGY RELIEF
Teldrin®
chlorpheniramine maleate TIMED-RELEASE CAPSULES

Relieves
runny nose,
sneezing and itchy,
watery eyes

12 CAPSULES   8 mg.

**TELDRIN®
TIMED-RELEASE CAPSULES**
(chlorpheniramine maleate)

Menley & James

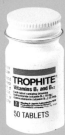

TROPHITE
Vitamins B₁ and B₁₂

50 TABLETS

4 oz. liquid and
50 tablet bottle

**TROPHITE® LIQUID AND
TABLETS**
Vitamins B1, B12

Miles Laboratories, Inc.

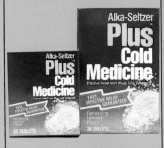

**ALKA-SELTZER PLUS®
COLD MEDICINE**

Miles Laboratories, Inc.

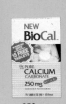

250 mg

chewable

500 mg

**BIOCAL™
CALCIUM SUPPLEMENT**
(Calcium Carbonate)

Menley & James

In 12 and 24
packages; in
bottles of 50

12 mg.

12-HOUR ALLERGY RELIEF
Teldrin®
chlorpheniramine maleate TIMED-RELEASE CAPSULES

Relieves
runny nose,
sneezing and itchy,
watery eyes

MAXIMUM
STRENGTH

12 CAPSULES   12 mg.

**TELDRIN®
TIMED-RELEASE CAPSULES**
(chlorpheniramine maleate)

MERRICK

**PERCY
MEDICINE**

PERCY MEDICINE®
(bismuth subnitrate NF & calcium
hydroxide USP)

Miles Laboratories, Inc.

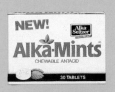

**NEW!
Alka-Mints**
CHEWABLE ANTACID

30 TABLETS

**ALKA-MINTS® Chewable
Antacid**
(Calcium Carbonate 850 mg)

Miles Laboratories, Inc.

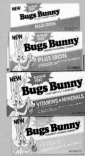

**BUGS® BUNNY BRAND SUGAR FREE
CHILDREN'S CHEWABLE VITAMINS
WITH EXTRA C, REGULAR,
AND PLUS IRON**

Menley & James

Packages of 20 and 40
capsules

**Teldrin
MULTI-SYMPTOM
ALLERGY
RELIEVER**

20 CAPSULES

**TELDRIN®
MULTI-SYMPTOM ALLERGY
RELIEVER CAPSULES**

MILES

**ORIGINAL
Alka-Seltzer®
BRAND
FAST RELIEF**

**EFFERVESCENT
ANTACID &
PAIN RELIEVER**

**ALKA-SELTZER® BRAND
EFFERVESCENT
PAIN RELIEVER & ANTACID**

Miles Laboratories, Inc.

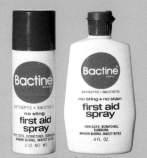

Bactine
ANTISEPTIC · ANESTHETIC
no sting · no stain
first aid
spray

**BACTINE® BRAND
ANTISEPTIC · ANESTHETIC
FIRST AID SPRAY**
Aerosol and Liquid

Miles Laboratories, Inc.

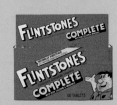

FLINTSTONES COMPLETE

**FLINTSTONES® COMPLETE
CHILDREN'S CHEWABLE VITAMINS**
Complete with Iron, Calcium & Minerals

Menley & James

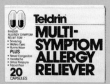

TROPH-IRON
Vitamins B₁, B₁₂ and Iron

4 oz. liquid

TROPH-IRON®
Vitamins B1, B12 and Iron

Miles Laboratories, Inc.

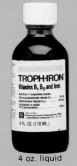

**Alka-Seltzer®
BRAND
Special Antacid Formula**

**For ACID INDIGESTION
HEARTBURN · SOUR STOMACH**
36 TABLETS IN 18 FOIL PACKS

**ALKA-SELTZER® BRAND
EFFERVESCENT ANTACID**

Miles Laboratories, Inc.

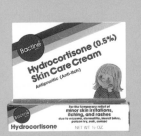

**Hydrocortisone (0.5%)
Skin Care Cream**
Antipruritic (Anti-itch)

**BACTINE® BRAND
HYDROCORTISONE (0.5%)
SKIN CARE CREAM**

Miles Laboratories, Inc.

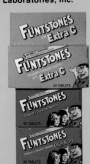

**FLINTSTONES
Extra C**

**FLINTSTONES® BRAND
CHILDREN'S CHEWABLE VITAMINS
WITH EXTRA C, REGULAR,
AND PLUS IRON**

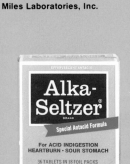
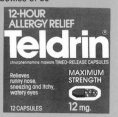

Miles Laboratories, Inc.

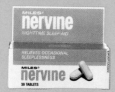

MILES® NERVINE
NIGHTTIME SLEEP-AID
(Diphenhydramine HCl 25 mg)

Miles Laboratories, Inc.

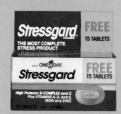

STRESSGARD®
STRESS FORMULA VITAMINS

Norcliff Thayer

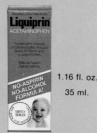

1.16 fl. oz.
35 ml.

LIQUIPRIN®

Norcliff Thayer

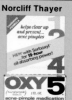

1 fl. oz.
OXY-5® LOTION

1 fl. oz.
OXY-10® LOT

OXY 10® COVER
LOTION

Miles Laboratories, Inc.

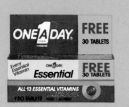

ONE A DAY® BRAND VITAMINS

Miles Laboratories, Inc.

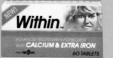

ONE-A-DAY® WITHIN™
Advanced Multivitamin
For Women With Calcium &
Extra Iron

Norcliff Thayer

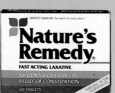

60 tablets

NATURE'S REMEDY®

Also available:
Box 12s and 30s

Norcliff Thayer

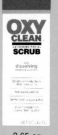

2.65 oz.

OXY CLEAN™
SCRUB
Lathering
Facial Scrub

4 fl. oz.

OXY 10® WAS

Miles Laboratories, Inc.

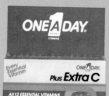

ONE A DAY™ PLUS EXTRA C
BRAND VITAMINS

All 13 essential vitamins
With high potency
500 mg Vitamin C

NATREN

Refer to page 616 for description of
Natren's BIFIDO FACTOR (not shown).

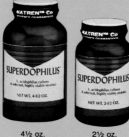

4½ oz.   2½ oz.

SUPERDOPHILUS™
L. acidophilus culture

Norcliff Thayer

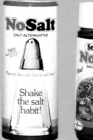

11 oz.   8 oz.

NOSALT™   **SEASONED**
Salt Alternative   **NOSALT™**
     Salt Alternative

Norcliff Thayer

Bottle 75s,
Peppermint

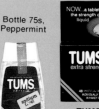

Carton 4

NOW...a tablet with
the strength of a
liquid

TUMS. E-X
extra strength antac

TUMS®

TUMS E-X™
Also availab
in blister-pac
of 12s

Also available: Tums Single Roll
Three Roll Wrap, Peppermint
Assorted Flavors; Tums Bottle
Assorted Flavors; Tums Bottle 1
Peppermint and Assorted Flavors.

Miles Laboratories, Inc.

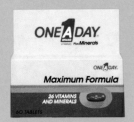

ONE A DAY® BRAND
MAXIMUM FORMULA
THE MOST COMPLETE
LEADING BRAND

NORCLIFF THAYER

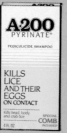

A.200
PYRINATE®
PEDICULICIDE SHAMPOO

KILLS
LICE
AND THEIR
EGGS
ON CONTACT

4 fl. oz.

A-200 PYRINATE® LIQUID

Also available:
A-200 Pyrinate Liquid, 2 fl. oz.
A-200 Pyrinate Gel, 1 oz.

Norcliff Thayer

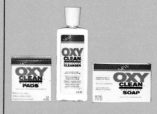

Medicated   Medicated   Medicated
Pads   Cleanser   Soap
50 pads   4 fl. oz.   3.25 oz.

OXY CLEAN™

NOXELL

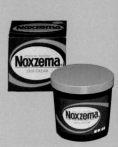

NOXZEMA®
Greaseless   Medicated
Skin Cream

NUTRITIONAL SPECIALTY

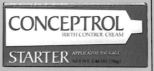

GERIAVIT PHARMATON®

Multivitamin and mineral food supplement +Ginseng Extract-G115®

FOREST

formerly O'Neal, Jones & Feldman

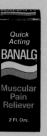

Quick Acting BANALG Muscular Pain Reliever 2 Fl. Ozs.

Banalg Hospital Strength Arthritic Pain Reliever 2 Fl. Ozs.

BANALG®
Analgesic Lotions

OPTIMOX, INC.

OPTIVITE for Women
Multivitamin & Multimineral Supplement

OPTIVITE for Women

ORTHO—

Ortho—Advanced Care Prods.

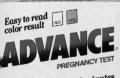

Easy to read color result
Accurate results in 30 minutes
ONE TEST

Accurate results in 30 minutes
ADVANCE®
Pregnancy Test

Ortho—Advanced Care Prods.

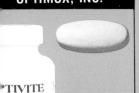

Applicator Package (2.46 oz. tube w/applicator package)

CONCEPTROL® Birth Control Cream
(nonoxynol 9, 5%)

Ortho—Advanced Care Prods.

CONCEPTROL Contraceptive Gel
APPLICATOR PACKAGE
NET WT. 2.46 OZ. (70g)
UNSCENTED GEL

Applicator Package (2.46 oz. tube w/applicator package)

CONCEPTROL® Contraceptive Gel
(nonoxynol 9, 4%)

Ortho—Advanced Care Prods.

CONCEPTROL DISPOSABLE Contraceptive Gel Prefilled Applicators
UNSCENTED GEL
10 APPLICATORS 0.09 OZ. EACH

6's (6 disposable prefilled applicators)
10's (10 disposable prefilled applicators)

CONCEPTROL® Disposable Contraceptive Gel
(nonoxynol 9, 4%)

Ortho—Advanced Care Prods.

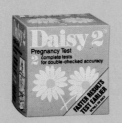

Daisy 2 Pregnancy Test
complete tests for double-checked accuracy
FASTER RESULTS TEST EARLIER

Two complete tests in each kit.

DAISY 2®
Pregnancy Test Kit

Ortho—Advanced Care Prods.

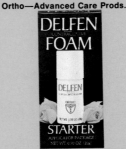

DELFEN FOAM
STARTER APPLICATOR PACKAGE
NET WT. 0.70 OZ. (20g)

Starter (0.70 oz. vial w/applicator package)
Refill (0.70 oz. and 1.75 oz. vial only packages)

DELFEN® Contraceptive Foam
(nonoxynol 9, 12.5%)

Ortho—Advanced Care Prods.

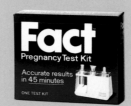

Dimensyn
Maximum Strength Menstrual Discomfort Relief
• Relieves irritability and nervous tension
• pain of cramps
• swelling

24 and 48 capsules

DIMENSYN™
Maximum Strength Menstrual Discomfort Relief
(acetaminophen 500mg., pamabrom 25mg., pyrilamine maleate 15mg.)

Ortho—Advanced Care Prods.

Fact
Pregnancy Test Kit
Accurate results in 45 minutes
ONE TEST KIT

Accurate results in 45 minutes

FACT™
Pregnancy Test Kit

Ortho—Advanced Care Prods.

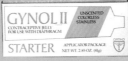

GYNOL II CONTRACEPTIVE JELLY FOR USE WITH DIAPHRAGM
UNSCENTED COLORLESS STAINLESS
STARTER APPLICATOR PACKAGE
NET WT. 2.85 OZ. (81g)

Gynol II is intended for use with a diaphragm

Starter (2.85 oz. tube with applicator package)
Refill (2.85 oz. and 4.44 oz. tube only packages)

GYNOL II®
Contraceptive Jelly
(nonoxynol 9, 2%)

Ortho—Advanced Care Prods.

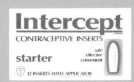

Intercept
CONTRACEPTIVE INSERTS
starter
safe effective convenient
12 INSERTS WITH APPLICATOR

Starter (12 inserts w/applicator package)
Refill (12 inserts)

INTERCEPT®
Contraceptive Inserts
(nonoxynol 9, 5.56%)

Ortho—Advanced Care Prods.

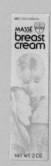

MASSE breast cream
NET WT. 2 OZ

2 oz. tube
MASSÉ® Breast Cream

Ortho—Advanced Care Prods.

Micatin ANTIFUNGAL SPRAY LIQUID CURES ATHLETE'S FOOT
Micatin ANTIFUNGAL CREAM CURES ATHLETE'S FOOT
Micatin ANTIFUNGAL POWDER CURES ATHLETE'S FOOT

Spray Liquid (3.5 oz.)
Cream (½ oz. and 1 oz.)
Powder (1.5 oz.)

Also Spray Powder (3.0 oz.)

MICATIN® Antifungal
For Athlete's Foot

Ortho—Advanced Care Prods.

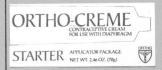

ORTHO-CREME CONTRACEPTIVE CREAM FOR USE WITH DIAPHRAGM
STARTER APPLICATOR PACKAGE
NET WT. 2.46 OZ. (70g)

Ortho-Creme is intended for use with a diaphragm

Starter (2.46 oz. tube w/applicator package). Refill (2.46 oz. and 4.05 oz. tube only packages).

ORTHO-CREME®
Contraceptive Cream
(nonoxynol 9, 2.00%)

Ortho—Advanced Care Prods.

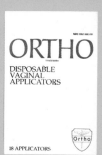

Packages of 18 applicators each

ORTHO®
Disposable Vaginal Applicators

Ortho—Derm. Div.

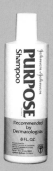

PURPOSE™
SHAMPOO

Parke-Davis

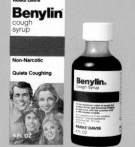

Available in 4 Oz. and 8 Oz. Packages

BENYLIN®
Cough Syrup

Parke-Davis

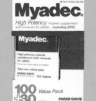

Available in bottles of 130 and 250 tablets

MYADEC®

High potency vitamin supplement with minerals

Ortho—Advanced Care Prods.

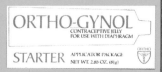

Ortho-Gynol is intended for use with a diaphragm

Starter (2.85 oz. tube w/applicator package). Refill (2.85 oz. and 4.44 oz. tube only packages).

ORTHO-GYNOL® Contraceptive Jelly
(diisobutylphenoxypolyethoxyethanol, 1.00%)

Ortho—Derm. Div.

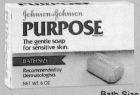

Bath Size

PURPOSE™
SOAP

Parke-Davis

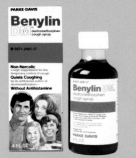

Available in 4 Oz. and 8 Oz. Packages

BENYLIN®
Cough Syrup

Parke-Davis

100 pads

40 pads

TUCKS®
Pre-Moistened Pads

Ortho—Advanced Care Prods.

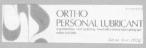

2 oz. and 4 oz. tubes

ORTHO® PERSONAL LUBRICANT

PARKE-DAVIS

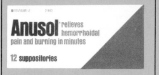

Available in boxes of 12, 24 and 48

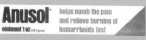

Available in 1 Oz. and 2 Oz. Tubes

ANUSOL®
Suppositories and Ointment

Parke-Davis

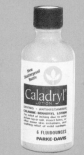

Available in 2½ and 6 Fl. Oz.

CALADRYL® LOTION

Parke-Davis

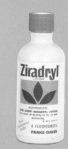

6 Fl. Oz.

ZIRADRYL® LOTION

ORTHO—DERM. DIV.

PURPOSE™
DRY SKIN CREAM

Parke-Davis

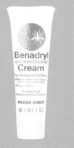

Available in 1 Oz. and 2 Oz. Tubes

BENADRYL®
Antihistamine Cream

Parke-Davis

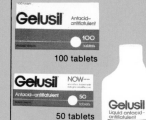

100 tablets

50 tablets

Also available:
165 tablets

GELUSIL®
Antacid-Anti-gas   12 Fl. Oz.

PFIPHARMECS

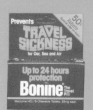

25 mg.

8 Chewable Tablets
per pack

BONINE® TABLETS
(meclizine HCl)

armecs

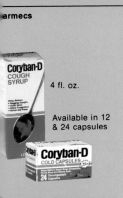

Coryban-D COUGH SYRUP

4 fl. oz.

Available in 12 & 24 capsules

Coryban-D COLD CAPSULES

RYBAN-D® COLD CAPSULES & COUGH SYRUP

PHARMACRAFT

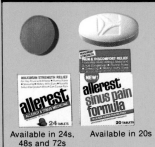

allerest ALLERGY & SINUS MEDICINE

NEW! allerest sinus pain formula

Available in 24s, 48s and 72s

Available in 20s

ALLEREST® ALLERGY TABLETS and SINUS PAIN FORMULA TABLETS

Pharmacraft

1.5 oz.

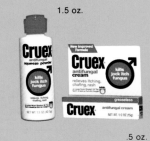

Cruex antifungal squeeze powder — kills jock itch fungus

Cruex antifungal cream — kills jock itch fungus — greaseless

Cruex antifungal cream

.5 oz.

Also available: 1.8, 3.5 and 5.5 oz. spray powder

CRUEX® ANTIFUNGAL POWDER and CREAM

Plough, Inc.

Aerosol Powder

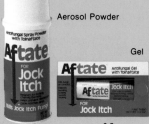

Gel

Aftate FOR Jock Itch — Kills Jock Itch Fungus

Aftate Antifungal Gel with Tolnaftate

3.5 oz.   0.5 oz.

Also available in 1.5 oz. shaker powder.

AFTATE® FOR JOCK ITCH (tolnaftate)

---

armecs

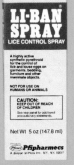

LI-BAN SPRAY LICE CONTROL SPRAY

A highly active synthetic pyrethroid for the control of lice and louse eggs on garments, bedding, furniture and other inanimate objects.

NOT FOR USE ON HUMANS OR ANIMALS

CAUTION: KEEP OUT OF REACH OF CHILDREN

Net Wt 5 oz (147.8 ml)

Pfipharmecs
A division of Pfizer Inc., N.Y., N.Y. 10017

LI-BAN® SPRAY

Pharmacraft

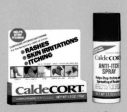

CaldeCORT — RASHES, SKIN IRRITATIONS, ITCHING

CaldeCORT ANTI-ITCH SPRAY — Helps Stop Itching and Spreading of Redness

Available in ½ oz. and 1 oz.

1.5 oz.

CaldeCORT® CREAM and SPRAY (hydrocortisone acetate .5%)

Pharmacraft

2.7 and 5.5 oz.

1.5 and 3.0 oz.

.5 oz.

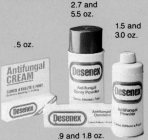

Antifungal CREAM — CURES ATHLETE'S FOOT

Desenex Antifungal Spray Powder — Cures Athlete's Foot

Desenex Antifungal Ointment — Cures Athlete's Foot

Desenex Antifungal Powder — Cures Athlete's Foot

.9 and 1.8 oz.

DESENEX® ANTIFUNGAL CREAM, OINTMENT AND POWDER

Plough, Inc.

Aspergum — CHERRY FLAVOR — sore throat pain — 16 GUM TABLETS

Cherry 16 Tablet Size

Orange 16 Tablet Size

Aspergum — ORANGE FLAVOR — sore throat pain — 16 GUM TABLETS

Also available in Orange and Cherry flavors, 40 tablet sizes.

ASPERGUM® (3½ grs. aspirin per tablet)

---

armecs

4 fl. oz.

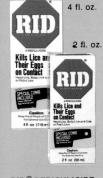

RID — Kills Lice and Their Eggs on Contact — Head Lice, Body Lice and Crabs or Pubic Lice

SPECIAL COMB INCLUDED

2 fl. oz.

RID — Kills Lice and Their Eggs on Contact

RID® PEDICULICIDE

Pharmacraft

4 oz.

2 oz.

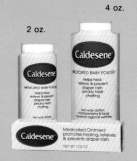

Caldesene MEDICATED BABY POWDER — helps heal, relieve & prevent diaper rash, prickly heat, chafing — two way action — kills bacteria & fungi — protects against wetness

Caldesene Medicated Ointment — promotes healing, relieves & prevents diaper rash.

1.25 oz.

CALDESENE® MEDICATED POWDER and OINTMENT

PHARMADERM

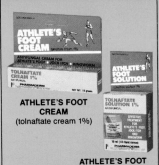

ATHLETE'S FOOT CREAM — ANTIFUNGAL CREAM FOR ATHLETE'S FOOT, JOCK ITCH, RINGWORM — TOLNAFTATE CREAM 1% ANTIFUNGAL — PHARMADERM — NET WT. 15 grams

ATHLETE'S FOOT SOLUTION — TOLNAFTATE SOLUTION 1% ANTIFUNGAL — EFFECTIVE TREATMENT FOR ATHLETE'S FOOT, JOCK ITCH AND RINGWORM — PHARMADERM

ATHLETE'S FOOT CREAM (tolnaftate cream 1%)

ATHLETE'S FOOT SOLUTION (tolnaftate solution 1%)

Plough, Inc.

Correctol LAXATIVE — The Woman's Gentle Laxative — 30 TABLETS

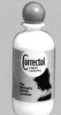

Correctol LAXATIVE — The Woman's Gentle Laxative

Available in 15, 30, 60 and 90 tablet sizes.

Available in 8 and 16 fl. oz. liquid sizes.

CORRECTOL® LAXATIVE (Tablet contains 100 mg. docusate sodium and 65 mg. phenolphthalein. Liquid contains 65 mg. phenolphthalein per tablespoon.)

---

armecs

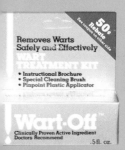

50¢ Rebate — See coupon on free side

Removes Warts Safely and Effectively

WART TREATMENT KIT
• Instructional Brochure
• Special Cleaning Brush
• Pinpoint Plastic Applicator

Wart-Off
Clinically Proven Active Ingredient Doctors Recommend

.5 fl. oz.

WART-OFF™

Pharmacraft

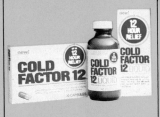

new! 12 HOUR RELIEF — COLD FACTOR 12 — 10 CAPSULES

12 HOUR RELIEF — COLD FACTOR 12 LIQUID

COLD FACTOR 12™ LIQUID AND CAPSULES

PLOUGH, INC.

Aerosol Liquid

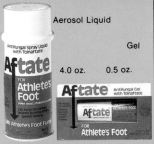

Gel

Aftate Antifungal Spray Liquid with Tolnaftate — FOR Athlete's Foot — Kills Athlete's Foot Fungus

4.0 oz.   0.5 oz.

Aftate Antifungal Gel with Tolnaftate — FOR Athlete's Foot

Also available in 3.5 oz. spray powder and 2.25 oz. shaker powder.

AFTATE® FOR ATHLETE'S FOOT (tolnaftate)

Plough, Inc.

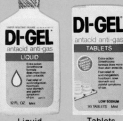

DI-GEL antacid anti-gas LIQUID — Extra-action Simethicone formula does more than plain antacids — Fast relief of acid indigestion, heartburn, sour stomach and painful symptoms of gas — LOW SODIUM — 12 FL. OZ. Mint

DI-GEL antacid anti-gas TABLETS — Extra-action Simethicone formula does more than plain antacids — Fast relief of acid indigestion, heartburn, sour stomach and painful symptoms of gas — LOW SODIUM — 90 TABLETS Mint

Liquid   Tablets

Mint and Lemon/Orange flavors, 6 fl. oz. and 12 fl. oz. liquid plus 30, 60 and 90 tablet sizes.

DI-GEL® (simethicone, aluminum hydroxide, magnesium hydroxide)

Plough, Inc.

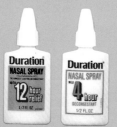

Available in ½ fl. oz.,
1 fl. oz. and ½ fl. oz.
mentholated.
(oxymetazoline HCl)

½ fl. oz.
(phenylephrine HCl)

**DURATION®
NASAL SPRAYS**

Plough, Inc.

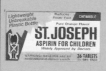

36 tablets per bottle

**ST. JOSEPH® ASPIRIN FOR
CHILDREN**
(1¼ grs. aspirin per tablet)

Plough, Inc.

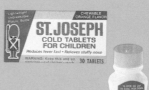

30 tablets per bottle

**ST. JOSEPH® COLD TABLETS
FOR CHILDREN**
(1¼ grs. aspirin and 3.125 mg.
phenylpropanolamine HCl per tablet)

Plough, Inc.

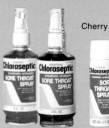

3 fl. oz.   3 oz.
Also available in 6 fl. oz. lotion,
5 oz. spray and 1 oz. First Aid
Cream
**SOLARCAINE® FIRST AID
PRODUCTS**
(benzocaine and triclosan)

Plough, Inc.

Pill
Available in 15,
30 and 60's

Gum
Available in 5,
16 and 40's

FEEN-A-MINT® LAXATIVE
Gum contains:
97.2 mg. phenolphthalein.
Pills contain: 100 mg. docusate
sodium and 65 mg. phenolphthalein.

Plough, Inc.

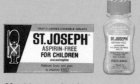

30 tablets per bottle

**ST. JOSEPH® ASPIRIN-FREE
Children's Sugar-Free
Chewable Tablets**
(80 mg. acetaminophen per tablet)

Plough, Inc.

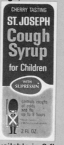
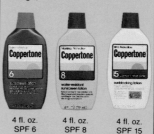

Available in 2 fl. oz. and 4 fl. oz.
sizes.

**ST. JOSEPH® COUGH SYRUP
FOR CHILDREN**
(dextromethorphan hydrobromide)

PROCTER & GAMBLE

Cherry   Menthol

Cherry   Menthol

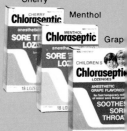

Available: 6 oz. with sprayer, 12 oz.
refill, 1.5 oz. nitrogen pressurized
pocket spray.

CHLORASEPTIC® LIQUID

Plough, Inc.

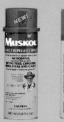

Available in
6 oz. size

Available in
1¼ fl. oz. &
2 fl. oz. sizes

**MUSKOL® INSECT
REPELLENT**

Plough, Inc.

Available in 2 fl. oz. and
4 fl. oz. sizes
**ST. JOSEPH®
ASPIRIN-FREE
Liquid for Children
Alcohol-Free,
Sugar-Free**
(80 mg. acetaminophen per
½ teaspoonful)

Plough, Inc.

4 fl. oz.
SPF 6

4 fl. oz.
SPF 8

4 fl. oz.
SPF 15

**COPPERTONE®
Sunscreens**

Procter & Gamble

Cherry

Menthol

Grape

Chloraseptic
SORE THROAT
LOZENGES

Chloraseptic
SORE THROAT
LOZENGES

CHILDREN'S
Chloraseptic
LOZENGES
ANESTHETIC
GRAPE FLAVORED

Available: all flavors in
cartons of 18; Menthol &
Cherry available in
cartons of 45 lozenges.

CHLORASEPTIC® LOZENGES

Plough, Inc.

Available in 30, 60 and 90
tablet sizes.

**REGUTOL®
STOOL SOFTENER**
(100 mg. docusate sodium per tablet)

Plough, Inc.

**ST. JOSEPH® ASPIRIN-FREE
Infant Drops
Alcohol-Free, Sugar-Free**
(80 mg. acetaminophen per
0.8 ml. dropperful)

Plough, Inc.

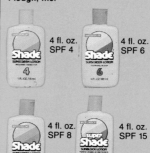

4 fl. oz.
SPF 4

4 fl. oz.
SPF 6

4 fl. oz.
SPF 8

4 fl. oz.
SPF 15

**SHADE® WATERPROOF
SUNSCREEN LOTIONS**

Procter & Gamble

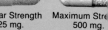

Regular Strength
325 mg.

Maximum Strength
500 mg.

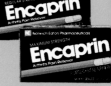
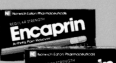

ENCAPRIN® CAPSULES
(Enteric-coated micrograins of
aspirin, USP)

Procter & Gamble

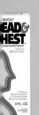

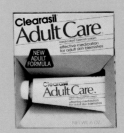
Tablets

Liquid

Capsules

See Product Information for sizes.

HEAD & CHEST™
DECONGESTANT/EXPECTORANT
Liquid, Capsules & Tablets

REED & CARNRICK

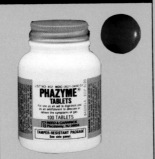

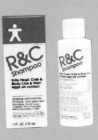

PHAZYME® TABLETS
Aid to digestion and an antiflatulent to
alleviate or relieve symptoms of gas

Reed & Carnrick
Available in 2 and 4 fl. oz. sizes

R&C SHAMPOO®
Kills head, crab and body lice
and their eggs on contact.

Richardson-Vicks
Personal Care Products Div.

CLEARASIL® ADULT CARE™
(sulfur, resorcinol)

Procter & Gamble

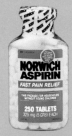

5 grains—325 mg.

NORWICH® ASPIRIN

Available in bottles of 100, 250
and 500 tablets.

Reed & Carnrick

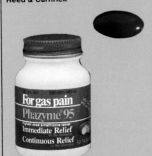

PHAZYME 95®
Immediate relief in the stomach and
continuous relief in the intestines

Reed & Carnrick
Available in 5 and 10 oz. sizes

R&C SPRAY"
Controls lice and their eggs
in the home. Insecticide: not
for use on humans or animals.

Richardson-Vicks
Personal Care Products Div.

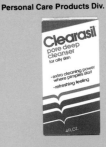

4 and 8 oz. sizes

CLEARASIL®
Pore Deep Cleanser
For Oily Skin
(0.5% salicylic acid)

Procter & Gamble

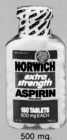

500 mg.

NORWICH® EXTRA STRENGTH
ASPIRIN

Available in bottles of 150 tablets

Reed & Carnrick

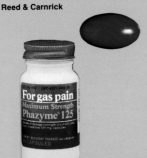

MAXIMUM STRENGTH
PHAZYME® 125
For gas pain

Reed & Carnrick

R&C LICE TREATMENT KIT
Contains 4 oz. R&C SHAMPOO,
5 oz. R&C SPRAY and nit comb.

For more detailed in-
formation on products
illustrated in this sec-
tion, consult the Prod-
uct Information Sec-
tion or manufacturers
may be contacted di-
rectly.

Procter & Gamble

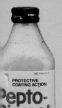

PEPTO-BISMOL® LIQUID AND
TABLETS

Liquid available in
4 oz., 8 oz., 12 oz.
and 16 oz. bottles

Tablets available
in cartons of
24 and 42

Reed & Carnrick

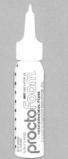

PROCTOFOAM®
(pramoxine hydrochloride) 1%

RICHARDSON-VICKS

Personal Care Products Div.

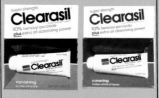

.65 and 1.0 oz. sizes available

CLEARASIL®
Acne Treatment Cream
(10% benzoyl peroxide)

A. H. ROBINS

Consumer
Products
Division

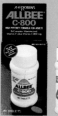

Available in bottles of 60

ALLBEE® C-800 TABLETS

A. H. Robins

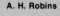

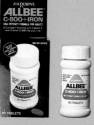

Available in bottles of 60

ALLBEE® C-800 PLUS IRON TABLETS

A. H. Robins

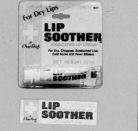

For Dry Lips
LIP SOOTHER
MEDICATED LIP CREAM
For Dry, Chapped, Sunburned Lips,
Cold Sores and Fever Blisters.

NET WEIGHT .12 oz.

LIP SOOTHER

LIP SOOTHER

LIP SOOTHER
Medicated Lip Cream
by CHAP STICK®

A. H. Robins

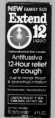

PRODUCT INSIDE
SEALED FOR YOUR PROTECTION
New
Dimetane
Extentabs® 8 mg
(Brompheniramine Maleate, USP)
ANTIHISTAMINE
LONG-ACTING Allergy Tablets
8- to 12-hour relief of hay fever symptoms:
• Itching of the nose or throat
• Itchy, watery eyes
• Sneezing
• Running nose
12 TABLETS

Available in consumer cartons of 12
and bottles of 100 and 500

DIMETANE EXTENTABS® 8 MG

A. H. Robins

NEW FAMILY SIZE
Extend 12
LIQUID
(Dextromethorphan Resin Complex)
Antitussive
12-Hour relief
of cough
due to minor throat
& bronchial irritation
Nonnarcotic • Nonalcoholic
CARTON SEALED. IF SEAL
IS BROKEN. DO NOT USE.

Available in bottles of
2 Fl. Oz. and 4 Fl. Oz.

EXTEND 12® LIQUID
(Dextromethorphan Polistirex)

A. H. Robins

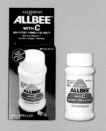

Available in bottles of 100 and 1000
ALLBEE® WITH C CAPSULES

A. H. Robins

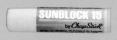

Relieves stuffy nose
Reduces chest congestion
Controls cough
Contains no sedatives
From the makers of Robitussin®
Dimacol
COLD & COUGH CAPSULES
24
CAPSULES
Not recommended for
children 12 and under

Available in consumer cartons of 12
and 24 and bottles of 100 and 500

DIMACOL® CAPSULES

A. H. Robins

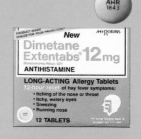

PRODUCT INSIDE
SEALED FOR YOUR PROTECTION
New
Dimetane
Extentabs® 12 mg
(Brompheniramine Maleate, USP)
ANTIHISTAMINE
LONG-ACTING Allergy Tablets
12-hour relief of hay fever symptoms:
• Itching of the nose or throat
• Itchy, watery eyes
• Sneezing
• Running nose
12 TABLETS

Available in consumer cartons of 12
and bottles of 100 and 500

DIMETANE EXTENTABS® 12 MG

A. H. Robins

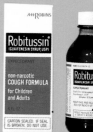

Robitussin®
(GUAIFENESIN SYRUP, USP)
EXPECTORANT
non-narcotic
COUGH FORMULA
for Children
and Adults
CARTON SEALED. IF SEAL
IS BROKEN. DO NOT USE.

Available in bottles of 4 Fl. Oz.
8 Fl. Oz., 16 Fl. Oz. and 128 Fl. Oz.

ROBITUSSIN® SYRUP
(Guaifenesin Syrup, USP)

A. H. Robins

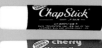

SUNBLOCK 15
by ChapStick®

Ultra sunscreen protection (SPF-15)

Aids prevention and healing of dry,
chapped, sun- and windburned lips.

CHAP STICK®
SUNBLOCK 15 Lip Balm

A. H. Robins

PLEASANT TASTING
Dimetane
Elixir
ALLERGY MEDICINE
For effective, temporary
relief of hay fever/
upper respiratory allergy
symptoms:
• Itchy, watery eyes
• Sneezing
• Itching nose or throat
CARTON SEALED. IF SEAL
IS BROKEN. DO NOT USE.
4 FL. OZ.

Dimetane
ALLERGY MEDICINE
4 FL. OZ.

4 Fl. Oz.

DIMETANE® ELIXIR
(Brompheniramine Maleate Elixir, USP)

A. H. Robins

Dimetane
Decongestant
ELIXIR
NASAL DECONGESTANT/ANTIHISTAMINE
For effective temporary relief of:
Colds & Allergies
• Stuffy nose
• Runny nose
• Hay fever symptoms
• Itchy, watery eyes
• Itching nose or throat
Red
Grape
Flavor
4 FL. OZ.

Dimetane
Decongestant
ELIXIR
Colds & Allergies
4 FL. OZ.

4 Fl. Oz.

DIMETANE®
DECONGESTANT ELIXIR

A. H. Robins

Robitussin
CF
EXPECTORANT
NASAL DECONGESTANT
COUGH SUPPRESSANT
COUGH FORMULA
for Children
and Adults
4 FL. OZ.
CARTON SEALED. IF SEAL
IS BROKEN. DO NOT USE.

Robitussin-CF

Available in bottles of 4 Fl. Oz.,
8 Fl. Oz. and 16 Fl. Oz.

ROBITUSSIN-CF® SYRUP

A. H. Robins

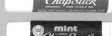
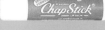

ChapStick®

cherry
ChapStick®

orange
ChapStick®

strawberry
ChapStick®

mint
ChapStick®

CHAP STICK®
Lip Balm

A. H. Robins

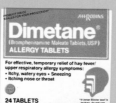

PRODUCT INSIDE
SEALED FOR YOUR PROTECTION
Dimetane®
(Brompheniramine Maleate Tablets, USP)
ALLERGY TABLETS
For effective, temporary relief of hay fever/
upper respiratory allergy symptoms:
• Itchy, watery eyes • Sneezing
• Itching nose or throat
24 TABLETS

Available in consumer cartons of
24 and bottles of 100 and 500

DIMETANE® TABLETS
(Brompheniramine Maleate Tablets, USP)

A. H. Robins

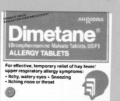

PRODUCT INSIDE
SEALED FOR YOUR PROTECTION
Dimetane
Decongestant
NASAL DECONGESTANT/ANTIHISTAMINE
For effective temporary relief of:
Colds & Allergies
• Nasal congestion • Hay fever symptoms
• Sinusitis • Itchy, watery eyes
• Runny nose • Itching nose or throat
• Sneezing
24 TABLETS

Available in consumer cartons of
24 and 48

DIMETANE® DECONGESTANT
TABLETS

A. H. Robins

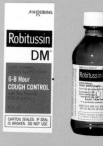

Robitussin
DM®
EXPECTORANT
6-8 Hour
COUGH CONTROL

Robitussin-DM

Available in bottles of 4 Fl. Oz.,
8 Fl. Oz., 16 Fl. Oz. and 128 Fl. Oz.

ROBITUSSIN-DM® SYRUP

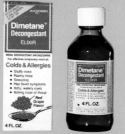
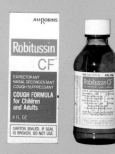

H. Robins	**Roche**	**William H. Rorer**	**William H. Rorer**

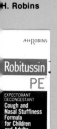 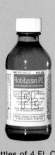

available in bottles of 4 Fl. Oz.,
8 Fl. Oz. and 16 Fl. Oz.

ROBITUSSIN-PE® SYRUP

0.6 cc
0.3 cc

VI-PENTA® MULTIVITAMIN DROPS

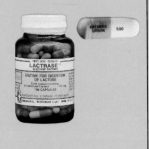

LACTRASE™
(lactase enzyme)

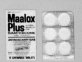 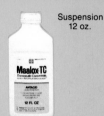

Tablets
12's & 50's

Suspension
12 oz.   Roll Pack

MAALOX® PLUS
Alumina, Magnesia and Simethicone
Oral Suspension and Tablets, Rorer

H. Robins	**RORER**	**William H. Rorer**	**William H. Rorer**

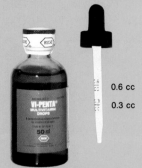

available in bottles of 4 Fl. Oz. and
. Oz. with convenient dosage cup.

ROBITUSSIN NIGHT RELIEF®

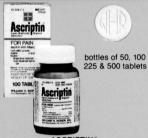

bottles of 50, 100
225 & 500 tablets

ASCRIPTIN®
Aspirin, Alumina and Magnesia
Tablets, Rorer (Aspirin: [5 grains] 325
mg. Maalox®: magnesium hydroxide,
75 mg and dried aluminum hydroxide
gel, 75 mg)

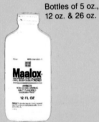

Bottles of 5 oz.,
12 oz. & 26 oz.

MAALOX® SUSPENSION
Magnesia and Alumina Oral
Suspension, Rorer
(225 mg Aluminum Hydroxide and
200 mg Magnesium Hydroxide)

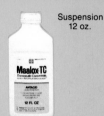

Suspension
12 oz.

MAALOX® TC
(Therapeutic Concentrate)

Magnesium and Aluminum Hydroxides
Oral Suspension, Rorer

(300 mg of magnesium hydroxide and
600 mg of aluminum hydroxide per 5 ml)

H. Robins	**William H. Rorer**	**William H. Rorer**	**William H. Rorer**

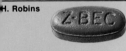 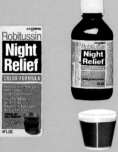

ailable in bottles of 60 and 500

Z-BEC® TABLETS

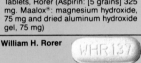

bottles of 100,
225 & 500 tablets

ASCRIPTIN® A/D
Aspirin, Alumina and Magnesia
Tablets, Rorer (Aspirin: [5 grains] 325
mg. Maalox®: magnesium hydroxide,
150 mg and dried aluminum hydroxide
gel, 150 mg)

bottles of 100

MAALOX® NO. 1 TABLETS
Magnesia and Alumina Tablets, Rorer
(200 mg of magnesium hydroxide
and 200 mg of aluminum hydroxide)

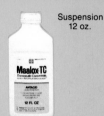

MAALOX® TC TABLETS
Magnesium and Aluminum Hydroxides
Tablets, Rorer
(300 mg magnesium hydroxide and
600 mg aluminum hydroxide)

ROCHE	**William H. Rorer**	**William H. Rorer**	**William H. Rorer**

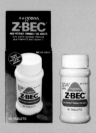

0.6 cc
0.3 cc

VI-PENTA® INFANT DROPS

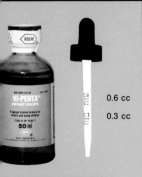

3 oz.
16 oz.

EMETROL®
(levulose [fructose], dextrose
[glucose] and phosphoric acid)

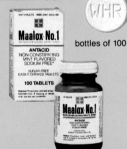 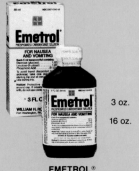

bottles of 50's
& 250's
strips of 24's
& 100's

MAALOX® NO. 2 TABLETS
Magnesia and Alumina Tablets, Rorer
(400 mg of magnesium hydroxide
and 400 mg of aluminum hydroxide)

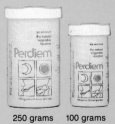

250 grams   100 grams

Granules

PERDIEM®
82 percent psyllium (Plantago Hydrocolloid)
18 percent senna (Cassia Pod Concentrate)

William H. Rorer

Also available in 100 gram canister

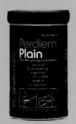

250 grams
Granules
PERDIEM® PLAIN
100% Psyllium
(Plantago Hydrocolloid)

Ross

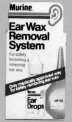

**MURINE® EAR
WAX REMOVAL
SYSTEM**
0.5 Fl. Oz.

**MURINE®
EAR DROPS**
0.5 Fl. Oz.

RYDELLE

Orange   Natural

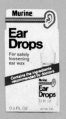

Powder 5 oz., 10 oz., and 15 oz.

**Sugar Free
FIBERALL™**
Natural Fiber Laxative
Psyllium Hydrophilic Mucilloid

Schering

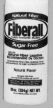

Afrinol® Repetabs® TABLETS
LONG-ACTING NASAL DECONGESTANT

up to 12 hour temporary relief of nasal congestion...helps decongest sinus openings, sinus passages ...without drowsiness

12 Repetabs TABLETS

AFRINOL® REPETABS® TABLET
(pseudoephedrine sulfate)

ROSS

0.5 Fl. Oz.

CLEAR EYES®
For Immediate Redness
Removal
Also available in 1.5 Fl. Oz.

Ross

4 Fl. Oz.

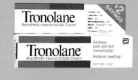

For Oily Hair   For Dry Hair   For Normal Hair

SELSUN BLUE®
Dandruff Shampoo
Also available in 7 and 11 Fl. Oz.

SCHERING

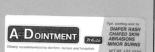

WMJ

A and D Reg. ™ **OINTMENT**

Schering

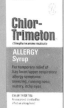

Chlor-Trimeton
ALLERGY Syrup

4 FL. OZ. (118 ml)

**CHLOR-TRIMETON®
ALLERGY SYRUP**
(chlorpheniramine maleate, USP)

Ross

0.5 Fl. Oz.

MURINE® REGULAR FORMULA
Soothes & Moisturizes Irritated Eyes
Also available in 1.5 Fl. Oz.

Ross

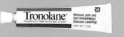

1 Oz. Tube With Applicator

TRONOLANE™
Anesthetic Hemorrhoidal Cream
Also available in a 2 oz. tube.

Schering

Afrin
NASAL SPRAY

Afrin
MENTHOL
NASAL SPRAY

**AFRIN®
NASAL SPRAY
0.05%**

**AFRIN® MENTHOL
NASAL SPRAY
0.05%**

(oxymetazoline hydrochloride, USP)

Schering

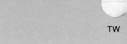
TW

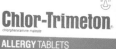

Chlor-Trimeton®
ALLERGY TABLETS

24 TABLETS 4mg

**CHLOR-TRIMETON®
ALLERGY TABLETS**
(4 mg chlorpheniramine maleate, USP)

Ross

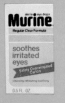

0.5 Fl. Oz.

MURINE® PLUS
For **Faster** Redness Removal
Also available in 1.5 Fl. Oz.

Ross

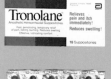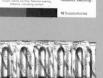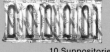

10 Suppositories

TRONOLANE™
Anesthetic Hemorrhoidal
Suppositories
Also available in size 20's.

Schering

Afrin
NOSE DROPS

Afrin
PEDIATRIC
NOSE DROPS

Nose Drops
0.05%

Pediatric
Nose Drops
0.025%

AFRIN® NOSE DROPS
(oxymetazoline hydrochloride, USP)

Schering

374

**LONG ACTING
Chlor-Trimeton**
ALLERGY Repetabs‡TABLETS

up to 12 hour continuous relief

24 Repetabs TABLETS 8mg

**CHLOR-TRIMETON®
LONG ACTING ALLERGY
REPETABS® TABLETS**
(8 mg chlorpheniramine maleate, USP)

Schering

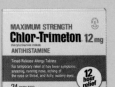

MAXIMUM STRENGTH Chlor-Trimeton 12 mg
ANTIHISTAMINE
Timed-Release Allergy Tablets
For temporary relief of hay fever symptoms; sneezing, running nose, itching of the nose or throat, and itchy, watery eyes.
12 hour relief
24 TABLETS

**CHLOR-TRIMETON®
MAXIMUM STRENGTH
TIMED RELEASE
ALLERGY TABLETS**
(lorpheniramine maleate, 12 mg, USP)

Schering

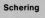

PKD
or
SN
or
171

Coricidin TABLETS
For cold and flu symptoms
60 TABLETS

New aspirin-free
formula, May 1985

**CORICIDIN®
TABLETS**

Schering

Dermolate

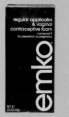

NEW Dermolate
HYDROCORTISONE ANTI-ITCH SPRAY
Temporary relief of ITCHING and MINOR SKIN IRRITATION due to:
45 ml (1.5 fl oz)

**DERMOLATE®
ANTI-ITCH CREAM AND SPRAY**
(hydrocortisone 0.5%)

Schering/Emko Product Line

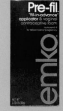

emko
regular applicator & vaginal contraceptive foam
for prevention of pregnancy
NET WT. 1.41 OZ (40g)

Pre-fil
fill-in-advance applicator & vaginal contraceptive foam
for prevention of pregnancy
emko
NET WT. 2.75 OZ (78g)

**EMKO®
CONTRACEPTIVE
FOAM**

**EMKO® PRE-FIL®
CONTRACEPTIVE
FOAM**

(nonoxynol-9)

Schering

901

NDC-0085-0901-03
**Chlor-Trimeton
DECONGESTANT
Allergy/Sinus Congestion Tablets**
For temporary relief of nasal/sinus passage congestion due to hay fever or sinusitis.
24 TABLETS

**CHLOR-TRIMETON®
DECONGESTANT TABLETS**
(mg chlorpheniramine maleate, USP and 60 mg pseudoephedrine sulfate)

Schering

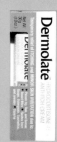

871
or
524

Coricidin 'D' DECONGESTANT TABLETS
For congested cold, flu, and sinus symptoms
50 TABLETS

New aspirin-free
formula, May 1985

**CORICIDIN 'D'®
DECONGESTANT TABLETS**

Schering

Dermolate

Dermolate
HYDROCORTISONE 0.5%
ANAL-ITCH OINTMENT
Temporary relief of ANAL ITCHING

Dermolate
HYDROCORTISONE 0.5%
SCALP-ITCH LOTION
Temporary relief of ITCHING and MINOR SCALP IRRITATION due to Scalp Dermatitis

**DERMOLATE®
ANAL-ITCH OINTMENT AND
SCALP-ITCH LOTION**
(hydrocortisone 0.5%)

Schering/White Product Line

**Chronosule®
Capsules**

Tablets

with Vitamin C
Tablets

MOL-IRON®

Schering

**LONG ACTING
Chlor-Trimeton
DECONGESTANT**
REPETABS® Tablets
Antihistamine/Nasal Decongestant
For temporary relief of nasal congestion due to hay fever and associated with sinusitis.
Up to 12 hour combination allergy relief
NDC-0085-0484-02
12 TABLETS

**LONG ACTING
CHLOR-TRIMETON®
DECONGESTANT REPETABS®**
(mg chlorpheniramine maleate, USP and 120 mg pseudoephedrine sulfate)

Schering

FOR YOUR CHILD'S CONGESTED COLD, FLU & SINUS SYMPTOMS
NEW REFORMULATED
Coricidin DEMILETS TABLETS
ASPIRIN-FREE 24 chewable tablets

**CORICIDIN® DEMILETS®
TABLETS**

Schering

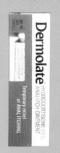

DRIXORAL
ANTIHISTAMINE/NASAL DECONGESTANT
12 hour relief
Temporarily relieves nasal congestion due to the common cold and associated with sinusitis. Alleviates running nose and sneezing due to hay fever.
20 SUSTAINED-ACTION TABLETS

**DRIXORAL®
SUSTAINED-ACTION TABLETS**
(6 mg dexbrompheniramine maleate and 120 mg pseudoephedrine sulfate)

Schering

KILLS ATHLETE'S FOOT and JOCK ITCH FUNGI
Tinactin ANTIFUNGAL CREAM

Tinactin ANTIFUNGAL SOLUTION
Kills ATHLETES FOOT and JOCK ITCH Fungi
10 ml (1/3 fluid ounce)

**TINACTIN®
CREAM AND SOLUTION**
(tolnaftate 1%)

Schering/White Product Line

**COD LIVER OIL CONCENTRATE
CAPSULES**

**COD LIVER OIL CONCENTRATE
TABLETS**

**COD LIVER OIL CONCENTRATE
TABLETS W/VITAMIN C**

Schering

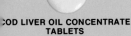

ADD
or
133

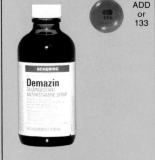

**SCHERING
Demazin
DECONGESTANT
ANTIHISTAMINE SYRUP**
4 FLUID OUNCES (118 ml)

**DEMAZIN® DECONGESTANT-
ANTIHISTAMINE REPETABS®
TABLETS AND SYRUP**

Schering/Emko Product Line

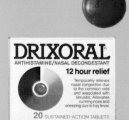

Because
portable six-use applicator containing vaginal contraceptive foam
for prevention of pregnancy
NET WT 0.35 OZ (10g)

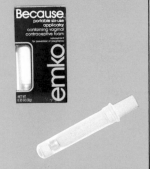

BECAUSE® CONTRACEPTOR®
(nonoxynol-9)

Schering

Tinactin
JOCK ITCH CREAM
KILLS JOCK ITCH FUNGI
ANTIFUNGAL
Tinactin JOCK ITCH CREAM

Tinactin
ANTIFUNGAL
JOCK ITCH
Spray POWDER
KILLS JOCK ITCH FUNGI

**TINACTIN® JOCK ITCH
CREAM AND SPRAY POWDER**

Schering

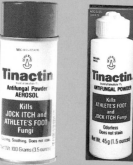

TINACTIN®
POWDER AEROSOL AND POWDER

Kills JOCK ITCH and ATHLETE'S FOOT Fungi

Searle Consumer Products

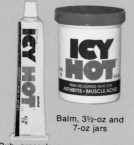

Balm, 3½-oz and 7-oz jars

Rub, greaseless, 1¼-oz and 3-oz tubes

ICY HOT®
Analgesic Balm and Rub for Arthritis and Muscle Aches

Searle Consumer Products

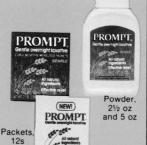

Packets, 12s

Powder, 2½ oz and 5 oz

PROMPT™
Gentle overnight laxative

STELLAR

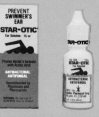

Prevent Swimmer's Ear

STAR-OTIC®
Antibacterial • Antifungal

Schering

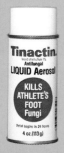

TINACTIN®
LIQUID AEROSOL
(toinaftate)

KILLS ATHLETE'S FOOT Fungi

Searle Consumer Products

Regular Flavor   Sugar Free Regular Flavor

Power, 7 oz, 14 oz, and 21 oz

Powder, 3.7 oz, 7.4 oz, and 11.1 oz

METAMUCIL®
A Natural-Fiber Laxative

SOLGAR

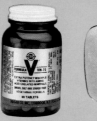

FORMULA VM-75
Extra Potency Multiple Vitamins with Amino Acid Chelated Minerals
Vegetarian Formula
Sugar, Salt and Starch Free

STUART

All Stuart products are packaged with tamper-resistant features as required by applicable Federal Regulations.

12 oz.

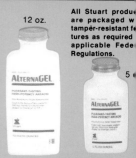

5

ALternaGEL®
High Potency Aluminum Hydroxide Antacid

SEARLE

DRAMAMINE®
(dimenhydrinate)
Tablets, packets of 12, and bottles of 36 and 100 (as shown).

DRAMAMINE® LIQUID
(dimenhydrinate syrup USP)
Liquid, 3 fl oz

Searle Consumer Products

Orange Flavor   Strawberry Flavor

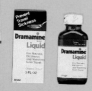

Powder, 7 oz, 14 oz and 21 oz
METAMUCIL®
A Natural-Fiber Laxative

SQUIBB

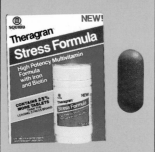

THERAGRAN® STRESS FORMULA
High Potency Multivitamin Formula with Iron and Biotin

Stuart

Available in bottles of 9 and 16 oz.

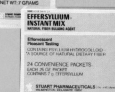

Convenience Packet

Searle Consumer Products

Pocket-Pak, 100 sweet-tabs*

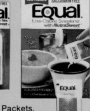

Packets, 50s and 100s

*One sweet-tab equals the sweetness of 1 teaspoon of sugar
EQUAL®
Low-calorie sweetener

Searle Consumer Products

Regular   Orange Flavor

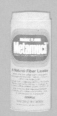
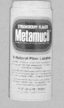

Single-dose packets, cartons of 16 and 30

INSTANT MIX METAMUCIL®
A Natural-Fiber Laxative

E. R. Squibb & Sons

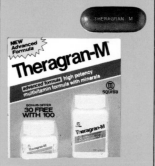

THERAGRAN-M®
Advanced Formula High Potency
Multivitamin Formula with Minerals

Available in boxes of 12 and 24 Convenience Packets

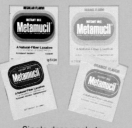

EFFERSYLLIUM® INSTANT MIX
Bulk Laxative containing
Natural Dietary Fiber

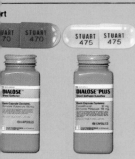

Stuart

DIALOSE DIALOSE PLUS

...les of 36, 100 and 500 capsules

DIALOSE
(...sate potassium,
100 mg.)

DIALOSE PLUS
(docusate potassium,
100 mg. and casan-
thranol, 30 mg.)

Stool Softeners

Stuart

Sodium Free

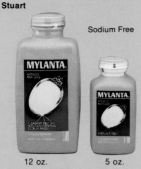

12 oz.   5 oz.

MYLANTA® LIQUID
Antacid/Anti-Gas

(magnesium and aluminum hydroxides
with simethicone)

Stuart

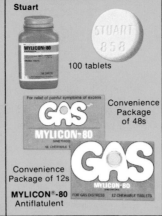

100 tablets

Convenience
Package
of 48s

Convenience
Package of 12s

MYLICON®-80
Antiflatulent

Stuart

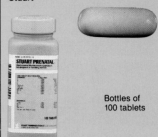

Bottles of
100 tablets

STUART PRENATAL® TABLETS
Multivitamin/Multimineral Supplement
for pregnant or lactating women

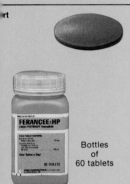

FERANCEE-HP

Bottles
of
60 tablets

FERANCEE®-HP
High Potency Hematinic

Stuart

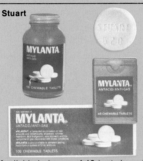

Available in boxes of 40 (not shown)
and 100, bottles of 180, and flip-top
Convenience Packs of 48

MYLANTA® TABLETS
Antacid/Anti-Gas

Stuart

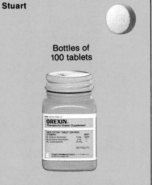

Bottles of
100 tablets

OREXIN

OREXIN®
Therapeutic Vitamin Supplement

Stuart

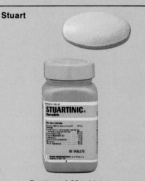

STUARTINIC

Bottles of 60 tablets

STUARTINIC®
Hematinic

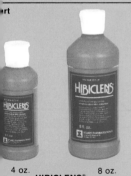

HIBICLENS

4 oz.   8 oz.

HIBICLENS®
(chlorhexidine gluconate)

Antiseptic Antimicrobial
Skin Cleanser

Stuart

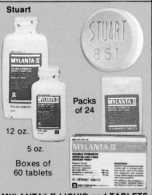

MYLANTA-II

12 oz.

5 oz.

Boxes of
60 tablets

Packs
of 24

MYLANTA®-II LIQUID and TABLETS
Double Strength Antacid/Anti-Gas

Stuart

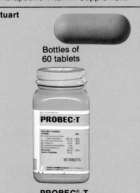

Bottles of
60 tablets

PROBEC-T

PROBEC®-T
High potency B complex supplement
with 600 mg. of vitamin C

SUNRISE & RAINBOW

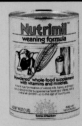

Nutrimil
weaning formula

NUTRIMIL™
Weaning Formula

Also available:
Nursamil Breastfeeding Formula and
Prenatamil Pregnancy Formula

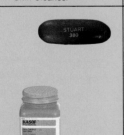

KASOF

Bottles of 30 and 60 capsules

KASOF®
(docusate potassium, 240 mg.)

High Strength Stool Softener

Stuart

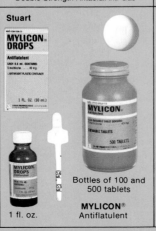

MYLICON
DROPS

MYLICON

MYLICON
DROPS

Bottles of 100 and
500 tablets

1 fl. oz.

MYLICON®
Antiflatulent

Stuart

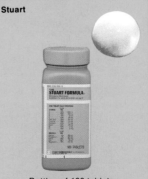

STUART FORMULA

Bottles of 100 tablets

STUART FORMULA® TABLETS
Multivitamin/Multimineral Supplement

For more detailed in-
formation on products
illustrated in this sec-
tion, consult the Prod-
uct Information Sec-
tion or manufacturers
may be contacted di-
rectly.

THOMPSON MEDICAL

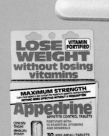

Available in 30 & 60 tablet sizes.

APPEDRINE®
APPETITE CONTROL TABLETS

Thompson Medical Company, Inc.

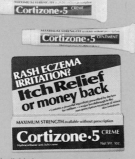

Available in 1 oz. creme 1 oz. ointment
CORTIZONE-5
(Hydrocortisone .05%)

Thompson Medical Company, Inc.

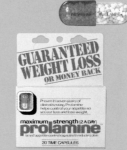

Available in 20 & 50 capsule sizes.
PROLAMINE™
APPETITE CONTROL CAPSULES

Upjohn

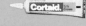

½ oz
&
1 oz

CORTAID® Cream

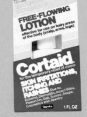

1 oz
&
2 oz

CORTAID® Lotion

½ oz
&
1 oz

CORTAID® Ointment
hydrocortisone acetate
(equivalent to hydrocortisone 0.5%)

Thompson Medical Company, Inc.

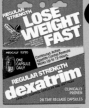

DEXATRIM®
APPETITE CON-
TROL CAPSULES

Available in
28 & 56
capsule sizes.

EXTRA-STRENGTH
DEXATRIM®

Available in
10, 20 & 40
capsule sizes.

CAFFEINE-FREE
EXTRA-STRENGTH
DEXATRIM®

Available in
10, 20 & 40
capsule sizes.

DEXATRIM®
EXTRA-STRENGTH
PLUS VITAMINS

Available in
16 & 32
capsule sizes.

Thompson Medical Company, Inc.

AQUA-BAN®
Diuretic

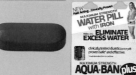

AQUA-BAN® PLUS
Diuretic Plus
Iron

Thompson Medical Company, Inc.

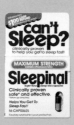

SLEEPINAL™
Night-time Sleep-aid Capsules

Thompson Medical Company, Inc.

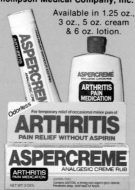

Available in 1.25 oz.,
3 oz., 5 oz. cream
& 6 oz. lotion.

ASPERCREME™

Thompson Medical Company, Inc.

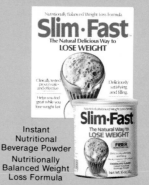

Instant
Nutritional
Beverage Powder

Nutritionally
Balanced Weight
Loss Formula

SLIM-FAST™

Upjohn

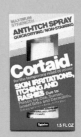
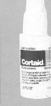

1.5 fl oz
CORTAID® Spray
(hydrocortisone 0.5%)

Thompson Medical Company, Inc.

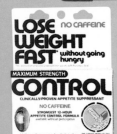

Available in 14, 28 & 56 capsule sizes

CONTROL®
APPETITE CONTROL CAPSULES

Thompson Medical Company, Inc.

Vaginal
Contraceptive
for
Prevention of
Pregnancy

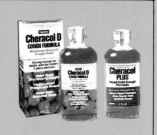

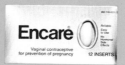

ENCARE®

UPJOHN

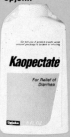

2 oz, 4 oz,
6 oz

CHERACOL D®
Cough Formula

4 oz, 6 oz

CHERACOL PLUS®
Head Cold/Cough
Formula

Upjohn

8, 12, 16 oz.
&
1 gallon

KAOPECTATE®

Anti-Diarrhea Medicine

8, 12 oz.

KAOPECTATE®
CONCENTRAT

John

Convenient Dose

aopectate

Tablet Formula

Easy-To-Swallow

Tablets

0 Tablets

Fast Relief **Convenient Dose**

NEW!
Kaopectate
Tablet Formula
Easy-To-Swallow
Tablets

12 Tablets

KAOPECTATE®
Tablet Formula

Upjohn

Bottles of
90, 120

UNICAP JR™
Chewable
Tablets

Bottles of
90, 120

UNICAP®
Senior
Tablets

Multivitamin Supplement

For more detailed information on products illustrated in this section, consult the Product Information Section or manufacturers may be contacted directly.

Vicks Health Care Div.

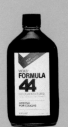
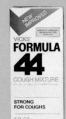

Available in 3 oz., 6 oz., 8 oz.

FORMULA 44®
Cough Mixture
(dextromethorphan hydrobromide,
doxylamine succinate)

John

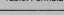

Mycitracin

TRIPLE ANTIBIOTIC FIRST AID OINTMENT
Aids in healing doesn't sting and helps prevent infection.
For burns, cuts, nicks, scrapes, scuffs and abrasions.

Mycitracin®

½ oz & 1 oz tubes
MYCITRACIN®
Triple Antibiotic Ointment
(acitracin-polymyxin-neomycin topical ointment)

Upjohn

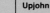
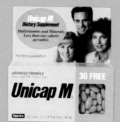

Unicap M
Dietary Supplement
Multivitamins and Minerals.
Less than one calorie per tablet.

ADVANCED FORMULA

30 FREE

Unicap M

Bottles of 30, 90, 120,
180, 500

UNICAP M® Tablets
Advanced Formula
Dietary Supplement

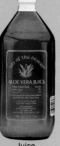

ALOE VERA

ALOE VERA JUICE

Gelly

Juice

Lily of the Desert®
ALOE VERA

Vicks Health Care Div.

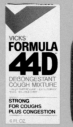
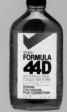

VICKS
FORMULA
44D
DECONGESTANT
COUGH MIXTURE
STRONG
FOR COUGHS
PLUS CONGESTION

Available in 3 oz., 6 oz., 8 oz.

FORMULA 44D®
Decongestant Cough Mixture
(dextromethorphan hydrobromide,
phenylpropanolamine hydrochloride,
guaifenesin)

John

Extra Strength
Pyrroxate
CAFFEINE & ASPIRIN-FREE CAPSULES
ra strength, single-capsule dose
multi-symptom relief of
olds, Allergies &
nus Congestion **24**
Capsules

Available in bottles of
24 and 500

sal Decongestant/Antihistamine/
Analgesic

PYRROXATE® Capsules

Upjohn

LOW IN SODIUM
30 FREE
Unicap
Plus Iron

Bottles of
90, 120

UNICAP®
Plus Iron
Tablets

Unicap T
Stress Formula
High-potency Multivitamin with Minerals including Zinc and Selenium.
ADVANCED FORMULA
Unicap T
Stress Formula

Bottles of
60, 500

UNICAP T®
Tablets
Stress Formula

VICKS HEALTH CARE DIV.

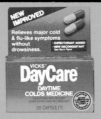

NEW IMPROVED
Relieves major cold & flu-like symptoms without drowsiness.
• EXPECTORANT ADDED
• NEW DECONGESTANT
See Back Panel

VICKS
DayCare
DAYTIME
COLDS MEDICINE
20 CAPSULES

Capsules imprinted DAYCARE
Blister Packs of 20 and 36

DAYCARE®
Daytime Colds Medicine
(acetaminophen, pseudoephedrine
hydrochloride, dextromethorphan
hydrobromide, guaifenesin)

Vick Health Care Div.

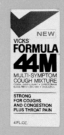
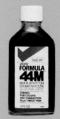

VICKS
FORMULA
44M
MULTI-SYMPTOM
COUGH MIXTURE
STRONG
FOR COUGHS
AND CONGESTION
PLUS THROAT PAIN

FORMULA 44M®
(dextromethorphan hydrobromide,
pseudoephedrine hydrochloride,
guaifenesin, acetaminophen)

John

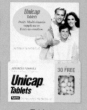

30 FREE
Unicap
Tablets

30 FREE
Unicap
Tablets

apsules
s of 90, 120,
0, 1000

Tablets
Bottles of
90, 120

UNICAP®
Capsules and Tablets
Multivitamin Supplement

UPSHER-SMITH

Lubrin

Lubrin

Lubrin

LUBRIN®
Vaginal Lubricating Inserts

Vicks Health Care Div.
Bottles of 6 oz. and 10 oz.

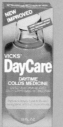

NEW IMPROVED
VICKS
DayCare
DAYTIME
COLDS MEDICINE

VICKS NEW IMPROVED
DayCare
DAYTIME
COLDS MEDICINE

DAYCARE®
Daytime Colds Medicine
(acetaminophen, pseudoephedrine
hydrochloride, dextromethorphan
hydrobromide, guaifenesin)

Vick Health Care Div.

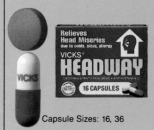

VICKS

Relieves
Head Miseries
due to colds, sinus, allergy
VICKS
HEADWAY
DECONGESTANT • ANALGESIC • ANTIHISTAMINE C
16 CAPSULES

Capsule Sizes: 16, 36

Also Available in Tablet Sizes:
20, 40

VICKS® HEADWAY®
(acetaminophen, phenylpropanolamine
hydrochloride and chlorpheniramine
maleate)

Vicks Health Care Div.

6 oz., 10 oz. and 14 oz.

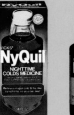

NYQUIL® NIGHTTIME COLDS MEDICINE
(acetaminophen, doxylamine succinate, pseudoephedrine hydrochloride, dextromethorphan hydrobromide)

Vicks Health Care Div.

1.5 oz., 3.0 oz., 6 oz.

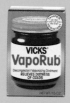

VICKS® VapoRub®
Decongestant Vaporizing Ointment

Special Vicks Medication
(menthol, camphor, eucalyptus oil, spirits of turpentine)

WALLACE

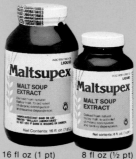

16 fl oz (1 pt)   8 fl oz (½ pt)
MALTSUPEX® LIQUID
(malt soup extract)

Wallace

1 pint (473 ml)

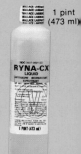

Also available: 4 fl oz (118 ml)
RYNA-CX® LIQUID
(antitussive-decongestant-expectorant)

Vicks Health Care Div.

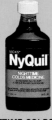

Available in ½ oz. and 1 oz. atomizers

SINEX™
Decongestant Nasal Spray
(phenylephrine hydrochloride, cetylpyridinium chloride)

Special Vicks Blend of Aromatics
(menthol, eucalyptol, camphor, methyl salicylate)

VICKS PHARMACY

Products Division

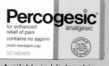

Available in blister strip boxes of 24 tablets and bottles of 50 and 90.

PERCOGESIC®
analgesic
(acetaminophen and phenyltoloxamine citrate)

Wallace

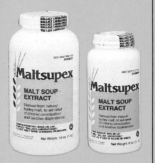

16 oz (1 lb)   8 oz (½ lb)
MALTSUPEX® POWDER
(malt soup extract)

Wallace

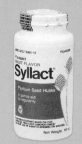

SYLLACT™
(powdered psyllium seed husks)

Vicks Health Care Div.

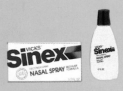

Available in ½ oz. and 1 oz. atomizers

SINEX™ LONG-ACTING
Decongestant Nasal Spray
(oxymetazoline hydrochloride)

VIDAL SASSOON, INC.

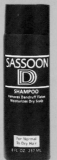

Available in 8 oz. & 12 oz.

For Normal to Dry Hair & Normal to Oily Hair

SASSOON D SHAMPOO

Removes loose dandruff flakes.
Moisturizes dry scalp.

Wallace

1 pint (473 ml)

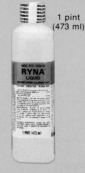

Also available: 4 fl oz (118 ml)
RYNA™ LIQUID
(antihistamine-decongestant)

WARNER-LAMBERT CO.

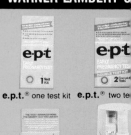

e.p.t.® one test kit   e.p.t.® two test kit

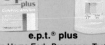

e.p.t.® plus
In-Home Early Pregnancy Test

Vicks Health Care Div.

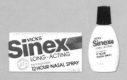

Available in ½ oz. and 1 oz. atomizers

SINEX™ LONG-ACTING

WAKUNAGA

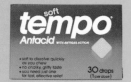

KYOLIC GARLIC®
Aged Garlic Extract

Super Formula 100
KYOLIC®
Capsules

Wallace

1 pint (473 ml)

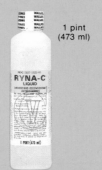

Also available: 4 fl oz (118 ml)
RYNA-C® LIQUID
(antitussive-antihistamine-decongestant)

Warner-Lambert Co.

Early Detector

EARLY DETECTOR™
In-Home Test
for Fecal Occult Blood

Vicks Health Care Div.

tempo
Antacid with antigas action

Available foil wrapped in boxes of 10, 30 and 60 soft drops.
TEMPO®
Antacid with antigas action
(calcium carbonate, aluminum hydroxide, magnesium hydroxide and simethicone)

Warner-Lambert Co.

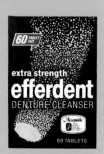

EXTRA STRENGTH EFFERDENT®

Denture Cleanser

Warner-Lambert Co.

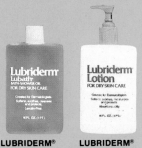

LUBRIDERM® LOTION

LUBRIDERM® LUBATH® BATH/SHOWER OIL

For Dry Skin Care

Warner-Lambert Inc.

Capsules

Tablets

**MAXIMUM STRENGTH SINUTAB®

Westwood

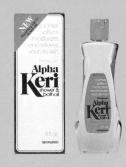

ALPHA KERI®
Shower & Bath Oil

Warner-Lambert Co.

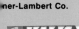
Sugar Free

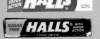

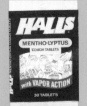

HALLS® Mentho-Lyptus®
Cough Tablets

Warner-Lambert Co.

12 squares

24 squares

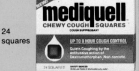

MEDIQUELL™
Chewy Cough Squares

Warner-Lambert Inc.

Capsules

Tablets

**MAXIMUM STRENGTH SINUTAB® II
**Product of Warner-Lambert Inc.,
Santurce, P.R. 00911

Westwood

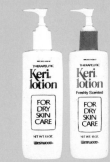

For dry skin

For dry skin (scented)

KERI® LOTION

Warner-Lambert Co.

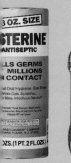

18 oz.

LISTERINE® ANTISEPTIC

Warner-Lambert Co.

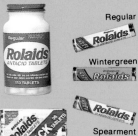

Regular

Wintergreen

Spearmint

ROLAIDS®

Fast, Safe, Lasting Relief from
Heartburn, Sour Stomach or Acid
Indigestion and Upset Stomach
Associated with these Symptoms.

FOSTEX®
5% benzoyl peroxide gel

FOSTEX®
10% benzoyl
peroxide gel
(vanishing)

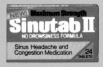

FOSTEX®
10% benzoyl
peroxide cream
(tinted)

Medicated Cleansing Bars

10% benzoyl peroxide

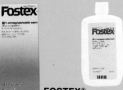

FOSTEX®
10% benzoyl peroxide wash

Westwood

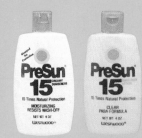

Creamy Sunscreen   Sunscreen Lotion
PRESUN® 15
15 Times Natural Protection

Westwood

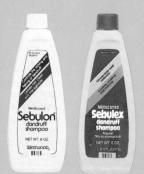

SEBULON®   **SEBULEX®**
Medicated Dandruff Shampoos

Warner-Lambert Co.

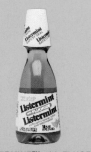

LISTERMINT™ with FLUORIDE
Anticavity Dental Rinse &
Mouth Wash

Easy-to-open package
(Non-child resistant)

Child-resistant package
**REGULAR SINUTAB®

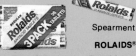

For more detailed information on products illustrated in this section, consult the Product Information Section or manufacturers may be contacted directly.

WHITEHALL

200 mg.    Advil

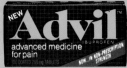

Coated Tablets in Bottles of
24, 50 and 100

ADVIL™
Ibuprofen Tablets, USP

Whitehall

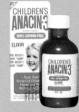 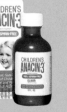
Front   Back
80 mg.

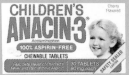

Bottles of 30 tablets.
CHILDREN'S ANACIN-3®
Acetaminophen Chewable Tablets

2 and 4 fl. oz. bottles with convenient
dosage cup.

CHILDREN'S ANACIN-3®
Acetaminophen Elixir

Whitehall

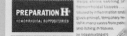
A
500

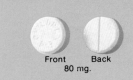

Available in Bottles of
24, 60 and 125
**Safety Coated
APF®
ARTHRITIS PAIN
FORMULA™**
by the makers of ANACIN®
Analgesic Tablets

Whitehall

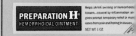

Ointment

Suppositories

PREPARATION H®
Hemorrhoidal Ointment
and Suppositories

Whitehall

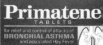

Lotion: 4 oz., 8 oz. and
12 oz. Bottles

Gel: 2 oz. and
4 oz. Tubes

DENOREX®
Medicated Shampoo

Whitehall

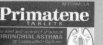

Available in 15
Inhaler Unit and
15 cc. and 22.5
Refills.

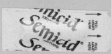

PRIMATENE® MIST

Asthma Remedy

Whitehall

Available in Tins of 12 and Bottles of
30, 50, 100, 200 and 300

ANACIN®
Analgesic Tablets

Whitehall

Liquid
.31 oz.
and
.74 oz.

Gel
.25 oz.

Baby Teething
Gel
.25 oz.

ANBESOL®
Antiseptic—Anesthetic

Whitehall

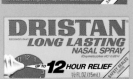

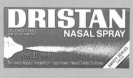

Both Available in Bottles of
15 ml. and 30 ml.

DRISTAN®
Nasal Spray

Whitehall   Front   Back

P FORMULA

for relief and control of attacks of
BRONCHIAL ASTHMA
and associated Hay Fever
60 TABLETS

P Formula

M Formula
Both Available in Bottles of 24
60 Tablets
PRIMATENE® TABLETS
Asthma Remedy

Whitehall

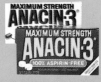
Front   Back
500 mg.

MAXIMUM STRENGTH
ANACIN-3

Coated Tablets: Tins of 12. Bottles of 30,
60, 100. Capsules: Bottles of 24, 50, 72.

MAXIMUM STRENGTH ANACIN-3®
Acetaminophen Tablets and Capsules

Whitehall

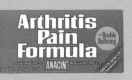

Available in Bottles of 40, 100 and
175 Tablets

ARTHRITIS PAIN FORMULA
by the makers of ANACIN®
Analgesic Tablets

Whitehall

Front   Back   DRISTAN   DRISTAN

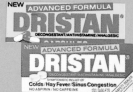

Capsules: Bottles of 20, 40
Tablets: Tins of 12; Bottles of 24 50, 100

DRISTAN® CAPSULES AND TABLETS
Decongestant/Antihistamine/Analgesic

Whitehall

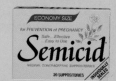

Available in Packages of 10 and 20

SEMICID®
Vaginal Contraceptive
Suppositories

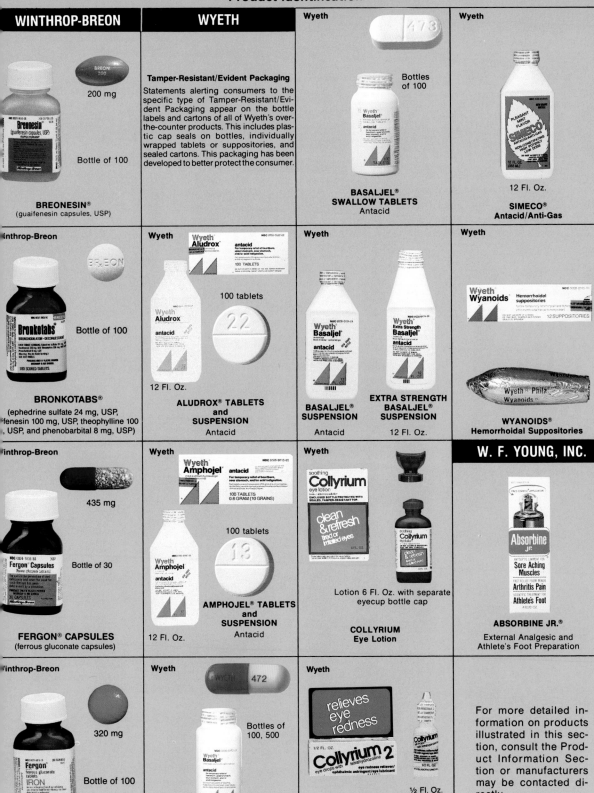

WINTHROP-BREON

BREONESIN®
(guaifenesin capsules, USP)

200 mg

Bottle of 100

Winthrop-Breon

BRONKOTABS®
(ephedrine sulfate 24 mg, USP,
guaifenesin 100 mg, USP, theophylline 100
mg, USP, and phenobarbital 8 mg, USP)

Bottle of 100

Winthrop-Breon

FERGON® CAPSULES
(ferrous gluconate capsules)

435 mg

Bottle of 30

Winthrop-Breon

FERGON® TABLETS
(ferrous gluconate tablets)

320 mg

Bottle of 100

WYETH

Tamper-Resistant/Evident Packaging
Statements alerting consumers to the specific type of Tamper-Resistant/Evident Packaging appear on the bottle labels and cartons of all of Wyeth's over-the-counter products. This includes plastic cap seals on bottles, individually wrapped tablets or suppositories, and sealed cartons. This packaging has been developed to better protect the consumer.

Wyeth

100 tablets

**ALUDROX® TABLETS
and
SUSPENSION**

Antacid

12 Fl. Oz.

Wyeth

100 tablets

**AMPHOJEL® TABLETS
and
SUSPENSION**

Antacid

12 Fl. Oz.

Wyeth

Bottles of
100, 500

BASALJEL® CAPSULES

Antacid

Wyeth

Bottles
of 100

**BASALJEL®
SWALLOW TABLETS**

Antacid

Wyeth

**BASALJEL®
SUSPENSION**

Antacid

**EXTRA STRENGTH
BASALJEL®
SUSPENSION**

12 Fl. Oz.

Wyeth

**COLLYRIUM
Eye Lotion**

Lotion 6 Fl. Oz. with separate
eyecup bottle cap

Wyeth

relieves
eye
redness

Collyrium 2
eye redness reliever/
ophthalmic astringent/eye lubricant

½ Fl. Oz.

COLLYRIUM₂™

Eye Drops with
Tetrahydrozoline

Wyeth

**SIMECO®
Antacid/Anti-Gas**

12 Fl. Oz.

Wyeth

**WYANOIDS®
Hemorrhoidal Suppositories**

W. F. YOUNG, INC.

Absorbine Jr.
Sore Aching
Muscles
Arthritis Pain
Athlete's Foot

ABSORBINE JR.®

External Analgesic and
Athlete's Foot Preparation

For more detailed information on products illustrated in this section, consult the Product Information Section or manufacturers may be contacted directly.

Product Information Section

This section is made possible through the courtesy of the manufacturers whose products appear on the following pages. The information concerning each product has been prepared, edited and approved by the manufacturer.

Products described in this edition comply with labeling regulations. Copy may include all the essential information necessary for informed usage such as active ingredients, indications, actions, warnings, drug interactions, precautions, symptoms and treatment of oral overdosage, dosage and administration, professional labeling, and how supplied. In some cases additional information has been supplied to complement the foregoing. The Publisher has emphasized to manufacturers the necessity of describing products comprehensively so that all information essential for intelligent and informed use is available. In organizing and presenting the material in this edition the Publisher is providing all the information available by manufacturers.

In presenting the following material to the medical profession, the Publisher is not necessarily advocating the use of any product.

Abbott Laboratories—

Abbott Pharmaceuticals, Inc.

Pharmaceutical Products Division
NORTH CHICAGO, IL 60064

OPTILETS®–500
High potency multivitamin
for use in treatment of
multivitamin deficiency.*

OPTILETS–M–500®
High potency multivitamin
for use in treatment of
multivitamin deficiency.*
Mineral supplementation added.**

Description: A therapeutic formula of
ten important vitamins, with and without minerals, in a small tablet with the
Abbott Filmtab® coating. Each Optilets-
500 tablet provides:

Vitamin C
　(as sodium ascorbate) ....500 mg
Niacinamide ....100 mg
Calcium Pantothenate ....20 mg
Vitamin B₁
　(thiamine mononitrate) ....15 mg
Vitamin B₂ (riboflavin) ....10 mg
Vitamin B₆
　(pyridoxine hydrochloride) ....5 mg
Vitamin A (as palmitate
　1.5 mg, as acetate 1.5 mg—
　total 3 mg) ....10,000 IU
Vitamin B₁₂
　(cyanocobalamin) ....12 mcg
Vitamin D
　(cholecalciferol) ....(10 mcg) 400 IU
Vitamin E (as dl-alpha
　tocopheryl acetate) ....30 IU
Each Optilets-M-500 Filmtab contains
all the vitamins (vitamin C—ascorbic
acid) in the same quantities provided in
Optilets-500, plus the following minerals:
Magnesium (as oxide) ....80 mg**
Iron (as dried ferrous sulfate) ..20 mg
Copper (as sulfate) ....2 mg
Zinc (as sulfate) ....1.5 mg**
Manganese (as sulfate) ....1 mg
Iodine (as calcium iodate) ......0.15 mg
* These products contain no folic acid
and only dietary supplement levels of
vitamins D and E.
** Below USRDA levels.

Dosage and Administration: Usual
adult dosage is one Filmtab tablet daily,
or as directed by physician.

How Supplied: Optilets-500 tablets
are supplied in bottles of 100 (**NDC** 0074-
4287-13). Optilets-M-500 tablets are supplied in bottles of 30 (**NDC** 0074-4286-30)
and 100 (**NDC** 0074-4286-13).
Abbott Laboratories
North Chicago, IL 60064

SURBEX–T®
High-potency vitamin B-complex*
with 500 mg of vitamin C

Description: Each Filmtab® tablet
provides:
Vitamin C (ascorbic acid) ....500 mg
Niacinamide ....100 mg
Calcium Pantothenate ....20 mg

Vitamin B₁ (thiamine
　mononitrate) ....15 mg
Vitamin B₂ (riboflavin) ....10 mg
Vitamin B₆ (pyridoxine
　hydrochloride) ....5 mg
Vitamin B₁₂ (cyanocobalamin) ...10 mcg

Indications: For use in treatment of
Vitamin B-Complex* with Vitamin C
deficiency.
* Contains no folic acid; not for treatment of folate deficiency.

Dosage and Administration: Usual
adult dosage is one Filmtab tablet daily,
or as directed by physician.

How Supplied: Orange-colored tablets
in bottles of 50 (**NDC** 0074-4878-50), 100
(**NDC** 0074-4878-13), and 500 (**NDC** 0074-
4878-53). Also supplied in Abbo-Pac®
unit dose packages of 100 tablets in strips
of 10 tablets per strip (**NDC** 0074-4878-
11). ®Filmtab—Film-sealed Tablets, Abbott.
Abbott Pharmaceuticals, Inc.
North Chicago, IL 60064
Ref. 03-1074-5/R7

SURBEX®–750 with IRON
High-potency B-complex with iron,
vitamin E and 750 mg vitamin C

Description: Each Filmtab® tablet
provides:
VITAMINS
Vitamin C (as sodium ascorbate)　750 mg
Niacinamide .... 100 mg
Vitamin B₆ (pyridoxine
　hydrochloride) .... 25 mg
Calcium Pantothenate .... 20 mg
Vitamin B₁ (thiamine
　mononitrate) .... 15 mg
Vitamin B₂ (riboflavin) .... 15 mg
Vitamin B₁₂ (cyanocobalamin)　12 mcg
Folic Acid ....400 mcg
Vitamin E (as dl-alpha tocopheryl
　acetate) .... 30 IU
MINERAL
Elemental Iron (as dried
　ferrous sulfate) .... 27 mg
　equivalent to 135 mg ferrous sulfate

Indications: For the treatment of vitamin C and B-complex deficiencies and to
supplement the daily intake of iron and
vitamin E.

Dosage and Administration: Usual
adult dosage is one tablet daily or as directed by physician.

How Supplied: Bottles of 50 tablets
(**NDC** 0074-8029-50)
Abbott Pharmaceuticals, Inc.
North Chicago, IL 60064
Ref. 03-1120-3/R5

SURBEX®–750 with ZINC
High-Potency B-Complex with zinc,
vitamin E and 750 mg of vitamin C.
For persons 12 years of age or older

Description: Daily dose (one Film-
tab® tablet) provides:

	%U.S.
VITAMINS	**R.D.A.***
Vitamin E .... 30 IU 100%	
Vitamin C ....750 mg ... 1250%	
Folic Acid .... 0.4 mg ... 100%	
Thiamine (B₁) .... 15 mg 1000%	
Riboflavin (B₂) .... 15 mg 882%	
Niacin ....100 mg 500%	
Vitamin B₆ .... 20 mg 1000%	
Vitamin B₁₂ .... 12 mcg 200%	
Pantothenic Acid ..... 20 mg 200%	

MINERAL
Zinc** ....22.5 mg 150%
* % U.S. Recommended Daily Allow-
ance for Adults.
** Equivalent to 100 mg of zinc sulfate.

Ingredients: Ascorbic acid, niacinamide, cellulose, dl-alpha tocopheryl acetate, zinc sulfate, povidone, pyridoxine
hydrochloride, calcium pantothenate,
riboflavin, thiamine mononitrate,
cyanocobalamin, magnesium stearate,
colloidal silicon dioxide, folic acid, in a
film-coated tablet with vanillin flavoring
and artificial coloring added.
Usual Adult Dose: One tablet daily.

How Supplied: Bottles of 50 tablets
(**NDC** 0074-8152-50).
Abbott Pharmaceuticals, Inc.
North Chicago, IL 60064
Ref. 03-1121-4/R8

*If desired, additional information on
any Abbott Product will be provided
upon request to Abbott Laboratories.*

Adria Laboratories
Division of Erbamont Inc.
5000 POST ROAD
DUBLIN, OH 43017

MODANE®
(danthron)
Tablets and Liquid

Description: MODANE® Tablets
(yellow)—Each tablet contains danthron
75 mg.
MODANE® MILD Tablets—Each tablet
contains danthron 37.5 mg.
MODANE® Liquid—Each 5 ml (teaspoonful) contains danthron 37.5 mg and
alcohol 5%.
Danthron is classified as a stimulant laxative and is chemically 1,8-dihydroxy-
anthraquinone. Its chemical structure is:

danthron

The empirical formula is $C_{14}H_8O_4$ and
the molecular weight is 240.21. It is practically insoluble in water.

Clinical Pharmacology: Stimulant
cathartics act on the intestinal mucosa
and have effects both on the net absorption of electrolytes and water and on motility. This group includes danthron, the
docusates, castor oil, and bile acids. Despite similarity of their mechanism of
action, there are differences among these
drugs which are due, for the most part, to

dosage and the major site of action, i.e. small intestine or colon.

Anthraquinone cathartics vary in their effects depending upon their anthraquinone content and the ease of liberation of the active constituents from their inactive precursor glycosides. Danthron, although a free anthraquinone, is similar to the pro-drug glycosides in its pharmacological properties. A soft or semifluid stool is passed 6 to 8 hours after administration of an anthraquinone glycoside cathartic such as danthron.

Danthron is absorbed from the small intestine to a limited extent, circulated through the portal system and into the general circulation and excreted in the bile, urine, saliva, colonic mucosa and milk.

Indications and Usage: MODANE is indicated for the management of constipation. It may be useful in the management of constipation in geriatric, cardiac, surgical and postpartum patients. MODANE may be useful in the management of constipation which may occur with or during the concomitant use of antihypertensive agents, ganglionic blocking agents, antihistamines, tranquilizers, sympathomimetics and anticholinergics. A soft or semifluid stool is passed 6 to 8 hours after administration. Adequate bulk should be provided in the diet and, if the diet does not provide sufficient bulk, by hydrophilic bulking agents. Poor bowel habits should be corrected.

Contraindications: Should not be used when abdominal pain, nausea, vomiting or other signs and/or symptoms of appendicitis are present.

Precautions: *General*—MODANE may cause harmless pink discoloration of urine (the urine may be pink-red, redviolet or red-brown if alkaline).
As with all laxatives, frequent or prolonged use may result in dependence.
Drug Interactions—The absorption of danthron from the gastrointestinal tract and/or its uptake by hepatic cells may be increased by the co-administration of docusate.
Carcinogenesis, Mutagenesis, Impairment of Fertility—There have been no long term studies of MODANE to evaluate carcinogenic potential. There have been no studies to evaluate mutagenic potential or whether MODANE has the potential to impair fertility.
Teratogenic Effects—Pregnancy Category C. Animal reproduction studies have not been conducted with danthron. It is also not known whether danthron can cause fetal harm when administered to a pregnant woman or can affect reproductive capacity. MODANE should be given to a pregnant woman only if clearly needed.
Nursing Mothers—Danthron is excreted in human milk and has been reported to increase bowel activity in infants nursed by women taking it. Caution should be exercised when MODANE is administered to a nursing woman.

Pediatric Use—In general stimulant cathartics should seldom be used in children.

Adverse Reactions: Adverse reactions are uncommon. These are in order of frequency: excessive bowel activity (griping, diarrhea, nausea, vomiting), peri-anal irritation, weakness, dizziness, palpitations and sweating. Temporary brownish mucosal staining has occurred with prolonged use. There has also been reported a suspected allergic reaction with facial swelling, redness and discomfort.

Overdosage: The lowest reported lethal dose in mice and rats is 500 mg/kg. Overdosage may be expected to result in excessive bowel activity. Treatment is symptomatic when the duration of effects is prolonged.

Dosage and Administration: MODANE Tablet (yellow)–Adults—1 tablet with evening meal.
MODANE MILD Tablets (half-strength, pink)–Adults—1 or 2 tablets with the evening meal. For adults who have previously responded with excessive bowel activity to a mild laxative or who are diet-restricted or who are bedfast and for children 6–12 years of age—1 tablet with the evening meal.
MODANE Liquid–Adults—1 to 2 teaspoonfuls with the evening meal. For adults who have previously responded with excessive bowel activity to a mild laxative or who are diet-restricted or who are bedfast and children who are 6–12 years of age—1 teaspoonful with the evening meal.

How Supplied: Each MODANE Tablet contains danthron 75 mg in a yellow, round, sugar coated tablet, coded 13 501.
NDC 0013-5011-17 Bottle of 100 Tablets
NDC 0013-5011-23 Bottle of 1000 Tablets
NDC 0013-5011-18 STAT-PAK® (unit dose) 100 Tablets
NDC 0013-5011-07 Package of 10 Tablets
NDC 0013-5011-13 Package of 30 Tablets
Store at room temperature.
Each MODANE MILD Tablet contains danthron 37.5 mg in a pink, round, sugar coated tablet, coded 13 502.
NDC 0013-5021-17 Bottle of 100 tablets
Store at room temperature.
Each 5 ml (teaspoonful) of MODANE Liquid contains danthron 37.5 mg in a red liquid.
NDC 0013-5033-51 Pint Bottles
Protect from cold.
Shown in Product Identification Section, page 403

MODANE® BULK
(psyllium and dextrose)

Description: MODANE BULK is a powdered mixture of equal parts of psyllium, a bulking agent, and dextrose, as a dispersing agent. Psyllium is a highly efficient dietary fiber derived from the husk of the seed of *Plantago ovata*. Each rounded teaspoonful contains approximately 3.5 g psyllium, 3.5 g dextrose, 2 mg sodium and 37 mg potassium, and provides 14 calories.

Clinical Pharmacology: Psyllium absorbs water and expands. When taken with adequate amounts of water, it increases the water content and bulk volume of the stool. The initial response usually occurs in 12 to 24 hours but, in patients who have used laxatives chronically, up to three days may elapse before the initial response.

Indications and Usage: MODANE BULK is indicated in the treatment of constipation resulting from a diet low in residue. It is used also as adjunctive therapy in patients with diverticular disease, spastic or irritable colon, hemorrhoids, in pregnancy, and in convalescent and senile patients.

Contraindications: Intestinal obstruction, fecal impaction.

Precautions: *General*—Impaction or obstruction may occur if the bulk-forming agent is temporarily arrested in its passage through parts of the alimentary canal. In this case, water is absorbed and the bolus may become inspissated. Use of this product in patients with narrowing of the intestinal lumen may be hazardous. Inspissation should not occur in a normal gastrointestinal tract if the product is taken with one or more glasses of water.
Drug Interactions—Psyllium may combine with certain other drugs. Products containing psyllium should not be taken with salicylates, digitalis and other cardiac glycosides, or nitrofurantoin.

Adverse Reactions: Adverse reactions are uncommon, and most often have resulted from inadequate intake of water or from underlying organic disease. Esophageal, gastric, small intestinal and rectal obstruction have resulted from the accumulation of the mucilaginous components of psyllium.

Dosage and Administration: Adults and children over 12 years of age—ONE ROUNDED TEASPOONFUL ONE TO THREE TIMES DAILY STIRRED INTO AN 8 OUNCE GLASS OF WATER, JUICE OR OTHER SUITABLE LIQUID AND PREFERABLY FOLLOWED BY A SECOND GLASSFUL OF LIQUID. Children 6 to 12 years of age—one-half the adult dose in 8 ounces of liquid.

How Supplied: Each rounded teaspoonful of MODANE BULK powder contains approximately 3.5 g psyllium.
NDC 0013-5025-72 14 oz. container.
Store at room temperature.

MODANE® PLUS
(danthron and docusate sodium)
Tablets

Description: Each MODANE PLUS tablet contains danthron 50 mg and docusate sodium 100 mg. Danthron is classified as a stimulant cathartic and docusate sodium is a stool softener. Chemically, docusate sodium is sulfobutanedioic acid 1,4-bis (2-ethylhexyl) ester sodium salt and danthron is 1,8-

Continued on next page

Adria—Cont.

dihydroxyanthraquinone. The empirical formula of docusate sodium is $C_{20}H_{37}O_7SNa$ and its molecular weight is 444.56. The empirical formula of danthron is $C_{14}H_8O_4$ and its molecular weight is 240.21.

$$COOCH_2CH(CH_2)_3CH_3$$
$$CH_2$$
$$CH-SO_3Na$$
$$COOCH_2CH(CH_2)_3CH_3$$

danthron   docusate sodium

Danthron is practically insoluble in water. At 25°C the solubility of docusate sodium in water is 15 g/1.

Clinical Pharmacology: Contact cathartics act on the intestinal mucosa and have effects both on the net absorption of electrolytes and water and on motility. This group includes danthron, the docusates, castor oil, and bile acids. Despite similarity of their mechanism of action, there are differences among these drugs which are due, for the most part, to dosage and the major site of action, i.e. small intestine or colon.

Anthraquinone cathartics vary in their effects depending upon their anthraquinone content and the ease of liberation of the active constituents from their precursor glycosides. Danthron, although a free anthraquinone, is similar to the prodrug glycosides in its pharmacological properties. A soft or semifluid stool is passed 6 to 8 hours after administration of an anthraquinone glycoside cathartic or danthron.

Hydration of the stool has been attributed to docusate sodium's surfactant effect on the intestinal contents which was assumed to facilitate penetration of the fecal mass by water and lipids. Although this emollient effect may exist, there is evidence that mucosal permeability is increased and water absorption is inhibited in the jejunum. Similar concentrations inhibit colonic absorption and/or increase intraluminal water and electrolytes. In these respects docusate sodium is similar to bile salts and in this manner may also be considered as a stimulant laxative.

Danthron is absorbed from the small intestine to a limited extent, circulated through the portal system and into the general circulation and excreted in the bile, urine, saliva, colonic mucosa and milk.

Docusate sodium is absorbed to some extent in the duodenum and proximal jejunum. It appears in the bile.

Indications and Usage: MODANE PLUS is indicated for the management of constipation where a combination of a stimulant plus a stool softener is needed. It may be useful in geriatric or inactive patients, following surgery, and in patients refractory to other laxatives (see MODANE, MODANE SOFT and MODANE BULK). Adequate bulk should be provided in the diet and, if the diet does not provide sufficient bulk, by hydrophilic bulking agents (MODANE BULK). Poor bowel habits should be corrected.

Contraindications: Mineral oil administration, or when abdominal pain, nausea, vomiting or other signs and/or symptoms of appendicitis are present.

Precautions: *General*—It may cause harmless discoloration of urine (the urine may be pink-red, red-violet or red-brown if alkaline).

As with all laxatives, frequent or prolonged use may result in dependence.

Drug Interactions—Docusate sodium may increase the intestinal absorption and/or hepatic uptake of other drugs administered concurrently.

Carcinogenesis, Mutagenesis, Impairment of Fertility—There have been no long term studies of MODANE PLUS to evaluate carcinogenic potential. There have been no studies to evaluate mutagenic potential or to determine whether MODANE PLUS has the potential to impair fertility.

Teratogenic Effects—Pregnancy Category C. Animal reproduction studies have not been conducted with danthron and docusate sodium. It is also not known whether MODANE PLUS can cause fetal harm when administered to a pregnant woman or can affect reproductive capacity. MODANE PLUS should be given to a pregnant woman only if clearly needed.

Nursing Mothers—Danthron is excreted in human milk and has been reported to increase bowel activity in infants nursed by women taking it. Caution should be exercised when MODANE PLUS is administered to a nursing woman.

Pediatric Use—Because of its dosage size, MODANE PLUS is not recommended for use by children less than 12 years.

Adverse Reactions: Adverse reactions are uncommon. These are in order of frequency: Excessive bowel activity (griping, diarrhea, nausea, vomiting), peri-anal irritation, weakness, dizziness, palpitations and sweating. Temporary brownish mucosal staining has occurred with prolonged use. There have also been reports of rash and a report of facial swelling, redness and discomfort.

Overdosage: Docusates and danthron have low potential for toxicity. The oral LD_{50} values of danthron, docusate sodium and danthron—docusate sodium combination in mice were greater than 7 g/kg, 2.64 g/kg and 3.44 g/kg, respectively. The lowest reported lethal dose of danthron in mice and rats is 500 mg/kg. Single doses of docusate sodium, as large as 50 mg/kg, have not produced adverse effects in children. Overdosage may be expected to result in anorexia, vomiting and diarrhea. Treatment is symptomatic when the duration of effects is prolonged.

Dosage and Administration: Adults and children over 12 years of age—1 tablet daily with evening meal.

How Supplied: Each MODANE PLUS tablet contains a combination of danthron 50 mg and docusate sodium 100 mg in a brown, round, sugar coated tablet coded 13 504.
NDC 0013-5041-13 30 Tablet Package
NDC 0013-5041-17 Bottle of 100 Tablets
Store at room temperature
AHFS 56:12
Shown in Product Identification Section, page 403

MODANE® SOFT
(docusate sodium)
Capsules

Description: Each MODANE SOFT capsule contains docusate sodium 100 mg. in a soft gelatin capsule. Docusate sodium is classified as a stool softener. Chemically, docusate sodium is sulfobutanedioic acid 1,4-bis (2-ethylhexyl) ester sodium salt. The chemical structure is:

$$COOCH_2CH(CH_2)_3CH_3$$
$$CH_2$$
$$CH-SO_3Na$$
$$COOCH_2CH(CH_2)_3CH_3$$

docusate sodium

The empirical formula is $C_{20}H_{37}O_7SNa$ and the molecular weight is 444.56. At 25°C the solubility of docusate sodium in water is 15 g/l.

Clinical Pharmacology: Hydration of the stool has been attributed to the drug's surfactant effect on the intestinal contents which was assumed to facilitate penetration of the fecal mass by water and lipids. Although this emollient effect may exist, there is evidence that mucosal permeability is increased and water absorption is inhibited in the jejunum. Similar concentrations inhibit colonic absorption and/or increase intraluminal water and electrolytes. In these respects, it is similar to bile salts and in this manner, may also be considered as a stimulant laxative.

Docusate sodium is absorbed to some extent in the duodenum and proximal jejunum. It appears in the bile.

Indications and Usage: MODANE SOFT is indicated for the management of functional constipation associated with dry hard stools. It is especially useful when it is desirable to lessen the strain of defecation (e.g. in persons with painful rectal lesions, hernia or cardiovascular disease). The effect on the stools may not be apparent until 1–3 days after the first dose.

Contraindications: Mineral oil administration or when abdominal pain, nausea, vomiting, or other signs and/or symptoms of appendicitis are present.

Precautions: *Drug Interactions*—MODANE SOFT may increase the intestinal absorption of mineral oil and may increase the intestinal absorption and/or hepatic uptake of other drugs administered concurrently.

Carcinogenesis, Mutagenesis, Impairment of Fertility—There have been no long term studies of docusate to evaluate carcinogenic potential. There have been no studies to evaluate mutagenic potential or to determine whether docusate has the potential to impair fertility.

Teratogenic Effects—Pregnancy Category C. Animal reproduction studies have not been conducted with docusate. It is also not known whether MODANE SOFT can cause fetal harm when administered to a pregnant woman or can affect reproductive capacity. MODANE SOFT should be given to a pregnant woman only if clearly needed.

Nursing Mothers—It is not known whether this drug is excreted in human milk. Caution should be exercised when MODANE SOFT is administered to a nursing woman.

Pediatric Use—Because of its dosage size, MODANE SOFT is not recommended for use by children less than 6 years of age.

Adverse Reactions: Adverse reactions are uncommon. Diarrhea, cramping pains and rash have been reported.

Overdosage: Docusates have a low potential for toxicity. Single doses as large as 50 mg/kg have not produced adverse effects in children. Anorexia, vomiting and diarrhea may result from overdosage.

Dosage and Administration: Adults and children over 12 years of age—1 to 3 capsules daily. Children 6–12 years of age—one capsule daily.

How Supplied: Each MODANE SOFT green, soft gelatin capsule contains docusate sodium 100 mg coded 13 503.

NDC 0013-5031-13 Package of 30 Capsules

Store at controlled room temperature (59°– 86°F, 15°–30°C).

MYOFLEX® CREME
(Trolamine Salicylate)

Description: Trolamine (formerly Triethanolamine) salicylate 10% in a nongreasy base is a nonirritating, nonburning, odorless, stainless, readily absorbed creme. Trolamine salicylate is a topical analgesic. The empirical formula of trolamine salicylate is $C_6H_{15}NO_3 \cdot C_7H_6O_3$, molecular weight 287.31. Its chemical structure is:

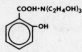

Trolamine salicylate is a light reddish viscous liquid with a faint odor. It is miscible in all proportions with water, glycerin, propylene glycol, and ethyl alcohol.

Clinical Pharmacology: Salicylic acid is the active moiety of MYOFLEX. Salicylic acid is enzymatically biotransformed to salicyluric acid and salicylphenolic glucuronide and eliminated in the urine. Salicylic acid is rapidly distributed throughout all body tissues, mainly by pH-dependent passive processes. It can be detected in synovial, spinal and peritoneal fluids, in saliva and in milk. It readily crosses the placental barrier. About 50% to 90% of salicylic acid is bound to plasma proteins, mainly to albumin.

The urinary excretion of salicylic acid equivalents was studied in 12 normal, healthy male subjects after MYOFLEX application. Salicylic acid was absorbed from MYOFLEX in 11 of 12 normal subjects over the 24-hour period post-application with a mean salicylic acid excretion of 13.5%.

Trolamine salicylate does not block neuronal membranes as do topical anesthetics. Some degree of percutaneous absorption occurs through the skin and blood levels have been demonstrated following topical application in animals and humans. Trolamine salicylate is not a counterirritant analgesic.

Indications: MYOFLEX is indicated as a topical analgesic for the temporary relief of minor aches and pains of muscles and joints due to muscle strains, sprains and bruises or overexertion. It is a useful topical adjunct in arthritis and rheumatism as a cream for patients with minor rheumatic stiffness or sore hands and feet.

Contraindications: MYOFLEX is contraindicated in patients sensitive to its ingredients and patients with advanced chronic renal insufficiency.

Warnings: For external use only. Avoid contact with eyes or mucous membranes. Keep out of the reach of children. If condition worsens, or if symptoms persist for more than 7 days, or clear up and occur again within a few days, discontinue use and consult a doctor.

As with any drug, if you are pregnant or nursing a baby, seek the advice of a health professional before using this product.

As with all salicylates, MYOFLEX should be avoided or used with caution in patients with liver damage, pre-existing hypoprothrombinemia, vitamin K deficiency and before surgery.

Precautions: General—Apply to affected parts only. Do not apply to broken or irritated skin.

Appropriate precautions should be taken by persons known to be sensitive to salicylates or with impairment of renal function. If a reaction develops, the drug should be discontinued.

Drug Interactions—There are no known drug interactions with MYOFLEX. However, salicylates may counteract the effects of uricosuric agents such as probenecid and enhance the effects of oral anticoagulants such as coumadin. Therefore, they must be used with caution in patients on anticoagulants that affect the prothrombin time. Caution should also be exercised in patients concurrently treated with a sulfo-nylurea hypoglycemic agent, methotrexate, barbiturates and diphenylhydantoin, because these drugs may be displaced from plasma protein binding sites by salicylate resulting in an enhanced effect. Diphenylhydantoin intoxication has been precipitated by concomitant use of aspirin. The diuretic action of spironolactone is inhibited by salicylates.

Usage in Pregnancy (Category C)—Studies have not been performed in animals or humans to determine whether this drug affects fertility in males or females, has mutagenic, carcinogenic or teratogenic potential or other adverse effects on the fetus. Aspirin causes testicular atrophy and inhibition of spermatogenesis in animals and has been shown to be teratogenic in animals and to increase the incidence of still births and neonatal deaths in pregnant women. As with other salicylates, MYOFLEX should be used during pregnancy only if the potential benefit justifies the potential risk to the fetus.

Chronic, high dose salicylate therapy of pregnant women increases the length of gestation and the frequency of post-maturity and prolongs spontaneous labor. It is, therefore, recommended that MYOFLEX be taken during the last three months of pregnancy only under the close supervision of a physician.

Nursing Mothers—Salicylates are excreted in the breast milk of nursing mothers. Caution should be therefore exercised when MYOFLEX is administered to a nursing woman.

Pediatric Use—Safety and effectiveness of MYOFLEX in children have not been established.

Adverse Reactions: If applied to large skin areas, the absorbed salicylate may cause typical salicylate side effects such as tinnitus, nausea, or vomiting.

Overdosage: Acute overdosage with MYOFLEX is unlikely. A 2 oz. MYOFLEX tube contains the salicylate equivalent of about 56 grains of aspirin. Early signs and symptoms from repeated large doses consist of headache, dizziness, tinnitus (which may be absent in children or the elderly), difficulty in hearing, dimness of vision, mental confusion, lassitude, drowsiness, sweating, thirst, hyperventilation, nausea, vomiting and occasionally diarrhea. Treatment of acute salicylate poisoning is a medical emergency and should be undertaken in a hospital.

Dosage and Administration: Adults—Rub into painful or sore area two or three times daily. Wrists, elbows, knees or ankles may be wrapped loosely with 2″ or 3″ elastic bandage after application.

How Supplied:
NDC 0013-5404-61 Tubes, 2 oz.
NDC 0013-5404-60 Tubes, 4 oz.
NDC 0013-5404-65 Jars, 8 oz.
NDC 0013-5404-74 Jars, 1 lb.
Store at controlled room temperature (15–30°C, 59–86°F) (jars).

Continued on next page

Adria—Cont.

Protect from freezing or excessive heat (tubes).

Shown in Product Identification Section, page 403

Alberto-Culver Company
2525 ARMITAGE AVENUE
MELROSE PARK, IL 60160

MRS. DASH™
Salt Alternative

Description: Mrs. Dash and Mrs. Dash Low Pepper/No Garlic are all natural blends of herbs and spices to be used as an alternative to salt (NaCl). Because these blends are made of all natural ingredients there is no bitter, metallic aftertaste often associated with salt substitutes.

Uses: Use Mrs. Dash at the table or in cooking. Season meats, poultry, fish, salads, anything without using salt. Mrs. Dash is a healthier way to great eating for the whole family. Approved for low sodium diets.

Ingredients: Onion, spices (peppers, celery seed, basil, bay, marjoram, oregano, savory, thyme, coriander, cumin, mustard and rosemary), garlic (dill is substituted for garlic in no garlic product), carrots, corn syrup solids, tomato granules, bell peppers, lemon juice powder, citric acid, orange peel, oil of lemon. Contains 5 mg. of sodium/tsp. or 140 mg./100 g., and 19 mg. of potassium/tsp. or 1130 mg./100 g.

How Supplied: 2.5 oz. plastic container with shaker top.

SUGARTWIN®
Low Calorie Sugar Replacement

Active Ingredient: Soluble Saccharin

Indications: SugarTwin is a low calorie alternative to sugar as a sweetener in coffee, tea, for baking or for wherever a sweetener is appropriate. Each equivalent teaspoon of SugarTwin contains only 1½ calories.
NOTE TO DIABETICS: This product may be useful in your diet on the advice of a physician. SugarTwin can be used in conjunction with your food exchange program. Usage of 8 packets per day equals one List 2 Vegetable Exchange in calories only (24 calories)—not in protein, vitamins or minerals.

Warnings: USE OF THIS PRODUCT MAY BE HAZARDOUS TO YOUR HEALTH. THIS PRODUCT CONTAINS SACCHARIN WHICH HAS BEEN DETERMINED TO CAUSE CANCER IN LABORATORY ANIMALS

Dosage and Administration: One SugarTwin packet contains the equivalent sweetness of two teaspoons of sugar. White and brown granulated SugarTwin pour and measure spoon for spoon like sugar.

How Supplied: SugarTwin packets are sold in 50, 100, 250 and 500 count sizes. White granulated SugarTwin is sold in 2 lb. and 5 lb. equivalent sizes. Brown granulated SugarTwin is sold in a 1 lb. equivalent size.

Allergan Pharmaceuticals, Inc.
2525 DUPONT DRIVE
IRVINE, CA 92715

LACRI–LUBE® S.O.P.®
Sterile Ophthalmic Ointment

Contains: White petrolatum 55%, mineral oil 42.5%, nonionic lanolin derivatives 2% with chlorobutanol (chloral derivative) 0.5%.

Indications: Dry eye conditions.

Actions: Ocular lubricant.

Warnings: Do not touch tube tip to any surface since this may contaminate the ointment. Keep out of the reach of children. Store away from heat.

Dosage and Administration: Apply a small amount of ointment to affected areas as needed or as directed by physician.

Professional Labeling: Same as outlined under Indications.

How Supplied: 3.5 g and 7 g tubes and packs of 24 0.7 g unit-dose containers.
Shown in Product Identification Section, page 403

LIQUIFILM® FORTE
Enhanced Artificial Tears

Contains: Polyvinyl alcohol 3.0%, with thimerosal 0.002% and edetate disodium in a buffered, sterile, balanced isotonic solution.

Indications: Dry eye conditions.

Actions: Soothes and lubricates dry eyes.

Warnings: If irritation persists or increases, discontinue use. Keep container tightly closed. Do not touch dropper tip to any surface to prevent contamination. This product contains thimerosal. Do not use if you are sensitive to mercury. Keep out of reach of children.

Dosage and Administration: 1 drop in the eye as needed, or as directed by physician.

Professional Labeling: Same as outlined under Indications.

How Supplied: ½ fl oz and 1 fl oz plastic dropper bottles.

LIQUIFILM® TEARS
Artificial Tears

Contains: Polyvinyl alcohol 1.4% with chlorobutanol (chloral derivative) 0.5% and sodium chloride in a sterile, hypotonic solution.

Indications: Dry eye conditions and hard contact lens wear discomfort.

Actions: Soothes and lubricates dry eyes and promotes comfort and longer wearing of hard contact lenses.

Warnings: If irritation persists or increases, discontinue use. Keep container tightly closed. Do not touch dropper tip to any surface to prevent contamination. Not for use with soft contact lenses. Keep out of reach of children.

Dosage and Administration: 1 drop in the eye as needed, or as directed by physician.

Professional Labeling: Same as outlined under Indications.

How Supplied: ½ fl oz and 1 fl oz plastic bottles.
Shown in Product Identification Section, page 403

PREFRIN™ LIQUIFILM®
Eye Drops For Red Eyes

Contains: Phenylephrine HCl 0.12%, Liquifilm® (polyvinyl alcohol) 1.4%, antipyrine 0.1% and benzalkonium chloride 0.004% in a sterile buffered isotonic solution.

Indications: Minor eye irritations.

Actions: Lubricates and whitens the eye; relieves and soothes minor eye irritations.

Warnings: Do not use in presence of narrow-angle glaucoma. Pupillary dilation may occur in some individuals. If irritation persists or increases, discontinue use. Keep container tightly closed; do not touch dropper tip to any surface to avoid contamination. Not for use with soft contact lenses.

Dosage and Administration: 1 or 2 drops in each eye; repeat in 3 to 4 hours as needed.

Professional Labeling: Same as outlined under Indications.

How Supplied: 0.7 fl oz plastic bottle.
Shown in Product Identification Section, page 403

TEARS PLUS®
Artificial Tears

Contains: Liquifilm® (polyvinyl alcohol) 1.4% and povidone, with chlorobutanol 0.5% (chloral derivative) and sodium chloride.

Indications: Dry eye conditions. Relieves irritation caused by hard contact lens wear.

Actions: Soothes and lubricates dry eyes.

Warnings: If irritation persists or increases, discontinue use. Keep container tightly closed. Do not touch dropper tip to any surface to prevent contamination. Not for use with soft contact lenses. Keep out of reach of children.

Dosage and Administration: 1 drop in the eye as needed or directed.

Professional Labeling: Same as outlined under Indications.

How Supplied: ½ fl oz and 1 fl oz plastic bottles.

Shown in Product Identification Section, page 403

American Hygienic Laboratories, Inc.
555 ARTHUR GODFREY ROAD
MIAMI, FL 33140

SHUTTLE BLEMISH DISCS®

Active Ingredients: Purified water, Propylene Glycol, Citrimonium Chloride, Stearalkonium Chloride, Methylparaben

Indications: For acne, pimples and blackheads. Unlocks pores, medicates and prevents infection

Administration: Wipe disc over washed face. Repeat four times daily

How Supplied: 65 medicated pads per jar

Shown in Product Identification Section, page 403

SHUTTLE FIRST AID SPRAY®

Active Ingredients: Benzocaine, aloe, menthol, phenol, benzylkonium chloride, chlorothymol, isopropyl alcohol, water, methylparaben.

Indications: Provides fast temporary relief of surface pain, itching and discomfort due to sunburn, minor abrasions, non-poisonous insect bites, minor burns, poison ivy.

Warnings: Keep out of eyes and other mucus membranes. Keep out of reach of children. Not for deep puncture wounds or serious burns. Not for prolonged use. Consult physicians if rash or irritation develops or if condition persists. Do not use on children under 3 years old.

Administration: For best results hold approximately 3–6 inches from affected area. Spray liberally. Reapply if necessary.

How Supplied: 4 fl. oz.

Shown in Product Identification Section, page 403

SHUTTLE LOTION®

Active Ingredients: ½% Menthol, ½% Phenol, ½% Benzocaine, Precipitated Sulphur, Zinc Oxide, Corn Starch, Glycerin, Milk of Magnesia, Lime Water, Magma Bentonite.

Indications: a soothing and protective lotion for the relief of discomfort caused by Prickly Heat, sunburn, mosquito and insect bites, chiggers, Sand fleas, Man-O-War, Poison Ivy, Poison Oak, Diaper Rash, juvenile acne and pimples, and itching.

Precautions: Keep out of reach of children. Do not use near the eyes. Not for prolonged use. If condition persists, discontinue use and consult physician.

Administration: Shake well. Daub on affected area several times daily. Do not bandage if applied to fingers and toes. For babies and children—dilute if desired with water or milk of magnesia. Does not stain.

How Supplied: 4 fl. oz. and 8 fl. oz.

Shown in Product Identification Section, page 403

Anabolic Laboratories, Inc.
17802 GILLETTE AVENUE
IRVINE, CA 92714

CHROMEASE
Chromium (glucose tolerance factor yeast) plus support factors

Description: Two tablets provide:
Chromium (GTF yeast) ....30 mcg
Zinc (zinc gluconate) ....15 mg
Manganese (manganese
  gluconate) ....10 mg
Magnesium (magnesium
  oxide) ....100 mg
Vitamin B1 (thiamine
  hydrochloride) ....20 mg

Indication: Chromium supplement.

Dosage and Administration: Two to four tablets daily to be taken with food.

How Supplied: Bottle of 60 tablets.

TRI–B–PLEX
Sustained release B-complex capsules

Description: TRI-B-PLEX is a complete, balanced, high-potency B-complex formula in sustained release pellet form designed to release over an eight hour period ensuring maximum and efficient utilization and effectiveness. Two capsules provide:
Vitamin B1
  (thiamine hydrochloride) ....100 mg
Vitamin B2
  (riboflavin) ....40 mg
Niacinamide ....200 mg
Vitamin B6
  (pyridoxine hydrochloride) ......50 mg
Folic acid ....400 mcg
Vitamin B12
  (cyanocobalamin) ....25 mcg
Biotin ....300 mcg
Pantothenic acid
  (calcium pantothenate) ....100 mg

Indication: For use as a complete B-complex supplement.

Dosage and Administration: One capsule after breakfast and one after dinner.

How Supplied: Bottle of 60 capsules.

Products are cross-indexed by generic and chemical names in the
YELLOW SECTION

Arco Pharmaceuticals, Inc.
105 ORVILLE DRIVE
BOHEMIA, NY 11716

MEGA–B®
(super potency vitamin B complex, sugar & starch free)

Composition: Each Mega-B Tablet contains the following Mega Vitamins:

B1 (Thiamine Mononitrate)	100 mg.
B2 (Riboflavin)	100 mg.
B6 (Pyridoxine Hydrochloride)	100 mg.
B12 (Cyanocobalamin)	100 mcg.
Choline Bitartrate	100 mg.
Inositol	100 mg.
Niacinamide	100 mg.
Folic Acid	100 mcg.
Pantothenic Acid	100 mg.
d-Biotin	100 mcg.
Para-Aminobenzoic Acid (PABA)	100 mg.

In a base of yeast to provide the identified and unidentified B-Complex Factors.

Advantages: Each Mega-B capsule-shaped tablet provides the highest vitamin B complex available in a single dose. Mega-B was designed for those patients who require truly Mega vitamin potencies with the convenience of minimum dosage.

Indications: Mega-B is indicated in conditions characterized by depletions or increased demand of the water-soluble B-complex vitamins. It may be useful in the nutritional management of patients during prolonged convalescence associated with major surgery. It is also indicated for stress conditions, as an adjunct to antibiotics and diuretic therapy, pre and post operative cases, liver conditions, gastro-intestinal disorders interfering with intake or absorption of water-soluble vitamins, prolonged or wasting diseases, diabetes, burns, fractures, severe infections, and some psychological disorders.

Warning: NOT INTENDED FOR TREATMENT OF PERNICIOUS ANEMIA, OR OTHER PRIMARY OR SECONDARY ANEMIAS.

Dosage: Usual dosage is one Mega-B tablet daily, or varied, depending on clinical needs.

Supplied: Yellow capsule shaped tablets in bottles of 30, 100 and 500.

MEGADOSE™
(multiple mega-vitamin formula with minerals, sugar and starch free)

Composition:

Vitamin A	25,000 USP Units
Vitamin D	1,000 USP Units
Vitamin C w/Rose Hips	250 mg.
Vitamin E	100 IU
Folic Acid	400 mcg.
Vitamin B1	80 mg.
Vitamin B2	80 mg.
Niacinamide	80 mg.

Continued on next page

Arco—Cont.

Vitamin B$_6$	80 mg.
Vitamin B$_{12}$	80 mcg.
Biotin	80 mcg.
Pantothenic Acid	80 mg.
Choline Bitartrate	80 mg.
Inositol	80 mg.
Para-Aminobenzoic Acid	80 mg.
Rutin	30 mg.
Citrus Bioflavonoids	30 mg.
Betaine Hydrochloride	30 mg.
Glutamic Acid	30 mg.
Hesperidin Complex	5 mg.
Iodine (from Kelp)	0.15 mg.
Calcium Gluconate*	50 mg.
Zinc Gluconate*	25 mg.
Potassium Gluconate*	10 mg.
Ferrous Gluconate*	10 mg.
Magnesium Gluconate*	7 mg.
Manganese Gluconate*	6 mg.
Copper Gluconate*	0.5 mg.

*Natural mineral chelates in a base containing natural ingredients.

Dosage: One tablet daily.

Supplied: Capsule shaped tablets in bottles of 30, 100 and 250.

Arizona Natural Products
7750 E. EVANS, No. 3
SCOTTSDALE, AZ 85260

Arizona Natural Odorless Garlic

Description: Soft gel capsules and tablets containing whole garlic clove.

Active Ingredients: Garlic, Allicin (allyl allythiosulfinate) Lecithin, & Selenium

Indications: Dietary Supplement

Suggested Use: 2–4 capsules daily for health maintenance, 6–8 daily for therpeutic uses

How Supplied:
CAPSULE—Arizona Natural #101 odorless garlic capsule has 345 mg. garlic from whole clove, 200 mg. soya oil, 10 mg. lecithin, 4 umoles Allicin.
100 and 250 ct. bottles.
Arizona Natural #105 Odorless garlic w/Lecithin capsule has 500 mg. garlic from whole clove, 500 mg. lecithin, 200 mg. soya oil, 6.3 umoles Allicin.
100 and 200 ct. bottles.
TABLETS—Arizona Natural #301 Odorless garlic tablet w/Lemon & Parsley has 100 mg. garlic concentrate, 50 mg. parsley, 100 mg. citrus solids, 3.8 umoles Allicin.
100 and 250 ct. bottles.
Arizona Natural #305 Odorless garlic w/Selenium Yeast, has 150 mg. Selenium Yeast, 100 mg. garlic concentrate, 100 mg. citrus solids, 50 mg. parsley, 50 mcg. selenium, 3.8 umoles Allicin.
100 ct. bottles.

B. F. Ascher & Company, Inc.
15501 WEST 109th STREET
LENEXA, KS 66219
Mailing address:
P.O. BOX 827
KANSAS CITY, MO 64141

AYR® Saline Nasal Mist and Drops

AYR Mist or Drops restores vital moisture to provide prompt relief for dry, crusted and inflamed nasal membranes due to chronic sinusitis, colds, low humidity, overuse of nasal decongestant drops and sprays, allergies, minor nose bleeds and other minor nasal irritations. AYR provides a soothing way to thin thick secretions and aid their removal from the nose and sinuses. AYR can be used as often as needed without the side effects associated with overuse of decongestant nose drops and sprays.

SAFE & GENTLE ENOUGH FOR CHILDREN AND INFANTS
AYR Drops are particularly convenient for easy application with infants and children. AYR is formulated to prevent stinging, burning and irritation of delicate nasal tissue, even that of babies.

Directions For Use: SPRAY—Squeeze twice in each nostril as often as needed. DROPS—Two to four drops in each nostril every two hours as needed, or as directed by your physician.
AYR contains sodium chloride 0.65% buffered to a neutral pH and benzalkonium chloride and EDTA as antibacterial and antifungal preservatives.

How Supplied:
AYR Mist in 50 ml spray bottles, AYR Drops in 20 ml dropper bottles.

MOBISYL® Analgesic Creme

Active Ingredient: Triethanolamine salicylate 10%

Description: MOBISYL is a greaseless, odorless, penetrating, non-burning, non-irritating analgesic creme.

Indications: For adults and children, 12 years of age and older, MOBISYL is indicated for the temporary relief of minor aches and pains of muscles and joints, such as simple backache, lumbago, arthritis, neuralgia, strains, bruises and sprains.

Actions: MOBISYL penetrates fast into sore, tender joints and muscles where pain originates. It works to reduce inflammation. Helps soothe stiff joints and muscles and gets you going again.

Warnings: For external use only. Avoid contact with the eyes. Discontinue use if condition worsens or if symptoms persist for more than 7 days, and consult a physician. Do not use on children under 12 years of age except under the advice and supervision of a physician. In case of accidental ingestion, seek professional assistance or contact a Poison Control Center immediately. Close cap tightly. Keep this and all drugs out of the reach of children. Store at room temperature.

Dosage and Administration: Place a liberal amount of MOBISYL Creme in your palm and massage into the area of pain and soreness three or four times a day, especially before retiring. MOBISYL may be worn under clothing or bandages.

How Supplied: MOBISYL is available in 1.25 oz tubes, 3.5 oz tubes, 8 oz jars.

Astra Pharmaceutical Products, Inc.
50 OTIS ST.
WESTBORO, MA 01581-4428

XYLOCAINE® (lidocaine) 2.5% OINTMENT

For temporary relief of pain and itching due to minor burns, sunburn, minor cuts, abrasions, insect bites and minor skin irritations.

Composition: Diethylaminoacet-2, 6-xylidide 2.5% in a water miscible ointment vehicle consisting of polyethylene glycols and propylene glycol.

Action and Uses: A topical anesthetic ointment for fast, temporary relief of pain and itching due to minor burns, sunburn, minor cuts, abrasions, insect bites and minor skin irritations. The ointment can be easily removed with water. It is ineffective when applied to intact skin.

Administration and Dosage: Apply topically in liberal amounts for adequate control of symptoms. When the anesthetic effect wears off additional ointment may be applied as needed.

Important Warning: *In persistent, severe or extensive skin disorders, advise patient to use only as directed. In case of accidental ingestion advise patient to seek professional assistance or to contact a poison control center immediately. Keep out of the reach of children.*

Caution: *Do not use in the eyes. Not for prolonged use. If the condition for which this preparation is used persists or if a rash or irritation develops, advise patient to discontinue use and consult a physician.*

How Supplied: Available in tube of 35 grams (approximately 1.25 ounces).
Shown in Product Identification Section, page 404

Ayerst Laboratories
Division of American Home
  Products Corporation
685 THIRD AVE.
NEW YORK, NY 10017

BEMINAL STRESS PLUS™
Stress potency replacement vitamins

BEMINAL STRESS PLUS™
with Iron

Each tablet contains:	% U.S. RDA*
Vitamin B1 as	1717%
thiamine mononitrate, U.S.P. 25.0 mg	
Vitamin B2 as	735%
riboflavin, U.S.P. 12.5 mg	
Vitamin B3 as	504%
niacinamide 100.0 mg	
Vitamin B5 as	184%
calcium pantothenate, U.S.P. 20.0 mg	
Vitamin B6 as	411%
pyridoxine hydrochloride, U.S.P. 10.0 mg	
Vitamin B12 as	417%
cyanocobalamin 25.0 mcg	
Vitamin Bc as	100%
folic acid, U.S.P. 400.0 mcg	
Vitamin C as	1166%
sodium ascorbate, U.S.P. 787.0 mg	
Vitamin E as	150%
dl-α-tocopheryl acetate 45.0 I.U.	
Iron as	150%
ferrous fumarate, U.S.P. 82.2 mg	

*percentage of U.S. recommended daily
allowance

BEMINAL STRESS PLUS™
with Zinc

Each tablet contains:	% U.S. RDA*
Vitamin B1 as	1717%
thiamine mononitrate, U.S.P. 25.0 mg	
Vitamin B2 as	735%
riboflavin, U.S.P. 12.5 mg	
Vitamin B3 as	504%
niacinamide 100.0 mg	
Vitamin B5 as	184%
calcium pantothenate, U.S.P. 20.0 mg	
Vitamin B6 as	411%
pyridoxine hydrochloride, U.S.P. 10.0 mg	
Vitamin B12 as	417%
cyanocobalamin 25.0 mcg	
Vitamin C as	1166%
sodium ascorbate, U.S.P. 787.0 mg	
Vitamin E as	150%
dl-α-tocopheryl acetate 45.0 I.U.	
Zinc as	300%
zinc sulfate 111.1 mg	

*percentage of U.S. recommended daily
allowance

Indication: Dietary supplement.

Action and Uses: The BEMINAL STRESS PLUS formulas can help replenish the vitamins and minerals depleted by the stress of sickness, infections, and surgery. BEMINAL STRESS PLUS formulas may also be used where the demand on the body's store of vitamins and minerals may be increased by dieting, lack of sleep, the use of alcohol or cigarettes, jogging and other strenuous physical exercise.

Recommended Intake: *12-year-olds and older*, one tablet daily.

How Supplied: BEMINAL STRESS PLUS with Iron—bottles of 60 tablets. BEMINAL STRESS PLUS with Zinc— bottles of 60 tablets.
*Shown in Product Identification
Section, page 404*

DERMOPLAST®
Topical Anesthetic First Aid Spray

Contains (exclusive of propellants) 20% benzocaine and 0.5% menthol in a water-dispersible base of TWEEN® 85 and polyethylene glycol 400 monolaurate with methylparaben as a preservative. A topical anesthetic and antipruritic spray providing soothing, temporary relief of skin pain, itching, and discomfort due to sunburn, minor cuts, insect bites, abrasions, burns and minor skin irritations. May be applied without touching sensitive affected areas. Widely used in hospitals for pain and itch of episiotomy, pruritus vulvae, postpartum hemorrhoids.

Warnings: FOR EXTERNAL USE ONLY. Avoid spraying in eyes. Contents under pressure. Do not puncture or incinerate. Do not expose to heat or temperatures above 120° F. Do not use near open flame. Use only as directed. Intentional misuse by deliberately concentrating and inhaling the contents can be harmful or fatal.
Do not take orally. Not for prolonged use. If the condition for which this preparation is used persists or if a rash or irritation develops, discontinue use and consult physician.

Directions for Use: Hold can in a comfortable position 6–12 inches away from affected area. Point spray nozzle and press button. To apply to face, spray in palm of hand. May be administered three or four times daily, or as directed by physician.

How Supplied: DERMOPLAST Aerosol Spray, in Net Wt 2¾ oz (78g)—NDC 0046-1008-02.
*Shown in Product Identification
Section, page 404*

KERODEX®
Skin Barrier Cream

Action and Uses: A specially formulated barrier hand cream to help protect against potentially irritating chemicals, compounds, and solutions in common use. When applied and used as directed, KERODEX provides a barrier film that helps to block contact with skin irritants. KERODEX No. 71 (water-repellent) is for use in handling or working with *wet* materials; No. 51 is for *dry* or *oily* work. KERODEX is greaseless and stainless.

Application: 1. Wash hands clean and dry *thoroughly*. 2. Squeeze out ½ inch of cream into palm of one hand. Rub hands together with a washing motion until cream is *lightly* and *evenly* distributed, leaving no excess. Make sure cream reaches under nails, around cuticles, between fingers, across wrists and backs of hands (forearms, if necessary). 3. A second application is recommended. **NOTE:** After applying KERODEX 71, "set" by holding hands under cold running water. Pat dry. After applying KERODEX 51, avoid contact with water. If hands become wet during work, reapply.

How Supplied: KERODEX (water-repellent cream for wet work), in 4 oz (113 g) tubes (NDC 0046-0071-04) and 1 lb jars (NDC 0046-0071-01). KERODEX (water-miscible cream for dry or oily work), in 4 oz (113 g) tubes (NDC 0046-0051-04) and 1 lb jars (NDC 0046-0051-01).
*Shown in Product Identification
Section, page 404*

RIOPAN®
magaldrate
Antacid

Each teaspoonful (5 ml) of Suspension contains:	
Magaldrate	540 mg
Each Chew Tablet contains:	
Magaldrate	480 mg
Each Swallow Tablet contains:	
Magaldrate	480 mg

RIOPAN is a chemical entity (not a physical mixture), providing the advantages of a true buffer-antacid (not simply a neutralizing agent): (1) rapid action; (2) uniform buffering action; (3) high acid-consuming capacity; (4) no alkalinization or acid rebound.

Low Sodium Content: Not more than 0.1 mg of sodium—per teaspoonful (5 ml) suspension—per chew tablet—per swallow tablet.

Acid-neutralizing Capacity— 15.0 mEq/5 ml suspension or 13.5 mEq per tablet.

Indications: For the relief of heartburn, sour stomach, acid indigestion, and upset stomach associated with these symptoms. For symptomatic relief of hyperacidity associated with the diagnosis of peptic ulcer, gastritis, peptic esophagitis, gastric hyperacidity, and hiatal hernia.

Directions: RIOPAN (magaldrate) Antacid *Suspension*—Recommended dosage, one or two teaspoonfuls, between meals and at bedtime, or as directed by the physician. RIOPAN Antacid *Chew Tablets*—Recommended dosage, one or two tablets, between meals and at bedtime, or as directed by the physician. Chew before swallowing. RIOPAN Antacid *Swallow Tablets*—Recommended dosage, one or two tablets, between meals and at bedtime, or as directed by the physician. Take with enough water to swallow promptly.

Drug Interaction Precaution: Do not use in patients taking a prescription antibiotic drug containing any form of tetracycline.

Warnings: Patients should not take more than 20 teaspoonfuls (or 20 tablets) in a 24-hour period nor use this maximum dosage for more than two weeks, nor use if they have kidney disease except under the advice and supervision of a physician.

How Supplied: RIOPAN Antacid *Suspension*—in 12 fl oz (355 ml) plastic bottles (NDC 0046-0765-12). Individual

Continued on next page

Ayerst—Cont.

Cups, 1 fl oz (30 ml) ea., tray of 10—10 trays per packer (NDC 0046-0765-99). RIOPAN Antacid *Chew Tablets*—in bottles of 60 (NDC 0046-0928-59) and 100 (NDC 0046-0928-80). Boxes of 60 (NDC 0046-0928-60) and 100 (NDC 0046-0928-81); in individual film strips (10 x 6 and 10 x 10, respectively). Also, single rollpacks of 12 tablets (NDC 0046-0941-12) and 3-roll rollpacks of 36 tablets (NDC 0046-0941-36). RIOPAN Antacid *Swallow Tablets*—Boxes of 60 (NDC 0046-0927-60) and 100 (NDC 0046-0927-81) in individual film strips (6 x 10 and 10 x 10, respectively).

Shown in Product Identification Section, page 404

RIOPAN PLUS®
magaldrate and simethicone
Antacid/Anti-Gas

Each teaspoonful (5 ml) of Suspension contains:
Magaldrate .... 540 mg
Simethicone .... 20 mg
Each Chew Tablet contains:
Magaldrate .... 480 mg
Simethicone .... 20 mg

Low Sodium Content: Not more than 0.1 mg per teaspoonful (5 ml) or Chew Tablet.

Acid-neutralizing Capacity— 15.0 mEq/5 ml suspension or 13.5 mEq per tablet.

Indications: For the relief of heartburn, sour stomach, acid indigestion, and upset stomach associated with these symptoms, accompanied by the symptoms of gas. For symptomatic relief of hyperacidity associated with the diagnosis of peptic ulcer, gastritis, peptic esophagitis, gastric hyperacidity, and hiatal hernia. For postoperative gas pain or for use in endoscopic examinations.

Directions: RIOPAN PLUS (magaldrate and simethicone) Antacid/Anti-Gas *Suspension*—Recommended dosage, one or two teaspoonfuls between meals and at bedtime, or as directed by the physician. RIOPAN PLUS Antacid/Anti-Gas *Chew Tablets*—Recommended dosage, one or two tablets, between meals and at bedtime, or as directed by the physician. Chew before swallowing.

Drug Interaction Precaution: Do not use in patients taking a prescription antibiotic drug containing any form of tetracycline.

Warnings: Patients should not take more than 20 teaspoonfuls (or 20 tablets) in a 24-hour period nor use this maximum dosage for more than two weeks, nor use if they have kidney disease except under the advice and supervision of a physician.

How Supplied: RIOPAN PLUS Antacid/Anti-Gas *Suspension*—in 12 fl oz (355 ml) plastic bottles (NDC 0046-0768-12). Individual Cups, 1 fl oz (30 ml) ea., tray of 10—10 trays per packer (NDC 0046-0937-99).

RIOPAN PLUS Antacid/Anti-Gas *Chew Tablets*—in bottles of 60 (NDC 0046-0930-60) and 100 (NDC 0046-0930-81). Also, single rollpacks of 12 tablets (NDC 0046-0930-12) and 3-roll rollpacks of 36 tablets (NDC 0046-0930-36).

Shown in Product Identification Section, page 404

EXTRA STRENGTH RIOPAN PLUS®
magaldrate and simethicone
Antacid/Anti-Gas

Each teaspoonful (5 ml) of Suspension contains:
Magaldrate .... 1080 mg
Simethicone .... 30 mg

Low Sodium Content: Not more than 0.3 mg per teaspoonful (5 ml).

Acid-neutralizing Capacity— 30.0 mEq/5 ml suspension.

Indications: For the relief of heartburn, sour stomach, acid indigestion, and upset stomach associated with these symptoms, accompanied by the symptoms of gas. For symptomatic relief of hyperacidity associated with the diagnosis of peptic ulcer, gastritis, peptic esophagitis, gastric hyperacidity, and hiatal hernia. For postoperative gas pain or for use in endoscopic examinations.

Directions: EXTRA STRENGTH RIOPAN PLUS (magaldrate and simethicone) *Suspension*—Recommended dosage, one or two teaspoonfuls between meals and at bedtime, or as directed by the physician.

Drug Interaction Precaution: Do not use in patients taking a prescription antibiotic drug containing any form of tetracycline.

Warnings: Patients should not take more than 9 teaspoonfuls in a 24-hour period nor use this maximum dosage for more than two weeks, nor use if they have kidney disease except under the advice and supervision of a physician.

How Supplied: EXTRA STRENGTH RIOPAN PLUS *Suspension*—in 12 fl oz (355 ml) plastic bottles (NDC 0046-0779-12).

Shown in Product Identification Section, page 404

Baker/Cummins
Div. of Key Pharmaceuticals, Inc.
P.O. BOX 693670
MIAMI, FLORIDA 33269-0670

COMPLEX 15™
Phospholipid Moisturizing Cream and Lotion

Cream Ingredients: Water - Mineral Oil - Glycerin - Lecithin - Cetyl Acetate - Glyceryl Stearate - Dimethicone - Stearic Acid - Glycol Stearate - Lanolin Alcohol Acetate - Triethanolamine - Cetyl Alcohol - Magnesium Aluminum Silicate - Imidazolidinyl Urea - Methylparaben - Carbomer 934 - Propylparaben - Tetrasodium EDTA

Lotion Ingredients: Water - Mineral Oil - Glycerin - Lecithin - Cetyl Acetate - Glyceryl Stearate - Dimethicone - Glycol Stearate - Lanolin Alcohol Acetate - Stearic Acid - Triethanolamine - Methylparaben - Imidazolidinyl Urea - Carbomer 934 - Cetyl Alcohol - Magnesium Aluminum Silicate - Propylparaben - Tetrasodium EDTA

COMPLEX 15 relieves and protects the driest, most sensitive skin with a moisturizing system modeled from nature. COMPLEX 15 contains the phospholipid lecithin, a water binding agent which occurs naturally in the deepest layers of skin. Each phospholipid molecule forms a complex with 15 molecules of water, creating a moisture reservoir which restores the skin's natural moisture balance. Revitalize your skin with COMPLEX 15—you will see and feel the difference!

Directions: Apply as often as needed to the face and body.

How Supplied: COMPLEX 15 Cream is available in 4 ounce jars. COMPLEX 15 Lotion is available in 8 fluid ounce bottles.

P&S® LIQUID

Ingredients: Mineral Oil - Water - Fragrance - Glycerin - Phenol - Sodium Chloride - D&C Yellow #11 - D&C Red #17 - D&C Green #6
P&S LIQUID, used regularly, helps loosen and remove crusts and scales on the scalp.

Directions: Apply liberally to scalp lesions each night before retiring. Massage gently to loosen scales and crusts. Leave on overnight and shampoo the next morning. Use daily as needed.

Caution: Do not apply to large portions of body surfaces. Discontinue use if excessive skin irritation develops. Avoid contact with eyes or mucous membranes. Keep out of reach of children.
FOR EXTERNAL USE ONLY.

How Supplied: P&S LIQUID is available in 4 and 8 fluid ounce bottles.

P&S® PLUS
Tar Gel for Psoriasis and Other Scaling Conditions

Active Ingredients: 8% Coal Tar Solution (1.6% Crude Coal Tar, 6.4% Ethyl Alcohol) - 2% Salicylic Acid.
P&S PLUS relieves the itching, irritation and skin flaking associated with seborrheic dermatitis, psoriasis and dandruff.

Directions: Apply to affected areas of skin and scalp daily or as directed by physician.

Warnings: For external use only. Avoid contact with eyes; flush with water if product gets into eyes. If irritation develops, discontinue use. If condition worsens or does not improve after regular use of this product as directed, consult a physician. Do not use on children under 2 years of age except as directed by a physician. Use caution in exposing skin to sunlight after applying this product; it may increase your tendency to sunburn for up to 24 hours after application. Do not use product in or around the rectum or in the genital area or groin except on the advice of a physician.

Caution: Keep this and all drugs out of the reach of children. In case of accidental ingestion, seek professional assistance or contact Poison Control Center immediately.

How Supplied: P&S PLUS is available in 3.5 ounce tubes.

P&S® SHAMPOO

Active Ingredient: 2% Salicylic Acid P&S SHAMPOO relieves the itching, irritation, and skin flaking associated with seborrheic dermatitis of the scalp. It also relieves the itching, redness and scaling associated with psoriasis of the scalp. P&S SHAMPOO may be used alone as well as following treatment with P&S LIQUID. It's rich conditioning formula improves hair's manageability and helps prevent tangles.

Directions: For best results use twice a week or as directed by your physician. Wet hair, apply to scalp and massage vigorously. Rinse and repeat.

Warnings: FOR EXTERNAL USE ONLY. Avoid contact with eyes or mucus membranes. If this occurs, rinse thoroughly with water. If condition worsens or does not improve after regular use of this product as directed, consult a physician. Do not use on children under 2 years of age except as directed by a physician. Keep out of reach of children.

How Supplied: P&S SHAMPOO is available in 4 fluid ounce bottles.

ULTRA MIDE 25™
Moisturizer with 25% Urea for Extra Dry Skin

Ingredients: Water - Urea - Mineral Oil - Lanolin Oil - Glycerin - Propylene Glycol - Petrolatum - Glyceryl Stearate - PEG-50 Stearate - Cetyl Alcohol - Propylene Glycol Stearate SE - Lactic Acid - Sorbitan Laurate - Fragrance - Potassium Sorbate - Tetrasodium EDTA ULTRA MIDE 25 is rich with softeners and moisturizers to make dry, rough, thickened skin such as elbows and knees soft and supple.

Directions: Apply up to four times daily unless otherwise directed by a physician.
FOR EXTERNAL USE ONLY
Keep out of reach of children. Store in a cool place.

How Supplied: ULTRA MIDE 25 is available in 8 fluid ounce bottles.

X·SEB® SHAMPOO

Active Ingredient: 4% Salicylic Acid X·SEB SHAMPOO relieves the itching and scalp flaking associated with dandruff. It's conditioning formula leaves hair more manageable, with more body.

Directions: For best results, use twice a week or as directed by a physician. Wet hair, apply to scalp and massage vigorously. Rinse and repeat.

Warnings: FOR EXTERNAL USE ONLY. Avoid contact with eyes or mucus membranes. If this occurs, rinse thoroughly with water. If condition worsens or does not improve after regular use of this product as directed, consult a physician. Do not use on children under 2 years of age except as directed by a physician. Keep out of the reach of children.

How Supplied: X·SEB SHAMPOO is available in 4 fluid ounce bottles.

X·SEB® T SHAMPOO

Active Ingredients: 10% Coal Tar Solution (2% Crude Coal Tar, 8% Ethyl Alcohol), 4% Salicylic Acid.

Indications: Relieves the itching, irritation and skin flaking associated with seborrheic dermatitis, psoriasis and dandruff.

Directions: For best results use twice weekly or as directed by a physician. Wet hair, apply to scalp and massage thoroughly. Rinse and repeat.

Warnings: For external use only. Avoid contact with eyes; flush with water if product gets into eyes. If irritation develops, discontinue use. If condition worsens or does not improve after regular use of this product as directed, consult a physician. Do not use on children under 2 years of age except as directed by a physician. Use caution in exposing skin to sunlight after applying this product; it may increase your tendency to sunburn for up to 24 hours after application.

Caution: Keep this and all drugs out of the reach of children. In case of accidental ingestion, seek professional assistance or contact a Poison Control Center immediately.

How Supplied: X·SEB T SHAMPOO is available in 4 fluid ounce bottles.

Beach Pharmaceuticals
Division of BEACH PRODUCTS, INC.
5220 SOUTH MANHATTAN AVE.
TAMPA, FL 33681

BEELITH Tablets
Magnesium Oxide with Vitamin B$_6$

Description: Each tablet contains magnesium oxide 600 mg and pyridoxine hydrochloride (Vitamin B$_6$) 25 mg equivalent to B$_6$ 20 mg.
Inert Ingredients: caster oil, hydroxypropyl methylcellulose, magnesium stearate, microcrystalline cellulose, polyethylene glycol NF, propylene glycol USP, sodium starch glycolate. Also, D & C yellow #10, FDC yellow #6, titanium dioxide.

Warning: Keep this and all drugs out of the reach of children. In case of accidental overdose seek professional assistance or contact a Poison Control Center immediately. As with any drug, if you are pregnant or nursing a baby, seek the advice of a health professional before using this product.

Actions and Uses: BEELITH is a dietary supplement for patients deficient in magnesium and/or pyridoxine. Each tablet yields approximately 362 mg of elemental magnesium & supplies 1000% of the Adult U.S. Recommended Daily Allowance (RDA) for Vitamin B$_6$ and 90% of the RDA for magnesium.

Dosage: The usual adult dose is one or two tablets daily.

Precaution: Excessive dosage might cause laxation.

Caution: Use only under the supervision of a physician. Use with caution in renal insufficiency.

Drug Interaction Precautions: Do not take this product if you are presently taking a prescription antibiotic drug containing any form of tetracycline.

Storage: Keep tightly closed. Store at controlled room temperature 15°C–30°C (59°F–86°F).

How Supplied: Golden yellow film coated tablet with the name BEACH and the number 1132 printed on each tablet. Bottles of 100 (NDC 0486-1132-01) and bottles of 500 (NDC 0486-1132-05) tablets.

Shown in Product Identification Section, page 404

Becton Dickinson
Consumer Products
365 W. PASSAIC STREET
ROCHELLE PARK, NJ 07662

B–D Glucose Tablets

Indications and Usage: For fast relief from hypoglycemia. B-D Glucose tablets contain D-Glucose (Dextrose), the most readily absorbed sugar, and are recommended for treatment of hypoglycemia. The tablets are chewable and dissolve quickly in the mouth to facilitate ingestion.

Adverse Reactions: No adverse reactions have been reported with appropriate use of glucose. Occasional reports of nausea may be due to the hypoglycemia itself.

Dosage and Administration: The recommended dosage is three (3) to (4) tablets (15.0 to 20.0 grams of dextrose) at the first sign of hypoglycemia. Repeat dosage as needed to counter additional hypoglycemic episodes caused by longer acting insulins. Dosage may be regulated by taking fewer or more tablets, depending on severity of the episode. Notify your physician of hypoglycemic episodes.

Continued on next page

Becton Dickinson—Cont.

Do not administer to anyone who is unconscious.

How Supplied: Box containing six chewable 5.0 gram tablets. Tablets are packaged in durable three tablet blister packs.

Ingredients: Each tablet contains 5.0 grams dextrose. Other ingredients are flavors and tabletting aids: Microcrystalline cellulose and stearic acid. Contains no preservatives.

CANKAID®
(carbamide peroxide 10%)
Oral Antiseptic

Active Ingredient: Carbamide peroxide 10% in specially prepared anhydrous glycerol. Artificial flavor added.

Indications and Actions: CANKAID gives quick, temporary relief from minor mouth irritations such as canker sores, sore or injured gums, and inflammation caused by dentures, mouth appliances (orthodontics), or dental procedures. CANKAID cleanses oral wounds and inflammation gently but thoroughly with its antiseptic, microfoaming action. CANKAID coats and clings to tissue, prolonging its soothing, protective effects.

Precaution: If severe or persistent symptoms occur in the mouth or throat, consult physician or dentist promptly. Do not administer to children under three years of age unless directed by physician or dentist. Keep out of reach of children.

Dosage and Administration: Do not dilute. Use four times daily, or as directed by physician or dentist. Apply directly onto affected area with painless, no touch tip. To treat widespread inflammation or hard to reach areas, apply 10 drops onto tongue; mix with saliva; swish thoroughly; expectorate.

How Supplied: CANKAID comes in liquid form, in ¾ fl. oz. plastic bottles.

MERCUROCHROME II™
Antiseptic/Double Anesthetic First
Aid Spray and Liquid

Active Ingredients: Lidocaine HCl, Menthol, Benzalkonium Chloride, Isopropyl Alcohol 5%

Actions and Indications: MERCUROCHROME II contains a safe and effective germ killing ingredient plus two pain relieving anesthetics. It is indicated for minor burns, cuts, scrapes, insect bites, and sunburn. It does not sting or irritate injured skin. MERCUROCHROME II is colorless; it will not stain clothes or skin.

Precaution: For external use only. In case of deep or puncture wounds, or serious burns, consult physician. If irritation or swelling develops or persists, or if infection occurs, discontinue use and consult physician. KEEP OUT OF REACH OF CHILDREN. Do not use near the

eyes. In case of accidental ingestion seek professional assistance. Do not use in large quantities, particularly over raw surfaces or blistered areas. Benzalkonium chloride is inactivated by contact with soap.

Dosage and Administration: SPRAY—Hold bottle 3 to 6 inches from skin surface; spray until affected area is completely wetted.
LIQUID—Apply directly onto affected area with attached applicator rod.

How Supplied: 2 fl. oz. and 4 fl. oz. pump spray bottle, 1 fl. oz. applicator bottle.

Beecham Products
DIVISION OF BEECHAM INC.
POST OFFICE BOX 1467
PITTSBURGH, PA 15230

B.F.I.®
Antiseptic First-Aid Powder

Active Ingredient: Bismuth-Formic-Iodide 16.0%. Other ingredients—Boric Acid, Bismuth Subgallate, Zinc Phenolsulfonate, Potassium Alum, Thymol, Amol (mono-n-amyl hydroquinone ether), Menthol, Eucalyptol, and inert diluents.

Indications: For cuts, abrasions, minor burns, skin irritations, athlete's foot and dermatitis due to poison ivy and poison oak.

Actions: B.F.I. First-Aid Powder promotes healing of cuts, scratches, abrasions and minor burns. Relieves itching, chafing and irritations from prickly heat, sunburn, mosquito bites, athlete's foot and poison ivy and oak.

Warnings: Keep out of reach of children. If redness, irritation, swelling or pain persists or increases or if infection occurs, discontinue use and consult physician. For deep or puncture wounds or serious burns, consult physician.

Symptoms and Treatment of Oral Overdosage: In the event of ingestion of large quantities, consult a physician, local poison control center, or the Rocky Mt. Poison Control Center at 303-592-1710 (Collect), 24 hours a day.

Dosage and Administration: Freely sprinkle B.F.I. on the injured area to completely cover the area. Avoid use on extensive denuded (raw) areas particularly on infants and children.

How Supplied: ¼ oz., 1¼ oz. and 8 oz. shaker top container.

CUPREX®
Pediculicide

Active Ingredient: Tetrahydronaphthalene—30.97%; Copper Oleate—.03%

Indications: For the elimination of head lice, crab lice, body lice and their nits.

Actions: Cuprex provides an effective treatment for the elimination of lice and nits in the forms indicated above.

Warnings: Keep out of reach of children. Flammable—keep away from heat and open flame. Harmful if swallowed. Keep away from eyes. Store out of direct sunlight. Do not use more than twice in 48 hour period. Where skin is raw, broken or infected, consult a physician.

Precaution: Excessive or prolonged contact with the skin may produce erythema, edema, itching, and burning. In the event of excessive contact with skin or eyes, flush with copious amounts of clear water.

Symptoms and Treatment of Oral Overdosage: If ingestion is suspected, consult your physician, your local poison control center, or the Rocky Mt. Poison Control Center at 303-592-1710 (Collect), 24 hours a day.

Dosage and Administration: For Head Lice and Nits: Apply gently but thoroughly to scalp and hair using small quantities at a time. After 15 minutes, wash hair and scalp thoroughly with soap and warm water. While still damp, comb hair with a fine comb. For Crab Lice and Nits: Apply thoroughly on effected hairy areas. After 15 minutes, wash thoroughly with soap and warm water; while still damp, comb hair with fine comb. It is not necessary to shave the hair in uncomplicated cases. Body Lice and Nits: Treat skin and hair as for crab lice. General Instructions: If repeat application is required, apply a bland ointment or oil between treatments to avoid drying of skin. All infested clothing should be deloused to prevent reinfestation.

How Supplied: 3 and 16 fl. oz. bottles.

DEEP–DOWN® Pain Relief Rub

Active Ingredients: Methyl salicylate 15%; menthol 5%; methyl nicotinate 0.7%; camphor 0.5%.

Indications: To relieve the pain of minor arthritis, sore joints, muscle aches and sprains, backache, lumbago.

Actions: Counterirritation: cutaneous stimulation for relief of pain in underlying structures.

Warnings: For external use only. Avoid getting in eyes or on mucous membranes, broken or irritated skin. Discontinue use if excessive skin irritation develops. If pain lasts more than 7 days, or redness is present, or in conditions affecting children under 12 years of age, consult a physician. Keep product out of children's reach. In case of accidental swallowing, call a physician or contact a poison control center immediately.

Dosage and Administration: Rub generously into painful area, then massage gently until ointment is absorbed and disappears. Reapply every 3 to 4 hours or as needed. Do not bandage.

How Supplied: Available in 1.25 and 3 oz collapsible tubes.

ENO®
Sparkling Antacid

Active Ingredient: When mixed with water, one level teaspoon of Eno produces 1620 mg. of sodium tartrate and 1172 mg. of sodium citrate. Contains 819 mg. of sodium per teaspoonful.

Indications: For relief from the symptoms of sour stomach, acid indigestion, and heartburn.

Actions: Eno is a good tasting, fast acting and effective antacid. It is free of aspirin or sugar and is 100% antacid.

Warnings: If under 60 years of age, don't take more than 6 teaspoonfuls in a 24 hour period. If over 60, don't take over 3 teaspoonfuls. Don't use maximum dosage for over 2 weeks, or use the product if on a sodium restricted diet, except under the advice of a physician. May have a laxative effect. Keep out of reach of children.

Symptoms and Treatment of Oral Overdosage: In case of a large overdose, consult your physician, your local poison control center, or the Rocky Mt. Poison Control Center at 303-592-1710 (Collect), 24 hours a day.

Dosage and Administration: Adults—1 level teaspoonful in 6 ozs. of water. May be repeated every 4 hours. Children 4–6—¼ level teaspoonful; children 7–15—½ level teaspoonful.

How Supplied: 3½ and 7 oz. bottles.

FEMIRON® Tablets

Active Ingredient: (Per Tablet) Iron (from ferrous fumarate) 20 mg.

Indications: For use as an iron supplement.

Actions: Supplements dietary iron intake; helps maintain iron stores.

Warnings: Keep out of reach of children.

Precaution: Alcoholics and individuals with chronic liver or pancreatic disease may have enhanced iron absorption with the potential for iron overload. NOTE: Unabsorbed iron may cause some darkening of the stool.

Drug Interaction Precaution: Taking with antacid or tetracycline may interfere with absorption.

Symptoms and Treatment of Oral Overdose: Toxicity and symptoms are primarily due to iron overdose. Abdominal pain, nausea, vomiting and diarrhea may occur, with possible subsequent acidosis and cardiovasular collapse with severe poisoning. **Treatment:** Induce vomiting immediately. Administer milk, eggs to reduce gastric irritation. Contact a physician immediately.

Dosage and Administration: Women: One tablet daily.

How Supplied: Bottles of 40 and 120 tablets.

FEMIRON® Multi-Vitamins and Iron

Active Ingredients: Iron (from ferrous fumarate) 20 mg; Vitamin A 5,000 I.U.; Vitamin D 400 I.U.; Thiamine (Vitamin B_1) 1.5 mg; Riboflavin (Vitamin B_2) 1.7 mg; Niacinamide 20 mg; Ascorbic Acid (Vitamin C) 60 mg; Pyridoxine (Vitamin B_6) 2 mg; Cyanocobalamin (Vitamin B_{12}) 6 mcg; Calcium Pantothenate 10 mg; Folic Acid .4 mg; and Tocopherol Acetate (Vitamin E) 15 I.U.

Indications: For use as an iron and vitamin supplement.

Actions: Helps insure adequate intake of iron and vitamins.

Warnings: Keep out of reach of children.

Precaution: Alcoholics and individuals with chronic liver or pancreatic disease may have enhanced iron absorption with the potential for iron overload. NOTE: Unabsorbed iron may cause some darkening of the stool.

Symptoms and Treatment of Oral Overdosage: Toxicity and symptoms are primarily due to iron overdose. Abdominal pain, nausea, vomiting and diarrhea may occur, with possible subsequent acidosis and cardiovascular collapse with severe poisoning. **Treatment:** Induce vomiting immediately. Administer milk, eggs to reduce gastric irritation. Contact a physician immediately.

Dosage and Administration: Women: One tablet daily.

How Supplied: Bottles of 35, 60, and 90 tablets.

GERITOL® Liquid
High Potency Iron & Vitamin Tonic

Active Ingredients Per Dose (½ fluid ounce): Iron (as ferric ammonium citrate) 50 mg; Thiamine (B_1) 2.5 mg; Riboflavin (B_2) 2.5 mg; Niacinamide 50 mg; Panthenol 2 mg; Pyridoxine (B_6) 0.5 mg; Cyanocobalamin (B_{12}) 0.75 mcg; Methionine 25 mg; Choline Bitartrate 50 mg.

Inactive Ingredients: Alcohol, Benzoic acid, Caramel color, Citric acid, Invert sugar, Sucrose, Water, Flavors.

Indications: For use as a dietary supplement.

Actions: Help treat and prevent iron deficiency.

Warnings: Keep out of reach of children.

Precaution: Alcohol accelerates absorption of ferric iron. Alcoholics and individuals with chronic liver or pancreatic disease may have enhanced iron absorption with the potential for iron overload.
NOTE: Unabsorbed iron may cause some darkening of the stool.

Symptoms and Treatment of Oral Overdose: Toxicity and symptoms are primarily due to iron overdose. Abdominal pain, nausea, vomiting and diarrhea

may occur, with possible subsequent acidosis and cardiovascular collapse with severe poisoning. If an overdose is suspected, immediately seek professional assistance by contacting your physician, the local poison control center, or the Rocky Mt. Poison Control Center at 303-592-1710 (Collect), 24 hours a day.

Dosage and Administration (Adults): As an iron supplement and for normal menstrual needs: One (1) tablespoonful (0.5 fl. oz.) daily at mealtime. For iron deficiency: One (1) tablespoonful (0.5 fl. oz.) three times daily at mealtime or as directed by a physician.

How Supplied: Bottles of 4 oz., and 12 oz.

7001M
11/14/83

GERITOL COMPLETE™ Tablets
Vitamin/Mineral Tablets
With High Potency Iron

Active Ingredients (Per Tablet): Vitamin A (5000 IU); Vitamin E (30 IU); Vitamin C (60 mg.); Folic Acid (400 mcg.); Vitamin B_1 (1.5 mg.); Vitamin B_2 (1.7 mg.); Niacinamide (20 mg.); Vitamin B_6 (2 mg.); Vitamin B_{12} (6 mcg.); Vitamin D (400 IU); Biotin (300 mcg.); Pantothenic Acid (10 mg.); Calcium (162 mg.); Phosphorus (125 mg.); Iodine (150 mcg.); Iron (50 mg.); Magnesium (100 mg.); Copper (2 mg.); Manganese (7.5 mg); Potassium (7.7 mg.); Chloride (7 mg.); Chromium (15 mcg.); Molybdenum (15 mcg.); Selenium (15 mcg.); Zinc (15 mg.); Nickel (5 mcg.); Silicon (10 mcg.); Tin (10 mcg.); Vanadium (10 mcg.)

Inactive Ingredients: Carnauba wax, Croscarmelose sodium, Flavors, Gelatin, Glycerides of Stearic and Palmitic acids, Hydroxypropyl cellulose, Hydroxypropyl methylcellulose, Magnesium stearate, Microcrystalline cellulose, Polyethylene glycol, Silicon dioxide, Soy poly-saccharides, Stearic acid, White wax, FD&C Red #40, FD&C Blue #2, FD&C Yellow #6, Titanium dioxide.

Indications: For use as a dietary supplement.

Actions: Help treat and prevent iron deficiency.

Warnings: Keep out of reach of children.

Precaution: Alcoholics and individuals with chronic liver or pancreatic disease may have enhanced iron absorption with the potential for iron overload. NOTE: Unabsorbed iron may cause some darkening of the stool.

Symptoms and Treatment of Oral Overdose: Toxicity and symptoms are primarily due to iron overdose. Abdominal pain, nausea, vomiting and diarrhea may occur, with possible subsequent acidosis and cardiovascular collapse with severe poisoning. If an overdose is suspected, immediately seek professional assistance by contacting your physician,

Continued on next page

Beecham—Cont.

the local poison control center, or the Rocky Mt. Poison Control Center at 303-592-1710 (Collect), 24 hours a day.

Dosage and Administration (Adults): One (1) tablet daily at mealtime.

How Supplied: Bottles of 14, 40, 100, and 180 tablets.

CHILDREN'S HOLD®
4 Hour Cough Suppressant and Decongestant Lozenge

Active Ingredient: 3.75 mg. dextromethorphan HBr and 6.25 mg. phenylpropanolamine HCl per lozenge.

Inactive Ingredients: Citric acid, corn syrup, glycerin, magnesium trisilicate, sucrose, flavors, FD&C Blue #1, FD&C Red #40.

Indications: Suppresses coughs for up to 4 hours and helps provide relief of nasal congestion up to 4 hours.

Actions: Dextromethorphan is the most widely-used, non-narcotic/non-habit forming antitussive. Taken in a 5-10 mg. dose, it has been recognized as being effective for children (3-12 years) in relieving the discomfort of coughs up to 4 hours by reducing coughing intensity and frequency. Phenylpropanolamine is also non-narcotic and non-habit forming, and works as a decongestant.

Warnings: Persons with diabetes, high blood pressure, heart or thyroid disease should use only as directed by a physician. If symptoms persist or are accompanied by high fever, consult a physician promptly. Do not administer to children under 3. Do not exceed recommended dosage. Keep this and all other medications out of the reach of children.

Drug Interaction: Avoid the use of medications containing phenylpropanolamine when under treatment with monoamine oxidase inhibitors unless under the advice and supervision of a physician. As with any drug, if you are pregnant or nursing a baby, seek the advice of a health professional before using this product.

Symptoms and Treatment of Oral Overdosage: The principal symptoms of overdose are restlessness, dizziness, anxiety and/or slowing of respiration. Should these symptoms appear or a large overdose be suspected, seek professional advice by contacting your physician, the local poison control center, or the Rocky Mt. Poison Control Center at 303-592-1710 (Collect), 24 hrs. a day.

Dosage and Administration: Children over 6 years: Take 2 suppressants one after the other, every 4 hours. Children 3-6 years: One suppressant every 4 hours. Let dissolve fully.

How Supplied: 10 individually wrapped lozenges come packaged in a plastic tube container.

HOLD®
4 Hour Cough Suppressant Lozenge

Active Ingredient: 5.0 mg. dextromethorphan HBr per lozenge.

Inactive Ingredients: Corn syrup, magnesium trisilicate, sucrose, vegetable oil, flavors, FD&C Yellow #10.

Indications: Suppresses coughs for up to 4 hours.

Actions: Dextromethorphan is the most widely used, non-narcotic/non-habit forming antitussive. A 10-20 mg. dose has been recognized as being effective in relieving the discomfort of coughs up to 4 hours by reducing cough intensity and frequency.

Warnings: If cough persists or is accompanied by high fever, consult a physician promptly. Do not administer to children under 6. Do not exceed recommended dose. Keep this and all other medications out of reach of children.

Drug Interaction: No known drug interaction. As with any drug, if you are pregnant or nursing a baby, seek the advice of a health professional before using this product.

Symptoms and Treatment of Oral Overdosage: The principal symptom of overdose with dextromethorphan HBr is slowing of respiration. Should a large overdose be suspected seek professional assistance by contacting your physician, the local poison control center, or The Rocky Mt. Poison Control Center at 303-592-1710 (Collect), 24 hrs. a day.

Dosage and Administration: Adults (12 years and older): Take 2 suppressants one after the other, every 4 hours as needed. Children (6-12 years): One suppressant every 4 hours as needed. Let dissolve fully.

How Supplied: 10 individually wrapped suppressants come packaged in a plastic tube container.

MASSENGILL®
Disposable Douches
MASSENGILL®
Liquid Concentrate
MASSENGILL® Powder

Ingredients:
DISPOSABLES: Vinegar & Water-Extra Mild—Water and Vinegar.
Vinegar & Water-Extra Cleansing—Water, Vinegar, Cetylpyridinium Chloride, Diazolidinyl Urea, Disodium EDTA.
Belle-Mai—Water, SD Alcohol 40, Lactic Acid, Sodium Lactate, Octoxynol-9, Cetylpyridinium Chloride, Imidazolidinyl Urea, Disodium EDTA, Fragrance, FD&C Blue No. 1.
Country Flowers—Water, SD Alcohol 40, Lactic Acid, Sodium Lactate, Octoxynol-9, Cetylpyridinium Chloride, Imidazolidinyl Urea, Disodium EDTA, Fragrance, D&C Red No. 28, FD&C Blue No. 1.
Mountain Herbs—Water, SD Alcohol 40, Lactic Acid, Sodium Lactate, Octoxynol-9, Cetylpyridinium Chloride, Imidazolidinyl Urea, Disodium EDTA, Fra-

grance, D&C Yellow #10, FD&C Blue #1.
LIQUID CONCENTRATE: Water, SD Alcohol 40, Lactic Acid, Sodium Lactate, Octoxynol-9, Methyl Salicylate, Eucalyptol, Menthol, Thymol, D&C Yellow No. 10, FD&C Yellow No. 6.
POWDER: Sodium Chloride, Ammonium alum, PEG-8, Phenol, Methyl Salicylate, Eucalyptus Oil, Menthol, Thymol, D&C Yellow No. 10, FD&C Yellow No. 6.
FLORAL POWDER: Sodium Chloride, Ammonium alum, SD Alcohol 23-A, Octoxynol-9, Fragrance, FD&C Yellow #6.

Indications: Recommended for routine cleansing at the end of menstruation, after use of contraceptive creams or jellies (check the contraceptive package instructions first) or to rinse out the residue of prescribed vaginal medication (as directed by physician).

Actions: The buffered acid solutions of Massengill Douches are valuable adjuncts to specific vaginal therapy following the prescribed use of vaginal medication or contraceptives and in feminine hygiene.

Directions:
DISPOSABLES: Twist off flat, wing-shaped tab from bottle containing premixed solution, attach nozzle supplied and use. The unit is completely disposable.
LIQUID CONCENTRATE: Fill cap ¾ full, to measuring line, and pour contents into douche bag containing 1 quart of warm water. Mix thoroughly.
POWDER: Dissolve two rounded teaspoonfuls in a douche bag containing 1 quart of warm water. Mix thoroughly.

Warning: Vaginal cleansing douches should not be used more than twice weekly except on the advice of a physician. If irritation occurs, discontinue use. Keep out of reach of children. In case of accidental ingestion, seek professional assistance by contacting your physician, the local poison control center, or the Rocky Mt. Poison Control Center at 303-592-1710 (Collect), 24 hours a day.

How Supplied: Disposable—6 oz. disposable plastic bottle.
Liquid Concentrate—4 oz., 8 oz., plastic bottles.
Powder—4 oz., 8 oz., 16 oz., 22 oz. Packettes—10's, 12's.

MASSENGILL® Medicated
Disposable Douche

Active Ingredient: Cepticin™ (0.23% povidone-iodine).

Indications: For symptomatic relief of minor irritation and itching associated with vaginitis due to Candida albicans, Trichomonas vaginalis and Gardnerella vaginalis.

Action: Povidone-iodine is widely recognized as an effective broad spectrum microbicide against both gram negative and gram positive bacteria, fungi, yeasts and protozoa. While remaining active in the presence of blood, serum or bodily secretions, it possesses virtually none of the irritating properties of iodine.

Warnings: If symptoms persist after seven days of use, or if redness, swelling or pain develop during treatment, consult a physician. Women with iodine-sensitivity should not use this product. Women may douche during menstruation if they douche gently. Do not douche during pregnancy unless directed by a physician. Douching does not prevent pregnancy. Keep out of reach of children. In case of accidental ingestion, seek professional assistance by contacting your physician, the local poison control center, or the Rocky Mt. Poison Control Center at 303-592-1710 (Collect), 24 hours a day.

Dosage and Administration: Dosage is provided as a single unit concentrate to be added to 6 oz. of sanitized water supplied in a disposable bottle. A specially designed nozzle is provided. After use, the unit is discarded. Use one bottle daily for seven days. Even if symptoms are relieved earlier, treatment should be continued for the full seven days.

How Supplied: 6 oz. bottle of sanitized water with 0.17 oz. vial of povidone-iodine and nozzle.

N'ICE® Medicated Sugarless Cough Lozenges

Active Ingredient:
Cherry—Each lozenge contains 5.0 mg. menthol in a sorbitol base.
Citrus—Each lozenge contains 3.0 mg. menthol in a sorbitol base.
Menthol Eucalyptus—Each lozenge contains 5.0 mg. menthol in a sorbitol base.
Menthol Mint—Each lozenge contains 6.0 mg. menthol in a sorbitol base.

Inactive Ingredients:
Cherry—Sorbitol, Tartaric acid, flavors, FD&C Blue #1, FD&C Red #40.
Citrus—Citric acid, sorbitol, flavors, FD&C Yellow #10.
Menthol Eucalyptus—Citric acid, sorbitol, flavors.
Menthol Mint—Citric acid, sorbitol, flavors, FD&C Blue #1, FD&C Yellow #10.

Indications: Soothes irritated throat tissue to provide temporary relief of minor sore throat pain and coughs due to colds, allergies, and smoking.

Actions: Menthol in a sorbitol base soothes irritated throat tissue and leaves the throat feeling cool.

Warnings: Persistent cough or sore throat accompanied by high fever may be serious. Consult a physician in such case, or if sore throat persists more than 2 days. Do not administer to children under 6 years of age unless directed by a physician. Keep this and all medications out of the reach of children.

Drug Interaction: No known drug interaction.

Symptoms and Treatment of Oral Overdosage: Should a large overdose of N'ICE (Cherry, Citrus, Menthol Eucalyptus, or Menthol Mint-flavored) be sus-

pected, with symptoms of nausea, vomiting and diarrhea, seek professional assistance. Contact your physician, the local poison control center, or the Rocky Mountain Poison Control Center at 303-592-1710 (Collect); 24 hours a day.

Dosage and Administration: Let lozenge dissolve slowly in the mouth. Repeat as needed, up to 10 lozenges per day.

Professional Labeling: Same as those outlined under INDICATIONS.

How Supplied: Available in packages of 8 and 16 lozenges.

SCOTT'S EMULSION®
Vitamin A and D Food Supplement

Active Ingredient: Cod Liver Oil which provides 5,000 International Units of Vitamin A per 4 teaspoons of Scott's Emulsion (100% of RDA) and 400 International Units of Vitamin D per 4 teaspoons (100% of RDA).

Indications: Provides daily requirements of Vitamin A and D.

Actions: Scott's Emulsion supplies natural Vitamins A and D from cod liver oil. The product is in a highly emulsified form for more rapid absorption by the body. Flavoring agents are included to help mask the flavor of cod liver oil.

Dosage and Administration: 4 teaspoons per day provides 100% of the adult RDA for Vitamins A and D.

How Supplied: 6¼ and 12½ fl. oz. bottles.

SERUTAN® Concentrated Powder
Natural-Fiber Laxative

Active Ingredient: Vegetable hemicellulose derived from Plantago Ovata 45%.

Indications: For aiding bowel regularity.

Actions: Softens stools, increases bulk volume and water content.

Warnings: Keep out of the reach of children.

Precaution: Patients with suspected intestinal disorders should consult a physician.

Dosage and Administration: Adults: Stir one heaping teaspoonful into an 8 oz. glass of water. Drink immediately. Take one to three times daily, preferably at mealtime.

How Supplied: 7 oz., 14 oz., and 21 oz. bottles.

SERUTAN® Concentrated Powder
—Fruit Flavored
Natural-Fiber Laxative

Active Ingredient: Vegetable hemicellulose derived from Plantago Ovata 45%.

Indications: For aiding bowel regularity.

Actions: Softens stools, increases bulk volume and water content.

Warnings: Keep out of the reach of children.

Precaution: Patients with suspected intestinal disorders should consult a physician.

Dosage and Administration: Adults: Stir one heaping teaspoonful into an 8 oz. glass of water. Drink immediately. Take one to three times daily, preferably at mealtime.

How Supplied: 6 oz., 12 oz., and 18 oz. bottles.

SERUTAN® Toasted Granules
Natural-Fiber Laxative

Active Ingredients: Vegetable hemicellulose derived from Plantago Ovata 39%.

Indications: For aiding bowel regularity.

Actions: Softens stools, increases bulk volume and water content.

Warnings: Keep out of the reach of children.

Precaution: Patients with suspected intestinal disorders should consult a physician. Not to be taken directly by spoon.

Dosage and Administration: Adults: Sprinkle one heaping teaspoonful on cereal or other food, one to three times daily.

How Supplied: Available in 6 oz., and 18 oz. plastic bottles.

SOMINEX® Pain Relief Formula

Active Ingredients: 25 mg. diphenhydramine HCl and 500 mg. acetaminophen per tablet.

Inactive Ingredients: Corn starch, crospovidone, silicon dioxide, stearic acid, FD&C Blue #1.

Indications: For sleeplessness with accompanying occasional minor aches, pains, and headaches.

Action: An antihistamine with sedative effects combined with an internal analgesic.

Warnings: Do not give to children under 12 years of age. If systoms persists continuously for more than 10 days, or if new ones occur, consult your physician. Do not exceed recommended dosage because severe liver damage may occur. Insomnia may be a symptom of serious underlying medical illness. Take this product with caution if alcohol is being consumed. Do not take this product for the treatment of arthritis, except under the advice and supervision of a physician. As with any drug, if you are pregnant or nursing a baby, seek the advice of a health professional before using this product. Keep this and all drugs out of the reach of children. In case of accidental overdose, seek professional assistance or contact a poison control center immediately.

Continued on next page

Beecham—Cont.

DO NOT TAKE THIS PRODUCT IF YOU HAVE ASTHMA, GLAUCOMA OR ENLARGEMENT OF THE PROSTATE GLAND, EXCEPT UNDER THE ADVICE AND SUPERVISION OF A PHYSICIAN.

Drug Interaction: Monoamine oxidase (MAO) inhibitors prolong and intensify the anticholinergic effects of antihistamines. The CNS depressant affect is heightened by alcohol and other CNS depressant drugs.

Symptoms and Treatment of Oral Overdosage: Antihistamine overdosage reactions may vary from central nervous system depression to stimulation. Stimulation is particularly likely in children. Atropine-like signs and symptoms, such as dry mouth, fixed and dilated pupils, flushing, and gastrointestinal symptoms, may also occur.

Dosage and Administration: Take two tablets once daily at bedtime or as directed by a physician.

How Supplied: Available in blister packs of 16, 32, and 72 tablets.

SOMINEX® 2

Active Ingredients: Diphenhydramine hydrochloride, 25 mg per tablet.

Inactive Ingredients: Dibasic calcium phosphate, magnesium stearate, microcrystalline cellulose, silicon dioxide, starch, FD&C Blue #1.

Indications: To induce drowsiness and assist in falling asleep.

Action: An antihistamine with anticholinergic and sedative effects.

Warnings: Do not give to children under 12 years of age. If sleeplessness persists continuously for more than 2 weeks, consult your physician. Insomnia may be a symptom of serious underlying medical illness. Take this product with caution if alcohol is being consumed. Keep this and all drugs out of the reach of children. Do not take this product if you have asthma, glaucoma or enlargement of the prostate gland except under the advice of a physician. In case of accidental overdose, seek professional assistance by contacting your physician, the local poison control center, or the Rocky Mountain Poison Control Center at 303-592-1710 (Collect); 24 hours a day. As with any drug, if you are pregnant or nursing a baby, seek the advice of a health professional before using this product.

Drug Interaction: Monoamine oxidase (MAO) inhibitors prolong and intensify the anticholinergic effects of antihistamines. The CNS depressant affect is heightened by alcohol and other CNS depressant drugs.

Symptoms and Treatment of Oral Overdosage: Antihistamine overdosage reactions may vary from central nervous system depression to stimulation. Stimulation is particularly likely in chil-

dren. Atropine-like signs and symptoms, such as dry mouth, fixed and dilated pupils, flushing, and gastrointestinal symptoms, may also occur.

Dosage and Administration: Take 2 tablets once daily at bedtime or as directed by a physician.

How Supplied: Available in blister packs of 16, 32, and 72 tablets.

S.T.37®
Antiseptic Solution

Active Ingredient: .1% hexylresorcinol in a glycerin-aqueous solution

Indications: For use on cuts, abrasions, burns, scalds, sunburn and the hygienic care of the mouth.

Actions: S.T.37 is a non-stinging, non-staining antiseptic solution that provides soothing protection and helps relieve pain of burns, cuts, abrasions and mouth irritations.

Warnings: If redness, irritation, swelling or pain persists or increases or if infection occurs, discontinue use and consult physician. In case of deep or puncture wounds or serious burns, consult physician. Keep out of reach of children.

Symptoms and Treatment of Oral Overdosage: In case of a large overdose of S.T. 37, seek professional assistance. Contact a physician, the local poison control center, or call the Rocky Mt. Poison Control Center at 303-592-1710 (Collect), 24 hours a day.

Dosage and Administration: For cuts, burns, scalds and abrasions apply undiluted, bandage lightly keeping bandage wet with S.T.37 antiseptic solution. For hygienic care of the mouth, dilute with 1 or 2 parts of warm water.

How Supplied: 5 and 12 fl. oz. bottles.

SUCRETS® (Regular and Mentholated)
Sore Throat Lozenges

Active Ingredient: Hexylresorcinol, 2.4 mg. per lozenge.

Inactive Ingredients: Citric acid, corn syrup, sucrose, flavors, FD&C Blue #1, D&C Yellow #10.

Indications: Temporary relief of minor sore throat pain and mouth irritations.

Actions: Hexylresorcinol's soothing anesthetic action quickly relieves minor throat irritations.

Warnings: Do not administer to children under 3 years of age unless directed by a physician. Keep all medications out of the reach of children. Persistent sore throat or sore throat accompanied by high fever, headache, nausea or vomiting usually indicates a severe infection and may be serious. Consult a physician promptly in such case, or if sore throat persists more than 2 days.

Drug Interaction: No known drug interaction

Symptoms and Treatment of Oral Overdosage: Should a large overdose of Sucrets (Regular or Mentholated) be suspected, with symptoms of profuse sweating, nausea, vomiting and diarrhea, seek professional assistance. Call your physician, local poison control center or the Rocky Mountain Poison Control Center at 303-592-1710 (Collect), 24 hrs. a day.

Dosage and Administration: Use as needed. For best results dissolve slowly—do not chew.

Professional Labeling: Same as those outlined under Indications.

How Supplied: Sucrets-Regular: Available in tins of 24 and 48 individually wrapped lozenges. Sucrets-Mentholated: Available in tins of 24 lozenges.

SUCRETS® Children's Cherry Flavored
Sore Throat Lozenges

Active Ingredient: Dyclonine Hydrochloride, 1.2 mg. per lozenge.

Inactive Ingredients: Citric acid, corn syrup, silicon dioxide, sucrose, flavor, FD&C Blue #1, FD&C Red #40.

Indications: Temporary relief of minor sore throat pain and mouth irritations.

Actions: Dyclonine Hydrochloride's soothing anesthetic action quickly relieves minor throat irritations.

Warnings: Do not exceed recommended dosage. Persistent sore throat or sore throat accompanied by high fever, headache, nausea or vomiting usually indicates a severe infection and may be serious. Consult a physician promptly in such case, or if sore throat persists more than 2 days. Discontinue use and consult a physician if irritation persists or increases or a rash appears on the skin.

Drug Interaction: No known drug interaction.

Symptoms and Treatment of Oral Overdosage: Reactions due to large overdosage are systemic and involve the central nervous system. Central nervous system reactions are characterized by excitation and/or depression. Nervousness, dizziness, blurred vision or tremors may occur. Reactions involving the cardiovascular system include depression of the myocardium, hypotension, or bradycardia. Should a large overdose be suspected, seek professional assistance. Call your physician, local poison control center or the Rocky Mountain Poison Control Center at 303-592-1710 (Collect), 24 hours a day.

Dosage and Administration: Children (3 years and over) and adults: dissolve one lozenge in the mouth. One additional lozenge every 2 hours, if necessary. For best results dissolve slowly—do not chew.

Professional Labeling: Same as those outlined under INDICATIONS.

How Supplied: Available in tins of 24 lozenges.

SUCRETS®–Cold Decongestant Formula
Decongestant Lozenges

Active Ingredient: Phenylpropanolamine hydrochloride, 25 mg. per lozenge.

Inactive Ingredients: Citric acid, corn syrup, sucrose, titanium dioxide, flavors, FD&C Yellow #6.

Indications: For fast temporary relief of nasal congestion.

Warnings: Do not exceed recommended dosage because at higher dosages nervousness, dizziness or sleeplessness may occur. If symptoms do not improve within 7 days or are accompanied by high fever, consult a physician before continuing use. Do not take this product if you have high blood pressure, heart disease, diabetes or thyroid disease except under the advice of a physician. As with any drug, if you are pregnant or nursing a baby, seek the advice of a health professional before using this product.

Drug Interaction: Avoid the use of medications containing phenylpropanolamine when under treatment with monamine oxidase inhibitors unless under the advice and supervision of a physician.

Symptoms and Treatment of Oral Overdosage: The principal symptoms of an overdose are restlessness, dizziness, anxiety. Should these symptoms appear or a large overdose be suspected, seek professional assistance. Call your physician, the local poison control center or the Rocky Mt. Poison Control Center at 303-592-1710 (Collect), 24 hours a day.

Dosage and Administration: Adults (12 years and over): Slowly dissolve one lozenge in the mouth. One additional lozenge every 4 hours, but do not exceed 6 lozenges in 24 hours. Do not exceed recommended dosage. Children (under 12 years): Only as directed by a physician.

Professional Labeling: Same as those outlined under Indications.

How Supplied: Available in tins of 24 lozenges.

SUCRETS® Cough Control Formula
Cough Control Lozenges

Active Ingredient: Dextromethorphan hydrobromide, 7.5 mg. per lozenge.

Inactive Ingredients: Corn syrup, magnesium trisilicate sucrose, vegetable oil, flavors, FD&C Blue #1, FD&C Red #2, D&C Yellow #10.

Indications: For temporary suppression of cough and relief of minor throat irritation.

Actions: Dextromethorphan is the most widely used non-narcotic/non-habit forming antitussive. A 10-20 mg. dose in adults (7.5 mg in children over 6) has been recognized as being effective in relieving the frequency and intensity of cough for up to 4 hours.

Warnings: If cough persists or is accompanied by high fever, consult a physician promptly. Do not use more than two days or administer to children under 6 unless directed by a physician. Keep out of the reach of children. As with any drug, if you are pregnant or nursing a baby, seek the advice of a health professional before using this product.

Drug Interaction: No known drug interaction.

Symptoms and Treatment of Oral Overdosage: Slowing of respiration is the principal symptom of dextromethorphan HBr overdose. Should a large overdose be suspected, seek professional assistance. Call your physician, the local poison control center or the Rocky Mt. Poison Control Center at 303-592-1710 (Collect), 24 hours a day.

Dosage and Administration: Adults (12 years and over): Take 2 lozenges every 4 hours as needed. Let dissolve fully in mouth. Children (6–12 years): One lozenge every 4 hours as needed. Let dissolve fully in mouth. Do not exceed recommended dosage.

Professional Labeling: Same as those outlined under Indications.

How Supplied: Available in tins of 24 lozenges.

SUCRETS® Maximum Strength
Sore Throat Lozenges

Active Ingredient: Dyclonine Hydrochloride, 3.0 mg. per lozenge.

Inactive Ingredients: Citric acid, corn syrup, silicon dioxide, sucrose, flavors, FD&C Yellow #10.

Indications: Temporary relief of minor sore throat pain and mouth irritations.

Actions: Dyclonine Hydrocloride's soothing anesthetic action quickly relieves minor throat irritations.

Warnings: Do not exceed recommended dosage. Persistent sore throat or sore throat accompanied by high fever, headache, nausea or vomiting usually indicates a severe infection and may be serious. Consult a physician promptly in such case, or if sore throat persists more than 2 days. Discontinue use and consult a physician if irritation persists or increases or a rash appears on the skin.

Drug Interaction: No known drug interaction.

Symptoms and Treatment of Oral Overdosage: Reactions due to large overdosage are systemic and involve the central nervous system and cardiovascular system. Central nervous system reactions are characterized by excitation and/or depression. Nervousness, dizziness, blurred vision or tremors may occur. Reactions involving the cardiovascular system include depression of the myocardium, hypotension or bradycardia.

Should a large overdose be suspected seek professional assistance. Call your physician, local poison control center or the Rocky Mountain Poison Control Center at 303-592-1710 (Collect), 24 hours a day.

Dosage and Administration: Adults (12 years and over): dissolve one lozenge in the mouth. One additional lozenge every 2 hours, if necessary. Not recommended for children under 12 years. For best results dissolve slowly—do not chew.

Professional Labeling: Same as those outlined under INDICATIONS.

How Supplied: Available in tins of 24 lozenges.

THERMOTABS®
Buffered Salt Tablets

Active Ingredient: Per tablet—sodium chloride—450 mg.; potassium chloride—30 mg.; calcium carbonate—18 mg.; dextrose—200 mg.

Indications: To minimize fatigue and prevent muscle cramps and heat prostration due to excessive perspiration.

Actions: Thermotabs are designed for tennis players, joggers, golfers and other athletes who experience excessive perspiration. Also for use in steel mills, industrial plants, kitchens, stores, or other locations where high temperatures cause heat fatigue, cramps or heat prostration.

Warnings: Keep out of reach of children.

Precaution: Individuals on a salt-restricted diet should use THERMOTABS only under the advice and supervision of a physician.

Symptoms and Treatment of Oral Overdosage: Signs of salt overdose include diarrhea and muscular twitching. If an overdose is suspected, contact a physician, the local poison control center, or call the Rocky Mt. Poison Control Center at 303-592-1710 (Collect), 24 hours a day.

Dosage and Administration: One tablet with a full glass of water, 5 to 10 times a day depending on temperature and conditions.

How Supplied: 100 tablet bottles.

VIVARIN® Stimulant Tablets

Active Ingredient: 200 mg. caffeine alkaloid per tablet.

Inactive Ingredients: Cornstarch, dextrose, magnesium stearate, microcrystalline cellulose, silicon dioxide, FD&C Yellow #6, FD&C Yellow #10.

Indications: Helps restore mental alertness or wakefulness when experiencing fatigue or drowsiness.

Actions: Stimulates cerebrocortical areas involved with active mental processes.

Warnings: Keep out of reach of children. For adult use only. Do not take

Continued on next page

Beecham—Cont.

more than 1 tablet in any 3–4 hour period. Product should not be substituted for normal sleep. Do not exceed recommended dose since side effects may occur which include increased nervousness, anxiety, irritability, difficulty in falling asleep and occasional disturbances in heart rate and rhythm called palpitations. For occasional use only. If fatigue or drowsiness persists continuously for more than 2 weeks, consult a physician. Do not give to children under 12 years of age. The recommended dose of this product contains about as much caffeine as two cups of coffee. Take this product with caution while taking caffeine containing beverages such as coffee, tea or cola drinks because large doses of caffeine may cause side effects as cautioned elsewhere on the label. As with any drug, if you are pregnant or nursing a baby, seek the advice of a health professional before using this product.

Drug Interaction: Use of caffeine should be lowered or avoided if drugs are being used to treat cardiovascular ailments, psychological problems, or kidney trouble.

Precaution: Higher blood glucose levels may result from caffeine use.

Symptoms and Treatment of Oral Overdosage: Convulsions may occur if caffeine is consumed in doses larger than 10 g. Emesis should be induced to empty the stomach. In case of accidental overdose, seek professional assistance by contacting your physician, the local poison control center, or the Rocky Mt. Poison Control Center at 303-592-1710 (Collect), 24 hours a day.

Dosage and Administration: Adults: 1 tablet every 3–4 hours, as needed.

How Supplied: Available in packages of 16, 40 and 80 tablets.

Beiersdorf, Inc.
BDF PLAZA
P.O. BOX 5529
NORWALK, CT 06856-5529

AQUAPHOR®
Ointment Base
NDC Number–10356-020-01

Composition: Petrolatum, mineral oil, mineral wax, wool wax alcohol.

Actions and Uses: Aquaphor is a stable, neutral, odorless, anhydrous ointment base. Miscible with water or aqueous solutions several times its own weight, Aquaphor forms smooth, creamy water-in-oil emulsions. Also, recommended for use as a topical preparation for extremely dry skin.

Administration and Dosages: Aquaphor will absorb many times its own weight of water or aqueous solution. Use Aquaphor in compounding virtually any ointment using aqueous solutions alone or in combination with other oil-based

substances, and all common topical medications.

Precautions: For external use only.

How Supplied:
1 lb. plastic jars—List Number 0020
5 lb. plastic jars—List Number 0021
45 lb. drum—List Number 0022

EUCERIN™
CLEANSING BAR

Active Ingredient: Eucerite®

Actions and Uses: Eucerin™ Cleansing Bar has been specially formulated for use on sensitive skin. The formulation contains Eucerite®, a special blend of ingredients that closely resemble the natural oils of the skin, thus providing excellent moisturizing properties. Additionally, the ph value of Eucerin Cleansing Bar is maintained at 5.5 in order to match the skin's normal acid mantle.

Directions: Use during shower or bath, or as directed by physician

How Supplied: 3 ounce bar.
List number 3854

EUCERIN® Creme
Unscented Moisturizing Formula
NDC Number–10356-090-01

Composition: Water, petrolatum, mineral oil, mineral wax, wool wax alcohol, 2-bromo-2 nitropropane-1, 3-diol.

Actions and Uses: A gentle, unscented water-in-oil emulsion. Eucerin helps alleviate excessive dry skin and may be helpful in conditions such as chapped or chafed skin, sunburn, windburn, and itching associated with dryness.

Administration and Dosages: Apply freely to affected areas of the skin as often as necessary or as directed by physician.

Precautions: For external use only.

How Supplied:
16 oz. jar—List Number 0090
4 oz. jar—List Number 3797

EUCERIN® Lotion
Unscented Moisturizing Formula

Composition: Water, Mineral Oil, Isopropyl Myristate, PEG-40 Sorbitan Peroleate, Lanolin Acid Glycerin Ester, Sorbitol, Propylene Glycol, Beeswax, Magnesium Sulfate, Aluminum Stearate, Lanolin Alcohol, BHT, Methylchloroisothiazolinone·Methylisothiazolinone.

Actions and Uses: Eucerin Lotion is a gentle, light moisturizing formula that works itself deep into the pores of the skin, to help replace lost moisture and augment the return of natural oils. Used daily, Eucerin Lotion keeps skin feeling soft, moist, and fresh all over.

Administration and Dosage: Apply Eucerin Lotion all over body—hands, arms, legs, and feet—to help moisturize, smooth and soothe rough, dry skin.

Precautions: For external use only.

How Supplied: 8 fluid oz. plastic bottles.
List Number 3793
16 fluid oz. plastic bottle.
List number 3794

GELOCAST®
GELOCAST® Unna Boot
NDC Number–10356-103-02

Composition: Water, glycerin, sorbitol, gelatin, magnesium aluminum silicate, zinc oxide, calamine, methylparaben, imidazolidinyl urea, propylparaben, and dimethicone.

Actions and Uses: For the compression treatment of venous insufficiency conditions such as stasis ulcers, stasis dermatitis, chronic lymphangitis, and varicose veins with ulceration. Also, indications for use in Orthopedics and in the treatment of post-fracture conditions and as an aid in helping prevent edema.

Administration and Dosage: Thoroughly wash the extremity with soap and water, towel dry, then sponge with alcohol. Remove Gelocast bandage from sealed, inner pouch.
Wrap the extremity by winding the bandage around knee or elbow. Maintain even pressure on the bandage, and avoid folds by molding to body contours. Allow Gelocast to dry, then cover with a layer of plain gauze to prevent adhering to other material (stocking or bed linen). Gelocast may be left in place from one to two weeks. To remove bandage, simply cut lengthwise with a pair of scissors.

Precautions: If skin sensitivity or irritation develops, discontinue use and consult a physician.

How Supplied:
4″ × 10 yards Unna Boot—List Number 1053
3″ × 10 yards Unna Boot—List Number 1052

MEDIPLAST®
40% Salicylic acid plaster
NDC Number–10356-703-03

Active Ingredient: 40% Salicylic Acid.

Indications: For removal of callous tissue.

Actions: Mediplast is a 40% salicylic acid plaster that is used for the softening of callous tissue and the removal of warts. Convenient to use, Mediplast is self-adhesive and can be cut to fit the affected area. Mediplast stays in place while it works to soften the calloused area.

Warnings
Caution: Not to be applied to healthy tissue. Do not use each application for more than 24 hours. If re-application to calloused part is necessary, allow time in between applications.
Upon evidence of irritation, remove plaster immediately and do not re-apply. Consult your physician. Do not use on

flamed sites or if diabetic or if circulatory impairments exist. Keep out of reach of children. For external use only.

Dosage and Administration: Cut out piece of plaster to dimension of calloused tissue. Remove backing paper and apply plaster. Use the envelope to store remaining plaster for next use. Store at room temperature 15-30 C (59-86F).

Professional Labeling: Same as those outlined under Indications.

How Supplied: 25 individually wrapped plasters per box. List Number 1496

Bigelow-Clark Inc.
360 MEACHAM AVE.
ELMONT, NY 11003

WORK OUT®
Athletic Rub

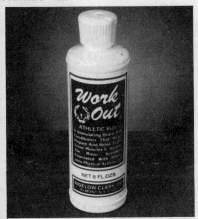

Active Ingredient: Thymol, Menthol, Methyl Salicylate, Capsicum, Salicylic Acid, Alcohol, Essential Oils and Tinctures.

Indications: A stimulating brace and conditioner that helps prepare and relax tight tense muscles and sooth the minor soreness associated with strenuous physical activity, allowing greater freedom of movement and increased muscle endurance.

Warnings: Work Out is a counter irritant and should be kept away from eyes and mucous membranes. Discontinue use if excessive irritation develops. Keep away from open flame and out of the reach of children.

Dosage and Administration: Apply in slow circular motion using direct pressure, kneading muscles with fingers until dry.

How Supplied: Direct from Bigelow Clark and drug wholesalers. 8 fl. oz. Bottles.

Products are cross-indexed by generic and chemical names in the
YELLOW SECTION

Bio Products, Inc.
55 POST ROAD WEST
WESTPORT, CT 06880

Q–VEL®
Muscle Relaxant Pain Reliever

Active Ingredient: Quinine Sulfate 1 gr. (64.8 mg).

Contains: Natural source vitamin E (400 I.U. d-alpha tocopheryl acetate) in a lecithin base.

Indications: Night leg cramps.

Actions: Muscle relaxant pain reliever for temporary relief of leg cramps.

Warnings: Do not take if pregnant or of childbearing potential. Discontinue use if ringing in the ears, deafness, skin rash or visual disturbances occur and consult your physician immediately. As with all medicine, keep out of reach of children. In case of accidental overdose, seek medical assistance or contact Poison Control Center at once.

Dosage and Administration: In acute attack, take 2 capsules at once, plus 2 capsules after ½ hour, if needed. To help prevent future attacks, 2 capsules after evening meal plus 2 capsules at bedtime for five days.

How Supplied: 30 and 50 capsule bottles.
Shown in Product Identification Section, page 404

Blistex Inc.
1800 SWIFT DRIVE
OAK BROOK, IL 60521

BLISTEX® LIP CONDITIONER™

Indications: Blistex Lip Conditioner is a medicated balm packaged in a plastic jar. The product is recommended for the prevention and relief of dry, chapped or cracked lips. Its MAXIMAL (SPF-12) sunscreen formula helps protect lips from the damaging effects of overexposure to the sun.

Ingredients:
Actives:
Petrolatum (skin protectant)
Octyl Dimethyl PABA 8.0% (sunscreen)
Benzophenone-3 2.0% (sunscreen)
Excipients:
An emollient base of Lanolin, Aloe Vera, and Cocoa Butter.

Mode of Action: Petrolatum serves as a skin protectant due to its emollient and lubricant properties. Petrolatum also excludes air, preventing evaporation and reducing pain.
The two sunscreen ingredients will block ultraviolet radiation which will reduce the sun's harmful effects on lip tissue. The emollient base helps prevent moisture loss from lip tissue and aids natural healing of dry and sunburned lips.

Directions: Dry, Chapped Lips: At first symptoms, apply and massage thoroughly. Continue to use as needed until lips are soft and smooth.
Protection from Sun, Wind, Cold: Apply thirty minutes before exposure to the elements and frequently (at least every two hours) thereafter.

Cautions: Avoid contact with the eyes. If signs of irritation or sensitization appear, the patient should discontinue use of the product.

Literature: Patient and professional pamphlets are available on request.

How Supplied: Blistex Lip Conditioner is available in a .38 oz. plastic jar (NDC 10157-0051-1).

BLISTIK®
Medicated Lip Balm

Indications: Blistik is a medicated lip balm in a plastic propel-repel container. The product is recommended for the prevention and relief of dryness and chapping from sun, wind and cold. Blistik has MAXIMAL (SPF-9) sunscreen protection. Liberal and regular use may help reduce the harmful effects of overexposure to the sun.

Ingredients:
Actives:
Octyl Dimethyl PABA 6.6% (sunscreen)
Oxybenzone 2.5% (sunscreen)
Allantoin 1.0% (skin protectant)
Excipients:
An emollient base with Petrolatum, Lanolin, and mixed waxes

Mode of Action: Allantoin affords protection of the lips against external irritants, since it forms complexes with a variety of sensitizing agents rendering them non-sensitizing. The emollient base helps prevent moisture loss from lip tissue, and aids healing of dry and sunburned lips. The two sunscreens will block ultraviolet radiation which will reduce the sun's harmful effects on lip tissue.

Directions: Dry, Chapped Lips: Apply frequently until lips are soft and smooth. Continue to use as needed.
Protection from Sun, Wind, Cold: Apply Blistik thirty minutes before exposure to the elements and frequently (at least every 2 hours) thereafter.

Cautions: Avoid contact with the eyes. If signs of irritation or sensitization appear, the patient should discontinue use of the product.

Literature Available: Patient and professional pamphlets available on request.

How Supplied: Blistik lip balm is available in .15 oz. containers in Regular (unflavored—NDC 10157-5197-1), Mint (NDC 10157-8065-1), and Berry (NDC 10157-8075-1) varieties.

Continued on next page

Blistex—Cont.

BLISTEX®
Medicated Lip Ointment

Indications: Blistex is a medicated ointment in a tube. The product is recommended for symptomatic relief of cold sores and for the prevention and relief of dry, chapped and sunburned lips.

Ingredients:
Actives:
  Camphor 1.0% (counter-irritant)
  Phenol 0.4% (antiseptic)
Excipients:
  An emollient base with Petrolatum, Lanolin, and Peppermint Oil

Mode of Action: Camphor is used to furnish slight local anesthetic and counter-irritant action to sore and chapped lips. Liquified Phenol will provide mild antiseptic action. The tissue cleansing properties for this product are contributed by the cationic soap produced in the preparation of finished product. The emollient and lubricant properties are produced by the lipid phase.

Directions: Dry, Chapped Lips: At first symptoms, apply and massage thoroughly. Repeat every half hour until condition is relieved.
Cold Sores: At the first sign of a cold sore, gently apply and massage Blistex into the immediate (sensitive) area.

Cautions: Do not use in the eyes. If the condition persists, or if inflammation develops, the patient should discontinue use and consult a physician. As with all products, a few individuals may prove to be allergic to ingredients contained in this ointment.

Literature Available: Patient and professional pamphlets available on request.

How Supplied: Blistex ointment is available in .14 oz. (NDC 10157-2549-1) and .5 oz. (NDC 10157-2549-3) tubes.
Shown in Product Identification Section, page 404

FOILLE®
First Aid Remedy in Aerosol, Liquid and Ointment forms

Indications: Foille is a line of medicated products recommended for relief of pain from sunburn, minor burns, abrasions, and non-poisonous insect bites.

Ingredients:
Actives:
  Benzocaine 5.0% (external analgesic)
  Chloroxylenol 0.1% (antiseptic)
Excipients:
  A bland vegetable oil base with Benzyl Alcohol and other ingredients.

Mode of Action: Foille combines antiseptic and analgesic properties and provides prompt relief of pain, burning, and itching. Foille is ideal for use on many local forms of skin irritation—particularly minor burns, sunburn, cuts, abrasions and non-poisonous insect bites.

Foille helps control the scratch reflex, and is not decomposed by perspiration.

Directions:
Burns: To stop heat damage, place affected area immediately in cold water and soak for several minutes. Apply Foille liberally over the burn and smooth into skin. If desired, surgical gauze or a clean white cloth can be placed gently over the injured area. Repeat application of Foille frequently to keep area moist.
Sunburn: Apply Foille immediately when first signs of inflammation appear. Reapply every two or three hours until pain and redness disappear.
Wounds/Abrasions: Apply Foille to the injured area. If desired, a light surgical dressing can be placed over the area.

Cautions: Do not use in the eyes. A physician should immediately be consulted in case of deep or puncture wounds or serious burns. If the condition persists, or if additional inflammation develops, the patient should discontinue use and consult a physician.

How Supplied: Foille is available in a 1 ounce ointment tube (NDC 0473-3014-04), a 3.25 ounce aerosol spray can (NDC 0473-1715-03), and a 1 ounce liquid bottle (NDC 0473-1715-02).
Shown in Product Identification Section, page 404

FOILLE® PLUS
First Aid Spray

Indications: Foille Plus is a water-washable first aid remedy in aerosol spray form. Foille Plus provides temporary relief of pain from minor burns, sunburn and abrasions, while helping to prevent infection.

Ingredients:
Actives:
  Benzocaine 5.0% (external analgesic)
  Chloroxylenol 0.6% (antiseptic)
Excipients:
  A non-staining base with Benzyl Alcohol and other ingredients. Alcohol 82.67% w/w.

Mode of Action: Benzocaine affords prompt, temporary relief of pain, burning and itching by creating surface anesthetic action on the affected area. Benzyl alcohol provides antiseptic and analgesic properties and helps prevent secondary infection due to bacteriostatic effects. The product is non-toxic, water-washable, and has a pleasant aromatic odor.

Directions: Minor Burns, Sunburn, and Abrasions: The patient should spray a liberal amount of Foille Plus over the injured area. Reapply every two or three hours to keep area moist. If desired, a light surgical dressing can be placed over the area.

Cautions: Patients with a known sensitivity to Benzocaine or to other para-amino compounds should avoid the use of this product. Avoid contact with the eyes. In case of deep puncture wounds, the patient should consult a physician. If the condition persists or if additional inflam-

mation develops, the patient should discontinue use and consult a physician.

How Supplied: Foille Plus is available in a 3.5 ounce aerosol spray can (NDC 10157-4887-2).
Shown in Product Identification Section, page 404

IVAREST®
Medicated Cream & Lotion

Indications: Ivarest is a medicated product for relief of inflammation from poison ivy, poison oak, and minor skin irritations.

Ingredients:
Actives:
  Calamine 14.0% (skin protectant)
  Benzocaine 5.0% (external analgesic)
Excipients:
  A water-washable base with Pyrilamine Maleate, Petrolatum and Lanolin oil.

Mode of Action: Benzocaine is used to relieve minor pain and itching caused by irritation from poison ivy, oak or sumac. The analgesic action of Benzocaine is almost entirely on nerve terminals. Calamine is used for its protective, antiseptic and antibacterial action against a wide variety of skin diseases.

Directions: Gently cleanse the affected area and apply a liberal amount of Ivarest. Repeat application 3 or 4 times daily until condition is relieved.

Cautions: Do not use in the eyes. If the condition persists, or if inflammation develops, the patient should discontinue use and consult a physician. The product is not designed for prolonged use.

How Supplied: Ivarest is available in a 1.25 ounce cream tube (NDC 0473-3012-03) and a 4 ounce lotion bottle (NDC 0473-3013-01).

KANK·A®
Medicated Liquid

Indications: Kank·a is a medicated liquid packaged in a plastic bottle. The product is recommended to relieve the pain of canker and mouth sores and to help protect against further irritation. Kank·a is accepted by the Council on Dental Therapeutics, American Dental Association.

Ingredients:
Actives:
  Compound Benzoin Tincture (oral mucosal protectant)
  Benzocaine 5.0% (oral mucosal analgesic)
  Cetylpyridinium Chloride 0.5% (antiseptic)
Excipients:
  A buffered vehicle with Castor Oil, Spirits of Ammonia, and flavoring

Mode of Action: Compound Benzoin Tincture is helpful when applied to painful vesiculobullous lesions of the oral mucosa, aphthous stomatitis and Vincent's infection.

Benzocaine, a local anesthetic virtually devoid of systemic toxicities, provides prompt, temporary relief of pain, itching, and soreness of mucous membrane. Cetylpyridinium Chloride reduces bacterial flora and helps prevent infection.

Directions: Dry the irritated area. Apply Kank·a (using the sponge applicator) directly to the mouth or canker sore and let dry. Repeat up to four times a day if necessary.

Cautions: Patients with a known sensitivity to Benzocaine or to other para-amino compounds should avoid use of this product. Do not apply to the area of recently extracted teeth. If irritation or inflammation persists, or if a fever develops, the patient should discontinue use of the product and consult a dentist or physician. Kank·a should not be used for a period exceeding seven days.

Literature Available: Patient and professional pamphlets available on request.

How Supplied: Kank·a is available in a ⅙ fl. oz. plastic bottle with a built-in sponge applicator (NDC 10157-0011-2).
Shown in Product Identification Section, page 404

Block Drug Company, Inc.
**257 CORNELISON AVENUE
JERSEY CITY, NJ 07302**

BC® POWDER

Active Ingredients: Aspirin 650 mg per powder, Salicylamide 195 mg per powder and Caffeine 32 mg per powder.

Indications: BC Powder is for relief of simple headache; for temporary relief of minor arthritic pain, neuralgia, neuritis and sciatica; for relief of muscular aches, discomfort and fever of colds; and for relief of normal menstrual pain and pain of tooth extraction.

Warnings: Do not exceed recommended dosage or administer to children under 12 years of age, unless a physician directs. If pain persists for more than 10 days or redness is present, consult a physician immediately. In case of accidental overdose, contact physician or poison control center immediately. Do not take this product if you are allergic to aspirin, have asthma, gastric ulcer, or are taking a medication that affects the clotting of blood, except under the advice and supervision of a physician. Keep this and all medication out of childrens' reach. As with any drug, if you are pregnant or nursing a baby, seek the advice of a physician before using this product.

Dosage and Administration: Stir one powder into a glass of water or other liquid, or, place powder on tongue and follow with liquid. May be used every 3 or 4 hours up to 4 times a day. For children under 12 consult a physician.

How Supplied: Available in tamper resistant cellophane wrapped envelopes of 2 or 6 powders, as well as tamper resistant boxes of 24 and 50 powders.

NYTOL® TABLETS

Active Ingredient: Diphenhydramine Hydrochloride, 25 mg per tablet.

Indications: Diphenhydramine Hydrochloride is an antihistamine with anticholinergic and sedative effects which induces drowsiness and helps in falling asleep.

Warnings: Do not give children under 12 years of age. If sleeplessness persists continuously for more than 2 weeks, consult your physician. Insomnia may be a symptom of serious underlying medical illness. If pregnant or nursing, consult your physician before taking this or any medicine. Do not take this product if you have asthma, glaucoma, or enlargement of the prostate gland except under the advice and supervision of a physician. Take this product with caution if alcohol is being consumed. Keep this and all drugs out of the reach of children. In case of accidental overdose, contact a physician immediately.

Drug Interaction: Alcohol and other drugs which cause CNS depression will heighten the depressant effect of this product. Monoamine oxidase (MAO) inhibitors will prolong and intensify the anticholinergic effects of antihistamines.

Symptoms and Treatment of Oral Overdosage: In adults overdose may cause CNS depression resulting in hypnosis and coma. In children CNS hyperexcitability may follow sedation; the stimulant phase may bring tremor, delirium and convulsions. Gastrointestinal reactions may include dry mouth, appetite loss, nausea and vomiting. Respiratory distress and cardiovascular complications (hypotension) may be evident. Treatment includes inducing emesis, and controlling symptoms.

Dosage and Administration: Take 2 tablets 20 minutes before bed or as directed by a physician.

How Supplied: Available in tamper resistant packages of 16, 32, and 72 tablets.

PROMISE® TOOTHPASTE

Active Ingredients: 5% Potassium Nitrate and 0.76% Sodium Monofluorophosphate in a pleasantly mint-flavored dentifrice.

Promise contains Potassium Nitrate for relief of dentinal hypersensitivity resulting from the exposure of tooth dentin due to periodontal surgery, cervical (gum-line) erosion, abrasion or recession which causes pain on contact with hot, cold, or tactile stimuli. Also contains fluoride as an aid in caries prevention.

Actions: Promise significantly reduces tooth hypersensitivity, with response to therapy evident after two weeks of use.

Controlled double-blind clinical studies provide substantial evidence of the safety and effectiveness of Promise. The mechanism of action of potassium nitrate in Promise is not well-defined at this time: it may function by blocking the dentinal tubules to obtund pain transmission or have a direct or indirect effect on neural transmission. Sodium Monofluorophosphate has been proven to help prevent dental caries.

Precaution: Should not be used by persons with identified idiosyncracies to dentifrice flavorants. If relief does not occur after 3 months, a dentist should be consulted.

Dosage and Administration: Use twice a day in place of regular toothpaste or as directed by a dental professional.

How Supplied: Promise Toothpaste is supplied in 1.6 oz. and 3.0 oz. tubes, which are contained in tamper resistant packages.

SENSODYNE® TOOTHPASTE
Desensitizing dentifrice

Description: Each tube contains strontium chloride hexahydrate (10%) in a pleasantly flavored cleansing/polishing dentifrice.

Actions/Indications: Tooth hypersensitivity is a condition in which individuals experience pain from exposure to hot, cold stimuli, from chewing fibrous foods, or from tactile stimuli (e.g. toothbrushing.) Hypersensitivity usually occurs when the protective enamel covering on teeth wears away (which happens most often at the gum line) or if gum tissue recedes and exposes the dentin underneath.
Running through the dentin are microscopic small "tubules" which, according to many authorities, carry the pain impulses to the nerve of the tooth.
Sensodyne provides a unique ingredient—strontium chloride which is believed to be deposited in the tubules where it blocks the pain. The longer Sensodyne is used, the more of a barrier it helps build against pain.
The effect of Sensodyne may not be manifested immediately and may require a few weeks or longer of use for relief to be obtained. A number of clinical studies in the U.S. and other countries have provided substantial evidence of Sensodyne's performance attributes. Complete relief of hypersensitivity has been reported in approximately 65% of users and measurable relief or reduction in hypersensitivity in approximately 90%. Sensodyne has been commercially available for over 17 years and has received wide dental endorsement.

Contraindications: Subjects with severe dental erosion should brush properly and lightly with any dentifrice to avoid further removal of tooth structure. Subjects with identified idiosyncracies to dentifrice flavorants may also react to those in Sensodyne.

Continued on next page

Block—Cont.

Dosage: Use regularly in place of ordinary toothpaste or as recommended by dental professional.

NOTE: Individuals should be instructed to use SENSODYNE frequently since relief from pain tends to be cumulative. If relief does not occur after 3 months, a dentist should be consulted.

How Supplied: SENSODYNE Toothpaste is supplied as a paste in tubes of 4 oz. and 2.1 oz.

(U.S. Patent No. 3,122,483)

SENSODYNE-F® TOOTHPASTE

Active Ingredients: 5% Potassium Nitrate and 0.76% Sodium Monofluorophosphate in a pleasant mixed mint-flavor dentifrice.

SENSODYNE-F contains Potassium Nitrate for relief of dentinal hypersensitivity resulting from the exposure of tooth dentin due to periodontal surgery, cervical (gumline) erosion, abrasion or recession which causes pain on contact with hot, cold, or tactile stimuli. Also contains fluoride as an aid in caries prevention.

Actions: SENSODYNE-F significantly reduces tooth hypersensitivity, with response to therapy evident after two weeks of use. Controlled double-blind clinical studies provide substantial evidence of the safety and effectiveness of SENSODYNE-F. The mechanism of action of potassium nitrate in SENSODYNE-F is not well-defined at this time: it may function by blocking the dentinal tubules to obtund pain transmission or have a direct or indirect effect on neural transmission. Sodium Monofluorophosphate has been proven to help prevent dental caries.

Precautions: Should not be used by persons with identified idiosyncracies to dentifrice flavorants. If relief does not occur after 3 months, a dentist should be consulted.

Dosage and Administration: Use twice a day in place of regular toothpaste or as directed by a dental professional.

How Supplied: SENSODYNE-F Toothpaste is supplied in 1.0, 2.4, and 4.6 oz. tubes, which are contained in tamper resistant packages.

TEGRIN® MEDICATED SHAMPOO

Highly effective shampoo for moderate-to-severe dandruff and the relief of flaking, itching, and scaling associated with eczema, seborrhea, and psoriasis. Two commercial product versions are available: a cream shampoo and a lotion shampoo, each in two scents.

Description: Each tube of cream shampoo or bottle of lotion shampoo contains 5% special alcohol extract of coal tar in a pleasantly scented, high-foaming, cleansing shampoo base with emollients, conditioners and other formula components.

Actions/Indications: Coal Tar is obtained in the destructive distillation of bituminous coal and is a highly effective agent for the local therapy of a number of dermatological disorders. The action of tar is believed to be keratolytic, antiseptic, antipruritic and astringent. The special extract of coal tar used in the Tegrin products is prepared in such a way as to reduce the pitch and other irritant components found in crude coal tar without reduction in therapeutic potency.

Coal tar extract has been used clinically for many years as a remedy for dandruff and for scaling associated with scalp disorders such as eczema, seborrhea, and psoriasis. Its mechanism of action has not been fully established, but it is believed to retard the rate of turnover of epidermal cells with regular use. A number of clinical studies have demonstrated the performance attributes of Tegrin Shampoo against dandruff and seborrheic dermatitis. In addition to relieving the above symptoms, Tegrin shampoo used regularly, maintains scalp and hair cleanliness and leaves the hair lustrous and manageable.

Contraindications: For External Use Only—Should irritation develop, discontinue use. Avoid contact with eyes. Keep out of reach of children.

Dosage: Use regularly as a shampoo. Wet hair thoroughly. Rub Tegrin liberally into hair and scalp. Rinse thoroughly. Briskly massage a second application of the shampoo into a rich lather. Rinse thoroughly.

How Supplied:

Tegrin Cream Shampoo is supplied in 2 oz. collapsible tubes.

Tegrin Lotion Shampoo is supplied in 3.75 and 6.6 oz. plastic bottles.

TEGRIN® for Psoriasis Lotion and Cream

Description: Each tube of cream or bottle of lotion contains special crude coal tar extract (5%) and allantoin (1.7%) in a greaseless, stainless vehicle.

Actions/Indications: Crude coal tar is obtained in the destructive distillation of bituminous coal and is a highly effective agent for the local therapy of a number of dermatological disorders. The action of tar is believed to be keratolytic, antiseptic, antipruritic and astringent. The special coal tar extract used in the Tegrin products is prepared in such a way as to reduce the pitch and other irritant components found in crude coal tar. Allantoin (5-Ureidohydantoin) is a debriding and dispersing agent for psoriatic scales and is believed to accelerate proliferation of normal skin cells. The combination of coal tar extract and allantoin used in Tegrin has been demonstrated in a number of controlled clinical studies to have a high level of efficacy in controlling the itching and scaling of psoriasis.

Contraindications: Discontinue medication should irritation or allergic reactions occur. Avoid contact with eyes and mucous membranes. Keep out of reach of children.

Dosage and Administration: Apply 2 to 4 times daily as needed, massaging thoroughly into affected areas. A hot bath before application will help to soften heavy scales. Once condition is under control, maintenance therapy should be individually adjusted. Occlusive dressings are not required.

How Supplied: Tegrin Lotion 6 fl. oz. Tegrin Cream 2 oz. and 4.4 oz. tubes.

Boehringer Ingelheim Pharmaceuticals, Inc.

90 EAST RIDGE
POST OFFICE BOX 368
RIDGEFIELD, CT 06877

DULCOLAX®
brand of bisacodyl USP
Tablets of 5 mg.................BI-CODE 12
Suppositories of 10 mg..BI-CODE 52
Laxative

Description: Dulcolax is a contact laxative acting directly on the colonic mucosa to produce normal peristalsis throughout the large intestine. Its unique mode of action permits either oral or rectal administration, according to the requirements of the patient. Because of its gentleness and reliability of action, Dulcolax may be used whenever constipation is a problem. In preparation for surgery, proctoscopy, or radiologic examination, Dulcolax provides satisfactory cleansing of the bowel, obviating the need for an enema.

The active ingredient in Dulcolax, bisacodyl, is a colorless, tasteless compound that is practically insoluble in water and alkaline solution. It is designated chemically bis(p-acetoxyphenyl)-2-pyridylmethane.

Dulcolax tablets and suppositories are sodium free.

Actions: Dulcolax differs markedly from other laxatives in its mode of action: it is virtually nontoxic, and its laxative effect occurs on contact with the colonic mucosa, where it stimulates sensory nerve endings to produce parasympathetic reflexes resulting in increased peristaltic contractions of the colon. Administered orally, Dulcolax is absorbed to a variable degree from the small bowel but such absorption is not related to the mode of action of the compound. Dulcolax administered rectally in the form of suppositories is negligibly absorbed. The contact action of the drug is restricted to the colon, and motility of the small intestine is not appreciably influenced. Local axon reflexes, as well as segmental reflexes, are initiated in the region of contact and contribute to the widespread peristaltic activity producing evacuation. For this reason, Dulcolax may often be employed satisfactorily in patients with ganglionic blockage or spinal cord damage (paraplegia, poliomyelitis, etc.).

Indications: *Acute Constipation:* Taken at bedtime, Dulcolax tablets are almost invariably effective the following morning. When taken before breakfast, they usually produce an effect within six hours. For a prompter response and to replace enemas, the suppositories, which are usually effective in 15 minutes to one hour, can be used.

Chronic Constipation and Bowel Retraining: Dulcolax is extremely effective in the management of chronic constipation, particularly in older patients. By gradually lengthening the interval between doses as colonic tone improves, the drug has been found to be effective in redeveloping proper bowel hygiene. There is no tendency to "rebound".

Preparation for Radiography: Dulcolax tablets are excellent in eliminating fecal and gas shadows from x-rays taken of the abdominal area. For barium enemas, no food should be given following the administration of the tablets, to prevent reaccumulation of material in the cecum, and a suppository should be given one to two hours prior to examination.

Preoperative Preparation: Dulcolax tablets have been shown to be an ideal laxative in emptying the G.I. tract prior to abdominal surgery or to other surgery under general anesthesia. They may be supplemented by suppositories to replace the usual enema preparation. Dulcolax will not replace the colonic irrigations usually given patients before intracolonic surgery, but is useful in the preliminary emptying of the colon prior to these procedures.

Postoperative Care: Suppositories can be used to replace enemas, or tablets given as an oral laxative, to restore normal bowel hygiene after surgery.

Antepartum Care: Either tablets or suppositories can be used for constipation in pregnancy without danger of stimulating the uterus.

Preparation for Delivery: Suppositories can be used to replace enemas in the first stage of labor provided that they are given at least two hours before the onset of the second stage.

Postpartum Care: The same indications apply as in postoperative care, with no contraindication in nursing mothers.

Preparation for Sigmoidoscopy or Proctoscopy: For unscheduled office examinations, adequate preparation is usually obtained with a single suppository. For sigmoidoscopy scheduled in advance, however, administration of tablets the night before in addition will result in adequate preparation almost invariably.

Colostomies: Tablets the night before or a suppository inserted into the colostomy opening in the morning will frequently make irrigations unnecessary, and in other cases will expedite the procedure.

Contraindication: There is no contraindication to the use of Dulcolax, other than an acute surgical abdomen.

Precaution: Dulcolax tablets contain FD&C Yellow No. 5 (tartrazine) which may cause allergic-type reactions (including bronchial asthma) in certain susceptible individuals. Although the over-all incidence of FD&C Yellow No. 5 (tartrazine) sensitivity in the general population is low, it is frequently seen in patients who also have aspirin hypersensitivity.

Do not use laxative products when abdominal pain, nausea or vomiting are present unless directed by a doctor. Frequent or continued use of this preparation may result in dependence on laxatives.

Adverse Reactions: As with any laxative, abdominal cramps are occasionally noted, particularly in severely constipated individuals.

Dosage:
Tablets
Tablets must be swallowed whole, not chewed or crushed, and should not be taken within one hour of antacids or milk.

Adults: Two or three (usually two) tablets suffice when an ordinary laxative effect is desired. This usually results in one or two soft, formed stools. Tablets when taken before breakfast usually produce an effect within 6 hours, when taken at bedtime usually in 8–12 hours.

Up to six tablets may be safely given in preparation for special procedures when greater assurance of complete evacuation of the colon is desired. In producing such thorough emptying, these higher doses may result in several loose, unformed stools.

Children: One or two tablets, depending on age and severity of constipation, administered as above. Tablets should not be given to a child too young to swallow them whole.

Suppositories
Adults: One suppository at the time a bowel movement is required. Usually effective in 15 minutes to one hour.

Children: Half a suppository is generally effective for infants and children under two years of age. Above this age, a whole suppository is usually advisable.

Combined
In preparation for surgery, radiography and sigmoidoscopy, a combination of tablets the night before and a suppository in the morning is recommended (see Indications).

How Supplied: Dulcolax, brand of bisacodyl: Yellow, enteric-coated tablets of 5 mg in boxes of 25, 50, 100 and bottles of 1000 and unit strip packages of 100; suppositories of 10 mg in boxes of 2, 4, 8, 50 and 500.

Note: Store Dulcolax suppositories and tablets at temperatures below 86°F (30°C). Avoid excessive humidity.

Also Available: Dulcolax® Bowel Prep Kit. Each kit contains:
1 Dulcolax suppository of 10 mg bisacodyl;
4 Dulcolax tablets of 5 mg bisacodyl;
Complete patient instructions.

Clinical Applications: Dulcolax can be used in virtually any patient in whom a laxative or enema is indicated. It has no effect on the blood picture, erythrocyte sedimentation rate, urinary findings, or hepatic or renal function. It may be safely given to infants and the aged, pregnant or nursing women, debilitated patients, and may be prescribed in the presence of such conditions as cardiovascular, renal, or hepatic diseases.

Shown in Product Identification Section, page 404

NŌSTRIL® Nasal Decongestant
phenylephrine HCl, USP

Active Ingredient: Contains phenylephrine HCl, USP, 0.25% (¼%-Mild strength) or phenylephrine HCl, USP, 0.5% (½%-Regular strength), preserved with benzalkonium chloride 0.004% in a buffered aqueous solution.

Indications: For temporary relief of nasal congestion due to the common cold, sinusitis, hay fever or other upper respiratory allergies.

Actions: NŌSTRIL®, the first metered one-way pump spray for nasal decongestion, constricts the smaller arterioles of the nasal passages, producing a gentle, predictable, decongestant effect. Nōstril® penetrates and shrinks swollen membranes, restoring freer breathing and unclogs sinus passages, bringing the effective medication in contact with inflamed, swollen tissues. It will not hurt tender membranes since it is formulated to match the pH of normal nasal secretions. The first one-way pump spray helps prevent draw-back contamination of the medication.

Warnings: Do not exceed recommended dosage because symptoms such as burning, stinging, sneezing, or increased nasal discharge may occur. Do not use for more than 3 days. If symptoms persist, consult a physician. Do not give Nōstril® 0.25% to children under 6 or Nōstril® 0.5% to children under 12 except under the advice and supervision of a physician. Nōstril® 0.5% for adult use only. Use of the dispenser by more than one person may spread infection. Keep out of reach of children.

Symptoms and Treatment of Oral Overdosage: In case of accidental ingestion, seek professional assistance or consult a poison control center immediately.

Dosage and Administration:
0.25% for adults and children 6 years and over: 1 to 2 sprays in each nostril not more frequently than every four hours.
0.5% for adults and children 12 years or older: 1 to 2 sprays in each nostril not more frequently than every four hours.

Remove protective cap. With head upright, insert metered pump spray nozzle in nostril. Hold bottle with thumb at base, nozzle between first and second fingers, depress pump once or twice, all the way down with a firm even stroke and sniff deeply.

Note: Before using for the first time, remove the protective cap from the tip and

Continued on next page

Boehringer Ingelheim—Cont.

depress the round tab firmly several times to prime the metering pump.

How Supplied: Metered one-way nasal pump spray in white plastic bottles of ½ fl. oz. (15 ml) packaged in tamper-resistant outer cartons.

0.25% (¼%-Mild strength): for children 6 years and over and adults who prefer a milder decongestant. (NDC #0597-0083-85)

0.5% (½%-Regular strength): for adults and children 12 years or older (NDC #0597-0084-85)

Shown in Product Identification Section, page 404

NŌSTRILLA™ Long Acting Nasal Decongestant
oxymetazoline HCl, USP

Active Ingredient: Contains oxymetazoline HCl, USP, 0.05% with benzalkonium Cl 0.02% as a preservative. (Mercury preservatives are not used in this product.)

Indications: For up to 12 hour relief of nasal congestion due to the common cold, sinusitis, hay fever or other upper respiratory allergies.

Actions: NŌSTRILLA™, the first metered one-way pump spray for nasal decongestion, constricts the smaller arterioles of the nasal passages, producing a prolonged (up to 12 hours), gentle, predictable, decongestant effect. Nōstrilla™ penetrates and shrinks swollen membranes, restoring freer breathing and unclogs sinus passages, bringing the effective medication in contact with inflamed, swollen tissues. It will not hurt tender membranes since it is formulated to match the pH of normal nasal secretions. Use at bedtime restores freer nasal breathing through the night.

Warnings: Do not exceed recommended dosage because symptoms such as burning, stinging, sneezing or increased nasal discharge may occur. Do not use for more than 3 days. If symptoms persist, consult a physician. Do not give this product to children under 6 except under advice and supervision of a physician. Use of the dispenser by more than one person may spread infection. Keep this and all drugs out of reach of children.

Symptoms and Treatment of Oral Overdosage: In case of accidental ingestion, seek professional assistance or contact a poison control center immediately.

Dosage and Administration: Adults and children 6 and over: 1 to 2 sprays in each nostril of 0.05% aqueous solution 2 times daily (in the morning and evening).

Remove protective cap. With head upright, insert metered pump spray nozzle in nostril. Hold bottle with thumb at base, nozzle between first and second fingers, depress pump once or twice, all the way down with a firm even stroke and sniff deeply.

Note: Before using for the first time, remove the protective cap from the tip and depress the round tab firmly several times to prime the metering pump.

How Supplied: Metered one-way nasal pump spray in white plastic bottles of ½ fl. oz. (15 ml.) packaged in tamper-resistant outer cartons. (NDC #0597-0085-85).

Shown in Product Identification Section, page 404

John A. Borneman and Sons, Inc.
1208 AMOSLAND ROAD
NORWOOD, PA 19074

OSCILLOCOCCINUM®

Active Ingredient: Anas Barbariae Hepatis et Cordis Extractum HPUS 200C.

Indications: For the relief of flu-like symptoms such as fever, chills, body aches and pains.

Actions: Like most Homeopathic remedies, Oscillococcinum® acts gently by stimulating the patient's natural defense mechanisms.

Warnings: If symptoms persist for more than three days or worsen, consult your physician. Keep all medication out of reach of children. As with any drug if you are pregnant or nursing a baby, seek professional advice before using this product.

Dosage and Administration: (Adults and Children over 2 years) Take the entire contents of one tube by mouth at the first appearance of symptoms. Repeat every 6 to 8 hours as necessary. For maximum results, Oscillococcinum® should be taken early, at the onset of symptoms. Should be taken at least 15 minutes before or 1 hour after meals.

How Supplied: boxes of 3 unit-doses of 0.04 oz. (1 Gram) each. (NDC 51979-9756-43) Tamper resistant package.
Manufactured by Boiron, France.
Distributor: John A. Borneman & Sons, Inc.

Shown in Product Identification Section, page 404

IDENTIFICATION PROBLEM?
Consult the
Product Identifcation Section
where you'll find
products pictured
in full color.

Bristol Laboratories
(Division of Bristol-Myers Co.)
SYRACUSE, NY 13221-4755

NALDECON-CX® SUSPENSION ©
Decongestant/Expectorant/Antitussive

Description: Each teaspoonful (5 ml) of Naldecon-CX Suspension contains:
Phenylpropanolamine
  hydrochloride .... 18 mg
Guaifenesin .... 200 mg
Codeine Phosphate .... 10 mg
  (Warning: May be Habit Forming)

Indications: Provide prompt relief from cough and nasal congestion due to the common cold, bronchitis, nasopharyngitis, and influenza. Codeine temporarily quiets non-productive coughing by its antitussive action while guaifenesin's expectorant action helps loosen phlegm and bronchial secretions. Phenylpropanolamine reduces swelling of nasal passages and shrinks swollen membranes. This combination production is antihistamine and alcohol free.

Contraindications: Hypersensitivity to guaifenesin, codeine or sympathomimetic amines.

Warnings: Nervousness, dizziness or sleeplessness may occur if recommended dosage is exceeded. Do not give this product to a child with high blood pressure, heart disease, diabetes or thyroid disease except under the advice and supervision of a physician. Do not give this product to a child presently taking a prescription drug containing a monoamine oxidase inhibitor except under the advice and supervision of a physician. Do not administer this product for persistent or chronic cough associated with asthma or emphysema or when cough is accompanied by excessive secretions, except under the care and advice of a physician. A persistent cough may be a sign of a serious condition. If cough persists for more than 1 week, tends to recur, or is accompanied by high fever, rash or persistent headaches, consult a physician.

Dosage and Administration: Children 2 to 6 years—½ teaspoon 4 times daily. 6 to 12 years—1 teaspoon 4 times daily. Over 12 years—2 teaspoons 4 times daily.

How Supplied: Naldecon-CX Suspension—4 oz. and pint bottles.

NALDECON–DX®
Pediatric Syrup

Description: Each teaspoonful (5 ml.) of Naldecon-DX Syrup contains:
dextromethorphan
  hydrobromide ....7.5 mg
phenylpropanolamine
  hydrochloride ....9 mg
guaifenesin ....100 mg
alcohol 5%

Indications: Provide prompt relief from cough and nasal congestion due to the common cold, bronchitis, nasopharyngitis and recurrent bronchial coughng. Dextromethorphan temporarily quiets non-productive coughing by its antitussive action while guaifenesin's expectorant action helps loosen phlegm and bronchial secretions. Phenylpropanolamine reduces swelling of nasal passages; shrinks swollen membranes. This combination product is antihistamine-free.

Contraindications: Hypersensitivity to guaifenesin, dextromethorphan or sympathomimetic amines.

Warnings: Nervousness, dizziness or sleeplessness may occur if recommended dosage is exceeded. Do not give this product to a child with high blood pressure, heart disease, diabetes or thyroid disease except under the advice and supervision of a physician. Do not give this product to a child presently taking a prescription drug containing a monoamine oxidase inhibitor except under the advice and supervision of a physician. Do not administer this product for persistent or chronic cough such as occurs with asthma or emphysema or when cough is accompanied by excessive secretions except under the care and advice of a physician. A persistent cough may be a sign of a serious condition. If cough persists for more than 1 week, tends to recur, or is accompanied by high fever, rash or persistent headaches, consult a physician.

Dosage and Administration: Children 2 to 6 years—1 teaspoonful 4 times daily. Over 6 years—2 teaspoons 4 times daily.

How Supplied: Naldecon-DX Syrup in 4 oz. and pint bottles.

(1) 8/80

NALDECON–EX®
Pediatric Drops

Description: Each 1 ml. dropperful of Naldecon-EX contains:
phenylpropanolamine
hydrochloride ....9 mg
guaifenesin ....30 mg
alcohol 0.6%

Indications: Combined decongestant/expectorant designed specifically to promptly reduce the swelling of nasal membranes and to help loosen phlegm and bronchial secretions through productive coughing. This dual action is of particular value in infants with common cold, acute bronchitis, bronchiolitis, tracheobronchitis, nasopharyngitis and croup. This combination product is antihistamine-free.

Contraindications: Hypersensitivity to guaifenesin or sympathomimetic amines.

Warnings: Nervousness, dizziness or sleeplessness may occur if recommended dosage is exceeded. Do not give this product to a child with high blood pressure, heart disease, diabetes or thyroid disease except under the advice and supervision of a physician. Do not give this product to a child presently taking a prescription drug containing a monoamine oxidase inhibitor except under the advice and

supervision of a physician. Do not administer this product for persistent or chronic cough such as occurs with asthma or emphysema or when cough is accompanied by excessive secretions except under the care and advice of a physician. A persistent cough may be a sign of a serious condition. If cough persists for more than 1 week, tends to recur, or is accompanied by high fever, rash or persistent headaches, consult a physician.

Dosage and Administration: Dose should be adjusted to age or weight and be given 4 times a day (see calibrations on dropper). Administer by mouth only.

1–3 Months: (8–12 lbs.)	¼ ml
4–6 Months: (13–17 lbs.)	½ ml
7–9 Months: (18–20 lbs.)	¾ ml
10 Months or over (21 lbs. or more)	1 ml

Bottle label dosage reads as follows: children under 2 years of age: use only as directed by a physician.

How Supplied: Naldecon-EX Pediatric Drops in 20 ml. bottles with calibrated dropper.

(1) 8/80

Bristol-Myers Products
(Div. of Bristol-Myers Co.)
345 PARK AVENUE
NEW YORK, NY 10154

ARTHRITIS STRENGTH
BUFFERIN®
Analgesic

Composition: Aspirin 7½ gr. (486 mg.) in a formulation buffered with Di-Alminate,® Bristol-Myers' brand of Aluminum Glycinate and Magnesium Carbonate.

Action and Uses: ARTHRITIS STRENGTH BUFFERIN is specially formulated to give temporary relief from the minor aches and pains, stiffness, swelling and inflammation of arthritis and rheumatism. ARTHRITIS STRENGTH BUFFERIN also reduces pain and fever of colds and "flu" and provides fast, effective pain relief for: simple headache, lower back muscular aches from fatigue, sinusitis, neuralgia, neuritis, tooth extraction, muscle strain, athletic soreness, painful distress associated with normal menstrual periods. The leading aspirin substitute, acetaminophen, cannot provide effective relief from inflammation.

Contraindications: Hypersensitivity to salicylates.

Caution: If pain persists for more than 10 days or redness is present or in arthritic or rheumatic conditions affecting children under 12, consult physician immediately. Do not take without consulting physician if under medical care.

WARNING: KEEP THIS AND ALL MEDICINES OUT OF CHILDREN'S REACH. IN CASE OF ACCIDENTAL

OVERDOSE, CONTACT A PHYSICIAN IMMEDIATELY. As with any drug, if you are pregnant or nursing a baby, seek the advice of a health professional before using this product.

Administration and Dosage: Two tablets with water. Repeat after four hours if necessary. Do not exceed 8 tablets in any 24 hour period. If dizziness, impaired hearing or ringing in ear occurs, discontinue use. Not recommended for children.

Overdose: In case of accidental overdose contact a physician or a regional poison control center immediately.

How Supplied: Tablets in bottles of 40 and 100. Samples available upon request.

Product Identification: White elongated tablet.

Literature Available: Upon request.
Shown in Product Identification
Section, page 405

BUFFERIN® Analgesic

Composition: Each tablet or capsule contains Aspirin 5 gr. (324 mg.). Tablets are buffered with Di-Alminate®, Bristol-Myers's brand of Aluminum Glycinate and Magnesium Carbonate. Capsules are buffered with Calcium Carbonate, Magnesium Oxide, and Magnesium Carbonate.

Action and Uses: Bufferin is for relief of simple headache; and for temporary relief of: toothache, minor arthritic pain, the painful discomforts and fever of colds and "flu", pain of menstrual cramps and muscular aches from fatigue.

Contraindications: Hypersensitivity to salicylates.

Caution: If pain persists for more than 10 days or redness is present or, in arthritic or rheumatic conditions affecting children under 12, consult physician immediately. Do not take without consulting physician if under medical care. Consult a dentist for toothache promptly.

Warning: KEEP THIS AND ALL MEDICINES OUT OF CHILDREN'S REACH. IN CASE OF ACCIDENTAL OVERDOSE, CONSULT A PHYSICIAN IMMEDIATLEY. As with any drug, if you are pregnant or nursing a baby, seek the advice of a health professional before using this product.

Dosage: Tablets or Capsules—2 every four hours as needed. Do not exceed 12 in 24 hours, unless directed by a physician. For children 6-12, one-half dose. Under 6, consult physician.

Overdose: In case of accidental overdose contact a physician or a regional poison control center immediately.

How Supplied: Tablets in bottles of 12, 36, 60, 100, 165, 225, and 375. For hospital and clinical use: bottle—1,000; boxed 200x2 tablet foil packets. Samples available on request.

Continued on next page

Bristol-Myers—Cont.

Product Identification Mark: Tablet is white with letter "B" on one surface. Capsule is white with BUFFERIN on four sides of outer half of capsule.

Literature Available: Upon request.
Shown in Product Identification Section, page 405

EXTRA-STRENGTH BUFFERIN®

Composition: Each tablet and capsule contains aspirin 500 mg. Tablets are buffered with Di-Alminate®, Bristol-Myers' brand of Aluminum Glycinate and Magnesium Carbonate.
Capsules are buffered with Calcium Carbonate, Magnesium Oxide and Magnesium Carbonate.

Action and Uses: Extra-Strength BUFFERIN provides fast extra-strength pain relief.
- Each 2 capsule or 2 tablet dose contains 1000 mg. of pain reliever, the maximum quantity recommended without a prescription.
- Provides relief of headaches, pain of menstrual cramps, toothache, muscular aches, painful discomforts and fever of colds or flu, and temporary relief from the minor aches, pain and inflammation of arthritis and rheumatism.

Contraindications: Hypersensitivity to salicylates.

Caution: If pain persists for more than 10 days, or redness is present, or in arthritic or rheumatic conditions affecting children under 12, consult a physician immediately. Do not take without consulting a physician if under medical care. Consult a dentist for toothache promptly.

Warning: KEEP THIS AND ALL MEDICINES OUT OF CHILDREN'S REACH. IN CASE OF ACCIDENTAL OVERDOSE, CONSULT A PHYSICIAN IMMEDIATELY. As with any drug, if you are pregnant or nursing a baby, seek the advice of a health professional before using this product.

Administration and Dosage: Tablets or Capsules—2 every 4 hours as needed. Do not exceed 8 in 24 hours, or give to children 12 or under, unless directed by a physician.

Overdose: In case of accidental overdose contact a physician or a regional poison control center immediately.

How Supplied: Bottles of 30, 60 and 100 tablets. Capsules in bottles of 24's, 50's and 75's. All sizes packaged in child resistant closures except 60's (for tablets); 50's (for capsules) which are sizes not recommended for households with young children.

Product Identification Mark: White, elongated tablets with "ESB" imprinted on one side. White and blue capsules with "EXTRA-STRENGTH BUFF-ERIN" imprinted on 3 sides.
Shown in Product Identification Section, page 405

COMTREX®
Multi-Symptom Cold Reliever

Composition: Each tablet, fluid ounce (30 ml.), or capsule contains:
[See table below].

Actions and Uses: COMTREX® contains safe and effective fast acting ingredients including a non-aspirin analgesic, a decongestant, an antihistamine and a cough reliever. COMTREX relieves these major cold symptoms: nasal and sinus congestion, coughing, fever, minor sore throat pain (systemically), headache, body aches and pain.

Contraindications: Hypersensitivity to acetaminophen or antihistamines.

Caution: Do not take without consulting a physician if under medical care. Do not drive a car or operate machinery while taking this cold remedy as it may cause drowsiness.

Warning: KEEP THIS AND ALL MEDICINE OUT OF CHILDREN'S REACH. IN CASE OF ACCIDENTAL OVERDOSE, CONSULT A PHYSICIAN IMMEDIATELY. Persistent cough may indicate the presence of a serious condition. Persons with a high fever or persistent cough, or with high blood pressure, diabetes, heart or thyroid disease, asthma, glaucoma or difficulty in urination due to enlargement of the prostate gland should not use this preparation unless directed by a physician. Do not use for more than 10 days unless directed by a physician. As with any drug, if you are pregnant or nursing a baby, seek the advice of a health professional before using this product.

Administration and Dosage:
Tablets or Capsules—Adults: 2 tablets or capsules every 4 hours as needed not to exceed 12 tablets or capsules in 24 hours. Children 6-12 years: ½ the adult dose. Under 6, consult a physician.
Liquid—Adults: 1 fluid ounce (30 ml.) every 4 hours as needed, not to exceed 6 fluid ounces (180 ml.) in 24 hours. Children 6-12 years: ½ the adult dose. Under 6, consult a physician.

Overdose: In case of accidental overdose contact a physician or a regional poison control center immediately.

How Supplied: Tablets in bottles of 12's, 24's, 50's, 100's. Capsules in bottles of 16's and 36's. Liquid in 6 oz. and 10 oz plastic bottles. Samples available on request.

Product Identification Mark: Yellow tablet with letter "C" on one surface. Orange and Yellow capsules with "Bristol-Myers" and "Comtrex" on one side. Liquid Comtrex is clear orange in color.

Literature Available: Upon request.
Shown in Product Identification Section, page 405

CONGESPIRIN® for Children
Cough Syrup

Composition: Each 5 ml teaspoon contains Dextromethorphan hydrobromide—5 mg.

Actions and Uses: Contains a non narcotic antitussive comparable in potency to codeine, in an orange flavored syrup. Reduces coughs due to colds and soothes minor throat irritations.

Warning: Do not administer without consulting a physician if child is under medical care. Persistent cough may indicate the presence of a serious condition. Children with a cough persisting for more than 10 days, with high fever, or with fever lasting more than 3 days should not be given this preparation unless directed by a physician. Do not administer to children under two years of age, except as directed by physician. KEEP THIS AND ALL MEDICINES OUT OF THE REACH OF CHILDREN.

Administration and Dosage: Children 2–6, one teaspoon every 4 hours as needed. Do not exceed 6 teaspoons in 24 hours. Children 6–12, two teaspoons every 4 hours as needed. Do not exceed 12 teaspoons in 24 hours.

Overdose: In case of accidental overdose contact a physician or a regional poison control center immediately.

How Supplied: Available in 3 oz plastic bottles

Product Identification: Clear Orange Liquid

Literature Available: Upon request.
Shown in Product Identification Section, page 405

CONGESPIRIN® Aspirin Free
Chewable Cold Tablets for Children

Composition: Each tablet contains 81 mg. (1¼ grains) acetaminophen, 1¼ mg phenylephrine hydrochloride.

Action and Uses: A non-aspirin analgesic/nasal decongestant that temporarily reduces fever and relieves aches, pains and nasal congestion associated with colds and flu.

Warnings: KEEP THIS AND ALL MEDICATIONS OUT OF CHILDREN'S REACH. IN CASE OF ACCIDENTAL OVERDOSE, CONTACT A PHYSICIAN IMMEDIATELY.

Caution: If child is under medical care, do not administer without consulting

	COMTREX Tablets	COMTREX Liquid	COMTREX Capsules
Acetaminophen	325 mg.	650 mg.	325 mg.
Phenylpropanolamine HCl.	12 ½ mg.	25 mg.	12 ½ mg.
Chlorpheniramine Maleate	1 mg.	2 mg.	1 mg.
Dextromethorphan HBr.	10 mg.	20 mg.	10 mg.
Alcohol:	—	20% by Volume	—

physician. Do not exceed recommended dosage. Consult your physician if symptoms persist or if high blood pressure, heart disease, diabetes or thyroid disease is present. Do not administer for more than 10 days unless directed by physician.

Dosage and Administration:
Under 2, consult your physician.

2–3 years	2 tablets
4–5 years	3 tablets
6–8 years	4 tablets
9–10 years	5 tablets
10–12 years	6 tablets
12 years	8 tablets

Repeat dose in four hours if necessary. Do not give more than four doses in any 24 hour period unless directed by your physician.

Overdose: In case of accidental overdose contact a physician or a regional poison control center immediately.

How Supplied: Tablets, in bottles of 24.
Shown in Product Identification Section, page 405

CONGESPIRIN®
Chewable Cold Tablets for Children

Composition: Each tablet contains aspirin 81 mg. (1¼ grains) phenylephrine hydrochloride (1¼ mg.). (Also available in an aspirin-free formula.)

Action and Uses: For the temporary relief of nasal congestion, fever, aches and pains of the common cold or "flu". Plus an effective nasal decongestant to help relieve stuffiness, runny nose and sneezing from colds.

Dosage and Administration:
Under Age 2 consult your physician

2–3 YRS.	2 TABLETS
4–5 YRS.	3 TABLETS
6–8 YRS.	4 TABLETS
9–10 YRS.	5 TABLETS
11 YRS	6 TABLETS
12 YRS	8 TABLETS

Repeat dose in four hours if necessary. Do not give more than four doses per day unless prescribed by your physician.

Overdose: In case of accidental overdose contact a physician or a regional poison control center immediately.

Caution: If child is under medical care, do not administer without consulting physician. Do not exceed recommended dosage. Consult your physician if symptoms persist or if high fever, high blood pressure, heart disease, diabetes or thyroid disease is present. Do not administer for more than 10 days unless directed by your physician.

Warning: KEEP THIS AND ALL MEDICINES OUT OF CHILDREN'S REACH. IN CASE OF ACCIDENTAL OVERDOSAGE, CONTACT A PHYSICIAN IMMEDIATELY.

How Supplied: Tablets in bottles of 36.

Product Identification Mark: Two layer (orange/white) circular tablet with letter "C" imprinted on the orange side.
Shown in Product Identification Section, page 405

CONGESPIRIN®
Liquid Cold Medicine

Composition: Each 5 ml. teaspoon contains Acetaminophen 130 mg., Phenylpropanolamine Hydrochloride 6 ¼ mg., Alcohol 10% by volume.

Action and Uses: Reduces fever and relieves aches and pains associated with colds and "flu". Contains an effective decongestant for the temporary relief of nasal congestion due to the common cold, hay fever or other respiratory allergies. Reduces swelling of nasal passages, shrinks swollen membranes, restores freer breathing.

Dosage and Administration:
Children 3–5, 1 teaspoon every 3–4 hours.
Children 6–12, 2 teaspoons every 3–4 hours.
Children under 3 years use only as directed by your physician.
Do not give more than 4 doses a day unless directed by your physician.

Overdose: In case of accidental overdose contact a physician or a regional poison control center immediately.

Caution: If child is under medical care, do not administer without consulting physician. Do not exceed recommended dosage. Consult your physician if symptoms persist or if high fever, high blood pressure, heart disease, diabetes or thyroid disease is present. Do not administer for more than 10 days unless directed by your physician.

Warning: KEEP THIS AND ALL MEDICINES OUT OF CHILDREN'S REACH. IN CASE OF ACCIDENTAL OVERDOSAGE, CONTACT A PHYSICIAN IMMEDIATELY.

How Supplied: In 3 oz. plastic, unbreakable bottles.
Shown in Product Identification Section, page 405

EXTRA–STRENGTH DATRIL®

Composition: Each tablet or capsule contains acetaminophen, 500 mg.

Actions and Uses: Extra-Strength DATRIL has been specially developed to provide fast, extra-strength pain relief. It contains a non-aspirin ingredient (acetaminophen) which is less likely to irritate the stomach than plain aspirin. Extra-Strength DATRIL is fast-acting. Extra-Strength DATRIL tablets are for the temporary relief of minor aches, pains, headaches and fever. For most persons with peptic ulcer Extra-Strength DATRIL may be used when taken as directed for recommended conditions.

Contraindications: There have been rare reports of skin rash or glossitis attributed to acetaminophen. Discontinue use if a sensitivity reaction occurs. However, acetaminophen is usually well tolerated by aspirin-sensitive patients.

Caution: Severe or recurrent pain or high or continued fever may be indicative of serious illness. Under these conditions consult a physician. Do not take without consulting a physician if under medical care.

Warning: Do not give to children 12 and under or use for more than 10 days unless directed by a physician. KEEP THIS AND ALL MEDICINES OUT OF REACH OF CHILDREN. IN CASE OF ACCIDENTAL OVERDOSE CONTACT A PHYSICIAN IMMEDIATELY. As with any drug, if you are pregnant or nursing a baby, seek the advice of a health professional before using this product.

Dosage: Adults: Two tablets or capsules. May be repeated in 4 hours if needed. Do not exceed 8 tablets in any 24 hour period.

Overdose: In case of accidental overdose contact a physician or a regional poison control center immediately.

How Supplied: Tablets in bottles of 24's, 50's and 72's. Samples available on request.

Product Identification Mark: White tablet with DATRIL on one surface. Green and white capsule with Bristol-Myers on green half and DATRIL 500 mg on white half.

Literature Available: Upon request.
Shown in Product Identification Section, page 405

EXCEDRIN® Analgesic

Composition: Each tablet and capsule contains Acetaminophen 250 mg.; Aspirin 250 mg.; and Caffeine 65 mg.

Action and Uses: Extra-Strength Excedrin provides fast, effective relief from pain of: headache, sinusitis, colds or 'flu', muscular aches and menstrual discomfort. Also recommended for temporary relief of toothaches and minor arthritic pains.

Contraindications: Hypersensitivity to salicylates or acetaminophen.

Caution: If sinus or arthritis pain persists for a week, or if skin redness is present, or in arthritic conditions affecting children under 12, consult physician immediately. Consult dentist for toothache promptly. Do not take without consulting physician if under medical care. Store at room temperature.

Warning: Do not exceed 8 tablets or capsules in 24 hours or use for more than 10 days unless directed, or give to children under 12. **Keep this and all medicines out of children's reach. In case of accidental overdose, contact a physician immediately.** As with any drug, if you are pregnant or nursing a baby, seek the advice of a health professional before using this product.

Continued on next page

Bristol-Myers—Cont.

Administration and Dosage: Tablets and Capsules—Individuals 12 and over, take 2 every 4 hours as needed.

Overdose: In case of accidental overdose contact a physician or a regional poison control center immediately.

How Supplied: Bottles of 12, 36, 60, 100, 165, 225, and 375 tablets. Capsules in bottles of 24's, 40's and 60's. A metal tin of 12 tablets. All sizes packaged in child resistant closures except 100's (for tablets); 60's (for capsules) which are sizes not recommended for households with young children.

Product Identification Mark: White, circular tablet with letter "E" imprinted on both sides. Red capsules with "EXCE-DRIN" printed on 2 sides.

Literature Available: Upon request.
Shown in Product Identification Section, page 405

EXCEDRIN P.M.®
Analgesic Sleeping Aid

Composition: Each tablet contains Acetaminophen 500 mg. and Diphenhydramine Hydrochloride 38 mg.

Action and Uses: For the temporary relief of occasional headaches and minor aches and pains with accompanying sleeplessness. Also for fever with accompanying sleeplessness.

Contraindications: Hypersensitivity to acetaminophen or antihistamines.

Caution: Do not drive a car or operate machinery while taking this medication. Do not take without consulting physician if under medical care. Store at room temperature.

Warning: Do not exceed 2 tablets in 24 hours, or give to children under 12 or use for more than 10 days unless directed by physician. KEEP THIS AND ALL MEDICINES OUT OF CHILDREN'S REACH. IN CASE OF ACCIDENTAL OVERDOSE, CONTACT A PHYSICIAN IMMEDIATELY. Consult your physician if symptoms persist or new ones occur or if fever persists more than 3 days (72 hours) or recurs or if sleeplessness persists continuously for more than two weeks. Insomnia may be a symptom of serious underlying medical illness. Take this product with caution if alcohol is being consumed. DO NOT TAKE THIS PRODUCT IF YOU HAVE ASTHMA, GLAUCOMA OR ENLARGEMENT OF THE PROSTATE GLAND EXCEPT UNDER THE ADVICE AND SUPERVISION OF A PHYSICIAN. As with any drug, if you are pregnant or nursing a baby, seek the advice of a health professional before using this product.

Administration and Dosage: Adults take two tablets at bedtime or as directed by a physician. Do not exceed recommended dosage.

Overdose: In case of accidental overdose contact a physician or a regional poison control center immediately.

How Supplied: Bottles of 10, 30, 50, and 80 tablets. All sizes packaged in child resistant closures except 50's, which is a size not recommended for households with young children.

Product Identification Mark: Blue/green circular tablet with letters "PM" imprinted on one side.
Shown in Product Identification Section, page 405

4–WAY® Cold Tablets

Composition: Each tablet contains aspirin 324 mg., phenylpropanolamine HCl 12½ mg., and chlorpheniramine maleate 2 mg.

Action and Uses: For temporary relief of minor aches and pains, fever, nasal congestion and runny nose as may occur in the common cold.

Dosage and Administration: Adults—2 tablets every 4 hours, if needed. Do not exceed 6 tablets in 24 hours. Children 6–12 years—1 tablet every 4 hours. Do not exceed 4 tablets in 24 hours. Under age 6, consult a physician.

Overdose: In case of accidental overdose contact a physician or a regional poison control center immediately.

Warning: Do not take without consulting a physician if under medical care. As with any drug, if you are pregnant or nursing a baby, seek the advice of a health professional before using this product. Individuals with high blood pressure, heart disease, diabetes, thyroid disease, asthma, glaucoma or difficulty in urination due to enlargement of the prostate gland should not use this preparation unless directed by a physician. Do not exceed recommended dosage. KEEP THIS AND ALL MEDICINES OUT OF CHILDREN'S REACH. IN CASE OF ACCIDENTAL OVERDOSE, CONTACT PHYSICIAN IMMEDIATELY.

Caution: This preparation may cause drowsiness. Do not drive or operate machinery while taking this medication.

How Supplied: Carded 15's and bottles of 36's and 60's.

Product Identification Mark: Pink and White tablet with number "4" on one surface.
Shown in Product Identification Section, page 406

4–WAY® Nasal Spray

Composition: Phenylephrine hydrochloride 0.5%, naphazoline hydrochloride 0.05%, pyrilamine maleate 0.2%, in a buffered isotonic aqueous solution with thimerosal, 0.005% added as a preservative. Also available in a mentholated formula.

Action and Uses: For relief of nasal congestion, runny nose, sneezing, itching nose, and watery eyes which may be symptoms of common cold, sinusitis, nasal allergies, or hay fever.

Dosage and Administration: With head in a normal upright position, put atomizer tip into nostril. Squeeze atomizer with firm, quick pressure while inhaling. Adults-spray twice into each nostril. Children 6-12-spray once. Under 6-consult physician. Repeat in three hours, if needed.

Overdose: In case of accidental overdose contact a physician or a regional poison control center immediately.

Warning: Overdosage in young children may cause marked sedation. Do not exceed recommended dosage because symptoms may occur such as burning, stinging, sneezing or increase of nasal discharge. Follow directions carefully. Do not use this product for more than 3 days. If symptoms persist, consult physician. The use of this dispenser by more than one person may spread infection. Keep out of children's reach. Store at room temperature.

How Supplied: Atomizers of ½ fluid ounce and 1 fluid ounce.
Shown in Product Identification Section, page 406

4–WAY® Long Acting Nasal Spray

Composition: Oxymetazoline Hydrochloride 0.05% in a buffered isotonic aqueous solution. Thimerosal, 0.005% added as a preservative.

Action and Uses: Provides temporary relief of nasal congestion due to the common cold, sinusitis, hayfever or other upper respiratory allergies.

Dosage and Administration: With head in a normal upright position, put atomizer tip into nostril. Squeeze atomizer with firm, quick pressure while inhaling. Adults: Spray 2 or 3 times in each nostril twice daily—once in the morning and once in the evening. For children under 12, consult physician.

Overdose: In case of accidental overdose contact a physician or a regional poison control center immediately.

Warning: For adult use only. Do not give this product to children under 12 years except under the advice and supervision of a physician. Do not exceed recommended dosage because symptoms may occur such as burning, stinging, sneezing, or an increase of nasal discharge. Do not use this product for more than 3 days. If symptoms persist, consult physician. The use of this dispenser by more than one person may spread infection. KEEP OUT OF CHILDREN'S REACH

How Supplied: Atomizers of ½ fluid ounce.
Shown in Product Identification Section, page 406

NO DOZ® TABLETS

Composition: Each tablet contains 100 mg. Caffeine.

Action and Uses: Helps restore mental alertness.

Dosage and Administration: For Adults: 2 tablets initially, thereafter, 1 tablet every three hours should be sufficient.

Overdose: In case of accidental overdose contact a physician or a regional poison control center immediately.

Caution: Do not take without consulting physician if under medical care. No stimulant should be substituted for normal sleep in activities requiring physical alertness.

Warning: KEEP THIS AND ALL MEDICINES OUT OF THE REACH OF CHILDREN. As with any drug, if you are pregnant or nursing a baby, seek the advice of a health professional before using this product.

How Supplied: Carded 15's and 36's and bottles of 60's.

Product Identification Mark: A white tablet with No Doz on one side.
Shown in Product Identification Section, page 406

PAZO® HEMORRHOID OINTMENT/SUPPOSITORIES

Composition: Ointment: Triolyte®, Bristol-Myers brand of the combination of benzocaine (0.8%) and ephedrine sulphate (0.21%)]; zinc oxide (4.0%); camphor (2.18%), in an emollient base.

Suppositories (per suppository): Triolyte® [Bristol-Myers brand of the combination of benzocaine (15.44 mg) and ephedrine sulfate (3.86 mg)]; zinc oxide (77.2 mg); camphor (42.07 mg), in an emollient base.

Action and Uses: Pazo helps shrink swelling of inflamed hemorrhoid tissue. Provides prompt, temporary relief of burning itch and pain in many cases.

Administration:

Ointment—Apply Pazo well up in rectum night and morning, and after each bowel movement. Repeat as often during the day as may be necessary to maintain comfort. Continue for one week after symptoms subside. When applicator is used, lubricate applicator first with Pazo. Insert slowly, then simply press tube.

Suppositories—Remove foil and insert one Pazo suppository night and morning, and after each bowel movement. Repeat as often during the day as may be necessary to maintain comfort. Continue for one week after symptoms subside.

Warning: If the underlying condition persists or recurs frequently, despite treatment, or if any bleeding or hard irreducible swelling is present, consult your physician. Keep out of children's reach. Keep in a cool place.

How Supplied:
Ointment—1-ounce and 2-ounce tubes with plastic applicator.
Suppositories—Boxes of 12 and 24 wrapped in silver foil.

Literature Available: Yes.

Burroughs Wellcome Co.
3030 CORNWALLIS ROAD RESEARCH TRIANGLE PARK, NC 27709

ACTIDIL® Syrup
ACTIDIL® Tablets

Description: Each scored tablet contains 2.5 mg triprolidine hydrochloride. Each 5 ml (1 teaspoonful) contains: 1.25 mg triprolidine hydrochloride
Alcohol 4%
Preservatives: Methylparaben 0.1%
Sodium benzoate 0.1%

Indications: For the temporary relief of running nose, sneezing, itching of the nose or throat and itchy and watery eyes as may occur in allergic rhinitis (such as hay fever).

Warnings: May cause excitability especially in children. May cause drowsiness. Do not take this product if you have asthma, glaucoma or difficulty in urination due to enlargement of the prostate gland except under the advice and supervision of a physician. Do not give this product to children under 6 years except under the advice and supervision of a physician. As with any drug, if you are pregnant or nursing a baby, seek the advice of a health professional before using this product.

Caution: Avoid driving a motor vehicle or operating heavy machinery. Avoid alcoholic beverages while taking this product. Store at 15°–30°C (59°–86°F) in a dry place and protect from light.
KEEP THIS AND ALL DRUGS OUT OF THE REACH OF CHILDREN. In case of accidental overdose, seek professional assistance or contact a Poison Control Center immediately.

Dosage: Tablets: Adults and children 12 years of age and over, 1 tablet every 4 to 6 hours. Children 6 to under 12 years of age, ½ tablet every 4 to 6 hours. Children under 6 years of age, consult a physician. Do not exceed 4 doses in 24 hours. Syrup: Adults and children 12 years of age and over, 2 teaspoonfuls every 4 to 6 hours. Children 6 to under 12 years of age, 1 teaspoonful every 4 to 6 hours. Children under 6 years of age, consult a physician. Do not exceed 4 doses in 24 hours.

How Supplied: Tablets, bottle of 100; Syrup, 1 pint.

ACTIFED® Tablets
ACTIFED® Syrup

Description: Each scored tablet contains pseudoephedrine hydrochloride 60 mg and tripolidine hydrochloride 2.5 mg. Each 5 ml syrup contains pseudoephedrine hydrochloride 30 mg and tripolidine hydrochloride 1.25 mg.

Indications: For temporary relief of nasal congestion due to the common cold, hay fever or other upper respiratory allergies. Helps decongest sinus openings, sinus passages. For temporary relief of running nose, sneezing, itching of the nose or throat and itchy and watery eyes as may occur in allergic rhinitis (such as hay fever).

Warnings: May cause excitability especially in children. Do not give this product to children under 6 years except under the advice and supervision of a physician. May cause drowsiness. Do not exceed recommended dosage because at higher doses nervousness, dizziness or sleeplessness may occur. If symptoms do not improve within 7 days or are accompanied by high fever, consult a physician before continuing use. Do not take this product if you have high blood pressure, heart disease, diabetes, thyroid disease, asthma, glaucoma or difficulty in urination due to enlargement of the prostate gland except under the advice and supervision of a physician. As with any drug, if you are pregnant or nursing a baby, seek the advice of a health professional before using this product.

Drug Interaction Precaution: Do not take this product if you are presently taking a prescription antihypertensive or antidepressant drug containing a monoamine oxidase inhibitor except under the advice and supervision of a physician.

Caution: Avoid driving a motor vehicle or operating heavy machinery. Avoid alcoholic beverages while taking this product.
KEEP THIS AND ALL DRUGS OUT OF THE REACH OF CHILDREN. In case of accidental overdose, seek professional assistance or contact a Poison Control Center immediately.

Store at 15°–30°C (59°–86°F) in a dry place and protect from light.

Dosage: To be given every 4 to 6 hours. Do not exceed 4 doses in 24 hours.
Tablets: Adults and children 12 years of age and over, 1 tablet. Children 6 to under 12 years of age, ½ tablet. Children under 6 years of age, consult a physician. Syrup: Adults and children 12 years of age and over, 2 teaspoonfuls. Children 6 to under 12 years of age, 1 teaspoonful. Children under 6 years of age, consult a physician.

How Supplied: Tablets, boxes of 12, 24, and 48; bottles of 100 and 1000, unit-of-use bottle of 90. Syrup, 4 fl. oz, 1 pint, 1 gallon.
Shown in Product Identification Section, page 406

Continued on next page

Burroughs Wellcome—Cont.

BOROFAX® Ointment

Description: Contains 5% boric acid in an emollient base with high lanolin content.

Indications: Relief of discomfort of chapped skin, chafed skin, diaper rash, dry skin, abrasions, sunburn, windburn, insect bites, other skin irritations.

Actions: Provides a water-resistant protective film which soothes affected area, promotes rapid healing. Keeps infant's tender skin soft, smooth, free from irritation, especially in diaper area.

Directions: *Not to be applied to the eye.* Apply to inflamed areas three or four times daily.

How Supplied: Tube, 1¾ oz.

EMPIRIN® ASPIRIN

Description: Each tablet contains 325 mg (5 grs) aspirin.

Indications: For relief of headache, minor muscular aches and pains, toothache, discomfort and fever of colds and flu, pain of the menstrual period, and temporary relief of minor arthritis pain (see CAUTION below).

Caution: For children under 3 years of age, consult your physician. In arthritic conditions, if pain persists for more than 10 days or redness is present, or in conditions affecting children under 12 years of age, consult a physician immediately.

Warnings: Keep this and all medicines out of children's reach. In case of accidental overdose, contact a physician immediately. High or continued fever, severe or persistent sore throat especially when accompanied by high fever, headache, nausea or vomiting, may be serious. Consult your physician. Do not exceed dose unless directed by a physician. Do not take this product if you are allergic to aspirin, have asthma, a gastric ulcer or its symptoms, or are taking a medication that affects the clotting of blood, except under the advice of a physician. As with any drug, if you are pregnant or nursing a baby, seek the advice of a health professional before using this product. Store at 15°–30°C (59°–86°F) in a dry place.

Dosage and Administration: Adults: 1 or 2 tablets with a full glass of water. Repeat every 4 hours as needed, up to 12 tablets a day.

Children: To be administered only under adult supervision. Take with a full glass of water. Indicated dosage may be repeated every 4 hours up to 5 times a day.

under 3 years ..consult your physician
3 to under 4 years .... ½ tablet
4 to under 6 years .... ¾ tablet
6 to under 9 years .... 1 tablet
9 to under 11 years .... 1¼ tablet
11 to under 12 years ....1½ tablet
12 and over ....same as adult

How Supplied: Bottles of 25, 50, 100, 250. Note: Bottles of 250 available without child-resistant cap for people who have no children in the house and for the elderly or handicapped.
Shown in Product Identification Section, page 406

FEDRAZIL® Tablets

Description: Each sugar-coated tablet contains

pseudoephedrine hydrochloride ....30 mg
chlorcyclizine hydrochloride..........25 mg

Indications: For temporary relief of nasal and sinus congestion associated with colds and hay fever.

Actions: Antihistamine/Nasal Decongestant.

Warnings: Do not use if pregnant or likely to become pregnant, unless directed by a physician. This drug may have the potentiality of being injurious to the unborn child. As with any drug, if you are pregnant or nursing a baby, seek the advice of a health professional before using this product.

Drug Interaction Precaution: Do not take this product if you are presently taking a prescription antihypertensive or antidepressant drug containing a monoamine oxidase inhibitor except under the advice and supervision of a physician.

Caution: Antihistamines may cause drowsiness. If it occurs, do not drive a car or operate machinery. Should not be used where there is high blood pressure, heart disease, diabetes or thyroid disease, unless directed by a physician. Do not exceed recommended dosage. If symptoms persist after 3 days, see your physician.
KEEP THIS AND ALL MEDICINES OUT OF CHILDREN'S REACH. In case of accidental overdose, seek professional assistance or contact a Poison Control Center immediately.

Dosage: Adults and children over 12: One tablet three times daily. Children 12 and under: As directed by a physician.

Store at 15°–30°C (59°–86°F) in a dry place.

How Supplied: Vials of 24 and bottles of 100 tablets.

MAREZINE® Tablets

Description: Scored tablets, cyclizine hydrochloride 50 mg.

Indication: For nausea and vomiting of motion sickness — land, sea, air.

Warnings: Drowsiness may occur; use caution in operating motor vehicles or other machinery. Do not take this product in the presence of glaucoma or enlargement of the prostate except under the advice and supervision of a physician. Do not give to children under 6 years of age except under the advice and supervision of a physician. As with any

drug, if you are pregnant or nursing a baby, seek the advice of a health professional before using this product.
KEEP THIS AND ALL MEDICINES OUT OF CHILDREN'S REACH. In case of accidental overdose, seek professional assistance or contact a Poison Control Center immediately. Store at 15°–30°C (59°–86°F) in a dry place and protect from light.

Dosage and Administration: Adults and children 12 years and older: one tablet ½ hour before departure, to be repeated every 4 to 6 hours if required. Not to exceed four tablets per day. Children 6–12, ½ tablet up to three times daily.

How Supplied: Boxes, 12 scored tablets. Bottle of 100.

NEOSPORIN® Ointment

Description: Contains three antibacterial components: polymyxin B, bacitracin, neomycin. Each gram contains Aerosporin® (polymyxin B sulfate) 5,000 units, bacitracin zinc 400 units, neomycin sulfate 5 mg (equivalent to 3.5 mg neomycin base), special white petrolatum qs.

Indications: For first aid: to help prevent bacterial infection of minor cuts, burns, abrasions; as an aid to healing.

Actions: Gentle occlusive base helps soften dry lesions. Low melting point of base enables ointment to spread quickly and evenly without caking. Won't sting burn or irritate skin.

Warning: In case of deep or puncture wounds or serious burns consult physician. If redness, irritation, swelling or pain persists or increases or if infection occurs, discontinue use and consult physician. Do not use in the eyes.

Directions: May be applied to affected area as needed, 2 to 5 times daily.

How Supplied: Tubes, ½ oz (with applicator tip), 1 oz.
Shown in Product Identification Section, page 406

POLYSPORIN® Ointment

Description: Contains two antibacterial components: polymyxin B and bacitracin. Each gram contains Aerosporin® (polymyxin B sulfate) 10,000 units, bacitracin zinc 500 units, special white petrolatum qs.

Indications: Helps prevent bacterial infection in minor cuts, burns, abrasions as an aid to healing.

Actions: Provides antibacterial protection; especially useful in patients sensitive to neomycin. Bland base won't sting or burn tender lesions. Works even under occlusive dressings or bandages.

Warning: In case of deep or puncture wounds or serious burns, consult physician. If redness, irritation, swelling or pain persists or increases or if infection occurs, discontinue use and consult physician. Do not use in the eyes.

Directions: May be applied to affected area as needed, 2 to 5 times daily.

How Supplied: Tubes, ½ oz with applicator tip, 1 oz.

SUDAFED® Cough Syrup
Cough Formula For Children and Adults

Description: Each 5 ml (1 teaspoonful) contains pseudoephedrine hydrochloride 15 mg, dextromethorphan hydrobromide 5 mg, guaifenesin 100 mg, alcohol 2.4%; added as preservatives sodium benzoate 0.1% and methylparaben 0.1%.

Indications: For temporary relief of cough due to minor throat and bronchial irritation as may occur with the common cold or inhaled irritants. For temporary relief of nasal congestion due to the common cold. Helps loosen phlegm and bronchial secretions and rid the bronchial passage ways of bothersome mucus.

Actions: Suppresses unproductive coughing; loosens thick mucosal secretions; decongests stuffy noses; doesn't cause drowsiness.

Warnings: Do not give to children under 2 years except as directed by a physician. Do not exceed recommended dosage because at higher doses nervousness, dizziness or sleeplessness may occur. If cough persists for more than 7 days, tends to recur or is accompanied by high fever, rash or persistent headache, consult a physician before continuing use. Do not take this product for persistent or chronic cough such as occurs with smoking, asthma or emphysema, or where cough is accompanied by excessive secretions, or if you have high blood pressure, heart disease, diabetes, difficulty in urination due to enlargement of the prostate gland, asthma, glaucoma or thyroid disease except under the advice and supervision of a physician. As with any drug, if you are pregnant or nursing a baby, seek the advice of a health professional before using this product.

Drug Interaction Precaution: Do not take this product if you are presently taking a prescription antihypertensive or antidepressant drug containing a monoamine oxidase inhibitor except under the advice and supervision of a physician. Store at 15°–30°C (59°–86°F). DO NOT REFRIGERATE.
KEEP THIS AND ALL DRUGS OUT OF THE REACH OF CHILDREN. In case of accidental overdose, seek professional assistance or contact a Poison Control Center immediately.

Dosage: To be given every 4 to 6 hours. Do not exceed 4 doses in 24 hours. Adults and children 12 years of age and over, 4 teaspoonfuls. Children 6 to under 12 years of age, 2 teaspoonfuls. Children 2 to under 6 years of age, 1 teaspoonful. For children under 2 years of age, consult a physician.

How Supplied: Bottles, 8 oz family size; bottles, 4 fl. oz.
Shown in Product Identification Section, page 406

SUDAFED® Tablets
30 mg, Sugar Coated
SUDAFED® Syrup
30 mg/5ml tsp, Raspberry Flavored

Description: Each tablet contains 30 mg pseudoephedrine hydrochloride. Each 5 ml teaspoonful contains 30 mg pseudoephedrine hydrochloride.

Indications: For temporary relief of nasal congestion due to the common cold, hay fever or other upper respiratory allergies, and nasal congestion associated with sinusitis; promotes nasal and/or sinus drainage.

Actions: Clears stuffy nose and head within 15–30 minutes; decongestant effect lasts for at least 4 hours.

Warnings: Do not exceed recommended dosage because at higher doses nervousness, dizziness or sleeplessness may occur. If symptoms do not improve within 7 days, or are accompanied by a high fever, consult a physician before continuing use. Do not take this preparation if you have high blood pressure, heart disease, diabetes, or thyroid disease, except under the advice and supervision of a physician. As with any drug, if you are pregnant or nursing a baby, seek the advice of a health professional before using this product.

Drug Interaction Precaution: Do not take this product if you are presently taking a prescription antihypertensive or antidepressant drug containing a monoamine oxidase inhibitor, except under the advice and supervision of a physician.

Dosage: To be given every 4 to 6 hours. Do not exceed 4 doses in 24 hours. Adults and children 12 years of age and over, 2 tablets or 2 teaspoonfuls of syrup. Children 6 to under 12 years of age, 1 tablet or 1 teaspoonful. Children 2 to under 6 years of age, use Sudafed Syrup, ½ teaspoonful every 4 to 6 hours. For children under 2 years of age, consult a physician. Store at 15°-30°C (59°-86°F) in a dry place and protect from light.
KEEP THIS AND ALL MEDICINES OUT OF CHILDREN'S REACH. In case of accidental overdose, seek professional assistance or contact a Poison Control Center immediately.

How Supplied: SUDAFED® Tablets, 30 mg, boxes of 24, 48. Bottles of 100. SUDAFED® Syrup, 30 mg/5ml teaspoonful, bottles of 4 fl. oz., 1 pint.
Shown in Product Identification Section, page 406

SUDAFED® Tablets
60 mg, Sugar Coated, Adult Strength

Description: Each tablet contains 60 mg pseudoephedrine hydrochloride.

Indications: For temporary relief of nasal congestion due to the common cold, hay fever or other upper respiratory allergies, and nasal congestion associated with sinusitis; promotes nasal and/or sinus drainge.

Actions: Opens up congested noses and sinuses, reaching places inaccessible to drops and sprays; makes breathing easier. No antihistamine so should not cause drowsiness; no analgesic so fever isn't masked.

Warning: Do not exceed recommended dosage because at higher doses nervousness, dizziness or sleeplessness may occur. If symptoms do not improve within 7 days or are accompanied by a high fever, consult a physician before continuing use. Do not take this preparation if you have high blood presssure, heart disease, diabetes, or thyroid disease, except under the advice and supervision of a physician. As with any drug, if you are pregnant or nursing a baby, seek the advice of a health professional before using this product.

Drug Interaction Precaution: Do not take this product if you are presently taking a prescription antihypertensive or antidepressant drug containing a monamine oxidase inhibitor, except under the advice and supervision of a physician.

Dosage: To be given every 4 to 6 hours. Do not exceed 4 doses in 24 hours. Adults and children 12 years of age and over, 1 tablet. Children 6 to under 12 years of age, use Sudafed 30 mg Tablets, 1 tablet every 4 to 6 hours. Children 2 to under 6 years of age, use Sudafed Syrup, ½ teaspoonful every 4 to 6 hours. For children under 2 years of age, consult a physician.

Store at 15°–30°C (59°–86°F) in a dry place and protect from light.
KEEP THIS AND ALL MEDICINES OUT OF CHILDREN'S REACH. In case of accidental overdose, seek professional assistance or contact a Poison Control Center immediately.

How Supplied: Bottles of 100, 1000.
Shown in Product Identification Section, page 406

SUDAFED® Plus Tablets
SUDAFED® Plus Syrup

Description: Each scored tablet contains pseudoephedrine hydrochloride 60 mg and chlorpheniramine maleate 4 mg. Each 5 ml syrup contains pseudoephedrine hydrochloride 30 mg and chlorpheniramine maleate 2 mg.

Indications: Decongestant *plus* antihistamine effect. Relieves nasal/sinus congestion associated with the common cold *PLUS* sneezing; watery, itchy eyes; runny nose and other hay fever/upper respiratory allergy symptoms.

Actions: Clears areas unreached by nose drops, sprays, inhalants. Provides longer relief than some nose drops and sprays.

Warnings: May cause excitability especially in children. Do not give to children under 6 years except as directed by

Continued on next page

Burroughs Wellcome—Cont.

a physician. May cause drowsiness. Do not exceed recommended dosage because at higher doses nervousness, dizziness or sleeplessness may occur. If symptoms do not improve within 7 days, or are accompanied by a high fever, consult a physician before continuing use. Do not take this product if you have high blood pressure, heart disease, diabetes, thyroid disease, asthma, glaucoma or difficulty in urination due to enlargement of the prostate gland except under the advice and supervision of a physician. As with any drug, if you are pregnant or nursing a baby, seek the advice of a health professional before using this product.

Drug Interaction Precaution: Do not take this product if you are presently taking a prescription antihypertensive or antidepressant drug containing a monoamine oxidase inhibitor except under the advice and supervision of a physician.

Caution: Avoid driving a motor vehicle or operating heavy machinery. Avoid alcoholic beverages while taking this product.

Store at 15°–30°C (59°–86°F) in a dry place and protect from light.

KEEP THIS AND ALL MEDICINES OUT OF CHILDREN'S REACH. In case of accidental overdose, seek professional assistance or contact a Poison Control Center immediately.

Dosage: Tablets: To be given every 4 to 6 hours. Do not exceed 4 doses in 24 hours. Adults and children 12 years of age and over, 1 tablet. Children 6 to under 12 years of age, ½ tablet. Children under 6 years of age, consult a physician.
Syrup: Adults and children 12 years of age and over, 2 teaspoonfuls every 4 hours. Children 6 to under 12 years of age, 1 teaspoonful every 4 hours. Children under 6 years of age, consult a physician. Do not exceed 4 doses in 24 hours.

How Supplied: Tablets, boxes of 24 and 48. Syrup, bottles, 4 fl. oz.
Shown in Product Identification Section, page 406

SUDAFED® S.A. Capsules
Sustained Action

Description: Each capsule contains: 120 mg pseudoephedrine hydrochloride.

Indications: For temporary relief of nasal congestion due to the common cold, hay fever or other upper respiratory allergies, and nasal congestion associated with sinusitis; promotes nasal and/or sinus drainage.

Actions: Clears stuffy nose and head—up to 12 hours relief. Contains no antihistamine so won't cause drowsiness—no analgesic so fever isn't masked.

Warnings: Do not exceed recommended dosage because at higher doses

nervousness, dizziness, or sleeplessness may occur. If symptoms do not improve within 7 days or are accompanied by high fever, consult a physician before continuing use. Do not take this preparation if you have high blood pressure, heart disease, diabetes, or thyroid disease except under the advice and supervision of a physician. As with any drug, if you are pregnant or nursing a baby, seek the advice of a health professional before using this product.

Drug Interaction Precaution: Do not take this product if you are presently taking a prescription antihypertensive or antidepressant drug containing a monoamine oxidase inhibitor except under the advice and supervision of a physician.
Store at 15°–30°C (59°–86°F) in a dry place and protect from light.
KEEP THIS AND ALL DRUGS OUT OF THE REACH OF CHILDREN. In case of accidental overdose, seek professional assistance or contact a Poison Control Center immediately.

Dosage: One capsule every 12 hours, not to exceed two capsules in 24 hours. Do not give to children under 12 years old.

How Supplied: Capsules of 120 mg (clear red top and clear body). Box of 10 capsules and bottles of 40 and 100 capsules.
Shown in Product Identification Section, page 406

WELLCOME® LANOLINE

Description: A highly purified lanolin obtained from the fat of lamb's wool.

Indications: For all ages. Replaces natural oils in skin and hair. Useful in foot care of diabetics when impaired circulation causes skin of feet to be dry, cracked, fissured.

Actions: Soothes chapped, irritated skin dried out by soaps, detergents, weather; alleviates scaliness and dryness of scalp.

Directions: May be applied to the face, hands, scalp, feet or other areas of the body's skin as often as needed. For best results, apply after washing while the skin is still damp. Massage gently into skin, removing excess Lanoline with a tissue.

How Supplied: Tubes, 1¾ oz (49.6 g).

Products are
indexed alphabetically
in the
PINK SECTION

Campbell Laboratories Inc.
300 EAST 51st STREET
P.O. BOX 812, F.D.R. STATION
NEW YORK, NY 10022

HERPECIN-L® Cold Sore Lip Balm

Composition: A soothing, emollient, cosmetically pleasant lip balm incorporating pyridoxine HCl; allantoin; the sunscreen, octyl p-(dimethylamino)-benzoate (Padimate O); and titanium dioxide in a balanced, acidic lipid system. (All ingredients appear on the package. Does not contain any "caines", antibiotics, phenol or camphor.) (NDC 38083-777-31)

Actions and Uses: HERPECIN-L® relieves dryness and chapping by providing a lipid barrier to help restore normal moisture balance to labial tissues. The sunscreen is effective in 2900-3200 AU range while titanium dioxide helps to block, scatter and reflect the sun's rays.

Administration: (1) *Recurrent "cold sores, sun and fever blisters"*: Simply put, users report the sooner and more often applied, the better the results. Frequent sufferers report that with *prophylactic* use (B.I.D./P.R.N.), their attacks are fewer and less severe. Most recurrent herpes labialis patients are aware of the *prodromal* symptoms: tingling, itching, burning. At this stage, or if the lesion has already developed, HERPECIN-L should be applied liberally as often as convenient—at least *every hour* (qq. hor.). The prodrome will often persist and remind the patient to continue to reapply HERPECIN-L. (2) *Outdoor sun/winter protection:* Apply during and after exposure (and after swimming) and again at bedtime (h.s.). (3) *Dry, chapped lips:* Apply as needed.

Note: HERPECIN-L is for peri-oral use only; not for "canker sores" (aphthous stomatitis). Primary attacks, usually in children and young adults, are normally intra-oral and accompanied by foul breath, pain and fever. Lasting up to six weeks, they are resistant to most treatments. Adjunctive therapy for pain, fever and infection may be indicated.

Adverse Reactions: A few, rare instances of topical sensitivity to pyridoxine HCl (Vitamin B_6) have been reported. Discontinue use if reaction develops.

Contraindications: HERPECIN-L Lip Balm does not contain any steroids. (Oral or topical corticosteroids are normally contraindicated in *herpes* infections.)

How Supplied: 2.8 gm. swivel tubes.

Products are cross-indexed by
generic and chemical names
in the
YELLOW SECTION

Carnation Company
5045 WILSHIRE BLVD.
LOS ANGELES, CA 90036

CARNATION® DO-IT-YOURSELF DIET PLAN™

Active Ingredients: Nonfat dry milk, multivitamins and minerals; and separately packaged multivitamins.

Indications: One 1.06-oz. serving of diet powder is to be mixed with 6 fl. oz. (178 ml) vitamin D 2% lowfat milk. It is to be used as a meal replacement to maintain or slowly lose weight, or as a complete dietary replacement for more rapid weight loss when at least four servings are consumed daily as the total diet. CARNATION Do-It-Yourself Diet Plan is intended for children ages 4 years and older and adults.

Actions: When consumed as directed, one serving of CARNATION Do-It-Yourself Diet Plan diet food supplies 200 kilocalories, 25% of the U.S. RDA for protein, and 25% U.S. RDA of all vitamins and minerals for which a U.S. RDA has been established. Safety, and efficacy for weight loss, for patients consuming four servings per day have been clinically demonstrated for a period of three weeks.

Drug Interaction: No known drug interaction.

Symptoms and Treatment of Oral Overdosage: No known symptoms exist. Overconsumption might lead to excessive kilocalorie intake. Based on medical judgment, not on actual clinical experience, persons with lactose intolerance might develop temporary G.I. gas or diarrhea, depending on degree of overdosage.

Dosage and Administration: One or more daily servings (up to four per day) of the diet food, and one multivitamin pill per day.

Professional Labeling: Same information as outlined under Indications and Actions.

How Supplied: Packaged in 12.72-oz. canisters. A separate pouch containing 6 multivitamin tablets are included in each canister, as well as a menu plan booklet and plastic scoop (two level scoops equal one serving). Available flavors are Chocolate and Vanilla.

CARNATION® INSTANT BREAKFAST

Active Ingredients: Protein sources (nonfat dry milk, whey, caseinate); multivitamins and minerals.

Indications: When one envelope of Carnation instant breakfast is mixed with 8 fl. oz. (237 ml) vitamin D milk as directed, it is to be used as a meal replacement or as a supplement to the regular diet by children ages 4 years and over and adults. As such, it is indicated for low fiber/roughage diets, for burn patients, for those who temporarily cannot chew solid food, and for athletes who desire supplemental nutrition or a fast-digesting pre-game meal. When prepared with 8 fl. oz. nonfat milk, the product is also indicated for low-fat, low-cholesterol, and low-calorie diets.

Actions: When mixed with vitamin D whole milk as directed, one serving provides 280 kilocalories, 30% U.S. RDA for protein, and at least 25% U.S. RDA for all vitamins and minerals for which a U.S. RDA has been established, except for biotin. Calcium content per serving ranges from 380–510 mg depending on flavor variety. When mixed with 8 fl. oz. nonfat milk, one serving provides 220 kilocalories.

Drug Interaction: No known drug interaction.

Symptoms and Treatment of Oral Overdosage: No known symptoms of overdosage. Overconsumption might lead to excessive kilocalorie intake. Based on medical judgment, not on actual clinical experience, persons with lactose intolerance might develop temporary G.I. gas or diarrhea, depending on degree of overdosage.

Dosage and Administration: One envelope is to be mixed with 8 fl. oz. vitamin D milk. May be taken orally or by stomach tube.

Professional Labeling: Same as those described under Indications and Actions.

How Supplied: Available in either 6- or 10-envelope cartons, each envelope containing 1.21 to 1.26 oz (34.3 to 35.7 g), depending on flavor variety: Vanilla, Chocolate, Strawberry, Eggnog, Chocolate Malt, and Coffee.

CARNATION® NONFAT DRY MILK

Active Ingredients: Nonfat dry milk, 2203 I.U. % vitamin A palmitate, 440 I.U. % vitamin D_2.

Indications: For use by individuals wishing to increase calcium or reduce fat and caloric intakes by replacing nonfat milk for regular full-fat milk in the diet.

Actions: When mixed according to package directions, one 8-fl.-oz. (237-ml) serving provides 80 kilocalories, 0.16 g fat, and 279 mg calcium. 100 g of the dry milk powder contains 1231 mg calcium; one tablespoon provides 52 mg calcium.

Warnings: Not recommended for use as a base for formula preparation for infants less than 6 months old.

Drug Interaction: No known drug interaction.

Dosage and Administration: After reconstituting Carnation nonfat dry milk with the appropriate amount of water (100 g by weight mixed with 950 ml water, or 350 ml by volume mixed with 950 ml water equals 1 litre), to be consumed orally, as an alternative to fresh whole milk in the diet. The product is also used in its dry form for adding to various foods and recipes.

How Supplied: Available either in 3.2 oz. (90.7 g) envelopes which reconstitute to one quart (in either 5- or 10-envelope cartons), or in boxes containing bulk powder in amounts which reconstitute to the following volumes of fluid milk: 3 qt, 8 qt, 14 qt, 20 qt, and 50 qt.

SLENDER® DIET FOOD FOR WEIGHT CONTROL (INSTANT)

Active Ingredients: Nonfat dry milk, multivitamins and minerals; 0.0009% BHA added to strawberry flavor as a preservative.

Indications: One envelope of Slender instant is to be mixed with 6 fl. oz. (178 ml) vitamin D 2% lowfat milk. It is to be used as a meal replacement to maintain or slowly lose weight, or as a complete dietary replacement for more rapid weight loss when at least four servings are consumed daily as the total diet. Slender instant is intended for children ages 4 years and older and adults.

Actions: When consumed as directed, one serving of Slender instant supplies 200 kilocalories, 25% of the U.S. RDA for protein, and 25% of U.S. RDA of all vitamins and minerals for which a U.S. RDA has been established. Safety, and efficacy for weight loss, for patients consuming four servings per day have been clinically demonstrated for a period of three weeks.

Drug Interaction: No known drug interaction.

Symptoms and Treatment of Oral Overdosage: No known symptoms exist. Overconsumption might lead to excessive kilocalorie intake. Based on medical judgment, not on actual clinical experience, persons with lactose intolerance might develop temporary G.I. gas or diarrhea, depending on degree of overdosage.

Dosage and Administration: Taken orally, one or more daily servings (up to four per day), each mixed with 6 fl. oz. vitamin D 2% lowfat milk.

Professional Labeling: Same information as outlined under Indications and Actions.

How Supplied: Available in 1.05 to 1.07 oz. envelopes (depending on flavor variety), which come in cartons containing 4 envelopes. Available flavors are Dutch Chocolate, Chocolate, Vanilla, Strawberry.

SLENDER® DIET MEAL FOR WEIGHT CONTROL (CANNED)

Active Ingredients: Skim milk, multivitamins, and minerals.

Indications: For use as a meal replacement to maintain or slowly lose weight, or as a complete dietary replacement for more rapid weight loss when at least four servings are consumed daily. Slender liquid is intended for children ages 4 years and older and adults.

Continued on next page

Carnation—Cont.

Actions: One serving of Slender liquid (one 10-fl.-oz. can) supplies 220 kilocalories, 25% of the U.S. RDA for protein, and 25% of U.S. RDA of all vitamins and minerals for which a U.S. RDA has been established. Safety, and efficacy for weight loss, for patients consuming four servings per day have been clinically demonstrated for a period of three weeks.

Drug Interactions: No known drug interaction.

Symptoms and Treatment of Oral Overdosage: No known symptoms exist. Overconsumption might lead to excessive kilocalorie intake. Based on medical judgment, not on actual clinical experience, persons with lactose intolerance might develop temporary G.I. gas or diarrhea, depending on degree of overdosage.

Dosage and Administration: Taken orally, one or more daily servings up to four servings per day.

Professional Labeling: Same information as outlined under Indications and Actions.

How Supplied: Available in 10-fl.-oz. (296-ml; 313-g) cans in the following varieties: Chocolate, Chocolate Fudge, Milk Chocolate, Chocolate Malt, Vanilla, Strawberry, Banana, Peach.

SLENDER® DIET MEAL BARS FOR WEIGHT CONTROL

Active Ingredients: Protein sources, including peanuts, whey, calcium caseinate, egg white, and soy; multivitamins and minerals.

Indications: For use as a meal replacement to maintain or slowly lose weight, or as a complete dietary replacement for more rapid weight loss when at least four servings are consumed daily. Slender bars are intended for children ages 4 years and older and adults.

Actions: One serving of two Slender diet meal bars supplies 270 kilocalories, 25% of the U.S. RDA for protein, and 25% of U.S. RDA of all vitamins and minerals for which a U.S. RDA has been established. Safety, and efficacy for weight loss, for patients consuming four servings per day have been clinically demonstrated for a period of three weeks.

Drug Interaction: No known drug interaction.

Symptoms and Treatment of Oral Overdosage: No known symptoms exist. Overconsumption might lead to excessive kilocalorie intake.

Dosage and Administration: Taken orally, one or more daily servings (of two bars), up to four servings per day.

Professional Labeling: Same information as outlined under Indications and Actions.

How Supplied: Available in two-bar pouches, four pouches per carton. Each bar weighs 0.98 to 1.00 oz. (27.6 to 28.6 g), depending on flavor variety. Available flavors are Chocolate, Chocolate Peanut Butter, Vanilla, Chocolate Chip.

Carter Products
Division of Carter-Wallace, Inc.
767 FIFTH AVENUE
NEW YORK, NY 10153

CARTER'S LITTLE PILLS®
A Stimulant Laxative

Active Ingredient: 5 mg bisacodyl, U.S.P. in each enteric coated pill.

Indications: For effective short-term relief of simple constipation (infrequent or difficult bowel movement).

Actions: Bisacodyl is a stimulant laxative that promotes bowel movement by one or more direct actions on the intestine.

Directions for Use: Adult dosage is 1 to 3 pills (usually 2) at bedtime. Children over 3 years of age, 1 pill at bedtime.

Warnings: Do not chew. Do not give to children under 3 years of age or to persons who cannot swallow without chewing. Do not use this product when abdominal pain, nausea, or vomiting are present. Do not take this product within one hour before or after taking an antacid and/or milk. This product may cause abdominal discomfort, faintness, rectal burning or mild cramps. Store in a cool place at temperatures not above 86°F (30°C).
Prolonged or continued use of this product can lead to laxative dependence and loss of normal bowel function. Serious side effects from prolonged use or overdose can occur.
If you have noticed a sudden change in bowel habits that persists over a period of two weeks, consult a physician before using a laxative. This product should be used only occasionally, but in any event, no longer than daily for one week, except on the advice of a physician.
As with any drug, if you are pregnant or nursing a baby, seek the advice of a health professional before using this product.

Drug Interaction Precaution: No known drug interaction.

Treatment of Overdosage: In case of accidental overdose seek professional assistance or contact a Poison Control Center immediately.

Professional Labeling: For effective short-term relief of simple constipation. For use in preparation of the patient for surgery or for preparation of the colon for x-ray and endoscopic examination.

How Supplied: Available in packages of 30 pills and 85 pills.
Shown in Product Identification Section, page 407

Chattem Consumer Products
Division of Chattem, Inc.
1715 WEST 38TH STREET
CHATTANOOGA, TN 37409

PREMESYN PMS™
Premenstrual Syndrome Capsules

Active Ingredients: Each capsule contains Acetaminophen 500 mg., Pamabrom 25 mg., and Pyrilamine Maleate 1 mg.

Indications: Specially formulated to relieve the major symptoms of premenstrual syndrome. PREMESYN PMS™ contains two special ingredients that have been clinically proven to safely and effectively relieve premenstrual tension, irritability, nervousness, backache, and the water weight gain and bloating that often accompany premenstrual syndrome. Additionally, PREMESYN PMS™ contains an aspirin-free analgesic to provide relief from dysmenorrhea.

Warning: KEEP THIS AND ALL DRUGS OUT OF THE REACH OF CHILDREN. In case of accidental overdose, seek professional assistance or contact a poison control center immediately.

Precautions: If drowsiness occurs, do not drive or operate machinery. As with any drug, if pregnant or nursing a baby, seek the advice of a health professional before using this product.

Dosage and Administration: Two capsules at first sign of premenstrual discomfort and repeat every three or four hours as needed not to exceed 8 capsules in a 24 hour period.

How Supplied: Tamper-resistant bottles of 20 and 40 capsules.
Shown in Product Identification Section, page 407

Church & Dwight Co., Inc.
469 N. HARRISON STREET
PRINCETON, NJ 08540

ARM & HAMMER®
Pure Baking Soda

Active Ingredient: Sodium Bicarbonate U.S.P.

Indications: For alleviation of acid indigestion, also known as heartburn or sour stomach. Not a remedy for other types of stomach complaints such as nausea, stomachache, abdominal cramps, gas pains, or stomach distention caused by overeating and/or overdrinking. In the latter case, one should not ingest solids, liquids or antacid but rather refrain from all physical activity and—if uncomfortable—call a physician.

Actions: ARM & HAMMER® Pure Baking Soda provides fast-acting, effective neutralization of stomach acids. Each level ½ teaspoon dose will neutralize 20.9 mEq of acid.

Warnings: Except under the advice and supervision of a physician: (1) do not take more than eight level ½ teaspoons per person up to 60 years old or four level ½ teaspoons per person 60 years or older in a 24-hour period, (2) do not use this product if you are on a sodium restricted diet, (3) do not use the maximum dose for more than two weeks, (4) do not ingest food, liquid or any antacid when stomach is overly full to avoid possible injury to the stomach.

Dosage and Administration: Level ½ teaspoon in ½ glass (4 fl. oz.) of water every two hours up to maximum dosage or as directed by a physician. Accurately measure level ½ teaspoon. Each level ½ teaspoon contains 20.9 mEq (.476 gm) sodium.

How Supplied: Available in 8 oz., 16 oz., 32 oz., and 64 oz. boxes.

CIBA Consumer Pharmaceuticals
Division of CIBA-GEIGY Corporation
RARITAN PLAZA III
EDISON, NJ 08837

MAXIMUM STRENGTH ACUTRIM™ PRECISION RELEASE™ TABLETS Delivers 16 Full Hours of Controlled, Even Appetite Suppressant To Curb Hunger and Aid Weight Loss—Without Caffeine

Description:
ACUTRIM™ Precision Release™ tablets deliver their maximum strength dosage of appetite suppressant at a precisely controlled, even rate.
This steady release is scientifically targeted to effectively distribute the appetite suppressant over a full 16 hours.
ACUTRIM tablets start fast, and deliver appetite suppressant for the 16 hours when you need it most, from early morning to bedtime.
ACUTRIM makes it easier to follow the kind of reduced calorie diet needed for best weight control results.
A diet plan developed by an expert dietitian is included in the package for your personal use as a further aid.
ACUTRIM 16 Hour *Breakfast to Bedtime*™ Appetite Suppressant Contains no caffeine.

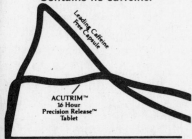

| Hours | 4 | 8 | 12 | 16 |

Formula: Each Precision Release™ tablet contains: Active Ingredient—

phenylpropanolamine HCl 75 mg. (appetite suppressant).
Inactive Ingredients—Cellulose compounds and stearic acid.

Dosage: For best results, take one tablet daily directly after breakfast. Do not take more than one tablet every 24 hours. Recommended dosage may be used up to three months.

Caution: Do not give this product to children under 12. Do not exceed recommended dosage. If nervousness, dizziness, or sleeplessness occurs, stop taking this medication and consult your physician. If you are being treated for high blood pressure or depression, or have heart disease, diabetes, or thyroid disease, do not take this product except under the supervision of a physician. If you are taking a cough/cold allergy medication containing any form of phenylpropanolamine, do not take this product. Recommended dosage may be used up to three months.

Warning: As with any drug, if you are pregnant or nursing a baby, seek the advice of a health professional before using this product.
KEEP THIS AND ALL MEDICATION OUT OF THE REACH OF CHILDREN. In case of accidental overdose, seek professional assistance or contact a poison control center immediately.
Tamper Resistant Blister Package. Do not use if individual seals are broken.

Drug Interaction Precaution: If you are taking any prescription drugs, or any type of nasal decongestant, antihypertensive or antidepressant drug, do not take this product except under the supervision of a physician.

How Supplied: Packages of 20 and 40 tablets.
Shown in Product Identification Section, page 407

CAFFEINE FREE/PRECISION RELEASE™ ACUTRIM® II MAXIMUM DURATION The longest lasting appetite suppressant. Helps you eat less and lose weight.

Description:
ACUTRIM® II Maximum Duration provides that extra measure of longer appetite suppressant delivery which many people need to help curb hunger and aid weight loss. It uses the science of Precision Release™ to deliver its maximum strength dosage evenly, steadily, longer than any other product.
ACUTRIM II Is specially designed to last longer and help you to avoid those after dinner and late evening snacks that can make sticking to your diet so difficult. And ACUTRIM II contains no caffeine.
ACUTRIM II makes it easier to follow the kind of reduced calorie diet needed for best weight control results. A diet plan is included in this package for your use as a further aid.

Formula: EACH PRECISION RELEASE™ TABLET CONTAINS: Active Ingredient—Phenylpropanolamine HCl 75 mg. (appetite suppressant). Inactive Ingredients—Cellulose compounds and stearic acid.

Dosage: For best results, take one tablet daily directly after breakfast. Do not take more than one tablet every 24 hours. Recommended dosage may be used up to three months.

Caution: Do not give this product to children under 12. Do not exceed recommended dosage. If nervousness, dizziness, or sleeplessness occurs, stop taking this medication and consult your physician. If you are being treated for high blood pressure or depression, or have heart disease, diabetes, or thyroid disease, do not take this product except under the supervision of a physician. If you are taking a cough/cold allergy medication containing any form of phenylpropanolamine, do not take this product.

Warning: As with any drug, if you are pregnant or nursing a baby, seek the advice of a health professional before using this product.
KEEP THIS AND ALL MEDICATION OUT OF THE REACH OF CHILDREN. In case of accidental overdose, seek professional assistance or contact a poison control center immediately.

Drug Interaction Precaution: If you are taking any prescription drugs, or any type of nasal decongestant, antihypertensive or antidepressant drug, do not take this product except under the supervision of a physician.

How Supplied: Packages of 20 and 40 tablets.

SLOW FE™
Slow Release Iron

Description: SLOW FE supplies ferrous sulfate, for the treatment of iron deficiency and iron deficiency anemia with a significant reduction in the incidence of common iron side effects. The wax matrix delivery system of SLOW FE is designed to maximize the release of ferrous sulfate in the duodenum and the jejunum where it is best tolerated and absorbed. SLOW FE is clinically shown to significantly reduce constipation, diarrhea and abdominal discomfort when compared to regular iron tablets and a leading capsule.

Formula: Each tablet contains 160 mg. dried ferrous sulfate USP, equivalent to 50 mg. elemental iron.

Dosage: ADULTS—one or two tablets daily or as recommended by a physician. A maximum of four tablets daily may be taken. CHILDREN—one tablet daily. Tablets must be swallowed whole.

Warning: The treatment of any anemic condition should be under the advice and supervision of a physician. As oral iron products interfere with absorption

Continued on next page

CIBA Consumer—Cont.

of oral tetracycline antibiotics, these products should not be taken within two hours of each other. As with any drug, if you are pregnant or nursing a baby, seek the advice of a health professional before using this product.

Keep this and all medicines out of reach of children. In case of accidental overdose, contact your physician or poison control center immediately.

Tamper Resistant Blister Package. Do not use if individual seals are broken.

How Supplied: Packages of 30 and 100.

CIBA Pharmaceutical Company
Division of CIBA-GEIGY Corporation
SUMMIT, NJ 07901

NUPERCAINAL®
Anesthetic Ointment
Pain-Relief Cream

Caution:
Nupercainal products are not for prolonged or extensive use and should never be applied in or near the eyes.
Consult labels before using.
Keep this and all medications out of reach of children.
NUPERCAINAL SHOULD NOT BE SWALLOWED. SWALLOWING OR USE OF A LARGE QUANTITY IS HAZARDOUS, PARTICULARLY TO CHILDREN. CONSULT A PHYSICIAN OR POISON CONTROL CENTER IMMEDIATELY.

Indications: Nupercainal Ointment and Cream are fast-acting, long-lasting pain relievers that you can use for a number of painful skin conditions. **Nupercainal Anesthetic Ointment** is for hemorrhoids and for general use. **Nupercainal Pain-Relief Cream** is for general use only. The **Cream** is half as strong as the **Ointment**.

How to use Nupercainal Anesthetic Ointment (for general use). This soothing Ointment helps lubricate dry, inflamed skin and gives fast, temporary relief of pain and itching. It is recommended for sunburn, nonpoisonous insect bites, minor burns, cuts and scratches. **DO NOT USE THIS PRODUCT IN OR NEAR YOUR EYES.**

Apply to affected areas gently. If necessary, cover with a light dressing for protection. Do not use more than 1 ounce of Ointment in a 24-hour period for an adult, do not use more than one-quarter of an ounce in a 24-hour period for a child. If irritation develops, discontinue use and consult your doctor.

How to use Nupercainal Anesthetic Ointment for fast, temporary relief of
pain and itching due to hemorrhoids (also known as piles).

Remove cap from tube and set it aside. Attach the white plastic applicator to the tube. Squeeze the tube until you see the Ointment begin to come through the little holes in the applicator. Using your finger, lubricate the applicator with the Ointment. Now insert the entire applicator gently into the rectum. Give the tube a good squeeze to get enough Ointment into the rectum for comfort and lubrication. Remove applicator from rectum and wipe it clean. Apply additional Ointment to anal tissues to help relieve pain, burning, and itching. For best results use Ointment morning and night and after each bowel movement. After each use detach applicator, and wash it off with soap and water. Put cap back on tube before storing. In case of rectal bleeding, discontinue use and consult your doctor.

Pain-Relief Cream for general use. This Cream is particularly effective for fast, temporary relief of pain and itching associated with sunburn, cuts, scratches, minor burns and nonpoisonous insect bites. **DO NOT USE THIS PRODUCT IN OR NEAR YOUR EYES.** Apply liberally to affected area and rub in gently. This Cream is water-washable, so be sure to reapply after bathing, swimming or sweating. If irritation develops, discontinue use and consult your doctor.

Nupercainal Anesthetic Ointment contains 1% (one percent) dibucaine USP in a lubricant base. Available in tubes of 1 and 2 ounces.

Nupercainal Pain-Relief Cream contains 0.5% (one-half of one percent) dibucaine USP in a water-soluble base. Available in 1 ½ ounce tubes.

Dibucaine USP is officially classified as a "topical anesthetic" and is one of the strongest and longest lasting of all pain relievers. It is not a narcotic.

C81-17 (5/81)

Shown in Product Identification Section, page 407

NUPERCAINAL™
Suppositories

Caution:
Nupercainal Suppositories are not for prolonged or extensive use. Contact with the eyes should be avoided.
Consult labels before using.
Keep this and all medications out of reach of children.
NUPERCAINAL SUPPOSITORIES SHOULD NOT BE SWALLOWED. SWALLOWING CAN BE HAZARDOUS, PARTICULARLY TO CHILDREN. IN THE EVENT OF ACCIDENTAL SWALLOWING CONSULT A PHYSICIAN OR POISON CONTROL CENTER IMMEDIATELY.

Indications: Nupercainal Suppositories are for the temporary relief from itching, burning, and discomfort due to hemorrhoids or other anorectal disorders.

How to use Nupercainal Suppositories for hemorrhoids (also known as piles) or other anorectal disorders.

Tear off one suppository along the perforated line. Remove foil wrapper. Insert the suppository, rounded end first, well into the anus until you can feel it moving into your rectum. For best results, use one suppository after each bowel movement and as needed, but not to exceed 6 in a 24-hour period. Each suppository is sealed in its own foil packet to reduce danger of leakage when carried in pocket or purse. **To prevent melting, do not store above 86°F (30°C).**

Nupercainal Suppositories contain 2.4 gram cocoa butter, .25 gram zinc oxide, .1 gram bismuth subgallate, and acetone sodium bisulfite as preservative.

Dist. by:
CIBA Pharmaceutical Company
Division of CIBA-GEIGY Corporation
Summit, New Jersey 07901

C82-56 (Rev. 12/82)

Shown in Product Identification Section, page 407

PRIVINE®
0.05% Nasal Solution
0.05% Nasal Spray

Caution: Do not use Privine if you have glaucoma. Privine is an effective nasal decongestant **when you use it in the recommended dosage.** If you use too much, too long, or too often, Privine may be harmful to your nasal mucous membranes and cause burning, stinging, sneezing or an increased runny nose.

Do not use Privine by mouth.

Keep this and all medications out of the reach of children. Do not use Privine with children under 6 years of age, except with the advice and supervision of a doctor.

OVERDOSAGE IN YOUNG CHILDREN MAY CAUSE MARKED SEDATION AND IF SEVERE, EMERGENCY TREATMENT MAY BE NECESSARY. IF NASAL STUFFINESS PERSISTS AFTER 3 DAYS OF TREATMENT, DISCONTINUE USE AND CONSULT A DOCTOR.

Privine is a nasal decongestant that comes in two forms: Nasal Solution (in a bottle with a dropper) and Nasal Spray (in a plastic squeeze bottle). Both are for prompt, and prolonged relief of nasal congestion due to common colds, sinusitis, hay fever, etc.

How to use Nasal Solution. Squeeze rubber bulb to fill dropper with proper amount of medication. For best results, tilt head as far back as possible and put two drops of solution into your right nostril. Then lean head forward, inhaling and turning your head to the left. Refill dropper by squeezing bulb. Now tilt head as far back as possible and put two drops of solution into your left nostril. Then lean head forward, inhaling, and turning your head to the right.

Use only 2 drops in each nostril. Do not repeat this dosage more than every 3 hours.

The Privine dropper bottle is designed to make administration of the proper dosage easy and to prevent accidental over-dosage. Privine will not cause sleeplessness, so you may use it before going to bed.

Important: After use, be sure to rinse the dropper with very hot water. This helps prevent contamination of the bottle with bacteria from nasal secretions. Use of the dispenser by more than one person may spread infection.

Note: Privine Nasal Solution may be used on contact with glass, plastic, stainless steel and specially treated metals used in atomizers. Do not let the solution come in contact with reactive metals, especially aluminum. If solution becomes discolored, it should be discarded.

How to use Nasal Spray. For best results do **not** shake the plastic squeeze bottle.

Remove cap. With head held upright, spray twice into each nostril. Squeeze the bottle sharply and firmly while sniffing through the nose.

For best results use every 4 to 6 hours. Do not use more often than every 3 hours. Avoid overdosage. Follow directions for use carefully.

Privine Nasal Solution contains 0.05% naphazoline hydrochloride USP with benzalkonium chloride as a preservative. Available in bottles of .66 fl. oz. (20 ml) with dropper, and bottles of 16 fl. oz. (473 ml). Privine Nasal Spray contains 0.05% naphazoline hydrochloride USP with benzalkonium chloride as a preservative. Available in plastic squeeze bottles of ½ fl. oz. (15 ml).

C80-5 (1/80)
*Shown in Product Identification
Section, page 407*

VIOFORM®
(clioquinol USP)

Listed in USP, a Medicare designated compendium.

Indications and Directions For Use: A soothing antifungal and antibacterial preparation for the treatment of inflamed conditions of the skin, such as eczema, athlete's foot and other fungal infections.

Apply to the affected area 2 or 3 times a day or use as directed by physician.

Caution: May prove irritating to sensitized skin in rare cases. If this should occur, discontinue treatment and consult physician. May stain.
KEEP OUT OF REACH OF CHILDREN.

How Supplied:
Ointment, 3% clioquinol in a petrolatum base; tubes of 1 ounce.
Cream, 3% clioquinol in a water-washable base; tubes of 1 ounce.

(7/80)

The full prescribing information for each CIBA drug is contained herein and is that in effect as of December 1, 1984.

Colgate-Palmolive Company
A Delaware Corporation
300 PARK AVENUE
NEW YORK, NY 10022

COLGATE MFP® FLUORIDE GEL

Active Ingredient: Sodium Monofluorophosphate (MFP®) 0.76% in a spearmint flavored gel toothpaste base.

Other Ingredients: Sorbitol, Glycerin, Hydrated Silica, Water, PEG-12, Sodium Lauryl Sulfate, Flavor, Sodium Benzoate, Cellulose Gum, Sodium Saccharin, Titanium Dioxide, FD&C Blue No. 1.

Indications: The gel toothpaste with the anti-cavity ingredient MFP® Fluoride providing maximum fluoride protection by a toothpaste and a fresh clean taste for the whole family.

Actions: Clinical tests have shown COLGATE® with MFP® Fluoride to be an effective aid in the reduction of the incidence of cavities. It is approved as a decay-preventive dentifrice by the American Dental Association.

Contraindications: Sensitivity to any ingredient in this product.

Directions: Brush regularly as part of a dental health program.

How Supplied: 1.4 oz., 2.6 oz., 4.6 oz., 6.4 oz., 8.2 oz. tubes. Also available in 4.5 oz. pump.
*Shown in Product Identification
Section, page 407*

COLGATE MFP® FLUORIDE TOOTHPASTE

Active Ingredient: Sodium Monofluorophosphate (MFP®) 0.76% in a doublemint flavored toothpaste base.

Other Ingredients: Dicalcium Phosphate Dihydrate, Water, Glycerin, Sodium Lauryl Sulfate, Cellulose Gum, Flavor, Sodium Benzoate, Tetrasodium Pyrophosphate, Sodium Saccharin.

Indications: The toothpaste with the anti-cavity ingredient MFP® Fluoride providing maximum fluoride protection by a toothpaste.

Actions: Clinical tests have shown COLGATE® with MFP® Fluoride to be an effective aid in the reduction of the incidence of cavities. It is approved as a decay-preventive dentifrice by the American Dental Association.

Contraindications: Sensitivity to any ingredient in this product.

Directions: Brush regularly as part of a dental health program.

How Supplied: 0.75 oz., 1.50 oz., 3.0 oz., 5.0 oz., 7.0 oz., 9.0 oz. tubes. Also available in 4.9 oz. pump.
*Shown in Product Identification
Section, page 407*

FLUORIGARD ANTI–CAVITY DENTAL RINSE

Fluorigard is accepted by the American Dental Association.

Active Ingredient: Sodium Fluoride (0.05%) in a neutral solution.

Other Ingredients: Water, Glycerin, SD Alcohol 38-B (6%), Poloxamer 338, Poloxamer 407, Sodium Benzoate, Sodium Saccharin, Benzoic Acid, Flavor, FD & C Blue No. 1, FD & C Yellow No. 5.

Indications: Good tasting Fluorigard Anti-Cavity Dental Rinse is fluoride in liquid form. It helps get cavity-fighting fluoride to back teeth, as well as front teeth; even floods those dangerous spaces between teeth where brushing might miss. 70% of all cavities happen in back teeth and between teeth.

Actions: Fluorigard Anti-Cavity Dental Rinse is a 0.05% Sodium Fluoride solution which has been proven effective in reducing cavities.

Contraindications: Sensitivity to any ingredient in this product.

Warnings: Do not swallow. For rinsing only. Not to be used by children under 6 years of age unless recommended by a dentist. Keep out of reach of young children. If an amount considerably larger than recommended for rinsing is swallowed, give as much milk as possible and contact a physician immediately.

Directions: Use once daily after thoroughly brushing teeth. For persons 6 years of age and over, fill measuring cap to 10 ml. level (2 teaspoons), rinse around and between teeth for one minute, then spit out. For maximum benefit, use every day and do not eat or drink for at least 30 minutes afterward. Rinsing may be most convenient at bedtime. This product may be used in addition to a fluoride toothpaste.

How Supplied:
6 oz.
10 oz.
16 oz.
1 Gallon Professional Size for use in dentists offices only.
*Shown in Product Identification
Section, page 407*

IDENTIFICATION PROBLEM?
Consult the
Product Identifcation Section
where you'll find
products pictured
in full color.

Combe Incorporated
**1101 WESTCHESTER AVENUE
WHITE PLAINS, NY 10604**

GYNECORT® Antipruritic
0.5% Hydrocortisone Acetate Creme

Active Ingredient: 0.5% Hydrocortisone Acetate

Indications: GYNECORT antipruritic creme medication was specifically formulated for effective relief of external vulval itching and itching associated with minor skin irritations. GYNECORT is a highly emollient white vanishing cream which is soothing to delicate external genital (vulval) tissue. It is hypoallergenic (contains no potentially irritating perfume), greaseless and non-staining.

Action: Hydrocortisone Acetate is an anti-inflammatory corticosteroid[1,2], whose mechanism of action has been widely investigated. Current thinking points to the following modes of action: (1) controlling the rate of protein synthesis; (2) reducing the amounts of prostaglandin substrate available for the enzyme.[3] Corticosteroids are also known to reduce immune hypersensitivity by reducing the inflammatory response.[1]

Warning: For external use only. Avoid contact with the eyes. If condition worsens or if symptoms persist for more than 7 days, or clear up and recur within a few days, discontinue use and consult a physician. Do not use if you have an unusual or abnormal vaginal discharge except under the supervision of your physician. Keep this and all drugs out of reach of children. In case of accidental ingestion, seek professional assistance or contact a Poison Control Center immediately.

Dosage and Administration: Adults and children 2 years of age and older: Apply to affected area not more than 3 or 4 times daily. Children under 2 years of age: Consult a physician.

How Supplied: Available in ½ oz. tubes.

References:
1. Goodman and Gilman, The Pharmacological Basis of Therapeutics, Page 1487, 5th Ed., MacMillan, 1975.
2. Su-Chen L. Hong, Lawrence Levine, J. Bio. Chem., Vol. 251, No. 18, pp. 5814-5816, 1976.
3. Ryszard J. Gryglewski, et al., Prostoglandins, Vol. 10, No. 2, pp. 343–35, August 1975.
Shown in Product Identification Section, page 406

LANABIOTIC® Neomycin,
Polymyxin B, Bacitracin
First Aid Ointment

Active Ingredients: Each gram contains Bacitracin 500 units, Neomycin Sulfate 5 mg., Polymyxin B Sulfate 5000 units.

Indications: LANABIOTIC® Ointment helps prevent infection and aids natural healing with the maximum strength triple antibiotic ingredients available without a prescription. Applied to minor cuts, scrapes, scratches, burns and other minor wounds, it aids healing, helps prevent infection. It is soothing to the minor wound site and will not sting.

Actions: The three ingredients provide broad spectrum topical antibiotic action against both gram positive and gram negative organisms. The gentle occlusive base helps soften dry lesions and provides temporary protection for the wound site. The low melting point of the base provides even, quick spreading without caking.

Warning: In case of deep or puncture wounds or serious burns, consult a physician. If redness, irritation, swelling or pain persists, or increases, or if infection occurs, discontinue use and consult a physician. Do not use in the eyes. Keep out of reach of children.

Directions: After gentle washing, apply a small amount (an amount equal to the surface area of the tip of a finger) directly to the affected areas and cover with sterile gauze if desired. May be applied 2 to 5 times daily as the condition indicates.

How Supplied: Available in ½ ounce and 1 ounce tubes.
Shown in Product Identification Section, page 406

LANACANE® Medicated Creme

Active Ingredients: Benzocaine; Resorcinol.

Indications: LANACANE® Creme Medication is specially formulated to give prompt, temporary relief from dry skin itching, external feminine and rectal itching, rashes, insect bites, sunburn, chafing, poison ivy, poison oak, chapping, sore detergent hands, minor burns and other irritated skin conditions. LANACANE checks bacteria to help speed natural healing.

Actions: Benzocaine is a local anesthetic of low toxicity considered to be one of the safest and most widely used of the over-the-counter topical anesthetics. Temporary anesthesia is elicited by penetrating the cutaneous barriers and blocking sensory receptors for the perception of pain and itching. Resorcinol activity is antipruritic, antimicrobial and mildly keratolytic.

Warnings: Not for prolonged use. Do not get into the eyes. If condition worsens, or if symptoms persist for more than 7 days or clear up and occur again within a few days, discontinue use of this product and consult a physician. Keep out of reach of children. In case of accidental ingestion, seek professional assistance or contact a Poison Control Center immediately.

Drug Interaction Precaution: Benzocaine has been known to occasionally cause allergic dermatitis. Cross-reactions have been reported with para-phenylenediamine, a hair dye, sulfonamide and sun screens containing para-aminobenzoic acid esters.

Dosage and Administration: Apply LANACANE Creme Medication liberally to the affected area. Repeat as needed three or four times daily.

How Supplied: Available in 1.0 and 2.0 oz. tubes.
Shown in Product Identification Section, page 406

LANACORT® Anti-Itch
Hydrocortisone Acetate 0.5% Creme
and Ointment with Aloe moisturizer

Active Ingredient: 0.5% Hydrocortisone Acetate.

Indication: Lanacort® blends hydrocortisone acetate with a soothing aloe-containing moisturizing creme (or ointment) to provide temporary relief of itching associated with minor skin irritations, inflammation and rashes due to eczema (symptoms are redness, itching, and flaking), soaps, detergents, insect bites, cosmetics, jewelry, poison ivy, poison oak, poison sumac and for external feminine and rectal itching.

Action: Hydrocortisone Acetate is an anti-inflammatory corticosteroid[1,2] whose mechanism of action has been widely investigated. Current thinking points to the following modes of action: (1) controlling the rate of protein synthesis; (2) reducing the amounts of prostaglandin substrate available for the enzyme.[3] Corticosteroids are also known to reduce immune hypersensitivity by reducing the inflammatory response.[1]

Warning: For external use only. Avoid contact with the eyes. If condition worsens or if symptoms persist for more than 7 days, or clear up and occur again within a few days, discontinue use of this product and consult a physician. Do not use for external feminine itching if an unusual or abnormal vaginal discharge is present. Consult a physician. Keep out of reach of children. In case of accidental ingestion, seek professional assistance or contact a Poison Control Center immediately.

Dosage and Administration: Adults and children 2 years of age and older: Apply to affected area not more than 3 to 4 times daily. Children under 2 years of age: Consult a physician.

How Supplied: Available in 0.5 and 1.0 oz. tubes. Ointment in 0.5 oz. tube.

References:
1. Goodman and Gilman, The Pharmacological Basis of Therapeutics, Page 1487, 5th Ed., MacMillan, 1975.
2. Su-Chen L. Hong, Lawrence Levine, J. Bio. Chem., Vol. 251, No. 18, pp. 5814–5816, 1976.
3. Ryszard J. Gryglewski, et al., Prostoglandins, Vol. 10, No. 2, pp. 343–35 August 1975.
Shown in Product Identification Section, page 406

VAGISIL® External Feminine Itching Medication

Active Ingredients: 5.0% Benzocaine; 2.0% Resorcinol.

Indications: VAGISIL Medication has been formulated to give prompt, effective relief from the discomfort of minor itching, burning, and other irritations in the external genital (vulval) area. VAGISIL forms a cooling, protective film over irritated tissues. Helps check bacteria to speed natural healing. Lightly scented, stainless, greaseless.

Actions: Benzocaine is a local anesthetic of low toxicity considered to be one of the safest and most widely used of the over-the-counter topical anesthetics. Temporary anesthesia is elicited by penetrating the cutaneous barriers and blocking sensory receptors for the perception of pain and itching. Resorcinol activity is antimicrobial, mildly keratolytic and antipyretic.

Warnings: For external use only. Avoid contact with the eyes. If condition worsens or if symptoms persist for more than 7 days, or clear up and recur within a few days, discontinue use and consult a physician. Keep this and all drugs out of reach of children. In case of accidental ingestion, seek professional assistance or contact a Poison Control Center immediately.

Drug Interaction Precaution: Benzocaine has been known to occasionally cause allergic dermatitis. Cross-reactions have been reported with para-phenylenediamine, a hair dye, sulfonamide and sun screens containing para-aminobenzoic acid esters.

Dosage and Administration: Apply VAGISIL Creme Medication liberally to the affected area. Repeat as needed three or four times daily.

How Supplied: Available in 1.0 and 2.0 oz. tubes.

Shown in Product Identification Section, page 407

Commerce Drug Company
Div. Del Laboratories, Inc.
565 BROAD HOLLOW ROAD FARMINGDALE, NY 11735

AURO® Ear Drops

Description: Safely dissolves hardened ear wax which may affect hearing. Gently relieves pressure pain caused by ear wax.

Active Ingredient: Carbamide peroxide 6.5% in a specially prepared base.

Indications: Auro Ear Drops dissolves ear wax which may impair hearing and cause pain. Regular use of Auro helps prevent wax accumulation.

Actions: The anti-bacterial properties of carbamide peroxide (urea hydrogen peroxide) are due to its release of nascent oxygen. The effervescence caused by the oxygen release mechanically removes debris from inaccessible regions. In otic preparations, the effervescence disorganizes wax accumulations. Carbamide (urea) helps debride the tissue. These actions soften the residue in the ear, and removal of the liquified cerumen may be assisted by warm water irrigation.

Warning: Keep this and all drugs out of the reach of children. For external use only. Do not use if tube tip is cut prior to opening.

Precaution: If redness, irritation, swelling or pain persists or increases, consult your physician. Protect package from direct sunlight and heat.

Directions: Cut open tip of tube on score mark. Use directly from tube. Tilt head sideways and squeeze tube gently. Allow 5–10 drops to flow into ear. Tip of tube should not enter ear canal. Keep drops in ear for several minutes while head remains tilted or by inserting cotton. Repeat twice daily for 3 or 4 days. Any remaining wax should be flushed out with warm water in a soft bulb ear syringe. Avoid excessive pressure.

How Supplied: ½ fl. oz. tube, with convenient dropper tube.

Baby ORAJEL®

Description: Baby Orajel is a soothing, pleasantly flavored product which quickly relieves teething pain.

Active Ingredient: Benzocaine 7.5% in a special base.

Indications: Baby Orajel is a soothing, pleasantly flavored product which helps to alleviate the pain of teething babies by its topical anesthetic effect on the gums.

Actions: Benzocaine is a topical, local anesthetic commonly used for pain, discomfort, or pruritis associated with wounds, mucous membranes and skin irritations. Local anesthetics inhibit conduction of nerve impulses from sensory nerves. This action results from an alteration of the cell membrane permeability to ions. These agents are poorly absorbed through the intact epidermis.

Warning: Keep this and all medications out of the reach of children. Do not use if tube tip is cut prior to opening.

Precaution: For persistent or excessive teething pain, consult your physician.

Directions: Wash hands. Cut open tip of tube on score mark. Apply a small amount with fingertip or cotton applicator to affected area.

How Supplied: Gel in ½ oz. (14.1 gram) tube.

Shown in Product Identification Section, page 408

Maximum Strength ORAJEL®

Description: Maximum Strength Orajel's longer lasting formula immediately relieves toothache pain.

Active Ingredient: Benzocaine 20% in a special base.

Indications: Maximum Strength Orajel is formulated to provide faster relief from toothache pain for hours.

Actions: Benzocaine is a topical, local anesthetic commonly used for pain, discomfort, or pruritis associated with wounds, mucous membranes and skin irritation. Local anesthetics inhibit conduction of nerve impulses from sensory nerves. This action results from an alteration of the cell membrane permeability to ions. These agents are poorly absorbed through the intact epidermis.

Warning: Keep this and all drugs out of the reach of children. Do not use if tube tip is cut prior to opening.

Precaution: This preparation is intended for use in cases of toothache only as a temporary expedient until a dentist can be consulted. Do not use continuously.

Directions: Cut open tip of tube on score mark. Squeeze a small quantity of Maximum Strength Orajel directly into cavity and around gum surrounding the teeth.

How Supplied: Gel in two sizes—3/16 oz. (5.3 gram) and ½ oz. (14.1 gram) tubes.

ORAJEL® Mouth-Aid

Description: Orajel Mouth-Aid helps provide immediate relief from cold sores, sun and fever blisters, gum sores, canker sores, severely chapped lips, and other minor mouth and lip irritations.

Active Ingredients: Benzocaine 20%, Benzalkonium Chloride 0.12%, Zinc Chloride 0.1% in a special emollient base.

Indications: Orajel Mouth-Aid combines a fast-acting maximum strength pain reliever, soothing ingredients which aid healing, a germicide and an astringent to help provide relief of minor mouth and lip irritations.

Actions: Benzocaine is a topical, local anesthetic commonly used for pain, discomfort, or pruritis associated with wounds, mucous membranes and skin irritations. Local anesthetics inhibit conduction of nerve impulses from sensory nerves. This action results from an alteration of the cell membrane permeability to ions. These agents are poorly absorbed through the intact epidermis. Benzalkonium chloride is a rapidly acting surface disinfectant and detergent. Zinc chloride provides an astringent effect.

Warning: Keep this and all medications out of reach of children. Do not use if tube tip is cut prior to opening.

Precaution: If condition persists, discontinue use and consult your physician or dentist. Not for prolonged use.

Continued on next page

Commerce Drug—Cont.

Directions: Cut open tip of tube on score mark. Apply directly to affected area as needed.

How Supplied: Gel in a ⅓ oz. (9.45 gm) tube.

Shown in Product Identification Section, page 408

STYE™ Ophthalmic Ointment

Description: Stye Ophthalmic Ointment relieves the soreness and discomfort of styes and minor infections of eyelids.

Active Ingredient: Sterile Yellow Mercuric Oxide 1.0% in a special ophthalmic base.

Indications: Stye Ophthalmic Ointment is indicated for the relief of discomfort of styes and for the treatment of irritation and minor infection of eyelids.

Actions: Yellow Mercuric Oxide has antibacterial properties. These properties are useful in the treatment of blepharitis, sty and conjunctivitis.

Warnings: Keep this and all drugs out of the reach of children. In case of accidental ingestion, seek professional assistance or contact a poison control center immediately.

Precaution: Do not use if rim of cap has been exposed prior to opening. In unopened tube, rim of cap is not exposed. Discontinue use if rash or irritation develops or if condition for which used persists. Use as indicated, but not for prolonged use.

Directions: Apply night and morning directly from the tube to the affected lid. If irritation persists, consult your physician.

How Supplied: In 0.125 oz. (3.54 gram) tube.

Shown in Product Identification Section, page 408

Consolidated Chemical, Inc.
3224 S. KINGSHIGHWAY BLVD.
ST. LOUIS, MO 63139

FORMULA MAGIC®
Antibacterial Nursing Lubricant

Composition: ACTIVE INGREDIENT: Benzethonium Chloride
INACTIVE INGREDIENTS: Talc, Mineral Oil, Magnesium Carbonate, Fragrance, DMDM Hydantoin NDC 46706-202

Action: Talc based body powder and nursing lubricant. Aids in preventing excoriation and friction chafing. Aids in controlling odor.

Precautions: Non-irritating to skin. Practically non-toxic. Slightly irritating to eyes. In case of eye contact flush with water.

Dosage and Administration: Apply liberally to body and rub gently into skin.

How Supplied: 4 oz., 12 oz.

PERINEAL/OSTOMY SPRAY CLEANER™

Composition: Water, Cocamidopropylamine Oxide, Witch Hazel, Coco Betaine, DMDM Hydantoin, Fragrance, D&C Red #33, FD&C Blue #1.

Action: A gentle, effective spray cleanser for cleaning, refreshing, and deodorizing the perineal area, stoma sites, and ostomy appliances.

Precautions: Non-irritating to skin. Practically non-toxic. May cause slight eye discomfort. In case of eye contact flush with water.

Dosage and Administration: Spray directly on the entire perineal area, or the peristomal skin and in the ostomy appliance for quick odor control and cleaning. See label for full instructions.

How Supplied: 8 oz., 1 gallon.

SATIN®
Antibacterial Skin Cleanser

Composition: ACTIVE INGREDIENT: Chloroxylenol
INACTIVE INGREDIENTS: Water, Sodium Laureth Sulfate, Cocamidoproply Betaine, PEG-8, Cocamide DEA, Glycol Stearate, Lanolin Oil, Fragrance, Citric Acid, Tetrasodium EDTA, D&C Yellow #10. NDC 46706-101

Action: Skin cleanser and shampoo for daily hygiene and odor control.

Precautions: Non-irritating to skin. Practically non-toxic. Moderate eye irritant. In case of eye contact flush with water.

Dosage and Administration: Apply directly to wet skin or hair or to a predampened washcloth. Wash in normal manner. Rinse thoroughly.

How Supplied: 4 oz., 8 oz., 16 oz., 1 gallon.

SKIN MAGIC™
Antibacterial Body Rub and Skin Lotion

Composition: ACTIVE INGREDIENT: Chloroxylenol
INACTIVE INGREDIENTS: Water, Stearic Acid, Mineral Oil, Propylene Glycol, Isostearyl Alcohol, Glycol Stearate, Stearamide DEA, Triethanolamine, Cetyl Alcohol, Myristyl Propionate, Lanolin Oil, Fragrance, Propylparaben, DMDM Hydantoin, Methylparaben, Carbomer 934. NDC 46706-201

Action: Emollient body rub and skin lotion. Soothes and moisturizes dry irritated skin.

Precautions: Non-irritating to skin. Practically non-toxic. Slight eye irritant. In case of eye contact flush with water.

Dosage and Administration: Apply liberally topically and massage into skin

How Supplied: 4 oz., 8 oz., 1 gallon.

Creighton Products Corporation
a Sandoz Company
(see also Ex-Lax Pharmaceutical Co., Inc.)
605 THIRD AVENUE
NEW YORK, NY 10158

BiCOZENE® Creme External Analgesic

Active Ingredients: Benzocaine 6% resorcinol 1.67% in a specially prepared cream base.

Indications: For the temporary relief of minor skin irritation and minor burns, sunburn, minor cuts, abrasions, and insect bites. For all kinds of external itching skin conditions; vaginal, rectal, poison ivy, heat rash, chafing, eczema, and common itching of the skin.

Actions: Benzocaine is a topical anesthetic and resorcinol is a topical antipruritic, at the concentrations used in BiCozene Creme. Both exert their actions by depressing cutaneous sensory receptors.

Warnings: Caution: Use only as directed. Keep away from the eyes. Not for prolonged use. If the condition for which this preparation is used persists, or if a rash or irritation develops, discontinue use and consult a physician. For external use only. KEEP ALL MEDICINES OUT OF THE REACH OF CHILDREN.

Drug Interaction Precautions: No known drug interaction.

Dosage and Administration: Apply liberally to affected area as needed, several times a day.

How Supplied: BiCozene Creme is available in 1-ounce tubes.

Shown in Product Identification Section, page 409

DENCLENZ® DENTURE CLEANSER

Indications: For daily cleaning of removable dentures.

Actions: Denclenz liquid works in combination with the mechanical action of the brush-applicator bottle. The combined action breaks up mineral deposits, plaque, and stain which adhere to dentures, and are responsible for denture odor and discoloration.

Caution: Not for use in mouth. Use with care. Keep away from eyes and out of children's reach. Contains dilute solution of hydrochloric acid. If spilled on eyes, skin, clothing, chrome or Formica® surfaces, rinse immediately with cold water.

Directions for use: Hold bottle upside down over sink. Squeeze bottle gently and brush Denclenz on dentures inside and out. Rinse thoroughly in running water (at least 30 seconds) to remove all of the Denclenz liquid. (Rinse brush too).

How Supplied: In bottles of 2 and 3.5 fluid ounce.

Shown in Product Identification Section, page 409

DIETENE®
Diet Shake Mix

Description: Dietene Diet Shake Mix is a good tasting high-nutrient, low-calorie supplement for use in the Dietene Diet Plan. The Dietene Plan provides reliable weight loss without chemical appetite suppressants or stimulants. Compliance is high because the Dietene plan provides 3 nutritionally balanced meals and two satisfying between meal diet shakes (Chocolate, Vanilla, or Strawberry).

Action: The 1000 calorie Dietene Plan allows 3 meals a day (from a list of provided menus) plus 2 Dietene Shakes for between-meal satisfaction. The Dietene Shakes are nutritionally balanced to prevent the tired, rundown feeling commonly reported by dieters. Each Dietene Shake (prepared with skim milk) provides more than $1/3$ of the U.S. recommended daily allowances (U.S. RDA) of essential vitamins, 9 minerals, and protein. The 1000-calorie Dietene Plan supplies approximately 18 grams of fiber.

Ingredients: Nonfat Milk, Fructose, Calcium Caseinate, Carrageenan, Magnesium Oxide, Artificial Flavor, Lecithin, Ascorbic Acid, Polysorbate 80, Ferrous Fumarate, Zinc Sulfate, Vitamin E Acetate, Niacinamide, Vitamin A Palmitate, Copper Gluconate, Calcium Pantothenate, Vitamin D, Pyridoxine Hydrochloride, Thiamine Hydrochloride, Biotin, Folic Acid.

Nutritional Information.
Serving Size: 1 oz.
Servings per 1 lb. can: 16

	1 OZ DIETENE POWDER	1 OZ DIETENE POWDER IN 1 CUP SKIM MILK**
CALORIES	100	190
PROTEIN	6G	15G
CARBOHYDRATE	17G	29G
FAT	0G	1G
SODIUM	110MG	240MG
POTASSIUM	290MG	650MG

PERCENTAGE OF U.S. RECOMMENDED DAILY ALLOWANCES (U.S. RDA)

PROTEIN	15	35
VITAMIN A	25	35
VITAMIN C	30	35
THIAMINE	30	35
RIBOFLAVIN	20	45
NIACIN	35	35
CALCIUM	20	50
IRON	35	35
VITAMIN D	25	50
VITAMIN E	35	35
VITAMIN B	30	35
FOLIC ACID	25	35
VITAMIN B	10	35
PHOSPHORUS	20	40
IODINE	20	50
MAGNESIUM	25	35
ZINC	30	35
COPPER	35	35
BIOTIN	50	50
PANTOTHENIC ACID	25	35

** VITAMIN A AND D FORTIFIED SKIM MILK

Directions: Mix 3 slightly rounded tablespoons (1 oz.) of Dietene Powder with 1 cup (8 fl. oz.) of cold skim milk (vitamin A and D fortified) by stirring vigorously in a tall glass or blender.

Fast Weight Loss: 1,000 Calorie Per Day Diet. Eat 3 complete Dietene Plan meals a day, plus 2 delicious Dietene shakes to prevent between-meal hunger. The Dietene Plan, in the booklet enclosed under plastic can top, includes instructions for Balanced Nutrition, Behavior Modification and Individualized Exercise, for successful permanent weight control. This is the weight loss program which has been proven in use and recommended by doctors for many years. Other programs are listed below.

Faster Weight Loss: 900 Calories Per Day Diet. Enjoy 2 delicious Dietene shakes a day in place of breakfast and lunch, and have two servings from Fruit list in the Dietene Plan. For dinner, have a complete Dietene Plan dinner from the enclosed Dietene Plan booklet with a 3rd Dietene shake, or have the 3rd Dietene shake later in the evening to help control the urge to snack. Use freely any of the items on the "Foods Allowed As Desired" list, and drink at least 4 to 5 (8 oz.) glasses of water or non-calorie beverage a day.

14 Day Fast Start Plan: 800 Calories Per Day Diet. Enjoy 4 Dietene shakes a day, with one serving from Fruit list in the Dietene Plan, as a total meal program, for no more than 2 weeks a month. Use freely any of the items on the "Foods Allowed As Desired" list, and drink at least 4 to 5 (8 oz.) glasses of water or non-calorie beverage a day.

For Weight Maintenance. Enjoy a Dietene shake in place of either breakfast or lunch. For other meals, select foods from the Dietene Plan lists, increasing quantities while watching your weight closely, until you find the intake level at which your weight is stable.

Caution. Anyone with high blood pressure, diabetes, pernicious anemia, heart, liver, kidney, thyroid, or other disease; during pregnancy, while nursing; anyone under the age of 18; anyone taking any prescription medications; consult a physician before starting any weight loss program.

Professional Labeling: A 1,000 calorie per day sodium restricted diet is available from Creighton Products. This diet is planned to restrict sodium intake to approximately 0.7 gram per day. You can lower the sodium content of this diet to 0.33 gram per day by specifying the use of low sodium bread, butter and milk.

How Supplied: 16 oz. (1 lb) cans in chocolate, vanilla and strawberry flavors.

Shown in Product Indentification Section, page 409

GAS–X® AND EXTRA STRENTH GAS-X®
High–Capacity Antiflatulent

Active Ingredients: GAS-X®—Each tablet contains 80 mg. simethicone. EXTRA STRENGHT GAS-X®—Each tablet contains 125 mg. simethicone.

Indications: For relief of the pain and pressure symptoms of excess gas in the digestive tract, which is often accompanied by complaints of bloating, distention, fullness, pressure, pain, cramps or excess anal flatus.

Actions: GAS-X acts in the stomach and intestines to disperse and reduce the formation of mucus-trapped gas bubbles. The GAS-X defoaming action reduces the surface tension of gas bubbles so that they are more easily eliminated.

Warning: Keep this and all medicines out of the reach of children.

Drug Interaction Precautions: No known drug interaction.

Dosage and Administration: Adults: Chew thoroughly and swallow one or two tablets as needed after meals and at bedtime. Do not exceed six GAS-X tablets or four EXTRA STRENGTH GAS-X tablets in 24 hours, except under the advice and supervision of a physician.

Professional Labeling: GAS-X may be useful in the alleviation of postoperative gas pain, and for use in endoscopic examination.

How Supplied: GAS-X is available in white, chewable, scored tablets in boxes of 30 tablets and convenience packages of 12 tablets.
EXTRA STRENGTH GAS-X is available in yellow, chewable, scored tablets in boxes of 18 tablets.

Shown in Product Identification Section, page 409

Daywell Laboratories Corporation
78 UNQUOWA PLACE
FAIRFIELD, CT 06430

VERGO® Cream

Composition: Vergo contains Pancin®, a special formulation of calcium pantothenate, ascorbic acid and starch.

Action and Uses: Vergo is a conservative, painless and safe treatment of warts. Vergo is very gentle, even for diabetics. It is not liquid. It is not caustic. It can be used on all parts of the body, even on the face. Vergo will not burn, blister, scar or injure surrounding tissue. Vergo is easily applied by finger. The ingredi-

Continued on next page

Daywell—Cont.

ents are essential to the soundness of tissues and skin and will relieve the pain of warts and promote healing. Vergo is not irritating and there are no contraindications to its use. The average treatment time is from 2 to 8 weeks depending on the size of the wart and the response of the patient. It is important that the directions be carefully followed and that treatment be continued without interruption as long as necessary. Mosaic-type warts are more resistant and usually require longer treatment for relief.

Administration and Dosage: Cleanse area with soap and water; rinse thoroughly. Apply Vergo liberally to wart. Do not massage or rub in. Cover with plain Band-Aid® or gauze and adhesive tape. Change dressing and apply Vergo twice a day, morning and evening.

Side Effects: None known.

How Supplied: In one-half ounce tubes.

Product   Identification   Mark: Vergo®.

Literature Available: Yes.

Dermik Laboratories, Inc.
500 VIRGINIA DRIVE
FT. WASHINGTON, PA 19034

FOMAC® FOAM
(medicated foam cleanser)

Description: Salicylic acid 2% in a soap-free, mild detergent system. Patent No. 4147782.

Indications: Acne and oily skin.

Directions: DO NOT SHAKE. Invert container and squeeze a puff of Fomac Foam into palm of hand and massage, gently but thoroughly, into affected area until foam disappears. For best results, do not wet skin. Leave on skin 3–5 minutes, then rinse well with lukewarm water and pat dry. Use once or twice daily, or as recommended by physician. Discontinue use of all soaps or other skin cleansers.

Precautions: If redness or irritation occurs or increases, reduce frequency of applications. If irritation persists, discontinue use and consult your physician. Keep away from eyes. For external use only. Keep out of reach of children. Keep tightly closed. Store at room temperature.

How Supplied: 3 fl oz non-aerosol bottle.

HYTONE® CREAM ½%
(hydrocortisone ½%)

Active   Ingredient: Hydrocortisone 0.5%.

Indications: For the temporary relief of minor skin irritations, itching, and

rashes due to eczema, dermatitis, insect bites, poison ivy, poison oak, poison sumac, soaps, detergents, cosmetics, jewelry, and for itchy genital and anal areas.

Actions: Provides temporary relief of itching and minor skin irritations.

Warnings: For External Use Only. Avoid contact with eyes. If condition worsens, or if symptoms persist for more than 7 days, discontinue use of this product and consult a physician. Do not use on children under 2 years of age except under the advice and supervision of a physician. KEEP OUT OF THE REACH OF CHILDREN.

Dosage   and   Administration: For adults and children 2 years of age and older: Apply to affected area not more than 3 or 4 times daily, or as directed by physician.

How Supplied: Tube, 1 ounce.

SHEPARD'S CREAM LOTION
Skin Lubricant—Moisturizer

Composition: Water, sesame oil, SD alcohol, 40-B, stearic acid, propylene glycol, ethoxydiglycol, glycerin, triethanolamine, glyceryl stearate, cetyl alcohol, may contain fragrance ("scented" only), simethicone, methylparaben, propylparaben, vegetable oil, monoglyceride citrate, BHT and citric acid.

Indications: For generalized dryness and itching, sunburn, "winter-itch", dry skin, heat rash.

Actions and Uses: Shepard's Cream Lotion is a rich lotion containing soothing Oil of Sesame.

Dosage and Administration: Apply as often as needed. Use particularly after bathing and exposure to sun, water, soaps and detergents.

How   Supplied: Scented   and   Unscented 8 oz bottle and 16 oz pump bottle.

SHEPARD'S SKIN CREAM
Concentrated
Moisturizer—Non-greasy Emollient

Composition: Water, glyceryl stearate, ethoxydiglycol, propylene glycol, glycerin, stearic acid, isopropyl myristate, cetyl alcohol, urea, lecithin, may contain fragrance ("scented" only) methylparaben and propylparaben.

Indications: For problem dry skin of the hands, face, elbows, feet, legs. Helps resist effects of soaps, detergents and chemicals.

Actions: Soothing, rich lubricant containing isopropyl myristate in a non-greasy or sticky base containing no lanolin or mineral oil. Shepard's Skin Cream helps retain moisture that makes skin feel soft, smooth, supple.

Dosage and Administration: A small amount is rubbed into dry skin areas as needed.

How   Supplied: Scented   and   Unscented, 4 oz jars.

SHEPARD'S MOISTURIZING SOAP
Cleanser for Dry Skin

Composition: Soap (Sodium Tallowate & Cocoate Types), Water, Glycerin, Fragrance, Coconut Acid, Sodium Chloride, Lanolin, Titanium Dioxide, BHT, Trisodium HEDTA

Indications: As a daily cleanser of dry skin of the face, hands, or in the bath or shower. Shepard's Soap helps to give the skin an overall smoothness.

Actions: A lightly scented, non-detergent moisturizing soap containing lanolin that cleanses the skin while helping to minimize the excessive drying inherent in most detergent-type soaps.

Dosage   and   Administration: Use regularly to cleanse face and hands as well as in the bath or shower.

How Supplied: 4 oz bars.

VANOXIDE® ACNE LOTION
(Dries Clear)
LOROXIDE® ACNE LOTION
(Flesh Tinted)

Description: Vanoxide® Lotion contains (as dispensed) benzoyl peroxide 5%, incorporated lotion that dries on clear. Loroxide® Lotion contains (as dispensed) benzoyl peroxide 5.5%, incorporated in a flesh-tinted lotion.

Actions: Provides keratolytic, peeling and drying action.

Indications: An aid in the treatment of acne and oily skin.

Contraindications: These products are contraindicated for use by patients having known hypersensitivity to benzoyl peroxide or any other component of these preparations.

Precautions: For external use only. Keep away from eyes. Do not add any other medicaments or substances to these lotions unless specifically directed by physician to do so. Patients should be observed carefully for possible local irritation or sensitivity during long-term topical therapy. If any irritation or sensitivity is observed, discontinue use and consult physician. Apply with caution on neck and/or other sensitive areas. There may be a slight, transitory stinging or burning sensation on initial application which invariably disappears on continued use. Ultraviolet and cold quartz light should be employed in lesser amounts as these lotions are keratolytic and drying. Harsh, abrasive cleansers should not be used simultaneously with these lotions. Colored or dyed garments may be bleached by the oxidizing action of benzoyl peroxide. Occurrence of excessive redness or peeling indicates that the amount and frequency of application should be reduced. Keep out of the reach of children.

Adverse Reactions: The sensitizing potential of benzoyl peroxide is low; but it can, on occasion, produce allergic reaction.

Directions: Shake well before using. Apply a thin film to affected areas with light massaging to blend in each application 1 or 2 times daily or in accordance with the physician's directions.

How Supplied: Vanoxide® Lotion—Bottles 25 grams (0.88 oz) and 50 grams (1.76 oz) net weights as dispensed. Loroxide® Lotion—Bottles, 25 grams (0.88 oz) net weight as dispensed. A "Dermik Color Blender™" is provided with Loroxide® Lotion which enables the patient to alter the basic shade of the lotion to match the skin color.

VLEMASQUE®
Acne Mask Treatment

Active Ingredient: Contains sulfurated lime topical solution 6%, S.D. alcohol 7% in a drying clay mask.

Indications: For the treatment of acne.

Warnings: Keep away from eyes. In case of contact, flush eyes thoroughly. For external use only. If any irritation appears, stop treatment immediately and consult physician.

Dosage and Administration: Daily, apply generous layer over entire face and neck, or as directed by physician. Avoid eyes, nostrils and lips. Leave on for 20–25 minutes. Remove with lukewarm water, using a gentle circular motion. Pat dry. U.S. Pat. No. 4,388,301

How Supplied: 4 oz Jars

ZETAR® SHAMPOO
(Antidandruff Shampoo)

Active Ingredients: WHOLE Coal Tar (as Zetar®) 1.0%, and parachlorometaxylenol 0.5% in a golden foam shampoo which produces soft, fluffy abundant lather.

Actions and Indications: Antiseptic, antibacterial, antiseborrheic. Loosens and softens scales and crusts. Indicated in psoriasis, seborrhea, dandruff, cradlecap and other oily, itchy conditions of the body and scalp.

Contraindications: Acute inflammation, open or infected lesions.

Precautions: If undue skin irritation develops or increases, discontinue use and consult physician. In rare instances, temporary discoloration of blond, bleached or tinted hair may occur. Avoid contact with eyes.

Dosage and Administration: Massage into moistened scalp. Rinse. Repeat; leave on 5 minutes. Rinse thoroughly.

How Supplied: 6 oz plastic bottles.

Products are cross-indexed by generic and chemical names in the **YELLOW SECTION**

DeWitt International Corporation
**5 N. WATSON ROAD
TAYLORS, SC 29687**

DEWITT'S PILLS FOR BACKACHE AND JOINT PAINS

Active Ingredients: Salicylamide, Potassium Nitrate, Uva Ursi, Buchu and Caffeine.

Indications: For backache and joint pains, muscular aches, headaches and mild urinary irritations caused by non-organic disturbances of a minor nature.

Actions: Analgesic ingredients help in relief of minor pains. Mild diuretic action helps eliminate retained fluids, flushes out bladder wastes and irritations that often cause physical distress including too frequent or difficult passage of urine.

Warnings: As with any drug, if you are pregnant or nursing a baby, seek the advice of a health professional before using this product. Keep this and all medicines out of the reach of children. In case of accidental overdose, seek professional assistance or contact a Poison Control Center immediately. Do not take for more than 10 consecutive days without consulting a physician.

Drug Interaction: No known drug interactions.

Precaution: A few pills will turn the urine blue or green because of the presence of Methylene Blue as a coloring agent.

Dosage and Administration: For adult use only. Take 3 pills before meals and 3 pills at bedtime, up to a maximum of 12 pills per day. Swallow with a glass of water. Drink plenty of water between meals.

Professional Labeling: Same as those outlined under indications.

How Supplied: Individual blistering of pills packaged in cartons of 20, 40 and 80 pills.

Dorsey Laboratories
**Division of Sandoz, Inc.
P.O. BOX 83288
LINCOLN, NE 68501**

ACID MANTLE® CREME and ACID MANTLE® LOTION

Description: A greaseless, water-miscible preparation containing buffered aluminum acetate.

Indications: A vehicle for compatible topical drugs. Restores and maintains protective acidity of the skin. Provides relief of mildly irritated skin due to exposure to soaps, detergents, chemicals, alkalis. Aids in the treatment of diaper rash, bath dermatitis, athlete's foot, anogenital pruritis, acne, winter eczema and dry, rough, scaly skin of varied causes.

Caution: Limited compatibility and stability with Vitamin A, neomycin and other water-sensitive antibiotics. For external use only. Not for ophthalmic use.

Directions: Apply several times daily, especially after wet work.

How Supplied: Creme: 1 oz tubes; 4 oz and 1 lb jars. Lotion: 4 oz bottles.
Shown in Product Identification Section, page 408

CAMA® ARTHRITIS PAIN RELIEVER

Description: Each CAMA Inlay-Tab® contains: aspirin, USP, 500 mg (7.7 grains); magnesium oxide, USP, 150 mg; aluminum hydroxide dried gel, USP, 150 mg.

Indications: For the temporary relief of minor arthritic pain.

Warning: If pain persists for more than 10 days, consult a physician immediately. As with any drug, if you are pregnant or nursing a baby, seek the advice of a health professional before using this product. Stop taking this product if ringing in the ears or dizziness occurs. Do not take this product if you are presently taking a prescription drug for anticoagulation (thinning the blood), gout or if you have an aspirin allergy.

Warning: Keep this and all medicines out of the reach of children. In case of accidental overdose, contact a physician immediately.

Directions For Use: Adults—2 tablets with a full glass of water every 6 hours. Not to exceed 8 tablets in 24 hours unless directed by a physican. Do not use in children under 12 years of age except under the advice and supervision of a physician.

How Supplied: CAMA Arthritis Pain Reliever Tablets (white with salmon inlay), imprinted "Cama 500" on one side, "Dorsey" on the other, in bottles of 100 and 250.
Shown in Product Identification Section, page 408

DORCOL® CHILDREN'S COUGH SYRUP

Description: Each teaspoonful (5 ml) of DORCOL Children's Cough Syrup contains pseudoephedrine hydrochloride 15 mg, guaifenesin 50 mg dextromethorphan hydrobromide 5 mg and alcohol 5%.

Indications: Temporarily relieves your child's cough due to minor throat and bronchial irritation as may occur with the common cold. Helps loosen phlegm (sputum) and bronchial secretions to rid the bronchial passageways of bothersome mucus. Relieves irritated membranes in the respiratory passageways by preventing dryness through increased mucus flow. Temporarily relieves nasal stuffiness due to the common

Continued on next page

Dorsey—Cont.

cold, hay fever or other upper respiratory allergies. Promotes nasal and/or sinus drainage.

Warning: EXCEPT UNDER THE ADVICE AND SUPERVISION OF A PHYSICIAN: DO NOT give your child more than the recommended dosage because at higher doses nervousness, dizziness or sleeplessness may occur. DO NOT give this preparation if your child has high blood pressure, heart disease, diabetes or thyroid disease. DO NOT give this product for persistent or chronic cough such as occurs with asthma or where cough is accompanied by excessive secretions. Keep this and all drugs out of the reach of children. In case of accidental overdose, seek professional assistance or contact a Poison Control Center immediately. A persistent cough may be a sign of a serious condition. If cough or other symptoms persist for more than one week, tend to recur or are accompanied by high fever, rash or persistent headache, consult a physician before continuing use. *Drug Interaction Precaution:* Do not give this product if your child is presently taking a prescription antihypertensive or antidepressant drug containing a monoamine oxidase inhibitor except under the advice and supervision of a physician.

Directions For Use: Children under 2 years—consult physician.
By age:
Children 2 to under 6 years: 1 teaspoonful every 4 hours.
Children 6 to under 12 years: 2 teaspoonfuls every 4 hours.
By weight:
Children 25 to 45 pounds: 1 teaspoonful every 4 hours.
Children 46 to 85 pounds: 2 teaspoonfuls every 4 hours.
Unless directed by a physician, do not exceed 4 doses in 24 hours.

How Supplied: DORCOL Children's Cough Syrup (grape colored) in 4 fl oz and 8 fl oz plastic bottles with tamper-evident band around child-resistant cap.
Shown in Product Identification Section, page 408

DORCOL™ CHILDREN'S DECONGESTANT LIQUID

Description: Each teaspoonful (5 ml) of DORCOL Children's Decongestant Liquid contains pseudoephedrine hydrochloride 15 mg.

Indications: For temporary relief of nasal congestion due to the common cold, hay fever or other upper respiratory allergies, or associated with sinusitis. Reduces swelling of nasal passages; shrinks swollen membranes.

Directions For Use: Children under 2 years—consult physician.
By age:
Children 2 to under 6 years: 1 teaspoonful every 4 to 6 hours.
Children under 6 years: 2 teaspoonfuls every 4 to 6 hours.
By weight:
Children 25 to 45 pounds: 1 teaspoonful every 4 to 6 hours.
Children 46 to 85 pounds: 2 teaspoonfuls every 4 to 6 hours.
Unless directed by a physician, do not exceed 4 doses in 24 hours.

Warnings: Do not give your child more than the recommended dosage because at higher doses nervousness, dizziness, or sleeplessness may occur. If symptoms do not improve within seven days or are accompanied by high fever, consult a physician before continuing use. Do not give this preparation if your child has high blood pressure, heart disease, diabetes, or thyroid disease except under the advice and supervision of a physician. Keep this and all drugs out of the reach of children. In case of accidental overdose, seek professional assistance or contact a Poison Control Center immediately.
Drug Interaction Precaution: Do not give this product if your child is presently taking a prescription antihypertensive or antidepressant drug containing a monoamine oxidase inhibitor except under the advice and supervision of a physician.

How Supplied: DORCOL Children's Decongestant Liquid (pale orange) in 4 fl oz bottles with tamper-evident band around child-resistant cap.
Shown in Product Identification Section, page 408

DORCOL™ CHILDREN'S FEVER & PAIN REDUCER

Description: Each teaspoonful (5 ml) of DORCOL Children's Fever & Pain Reducer contains acetaminophen 160 mg and alcohol 10%.

Indications: For temporary effective relief of your child's fever and occasional minor aches, pains and headache.

Directions For Use: Children under 2 years—consult physician.
By age:
Children 2 to under 4 years: 1 teaspoonful
Children 4 to under 6 years: 1½ teaspoonfuls
Children 6 years of age: 2 teaspoonfuls
By weight:
Children 25 to 35 pounds: 1 teaspoonful
Children 36 to 45 pounds: 1½ teaspoonfuls
Children 46 to 60 pounds: 2 teaspoonfuls
Give every 4 hours while symptoms persist or as directed by a physician. Unless directed by a physician do not exceed 5 doses in 24 hours.

Warnings: Do not give this product to your child for more than 5 days. Consult your physician if symptoms persist, new ones occur, or if fever persists for more than 3 days (72 hours) or recurs. DO NOT exceed recommended dosage. Keep this and all drugs out of the reach of children. In case of accidental overdose, seek professional assistance or contact a Poison Control Center immediately.

How Supplied: DORCOL Children's Fever & Pain Reducer (red) in 4 fl oz bottles with tamper-evident band around child-resistant cap.
Shown in Product Identification Section, page 408

DORCOL™ CHILDREN'S LIQUID CALCIUM SUPPLEMENT

Description: Each teaspoonful (5 ml) of DORCOL Children's Liquid Calcium Supplement contains glubionate calcium 1.8 gm (calcium content 115 mg).

Directions For Use: Children under one year of age—consult physician. Children 1 to 6 years: 1 to 2 teaspoonfuls three times daily. Dose may be taken undiluted or mixed with water or fruit juice.
[See table below].
Keep out of reach of children.

How Supplied: DORCOL Children's Liquid Calcium Supplement (straw colored) in 4 fl oz bottles with tamper-evident band around child-resistant cap.
Shown in Product Identification Section, page 408

DORCOL™ CHILDREN'S LIQUID COLD FORMULA

Description: Each teaspoonful (5 ml) of DORCOL Children's Liquid Cold Formula contains: pseudoephedrine hydrochloride 15 mg and chlorpheniramine maleate 1 mg.

Indications: For temporary relief of nasal congestion due to the common cold, hay fever or other upper respiratory allergies. Dries running nose and alleviates sneezing as may occur in allergic rhinitis (such as hay fever).

Directions For Use: Children under 6 years—consult physician.
By age:
Children 6 to under 12 years: 2 teaspoonfuls every 4 to 6 hours.

Dosage	Amount of Calcium Supplied Daily	Percentage of U.S. Recommended Daily Allowance (U.S. RDA)	
		Children 1 to under 4 (800 mg)	Children 4 to 6 (1000 mg)
1 teaspoonful 3 times daily	345 mg	45%	35%
2 teaspoonfuls 3 times daily	690 mg	90%	70%
(Part of need is supplied by diet)			

By weight:

Children 45 to 85 pounds: 2 teaspoonfuls every 4 to 6 hours.

Unless directed by a physician, do not exceed 4 doses in 24 hours.

Warnings: Do not give your child more than the recommended dosage because at higher doses nervousness, dizziness, or sleeplessness may occur. Do not give this preparation if your child has high blood pressure, heart disease, diabetes, thyroid disease, asthma, glaucoma, or difficulty in urination due to enlargement of the prostate gland except under the advice and supervision of a physician. If symptoms do not improve within 7 days or are accompanied by high fever, consult a physician before continuing use. May cause drowsiness. May cause excitability especially in children. Keep this and all drugs out of the reach of children. In case of accidental overdose, seek professional assistance or contact a Poison Control Center immediately.

Drug Interaction Precaution: Do not give this product if your child is presently taking a prescription antihypertensive or antidepressant drug containing a monoamine oxidase inhibitor except under the advice and supervision of a physician.

Caution: Avoid alcoholic beverages or operating a motor vehicle or heavy machinery while taking this product.

How Supplied: DORCOL Children's Liquid Cold Formula (light brown) in 4 fl oz bottles with tamper-evident band around child-resistant cap.

Shown in Product Identification Section, page 408

TOTAL ECLIPSE® SUNSCREEN LOTION, SPF 15
(Moisturizing Base and Alcohol Base)

Active Ingredient:

Total ECLIPSE (SPF 15) Sunscreen Lotion (Moisturizing Base): Padimate O (octyl dimethyl PABA), octyl salicylate, and oxybenzone (benzophenone-3).

Total ECLIPSE (SPF 15) Sunscreen Lotion (Alcohol Base): Oxybenzone (benzophenone-3), padimate O (octyl dimethyl PABA), and glyceryl PABA with alcohol (81%).

Indications: Prevention of harmful effects of sun.

Actions: Liberal and regular use may help reduce the chance of premature aging of the skin and skin cancer due to long-term overexposure to the sun.

Total ECLIPSE Sunscreen Lotion (Moisturizing and Alcohol Base) screens the sun's harsh and often harmful rays to prevent sunburn and tanning for the most sun-sensitive skin, either dry or oily, respectively.

Warnings: For external use only. Do not use if sensitive to PABA or related compounds (such as benzocaine, sulfonamides, aniline dyes or PABA esters). Avoid contact with eyes or eyelids. If contact occurs, rinse thoroughly with water. Discontinue use if signs of irritation or rash appear. May stain some fabrics.

Keep this and all drugs out of the reach of children. In case of accidental ingestion, seek professional assistance or contact a Poison Control Center immediately. Total ECLIPSE Sunscreen Lotion (Alcohol Base)—Avoid flame.

Drug Interaction: No known drug interaction.

Symptoms and Treatment of Oral Overdosage: Total ECLIPSE Sunscreen Lotion (Moisturizing Base): Push fluids.

Total ECLIPSE Sunscreen Lotion (Alcohol Base): Induce emesis by aspiration or gastric lavage. Then push fluids.

Directions: Apply liberally and evenly before sun exposure. Effective immediately upon application. ECLIPSE Sunscreens resist washoff from swimming and perspiration. Reapplication is recommended after 40 minutes in the water or after excessive sweating.

How Supplied: Total ECLIPSE Sunscreen Lotion: Moisturizing Base in 4 oz and 6 oz plastic bottles; Alcohol Base in 4 oz plastic bottles.

Shown in Product Identification Section, page 408

TRIAMINIC® ALLERGY TABLETS

Description: Each TRIAMINIC Allergy Tablet contains: phenylpropanolamine hydrochloride 25 mg, chlorpheniramine maleate 4.0 mg.

Indications: For the temporary relief of runny nose, nasal congestion, sneezing, itching of the eyes, nose or throat and watery eyes as may occur in hay fever or other upper respiratory allergies (allergic rhinitis).

Warning: Do not exceed the recommended dosage because at higher doses nervousness, dizziness or sleeplessness may occur. This preparation may cause drowsiness; this preparation may cause excitability especially in children. Do not take this preparation if you have high blood pressure, heart disease, diabetes, thyroid disease or are presently taking a prescription antihypertensive or antidepressant drug containing a monoamine oxidase inhibitor except under the advice and supervision of a physician. Do not give this preparation to children under 6 years except under the advice and supervision of a physician. Do not take this preparation if you have asthma, glaucoma or difficulty in urination due to enlargement of the prostate gland except under the advice and supervision of a physician. If symptoms do not improve within 7 days or are accompanied by high fever, consult a physician before continuing use. As with any drug, if you are pregnant or nursing a baby, seek the advice of a health professional before using this product. Keep this and all drugs out of the reach of children. In case of accidental overdose, seek professional assistance or contact a Poison Control Center immediately.

Caution: Avoid alcoholic beverages, operating a motor vehicle or heavy machinery while taking this product.

Dosage: Adults—1 tablet every 4 hours. Children 6–12 years—½ tablet every 4 hours. Unless directed by physician, do not exceed 4 doses in 24 hours or give to children under 6 years.

How Supplied: TRIAMINIC Allergy Tablets (yellow) scored, in blister packs of 24.

TRIAMINIC® CHEWABLES

Description: Each TRIAMINIC Chewable contains: phenylpropanolamine hydrochloride 6.25 mg, chlorpheniramine maleate 0.5 mg.

Indications: For prompt, temporary relief of children's nasal congestion due to the common cold or nasal allergies.

Caution: Unless directed by physician, do not exceed recommended dosage or give to children under 6 years. Individuals with high blood pressure, heart disease or thyroid disease should use only as directed by a physician. If drowsiness occurs, do not drive or operate machinery.

Warning: As with any drug, if you are pregnant or nursing a baby, seek the advice of a health professional before using this product. Keep this and all drugs out of the reach of children. In case of accidental overdose, seek professional assistance or contact a Poison Control Center immediately.

Dosage: Children 6 to 12 years—2 chewable tablets 4 times a day. For children under 6, consult your physician.

How Supplied: TRIAMINIC Chewables (hexagonal, yellow) in blister packs of 24.

TRIAMINIC® COLD SYRUP

Description: Each teaspoonful (5 ml) of TRIAMINIC Cold Syrup contains: phenylpropanolamine hydrochloride 12.5 mg and chlorpheniramine maleate 2 mg in a nonalcoholic vehicle.

Indications: Decreases running nose, sneezing, itching of the nose or throat and itchy and watery eyes as may occur in hay fever. Temporarily relieves nasal stuffiness due to the common cold, hay fever or other upper respiratory allergies. Promotes nasal and/or sinus drainage.

Warning: EXCEPT UNDER THE ADVICE AND SUPERVISION OF A PHYSICIAN: DO NOT exceed the recommended dosage because at higher doses nervousness, dizziness or sleeplessness may occur. DO NOT take this preparation if you have high blood pressure, heart disease, diabetes, thyroid disease or are presently taking a prescription antihypertensive or antidepressant drug containing a monoamine oxidase inhibitor. DO NOT take this product if you have asthma, glaucoma or difficulty in urination due to enlargement of the pros-

Continued on next page

Dorsey—Cont.

tate gland. This preparation may cause drowsiness or excitability (especially in children). If symptoms do not improve within 7 days or are accompanied by high fever, consult a physician before continuing use. As with any drug, if you are pregnant or nursing a baby, seek the advice of a health professional before using this product.

Keep this and all drugs out of the reach of children. In case of accidental overdose, seek professional assistance or contact a Poison Control Center immediately.

Caution: Avoid alcoholic beverages, operating a motor vehicle or heavy machinery while taking this product.

Dosage and Administration: Adults— 2 teaspoonfuls every 4 hours. Children 6–12 years—1 teaspoonful every 4 hours. Unless directed by physician, do not exceed 6 doses in 24 hours. Consult physician for dosage under 6 years of age.

How Supplied: TRIAMINIC Cold Syrup (orange) in 4 fl oz and 8 fl oz plastic bottles with tamper-evident band around child-resistant cap.

Shown in Product Identification Section, page 408

TRIAMINIC® COLD TABLETS

Description: Each TRIAMINIC Cold Tablet contains: phenylpropanolamine hydrochloride 12.5 mg and chlorpheniramine maleate 2 mg.

Indications: For temporary relief of nasal congestion due to the common cold, hay fever or other upper respiratory allergies and associated with sinusitis. Helps decongest sinus openings, sinus passages; promotes nasal and/or sinus drainage; temporarily restores freer breathing through the nose. For temporary relief of runny nose, sneezing, itching of the nose or throat and itchy and watery eyes as may occur in allergic rhinitis (such as hay fever).

Warnings: EXCEPT UNDER THE ADVICE AND SUPERVISION OF A PHYSICIAN: DO NOT exceed the recommended dosage because at higher doses nervousness, dizziness or sleeplessness may occur. DO NOT take this preparation if you have high blood pressure, heart disease, diabetes, thyroid disease or are presently taking a prescription antihypertensive or antidepressant drug containing a monoamine oxidase inhibitor. DO NOT take this product if you have asthma, glaucoma or difficulty in urination due to enlargement of the prostate gland. This preparation may cause drowsiness or excitability (especially in children). If symptoms do not improve within 7 days or are accompanied by high fever, consult a physician before continuing use.

Unless directed by physician, do not give this product to children under 6 years of age. As with any drug, if you are pregnant or nursing a baby, seek the advice of

a health professional before using this product. Keep this and all drugs out of the reach of children. In case of accidental overdose, seek professional assistance or contact a Poison Control Center immediately.

Caution: Avoid alcoholic beverages, operating a motor vehicle or heavy machinery while taking this product.

Dosage and Administration: Adults— 2 tablets every 4 hours. Children 6–12 years—1 tablet every 4 hours. Unless directed by physician, do not exceed 6 doses in 24 hours.

How Supplied: TRIAMINIC Cold Tablets (orange) imprinted "DORSEY" on one side, "TRIAMINIC" on the other, in blister packs of 24 and 48.

Shown in Product Identification Section, page 408

TRIAMINIC-DM® COUGH FORMULA

Description: Each teaspoonful (5 ml) of TRIAMINIC-DM Cough Formula contains: phenylpropanolamine hydrochloride 12.5 mg and dextromethorphan hydrobromide 10 mg in a nonalcoholic vehicle.

Indications: Temporarily relieves cough due to minor throat and bronchial irritation as may occur with the common cold or inhaled irritants. Promotes nasal and/or sinus drainage.

Warning: EXCEPT UNDER THE ADVICE AND SUPERVISION OF A PHYSICIAN: DO NOT exceed the recommended dosage because at higher doses nervousness, dizziness or sleeplessness may occur. DO NOT take this preparation if you have high blood pressure, heart disease, diabetes, thyroid disease or are presently taking a prescription antihypertensive or antidepressant drug containing a monoamine oxidase inhibitor. DO NOT take this product for persistent or chronic cough such as occurs with smoking, asthma or emphysema, or where cough is accompanied by excessive secretions. As with any drug, if you are pregnant or nursing a baby, seek the advice of a health professional before using this product.

Keep this and all drugs out of the reach of children. In case of accidental overdose, seek professional assistance or contact a Poison Control Center immediately.

Caution: A persistent cough may be a sign of a serious condition. If cough or other symptoms persist for more than one week, tend to recur or are accompanied by high fever, rash or persistent headache, consult a physician before continuing use.

Dosage and Administration: Adults— 2 teaspoonfuls every 4 hours. Children 6–12 years—1 teaspoonful every 4 hours. Children 2–6 years—½ teaspoonful every 4 hours. Unless directed by physician, do not exceed 6 doses in 24 hours or give to children under 2 years of age.

How Supplied: TRIAMINIC-DM Cough Formula (dark red) in 4 fl oz and 8 fl oz plastic bottles with tamper-evident band around child-resistant cap.

Shown in Product Identification Section, page 409

TRIAMINIC® EXPECTORANT

Description: Each teaspoonful (5 ml) of TRIAMINIC Expectorant contains: phenylpropanolamine hydrochloride 12.5 mg, guaifenesin 100 mg, alcohol 5%.

Indications: Helps loosen phlegm and bronchial secretions and rid the bronchial passageways of bothersome mucus. Relieves irritated membranes in the respiratory passageways by preventing dryness through increased mucus flow. Temporarily relieves nasal stuffiness due to the common cold, hay fever or other upper respiratory allergies. Promotes nasal and/or sinus drainage.

Warning: EXCEPT UNDER THE ADVICE AND SUPERVISION OF A PHYSICIAN: DO NOT exceed the recommended dosage because at higher doses nervousness, dizziness or sleeplessness may occur. DO NOT take this preparation if you have high blood pressure, heart disease, diabetes, thyroid disease or are presently taking a prescription antihypertensive or antidepressant drug containing a monoamine oxidase inhibitor. DO NOT take this product for persistent or chronic cough such as occurs with smoking, asthma or emphysema, or where cough is accompanied by excessive secretions. As with any drug, if you are pregnant or nursing a baby, seek the advice of a health professional before using this product.

Keep this and all drugs out of the reach of children. In case of accidental overdose, seek professional assistance or contact a Poison Control Center immediately.

Caution: A persistent cough may be a sign of a serious condition. If cough or other symptoms persist for more than one week, tend to recur or are accompanied by high fever, rash or persistent headache, consult a physician before continuing use.

Dosage and Administration: Adults— 2 teaspoonfuls every 4 hours. Children 6–12 years—1 teaspoonful every 4 hours. Children 2–6 years—½ teaspoonful every 4 hours. Unless directed by physician, do not exceed 6 doses in 24 hours or give to children under 2 years of age.

How Supplied: TRIAMINIC Expectorant (yellow) in 4 fl oz and 8 fl oz plastic bottles with tamper-evident band around child-resistant cap.

Shown in Product Identification Section, page 408

TRIAMINIC-12® TABLETS

Description: Each TRIAMINIC - 12 Tablet contains: phenylpropanolamine hydrochloride 75 mg and chlorpheniramine maleate 12 mg.

Product Information

TRIAMINIC-12 Tablets contain the nasal decongestant phenylpropanolamine, and the antihistamine chlorpheniramine, in a formulation providing 12 hours of symptomatic relief.

Indications: For the temporary relief of nasal congestion due to the common cold, hay fever or other upper respiratory allergies and associated with sinusitis. Helps decongest sinus openings, sinus passages; promotes nasal and/or sinus drainage; temporarily restores freer breathing through the nose. For temporary relief of running nose, sneezing, itching of the nose or throat and itchy and watery eyes as may occur in allergic rhinitis (such as hay fever).

Warning: Do not give this product to children under 12 years except under the advice and supervision of a physician. Do not take this preparation if you have high blood pressure, heart disease, diabetes, thyroid disease, asthma, glaucoma or difficulty in urination due to enlargement of the prostate gland except under the advice and supervision of a physician. Do not exceed the recommended dosage because at higher doses nervousness, dizziness, or sleeplessness may occur. This preparation may cause drowsiness; this preparation may cause excitability, especially in children. If symptoms do not improve within seven days or are accompanied by high fever, consult a physician before continuing use. As with any drug, if you are pregnant or nursing a baby, seek the advice of a health professional before using this product. Keep this and all drugs out of the reach of children. In case of accidental overdose, seek professional assistance or contact a Poison Control Center immediately.

Caution: Avoid driving a motor vehicle or operating heavy machinery. Avoid alcoholic beverages while taking this product.

Drug Interaction Precaution: Do not take this product if you are presently taking a prescription antihypertensive or antidepressant drug containing a monoamine oxidase inhibitor except under the advice and supervision of a physician.

Directions: Adults and children over 12 years of age—1 tablet swallowed whole every 12 hours. Unless directed by physician, do not exceed 2 tablets in 24 hours.

Note: The nonactive portion of the tablet that supplies the active ingredients may occasionally appear in your stool as a soft mass.

How Supplied: TRIAMINIC-12 Tablets (orange), imprinted "Dorsey" on one side, "TRIAMINIC 12" on the other, in blister packs of 10 and 20.
Shown in Product Identification Section, page 408

TRIAMINICIN® TABLETS

Description: Each TRIAMINICIN Tablet contains: phenylpropanolamine hydrochloride 25 mg, chlorpheniramine maleate 2 mg, aspirin 450 mg, caffeine 30 mg.

Indications: For prompt temporary relief of nasal congestion, simple headache and minor aches and pains due to the common cold, hay fever and similar conditions.

Warning: Individuals with high blood pressure, heart disease, diabetes or thyroid disease should use only as directed by physician. TRIAMINICIN Tablets should not be used by individuals sensitive to aspirin. If drowsiness occurs, do not drive or operate machinery. As with any drug, if you are pregnant or nursing a baby, seek the advice of a health professional before using this product. Keep this and all medicines out of the reach of children. In case of accidental overdose, seek professional assistance or contact a Poison Control Center immediately.

Dosage and Administration: Adults—1 tablet 4 times a day. Unless directed by a physician, do not exceed recommended dosage or give to children under 12 years.

How Supplied: TRIAMINICIN Tablets (yellow) imprinted "DORSEY" on one side, "TRIAMINICIN" on the other, in blister packs of 12, 24 and 48, and bottles of 100 tablets.
Shown in Product Identification Section, page 409

TRIAMINICOL® MULTI-SYMPTOM COLD SYRUP

Description: Each teaspoonful (5 ml) of TRIAMINICOL Multi-Symptom Cold Syrup contains: phenylpropanolamine hydrochloride 12.5 mg, chlorpheniramine maleate 2 mg, dextromethorphan hydrobromide 10 mg in a palatable non-alcoholic vehicle.

Indications: Decreases running nose, sneezing, itching of the nose or throat and itchy and watery eyes as may occur in hay fever. Promotes nasal and/or sinus drainage. Temporarily relieves cough due to minor throat and bronchial irritation as may occur with the common cold or inhaled irritants.

Warnings: EXCEPT UNDER THE ADVICE AND SUPERVISION OF A PHYSICIAN: DO NOT exceed the recommended dosage because at higher doses nervousness, dizziness, or sleeplessness may occur. DO NOT take this preparation if you have high blood pressure, heart disease, diabetes, thyroid disease or are presently taking a prescription antihypertensive or antidepressant drug containing a monoamine oxidase inhibitor. DO NOT take this product for persistent or chronic cough such as occurs with smoking, asthma or emphysema, or where cough is accompanied by excessive secretions. DO NOT take this preparation if you have asthma, glaucoma or difficulty in urination due to enlargement of the prostate gland. This preparation may cause drowsiness or excitability (especially in children). As with any drug, if

you are pregnant or nursing a baby, seek the advice of a health professional before using this product. Caution: May cause marked drowsiness. Keep this and all drugs out of the reach of children. In case of accidental overdose, seek professional assistance or contact a Poison Control Center immediately.

Caution: A persistent cough may be a sign of a serious condition. If cough or other symptoms persist for more than 1 week, tend to recur or are accompanied by high fever, rash or persistent headache, consult a physician before continuing use. Avoid alcoholic beverages, operating a motor vehicle or heavy machinery while taking this product.

Dosage and Administration: Adults—2 teaspoonfuls every 4 hours. Children 6–12 years—1 teaspoonful every 4 hours. Unless directed by physician, do not exceed 6 doses in 24 hours or give to children under 6 years of age.

How Supplied: TRIAMINICOL Multi-Symptom Cold Syrup (red) in 4 fl oz and 8 fl oz plastic bottles with tamper-evident band around child-resistant cap.
Shown in Product Identification Section, page 409

TRIAMINICOL® MULTI-SYMPTOM COLD TABLETS

Description: Each TRIAMINICOL Multi-Symptom Cold Tablet contains: phenylpropanolamine hydrochloride 12.5 mg, chlorpheniramine maleate 2 mg, dextromethorphan hydrobromide 10 mg.

Indications: For temporary relief of nasal congestion due to the common cold, hay fever or other upper respiratory allergies and associated with sinusitis. Helps decongest sinus openings, sinus passages; promotes nasal and/or sinus drainage; temporarily restores freer breathing through the nose. For temporary relief of runny nose, sneezing, itching of the nose or throat and itchy and watery eyes as may occur in allergic rhinitis (such as hay fever). For temporary relief of cough due to minor throat and bronchial irritation as may occur with the common cold or with inhaled irritants.

Warnings: EXCEPT UNDER THE ADVICE AND SUPERVISION OF A PHYSICIAN: DO NOT exceed the recommended dosage because at higher doses nervousness, dizziness, or sleeplessness may occur. DO NOT take this preparation if you have high blood pressure, heart disease, diabetes, thyroid disease or are presently taking a prescription antihypertensive or antidepressant drug containing a monoamine oxidase inhibitor. DO NOT take this product for persistent or chronic cough such as occurs with smoking, asthma or emphysema, or where cough is accompanied by excessive secretions. DO NOT take this preparation if you have asthma, glaucoma or dif-

Continued on next page

Dorsey—Cont.

ficulty in urination due to enlargement of the prostate gland. This preparation may cause drowsiness or excitability (especially in children).

Unless directed by physician, do not give this product to children under 6 years of age. As with any drug, if you are pregnant or nursing a baby, seek the advice of a health professional before using this product. Keep this and all drugs out of the reach of children. In case of accidental overdose, seek professional assistance or contact a Poison Control Center immediately.

Caution: May cause marked drowsiness. A persistent cough may be a sign of a serious condition. If cough or other symptoms persist for more than 1 week, tend to recur or are accompanied by high fever, rash or persistent headache, consult a physician before continuing use. Avoid alcoholic beverages, operating a motor vehicle or heavy machinery while taking this product.

Dosage and Administration: Adults—2 tablets every 4 hours. Children 6–12 years—1 tablet every 4 hours. For nighttime cough relief, give the last dose at bedtime. Unless directed by physician, do not exceed 6 doses in 24 hours or give to children under 6 years.

How Supplied: TRIAMINICOL Multi-Symptom Cold Tablets (cherry pink), imprinted "DORSEY" on one side, "TRIAMINICOL" on the other in blister packs of 24 and 48.

Shown in Product Identification Section, page 409

TUSSAGESIC® TABLETS and TUSSAGESIC® SUSPENSION

Description: Each TUSSAGESIC Timed Release Tablet contains: phenylpropanolamine hydrochloride 25 mg, pheniramine maleate 12.5 mg, pyrilamine maleate 12.5 mg, dextromethorphan hydrobromide 30 mg, terpin hydrate 180 mg, acetaminophen 325 mg. Each teaspoonful (5 ml) of TUSSAGESIC Suspension contains: phenylpropanolamine hydrochloride 12.5 mg, pheniramine maleate 6.25 mg, pyrilamine maleate 6.25 mg, dextromethorphan hydrobromide 15 mg, terpin hydrate 90 mg, acetaminophen 120 mg.

Indications: For prompt relief of symptoms associated with the common cold such as cough, nasal congestion, simple headache and minor muscular aches and pains. TUSSAGESIC contains the effective, nonnarcotic antitussive, dextromethorphan hydrobromide; a proven decongestant; an expectorant; and the well-tolerated analgesic, acetaminophen.

Precautions: Patients should be advised not to drive a car or operate dangerous machinery if drowsiness occurs. Use with caution in the presence of hypertension, hyperthyroidism, cardiovascular disease or diabetes. Use with caution in pregnant and nursing mothers.

Adverse Reactions: Occasional drowsiness, blurred vision, cardiac palpitations, flushing, dizziness, nervousness or gastrointestinal upsets.

Dosage and Administration: Tablets: Adults—1 tablet, swallowed whole, in morning, midafternoon and before retiring. Suspension: Children 1 to 6—½ teaspoonful every 4 hours; children 6 to 12—1 teaspoonful every 4 hours; adults—2 teaspoonfuls every 4 hours.

How Supplied: TUSSAGESIC Tablets (orange) in bottles of 100. TUSSAGESIC Suspension (orange) in pint bottles.

URSINUS® INLAY–TABS®

Description: Each URSINUS INLAY-TAB contains: Calurin® (calcium carbaspirin) equivalent to 300 mg aspirin; phenylpropanolamine hydrochloride 25 mg; pheniramine maleate 12.5 mg; pyrilamine maleate 12.5 mg.

Indications: For prompt, temporary relief of nasal congestion, simple headache and minor aches and pains due to sinusitis and the common cold.

Cautions: Individuals with high blood pressure, heart disease, diabetes, or thyroid disease should use only as directed by physician. Should not be used by individuals sensitive to aspirin. If drowsiness occurs, do not drive or operate machinery.

Warning: Keep this and all medicines out of the reach of children. In case of accidental overdose, contact a physician immediately.

Dosage and Administration: Adults—1 tablet 4 times a day. Unless directed by a physician, do not exceed recommended dosage or give to children under 12 years of age.

How Supplied: URSINUS INLAY-TABS (white with yellow inlay) in bottles of 24 and 100.

Ex-Lax Pharmaceutical Co., Inc.
a Sandoz Company
(see also Creighton Products Corporation)
605 THIRD AVENUE
NEW YORK, NY 10158

EX–LAX® Chocolated Laxative

Active Ingredient: Yellow phenolphthalein, 90 mg per tablet.

Indications: For short-term relief of constipation.

Actions: Yellow phenolphthalein was previously categorized as a "stimulant" laxative. Recent research appears to indicate that phenolphthalein acts primarily by its effect on intestinal absorption of water and electrolytes, thus causing propulsive activity.

Warnings: Caution: Do not take any laxative when abdominal pain, nausea, or vomiting are present. Frequent or prolonged use of this or any other laxative may result in dependence on laxatives. If skin rash appears, do not use this or any other preparation containing phenolphthalein.
Ex-Lax is a medicine, not a candy. **Warning:** Keep this and all other medicines out of the reach of children.

Drug Interaction Precautions: No known drug interaction.

Dosage and Administration: Adults: 1 to 2 tablets, preferably at bed time. Children over 6 years: ½ to 1 tablet. Adult dosage may be slightly increased or decreased to suit individual requirements. If slightly increased adult dose is necessary, take it the following day.

How Supplied: Available in boxes of 6, 18, 48, and 72 chewable chocolate-flavored tablets.

Shown in Product Identification Section, page 409

EX–LAX® Pills, Unflavored Laxative

Active Ingredient: Yellow phenolphthalein, 90 mg per tablet.

Indications: For short-term relief of constipation.

Actions: Yellow phenolphthalein was previously categorized as a "stimulant" laxative. Recent research appears to indicate that phenolphthalein acts primarily by its effect on intestinal absorption of water and electrolytes, thus causing propulsive activity.

Warnings: Caution: Do not take any laxative when abdominal pain, nausea, or vomiting are present. Frequent or prolonged use of this or any other laxative may result in dependence on laxatives. If skin rash appears, do not use this or any other preparation containing phenolphthalein.
Ex-Lax is a medicine, not a candy. **Warning:** Keep this and all other medicines out of the reach of children.

Drug Interaction Precautions: No known drug interaction.

Dosage and Administration: Adults: 1 to 2 tablets with a glass of water, preferably at bed time. Children over 6 years: 1 tablet. Adult dosage may be increased or decreased to suit individual requirements. If increased adult dose is necessary, take it the following day.

How Supplied: Available in boxes of 8, 30, and 60 unflavored strip packed pills.

Shown in Product Identification Section, page 409

EXTRA GENTLE EX-LAX

Active Ingredients: Docusate Sodium, 75 mg. and Yellow Phenolphthalein 65 mg. per tablet.

Indications: For short-term relief of constipation.

Actions: Docusate sodium is categorized as an emollient stool softener. It is an anionic surface-active agent whose effect is attributed to lowering surface tension. This action permits increased water and lipid absorption by the fecal mass, thus softening the feces. Yellow phenolphthalein was previously categorized as a "stimulant" laxative. Recent research appears to indicate that phenolphthalein acts primarily by its effect on intestinal absorption of water and electrolytes, thus causing propulsive activity.

Warnings: Caution: Not to be used when abdominal pain, nausea, or vomiting are present. Take only as needed. Frequent or prolonged use may result in dependence on laxatives. If a skin rash appears, do not take this or any other preparation containing phenolphthalein. Keep this and all medications out of reach of children.

Drug Interaction Precautions: No know drug interaction.

Dosage and Administration: Adults take 1 or 2 pills daily, with water, preferably at bedtime, or as directed by physician. Children over 6 years: 1 pill daily as needed.

How Supplied: Available in boxes of 24 and 48 strip packed pills.
Shown in Product Identification Section, page 409

Fiber-Up Inc.
P.O. BOX 288
CONVENT STATION, NJ 07961

"FIBER–UP!"

Description: Fiber-Up is a high fiber food supplement and is the most highly concentrated form of fiber available. **Fiber-Up** has more than 3 times as much dietary fiber compared to wheat bran. It's smooth texture and high concentration make it blend easily with many foods without any noticable change in taste or texture, and is extremely gentle to your system. Medical authorities have traced a relationship between the dwindling supply of fiber in our diet and the increase of certain diseases.
Dietary fiber is an intregal part of treatment for constipation, diverticulosis, irritable bowel syndrome and hemorrhoids. Lack of fiber in the diet is a recognized cause of constipation. Adequate fiber insures food wastes move through the body quickly, making elimination easier and more regular. Just one teaspoon of **Fiber-Up** can supply all the fiber needed to replace the missing part of an adult diet.

Nutritional Information:
  17 grams (1 tablespoon)

One serving (17g) contains:

Calories	8.5	
Carbohydrate	.807	gr
Moisture	1.13	g
Ash	.12	g
Protein	.98	g
Fat	.72	g
Crude Fiber	3.0	g
Dietary Fiber	15.0	g

Vitamins and Minerals

Vitamin C	3.57	mg
Thiamine	.007	mg
Riboflavin	.085	mg
Niacin	.29	mg
Calcium	13.8	mg
Iron	1.2	mg
Sodium	6.4	mg
Magnesium	15.6	mg
Phosphorous	19.4	mg

Ingredients: Corn, Rice, Soy Bran, Nonfat Dry Milk.

Usage:
For the Individual
1st week—1 level teaspoon of **Fiber-Up** once a day in juice, soup, eggs, milk, etc.
2nd week—1 level teaspoon of **Fiber-Up** twice a day
For The Family
½ to 1 tablespoon for 3 or more people. Add to mashed potatoes, meatloaf, stews, casseroles, cakes, sauces, gravy, soup, yogurt, etc.

Supplied: Fiber-Up is supplied in 16 oz (1 lb) containers, 7 ounce and 5 ounce sizes.

Fleming & Company
1600 FENPARK DR.
FENTON, MO 63026

IMPREGON Concentrate

Active Ingredient: Tetrachlorosalicylanilide 2%

Indications: Diaper Rash Relief, 'Staph' control, Mold inhibitor.

Actions: This is a bacteriostatic/fungistatic agent for home usage and hospital usage.

Warnings: Impregon should not be exposed to direct sunlight for long periods after applications.

Precaution: Addition of bleach prior to diaper treatment negates application effects.

Dosage and Administration: One capful (5ml) per gallon of water to impregnate diapers in the diaper pail. Dilutions for many home areas accompany the full package.

Note: for 'Pamper-type' diapers, add one teaspoonful to 8 oz of water to a 'Windex-type' sprayer. Spray inside area of diapers until damp, and allow to dry before using, to prevent rashes.

How Supplied: Four ounce amber plastic bottles.

MARBLEN Suspensions and Tablet

Composition: A modified 'Sippy Powder' antacid containing magnesium and calcium carbonates;

Action and Uses: The peach/apricot (pink) or unflavored (green) antacid suspensions are sugar-free and neutralize 18 mEq acid per teaspoonful with a low sodium content of 18mg per fl. oz. Each pink tablet consumes 18.0 mEq acid.

Administration and Dosage: One teaspoonful rather than a tablespoonful or one tablet to reduce patient cost by ⅔.

How Supplied: Plastic pints and bottles of 100 and 1000.

NEPHROX SUSPENSION
(aluminum hydroxide)
Antacid Suspension

Composition: A watermelon flavored aluminum hydroxide (320mg as gel)/mineral oil (10% by volume) antacid per teaspoonful.

Action and Uses: A sugar-free/saccharin-free pink suspension containing no magnesium and low sodium (19mg/oz). Extremely palatable and especially indicated in renal patients. Each teaspoon consumes 9 mEq acid.

Administration and Dosage: Two teaspoonfuls or as directed by a physician.

Caution: To be taken only at bedtime. Do not use at any other time or administer to infants, expectant women, and nursing mothers except upon the advice of a physician as this product contains mineral oil.

How Supplied: Plastic pints and gallons.

NICOTINEX Elixir
nicotinic acid

Composition: Contains niacin 50 mg./tsp. in a sherry wine base (amber color).

Action and Uses: Produces flushing when tablets fail. To increase micro-circulation of inner-ear in Meniere's, tinnitus and labyrinthine syndromes. For 'cold hands & feet', and as a vehicle for additives.

Administration and Dosage: One or two teaspoonsful on fasting stomach.

Side Effects: Patients should be warned of dermal flush. Ulcer and gout patients may be affected by 14% alcoholic content.

Contraindications: Severe hypotension and hemorrhage.

How Supplied: Plastic pints and gallons.

OCEAN MIST
(buffered saline)

Composition: Special isotonic saline, buffered with sodium bicarbonate to proper pH so as not to irritate the nose.

Action and Uses: Rhinitis medicamentosa, rhinitis sicca and atrophic rhinitis. For patients 'hooked on nose drops' and glaucoma patients on diuretics having dry nasal capillaries. OCEAN may be used as a mist or drop.

Administration and Dosage: One or two squeezes in each nostril.

Continued on next page

Fleming—Cont.

Supplied: Plastic 45cc spray bottles and pints.

PURGE
(flavored castor oil)

Composition: Contains 95% castor oil (USP) in a sweetened lemon flavored base that completely masks the odor and taste of the oil.

Indications: Preparation of the bowel for x-ray, surgery and proctological procedures, IVPs, and constipation.

Dosage: Infants—1–2 teaspoonfuls. Children—adjust between infant and adult dose. Adult—2–4 tablespoonfuls.

Precaution: Not indicated when nausea, vomiting, abdominal pain or symptoms of appendicitis occur. Pregnancy, use only on advice of physician.

Supplied: Plastic 1 oz. & 2 oz. bottles.

Forest Pharmaceuticals, Inc.
2510 METRO BLVD.
MARYLAND HEIGHTS, MO
63043

BANALG® HOSPITAL STRENGTH ARTHRITIC PAIN RELIEVER; BANALG® MUSCULAR PAIN RELIEVER

Composition: Banalg Hospital Strength Arthritic Pain Reliever contains high concentrations of Methyl salicylate and Menthol in a Blue colored non-greasy base.
Regular Banalg contains Methyl salicylate, Menthol, Camphor, and Eucalyptus oil in a Green colored non-greasy base.

Action and Uses: For temporary relief of minor pain caused by arthritis, sore muscles, low backpain, and soreness and stiffness caused by overexertion.
The high potency of Banalg Hospital Strength Arthritic Pain Reliever suggests its use when more intensive analgesic action, such as in arthritis, is required.

Administration: Several times a day, apply generously to painful areas and massage gently.

Caution: Discontinue use if excessive irritation of the skin develops. Avoid getting in the eyes or mucous membranes. If pain persists for more than 10 days or redness is present, or in conditions affecting children under 12 years of age, consult your physician immediately.

Warning: Keep this and all medicines out of the reach of children. If swallowed, induce vomiting and contact a physician or a poison control center immediately.

How Supplied: Banalg Hospital Strength Arthritic Pain Reliever, 2 oz.

bottle. Banalg liniment, 2 oz. and pint bottles.
Shown in Product Identification Section, page 419

E. Fougera & Company
Division of Altana Inc.
60 BAYLIS ROAD
MELVILLE, NY 11747

ANALGESIC BALM

Active Ingredient: Methyl Salicylate (wintergreen) and Menthol.

How Supplied: Available in 1 oz tubes and 1 lb jars.

ANTIFUNGAL CREAM and SOLUTION

Active Ingredient: Tolnaftate 1% in a base that will not stain the skin.

Indications: For the treatment of superficial fungus infections of the skin which cause tinea pedis (athlete's foot), tinea cruris (jock itch) and tinea corporis (body ringworm). For external use only. Do not use in the eyes.

Warnings: Not recommended for nail or scalp infections. Do not use in children under 2 years of age except under the advice and supervision of a physician. Keep this and all drugs out of the reach of children. In case of accidental ingestion, seek professional assistance or contact a Poison Control Center.

Precaution: If burning or itching do not improve within 10 days or if irritation occurs, discontinue use and consult your physician or podiatrist.

Dosage and Administration: Wash and dry infected area morning and evening. Apply cream or 2 or 3 drops of solution evenly to the infected area and gently rub in. To help prevent recurrence, continue treatment for two weeks after disappearance of all symptoms.

How Supplied: Antifungal Cream is available in 15 gram tubes. Antifungal Solution is available in 10 ml plastic squeeze bottles.

BACITRACIN OINTMENT, U.S.P.

Active Ingredient: Bacitracin 500 units per gram.

Indications: Bacitracin is a topical antibacterial ointment to help prevent infection in minor cuts, burns and abrasions.

Warnings: For external use only. Do not use in eyes. In case of accidental ingestion, seek professional assistance or contact a Poison Control Center immediately. Keep this and all drugs out of the reach of children.

Precaution: In case of deep or puncture wounds or serious burns, consult a physician. If redness, irritation, swelling or pain persists or increases or if infection occurs, discontinue use and consult a physician.

Dosage and Administration: Apply to affected area once or twice a day and cover with a dry, sterile gauze dressing.

How Supplied: Available in ½ oz and 1 oz tubes.

BACITRACIN–NEOMYCIN–POLYMYXIN OINTMENT
Triple Antibiotic Ointment

Active Ingredient: Bacitracin 400 units, neomycin sulfate 5mg, polymyxin B sulfate 5,000 units per gram.

Indications: A topical antibacterial to help prevent infection in minor cuts, burns and abrasions.

Warnings: For external use only. Do not use in eyes. Keep this and all drugs out of the reach of children. In case of accidental ingestion, seek professional assistance or conact a Poison Control Center immediately.

Precaution: In case of deep or puncture wounds or serious burns, consult a physician. If redness, irritation, swelling or pain persists or increases, or if infection occurs, discontinue use and consult a physician.

Dosage and Administration: Apply to affected area once or twice a day and cover with a dry, sterile gauze dressing.

How Supplied: Available in ½ oz and 1 oz tubes.

BACITRACIN–POLYMYXIN OINTMENT
Double Antibiotic Ointment

Active Ingredient: Bacitracin zinc 500 units, polymyxin B sulfate 10,000 units per gram.

Indications: A topical antibacterial to help prevent infection in minor cuts and abrasions.

Warnings: Keep this and all drugs out of the reach of children. In case of accidental ingestion, seek professional assistance or contact a Poison Control Center immediately. For external use only. Do not use in eyes.

Precaution: In case of deep or puncture wounds or serious burns, consult a physician. If redness, irritation, swelling or pain persists or increases, or if infection occurs, discontinue use and consult a physician.

Dosage and Administration: Apply to affected area 2–5 times a day, and cover with a dry sterile gauze dressing.

How Supplied: Available in ½ oz and 1 oz tubes.

BORIC ACID OINTMENT

Active Ingredient: Boric acid 10%.

Indications: A topical antiseptic dressing for minor cuts, scratches, abrasions, surface wounds and simple irritations of the skin.

Warnings: For external use only. Do not use in eyes. Keep this and all drugs out of the reach of children.

Precaution: In case of deep or puncture wounds or severe burns, consult physician. If irritation, swelling or pain persists, or if infection occurs, discontinue use and consult physician.

Dosage and Administration: Apply to the affected area once or twice daily, or as directed by a physician. Loose sterile bandage may be applied if desired.

How Supplied: Available in 1 oz and 2 oz tubes.

COLD CREAM, U.S.P.

Active Ingredient: White Wax USP (Bee's Wax) with other emollients.

How Supplied: Available in 1 oz tubes and 1 lb jars.

DIBUCAINE OINTMENT, U.S.P. 1%

Active Ingredient: Dibucaine 1% with acetone sodium bisulfate 0.5% as a preservative.

Indications: A topical anesthetic ointment for the temporary relief of pain and itching associated with hemminor burns, cuts, scratches, insect bites and sting.

Warnings: For external use only. Do not use in eyes. Keep this and other drugs out of the reach of children. In case of accidental ingestion, seek professional assistance or contact a Poison Control Center immediately.

Precaution: Not for prolonged use. Adults should not use more than one tube in 24 hours or ¼ tube for a child. If the condition for which this preparation is used persists or if rash or irritation develops, discontinue use and consult physician. In case of rectal bleeding, consult physician immediately.

Dosage and Administration: Apply to affected area 3 or 4 times daily and cover with a light dressing if necessary. For application to the anorectal area, use enclosed rectal applicator.

How Supplied: Available in 1 oz tubes.

HYDROCORTISONE CREAM and OINTMENT, U.S.P. 0.5%

Active Ingredient: Hydrocortisone, USP 0.5%.

Indications: For the temporary relief of minor skin irritations, itching and rashes due to dermatitis, insect bites, poison ivy, poison oak, poison sumac and itchy genital and anal areas.

Warnings: For external use only. Avoid contact with the eyes. Keep this and all drugs out of the reach of children. In case of accidental ingestion, seek professional assistance or contact a Poison Control Center immediately.

Precaution: Discontinue use if condition worsens or if symptoms persist for more than 7 days. Consult a physician. Do not use on children under 2 years except under the advice and supervision of a physician.

Dosage and Administration: Apply to the affected area 1–3 times daily.

How Supplied: 1 oz. tubes.

LANOLIN, U.S.P.

Composition: Lanolin anhydrous 72.5% with purified water 27.5%.

Indications: Topical lubricant. Also useful as an aid to chapped skin, sunburn and windburn.

Warnings: For external use only. Do not use in eyes. Keep this and all drugs out of the reach of children.

Dosage and Administration: Apply as needed to affected or exposed skin.

How Supplied: Available in 1 oz tubes and 1 lb jars.

PETROLATUM WHITE, U.S.P.

Composition: Petrolatum White, U.S.P. Pharmaceutical grade.

Indications: Topical lubricant, Useful as a soothing dressing for minor skin irritations such as burns, abrasions, scrapes, chafed or chapped skin, sunburn, diaper rash, detergent hands.

Precaution: This preparation is not intended for deep puncture wounds, serious burns or cuts. If redness, irritation, swelling or pain persists, discontinue use and consult your physician.

Dosage and Administration: Cleanse area with soap and water prior to application and apply petrolatum liberally to provide a continuous protective film.

How Supplied: Available in 1 oz tubes and 1 lb jars.

SWIM EAR®

Composition: Boric acid N.F. 2.75% in isopropyl alcohol.

Indications: To help prevent ear infections by drying out excess water after swimming, bathing, showering.

Warnings: Keep this and all drugs out of the reach of children. Keep away from open flame.

Precaution: Use as directed. Do not use on eyes, mucous membranes or broken skin.

Dosage and Administration: Put 3 to 6 drops in each ear after swimming or showering.

How Supplied: Available in plastic 1 oz squeeze bottles.

VITAMIN A + VITAMIN D OINTMENT

Composition: Vitamin A 1750 u/gm and Vitamin D 350 u/gm in a lanolin-petrolatum ointment base.

Indications: A topical emollient for first aid in minor burns, diaper rash, chafing, and abrasions.

Warnings: For external use only. Do not use in eyes. Keep this and all drugs out of the reach of children.

Precaution: If condition persists or worsens, consult your physician.

Dosage and Administration: Cleanse the affected area with mild soap and warm water. Dry thoroughly. Apply Vitamin A & Vitamin D ointment in a thin layer directly to the affected area or by spreading on sterile gauze or a clean cloth. Bandage loosely if necessary. In severe or extensive burns, call physician at once. Treatment of severe cuts or wounds should be under the direction of a physician.

How Supplied: Available in 2 oz and 4 oz tubes; 1 lb jars.

ZINC OXIDE OINTMENT, U.S.P.

Active Ingredient: Zinc Oxide 20%.

How Supplied: Available in 1 oz and 2 oz tubes; 1 lb jars.

Fox Pharmacal, Inc.
1750 W. McNAB ROAD
FT. LAUDERDALE, FL 33310

ODRINIL™ Natural Diuretic

Active Ingredients: Powdered Extract of Buchu; Powdered Extract of Uva Ursi; Powdered Extract of Corn Silk; Powdered Extract of Juniper; Caffeine.

Indications: To aid in the relief of simple water retention or "bloating" such as experienced in the premenstrual period and not associated with disease conditions.

Actions: Herbal extracts contained in this product have been recommended for centuries to aid in the excretion of excess sodium and thereby overcome excessive water retention that results from salt retention. Caffeine is widely recognized as having similar diuretic properties.

Warnings: This product is not indicated for water retention that results from kidney, heart or other systemic disease. It should not be used when such diseases or conditions are present except on the advice of a physician.

Drug Interaction Precautions: None.

Dosage and Administration: One tablet with a glass of water after each meal and before retiring when premenstrual bloating is experienced. The product has no value as a preventative, but is

Continued on next page

Fox—Cont.

only effective when water retention is present.

How Supplied: Packages of 60 tablets.

SUPER ODRINEX™ Reducing Aid

Active Ingredients:
Phenylpropanolamine HCl ....25 mg.

Indications: For use in short term (8–12 weeks) programs of weight reduction adjunctively to reduced caloric intake.

Actions: Phenylpropanolamine is a sympathomimetic amine with demonstrated appetite-suppressant effects. Clinical trials have shown that individuals on restricted caloric intake lose several times as much weight when taking SUPER ODRINEX adjunctively to the dietary restrictions as patients on the same dietary restrictions but receiving placebo tablets.

Warnings: Individuals being treated for high blood pressure, heart disease, diabetes, thyroid disease or depression or are pregnant or nursing, should not take this product except under the supervision of a physician. Do not exceed recommended dosage. Discontinue use when desired weight is attained. For adult use only. Do not administer this product to children under the age of 12 except on the advice of a physician.

Drug Interaction Precautions: Do not use concurrently with Cough, Cold or Allergy preparations which contain a decongestant.

Overdosage: Ingestion of marked overdoses is not usually life-threatening, but marked drowsiness or jitteryness may occur. The persistence of these symptoms is short-lived.

Dosage and Administration: One tablet with a glass of water three times daily, ½ hour before meals. For use by Adults only.

How Supplied: In packages of 50 or 110 tablets, each containing Phenylpropanolamine HCl 25 mg.

QUINTROL

Active Ingredient: Quinine Sulfate 1 gr (64.8 mg).
Contains: Vitamin E (200 I.U.) dl Alpha Tocopheryl Acetate.

Indications: Night leg cramps.

Actions: Relieves leg pain and relaxes spasms.

Warnings: Keep this and all medications out of children's reach. Do not give to children under 12.

Precaution: Discontinue use if diarrhea, skin rash, nausea, eye or ear problems occur.

Dosage and Administration: Take 2 capsules with water. If possible stand up

to relieve strain. ½ hour later take 2 more capsules.
To help prevent leg cramps—take 2 capsules after evening meal and 2 capsules prior to bed. Do not take more than 4 capsules a day for more than 5 consecutive days.

How Supplied: 30 capsules.

GEIGY Pharmaceuticals
Division of CIBA-GEIGY Corporation
ARDSLEY, NY 10502

OTRIVIN®
xylometazoline hydrochloride USP
Nasal Spray and Nasal Drops 0.1%
Pediatric Nasal Drops 0.05%

One application provides rapid and long-lasting relief of nasal congestion for up to 10 hours.
Quickly clears stuffy noses due to common cold, sinusitis, hay fever.
Nasal congestion can make life miserable—you can't breath, smell, taste or sleep comfortably. That is why Otrivin is so helpful. It clears away that stuffy feeling, usually within 5 to 10 minutes, and your head feels clear for hours.
Otrivin has been prescribed by doctors for many years. Here is how you use it:
Nasal Spray 0.1%—Spray 2 to 3 times into each nostril every 8–10 hours. With head upright, squeeze sharply and firmly while inhaling (sniffing) through the nose.
Nasal Drops 0.1%—for adults and children 12 years and older. Put 2 or 3 drops into each nostril every 8 to 10 hours. Tilt head as far back as possible. Immediately bend head forward toward knees, hold for a few seconds, then return to upright position.
Do not give Nasal Spray 0.1% or Nasal Drops 0.1% to children under 12 years except under the advice and supervision of a physician.
Pediatric Nasal Drops 0.05%—for children 2 to 12 years of age. Put 2 to 3 drops into each nostril every 8 to 10 hours. Tilt head as far back as possible. Immediately bend head forward toward knees, hold a few seconds, then return to upright position.
Do not give this product to children under 2 years except under the advice and supervision of a physician.
Otrivin Nasal Spray/Nasal Drops are available in unbreakable plastic spray package of ½ fl oz (15 ml) and in plastic dropper bottle of .66 fl oz (20ml).
Otrivin Pediatric Nasal Drops
Available in plastic dropper bottle of .66 fl oz (20ml).

Warnings: Do not exceed recommended dosage, because symptoms such as burning, stinging, sneezing, or increase of nasal discharge may occur. Do not use this product for more than 3 days. If symptoms persist, consult a physician. The use of this dispenser by more than one person may cause infection.
Keep this and all medicines out of the reach of children. In case of accidental

ingestion, seek professional assistance or contact a Poison Control Center immediately.

C80-47 (8/80)
Shown in Product Identification Section, page 409

PBZ®
tripelennamine hydrochloride
Antihistamine Cream

Description: PBZ Cream is a topical antihistaminic preparation containing 2% tripelennamine hydrochloride.

Indications: For the temporary relief of itching due to minor skin disorders, ivy and oak poisoning, hives, sunburn, insect bites (nonpoisonous), and stings.

Directions: Apply gently to the affected area 3 or 4 times daily or according to physician's directions.

Caution: If the condition persists or irritation develops, discontinue use and consult physician. Do not use in eyes. KEEP OUT OF REACH OF CHILDREN.

How Supplied: *Cream,* 2% tripelennamine hydrochloride in a water-washable base; tubes of 1 ounce.

(1/80)
Shown in Product Identification Section, page 409

The full prescribing information for each GEIGY drug is contained herein and is that in effect as of December 1, 1984.

Glenbrook Laboratories
Division of Sterling Drug Inc.
90 PARK AVENUE
NEW YORK, NY 10016

BAYER® ASPIRIN AND BAYER® CHILDREN'S CHEWABLE ASPIRIN
Aspirin (Acetylsalicylic Acid)

Composition: Bayer Aspirin—Aspirin 5 grains. (325 mg.) Contains a thin, inert, methylcellulose coating for easier swallowing. This is not an enteric coating and does not alter the onset of action of Bayer Aspirin.
Bayer Children's Chewable Aspirin—Aspirin 1¼ grains (81 mg.) per orange flavored chewable tablet.

Action and Uses: Analgesic antipyretic, anti-inflammatory. For relief of headache; painful discomfort, fever, muscular aches and pains, temporary relief of minor pains of arthritis, rheumatism, bursitis, lumbago, sciatica, toothache, teething pains, and pain following dental procedures; neuralgia and neuritic pain; functional menstrual pain; sleeplessness when caused by minor painful discomforts; painful discomfort and fever accompanying immunizations.

Administration and Dosage: The following dosages are those provided in the labelling, as appropriate for self-medication. Larger or more frequent dosage may be necessary as appropriate to the condition or needs of the patient.

The methylcellulose coating makes Bayer Aspirin particularly appropriate for those who must take frequent doses of aspirin and for those who have difficulty in swallowing uncoated tablets.

Bayer Aspirin—5 grain (325 mg.) tablets

Adult Dose: One or two tablets with water. May be repeated every four hours as necessary up to 12 tablets a day.

Children's Dose: To be administered only under adult supervision.

Under 2 years ....per physician
2 to under 4 years ....½ tablet
4 to under 6 years ....¾ tablet
6 to under 9 years ....1 tablet
9 to under 11 years ....1¼ tablets
11 to under 12 years ....1½ tablets
Over 12 years ....same as adult
Indicated dosage may be repeated every 4 hours, up to but not more than five times a day. Larger dosage may be prescribed per physician.

Bayer Children's Chewable Aspirin— 1¼ grain (81 mg.) tablets
DOSAGE

To be administered only under adult supervision. For children under 2, consult physician.

Age (years)	Weight (lbs)	Dosage
2 up to 4	27 to 35	2 tablets
4 up to 6	36 to 45	3 tablets
6 up to 9	46 to 65	4 tablets
9 up to 11	66 to 76	5 tablets
11 up to 12	77 to 83	6 tablets
12 and over	84 and over	8 tablets

Indicated dosage may be repeated every 4 hours, up to but not more than five times a day. Larger dosage may be prescribed per physician.

Contraindications: Consult a physician before giving this medicine to children, including teenagers, with chicken pox or flu. Hypersensitivity to salicylates. To be used with caution in presence of peptic ulcer, asthma, or with anticoagulant therapy.

How Supplied:
Bayer Aspirin 5 grains (325 mg.)—
NDC-12843-101-10, packs of 12 tablets
NDC-12843-101-11, bottles of 24 tablets
NDC-12843-101-17, bottles of 50 tablets
NDC-12843-101-12, bottles of 100 tablets
NDC-12843-101-20, bottles of 200 tablets
NDC-12843-101-13, bottles of 300 tablets
Child-resistant safety closures on 12s, 24s, 50s, 200s, 300s. Bottle of 100s available without safety closure for households without small children.
Bayer Children's Chewable Aspirin 1¼ grains (81 mg.)—
NDC-12843-131-05, bottle of 36 tablets with child-resistant safety closure.
Samples available on request.
Shown in Product Identification Section, page 409

BAYER® CHILDREN'S COLD TABLETS

Composition: Each tablet contains phenylpropanolamine HCl 3.125 mg., aspirin 1¼ gr. (81 mg.); the tablets are orange flavored and chewable.

Action and Uses: Bayer Children's Cold Tablets combine two effective ingredients: a gentle decongestant to relieve nasal congestion and ease breathing, and genuine Bayer Aspirin to reduce fever and relieve minor aches and pains of colds.

Administration and Dosage: The following dosage is provided in the packaging:

Age (yrs)	Weight (lbs)	Dosage
2 up to 6	27–45	2 tabs
6 up to 12	46–83	4 tabs
12 & over	84+	8 tabs

Indicated dosage may be repeated every four hours up to but not more than four times a day. Larger or more frequent dosage may be necessary as appropriate to the condition or needs of the patient.

Contraindications: Consult a physician before giving this medicine to children, including teenagers with chicken pox or flu. Side effects at higher doses may include nervousness, dizziness, sleeplessness. To be used with caution in presence of high blood pressure, heart disease, diabetes, asthma, or thyroid disease.

How Supplied: NDC-12843-181-01, bottles of 30 tablets with child-resistant safety closure.
Samples available on request.

BAYER® COUGH SYRUP FOR CHILDREN

Composition: Each 5 ml. (1 tsp.) contains phenylpropanolamine HCl 9 mg. and dextromethorphan hydrobromide 7.5 mg., alcohol 5% Cherry flavored.

Action and Uses: Bayer Cough Syrup for Children combines two effective ingredients in a syrup with a very appealing cherry flavor: a gentle nasal decongestant and a cough suppressant.

Administration and Dosage: The following dosage is provided on the packaging:
Dosage: For children under 2 consult physician.

Age (yrs)	Weight (lbs)	Dosage
2 up to 6	27–45	1 tsp.
6 up to 12	46–83	2 tsp.
12 & over	84+	4 tsp.

Dose may be repeated every 4 hrs., not more than 4 times/day.

Contraindications and Precautions: To be used with caution in presence of high blood pressure, heart disease, diabetes, asthma, or thyroid disease.

How Supplied: NDC–12843-401-02, 3.0 oz. bottles. Samples available on request.

Arthritis BAYER® TIMED–RELEASE ASPIRIN (aspirin)

Description: Each oblong white scored tablet contains 10 grains (650 mg.) of aspirin in microencapsulation form.

Indications: Bayer Timed-Release Aspirin is indicated for the temporary relief of low grade pain amenable to relief with salicylates, such as in rheumatoid arthritis, osteoarthritis, spondylitis, bursitis and other forms of rheumatism, as well as in many common musculoskeletal disorders. It possesses the same advantages for other types of prolonged aches and pains, such as minor injuries, dental pain and dysmenorrhea. Its long-lasting effectiveness should also make it valuable as an analgesic in simple headache, colds, grippe, flu and other similar conditions in which aspirin is indicated for symptomatic relief, either by itself or as an adjunct to specific therapy.

Dosage: Two Bayer Timed-Release Aspirin tablets q. 8 h. provide effective long-lasting pain relief. This two-tablet (20 grain or 1300 mg.) dose of timed-release aspirin promptly produces salicylate blood levels greater than those achieved by a 10-grain (650 mg.) dose of regular aspirin, and in the second 4 hour period produces a salicylate blood level curve which approximates that of two successive 10-grain (650 mg.) doses of regular aspirin at 4 hour intervals. The 10-grain (650 mg.) scored Bayer Timed-Release Aspirin tablets permit administration of aspirin in multiples of 5 grains (325 mg.), allowing individualization of dosage to meet the specific needs of the patient.

For the convenience of patients on a regular aspirin dosage schedule, two 10-grain (650 mg.) Bayer Timed-Release Aspirin tablets may be administered with water every 8 hours. Whenever possible, two tablets (20 grains or 1300 mg.) should be given before retiring to provide effective analgesic and anti-inflammatory action—for relief of pain throughout the night and lessening of stiffness upon arising. Do not exceed 6 tablets in 24 hours. Bayer Timed-Release Aspirin has been made in a special capsule-shaped tablet to permit easy swallowing. However, for patients who do have difficulty, Bayer Timed-Release Aspirin tablets may be gently crumbled in the mouth and swallowed with water without loss of timed-release effect. There is no bitter "aspirin" taste. For children under 12, per physician.

Side Effects: Side effects encountered with regular aspirin may be encountered with Bayer Timed-Release Aspirin. Tinnitus and dizziness are the ones most frequently encountered.

Contraindications and Precautions: Bayer Timed-Release Aspirin is contraindicated in patients with marked aspirin hypersensitivity, and should be given with extreme caution to any patient with a history of adverse reaction to salicylates. It may cautiously be tried in patients intolerant to aspirin because of gastric irritation, but the usual precautions for any form of aspirin should be observed in patients with gastric ulcers, bleeding tendencies, asthma, or hypoprothrombinemia.

Continued on next page

Glenbrook—Cont.

Supplied:
Tablets in Bottle of 30's
NDC-12843-191-72
Tablets in Bottle of 72's
NDC-12843-191-74
Tablets in Bottle of 125's
NDC-12843-191-76
All sizes packaged in child-resistant safety closure except 72's which is a size recommended for households without young children.
Samples available upon request.
Shown in Product Identification Section, page 410

MAXIMUM BAYER® ASPIRIN
Aspirin (Acetylsalicylic Acid)

Composition: Maximum Bayer Aspirin—Aspirin 500 mg. (7.7 grains) contains a thin, inert, methylcellulose coating for easier swallowing. This is not an enteric coating and does not alter the onset of action of Bayer Aspirin.

Actions and Uses: Analgesic, antipyretic, anti-inflammatory. For relief of headache; painful discomfort and fever of colds and flu; sore throats; muscular aches and pains, temporary relief of minor pains of arthritis, rheumatism, bursitis, lumbago, sciatica, toothache, teething pains, and pain following dental procedures; neuralgia and neurtic pain; functional menstrual pain; sleeplessness when caused by minor painful discomforts; painful discomfort and fever accompanying immunizations.

Administration and Dosage: The following dosages are those provided on the packaging, as appropriate for self-medication. Larger or more frequent dosage may be necessary as appropriate to the condition or needs of the patient.
The methyl-cellulose coating makes Maximum Bayer Aspirin particularly appropriate for those who must take frequent doses of aspirin and for those who have difficulty in swallowing uncoated tablets.
Maximum Bayer Aspirin—500 mg (7.7 grains) tablets
Usual Adult Dose: One or two tablets with water. May be repeated every four hours as necessary up to 8 tablets a day.

How Supplied: Maximum Bayer Aspirin 500 mg (7.7 grains)
NDC 12843-161-53 bottles of 30 tablets
NDC 12483-161-56 bottles of 60 tablets
NDC 12843-161-58 bottles of 100 tablets
Child-resistant safety closures on 30's and 100's. Bottle of 60's available without safety closure for households without small children.
Samples available on request.
Shown in Product Identification Section, page 410

COSPRIN® 325
ENTERIC RELEASE ASPIRIN

Composition: 325 mg. of Bayer Aspirin in an enteric release formulation. This formulation is designed to allow the aspirin to pass through the stomach into the intestine, thus protecting against stomach upset.

Actions and Uses: Cosprin is indicated for temporary relief of the minor pain and inflammation of rheumatoid arthritis, osteoarthritis, spondylitis, bursitis and other forms of rheumatism, as well as many common musculoskeletal disorders. Cosprin is also effective in relieving backaches, muscle aches and other aches and pains.

Administration and Dosage: Adult recommended dosage is two tablets with liquid every four hours (or 3 tablets every 6 hours), not to exceed 12 tablets a day unless directed by a physician. Children —as recommended by physician.

Contraindications: To be used with caution in presence of gastric ulcer, allergies, asthma, or anticoagulant therapy.

How Supplied: Cosprin 325 mg. (5 grains)
NDC-12843-184-44 bottles of 60 tablets
NDC-12843-184-46 bottles of 125 tablets
Shown in Product Identification Section, page 410

COSPRIN® 650
ENTERIC RELEASE ASPIRIN

Composition: 650 mg. of Bayer Aspirin in an enteric release formulation. This formulation is designed to allow the aspirin to pass through the stomach into the intestine, thus protecting against stomach upset.

Actions and Uses: Cosprin is indicated for temporary relief of the minor pain and inflammation of rheumatoid arthritis, osteoarthritis, spondylitis, bursitis and other forms of rheumatism, as well as many common musculoskeletal disorders. Cosprin is also effective in relieving backaches, muscle aches and other aches and pains.

Administration and Dosage: Adult recommended dosage is one tablet with liquid every four hours, not to exceed 6 tablets a day unless directed by a physician.

Contraindications: To be used with caution in presence of gastric ulcer, allergies, asthma, or anticoagulant therapy.

How Supplied: Cosprin 650 mg. (10 grains)
NDC-12843-184-52 bottles of 36 tablets
NDC-12843-184-54 bottles of 72 tablets
Shown in Product Identification Section, page 410

DIAPARENE® BABY POWDER

Description: Powder comprised of corn starch, magnesium carbonate, fragrance, and methylbenzethonium chloride.

Action and Uses: Diaparene Baby Powder has a corn starch base for high absorbency to help keep baby skin dry and for soothing diaper rash, prickly heat, and chafing.

Administration and Dosage: Apply liberally to baby's skin after bath and with each diaper change.

How Supplied: Canister sizes of 4 oz. 9 oz., 14 oz.
Shown in Product Identification Section, page 410

DIAPARENE™ BABY WASH CLOTHS

Description: Wash cloths are impregnated with a cleansing solution containing water, SD alcohol-40, propylene glycol, lanolin, sodium nonoxynol-9 phosphate, sorbic acid, citric acid, disodium phosphate, oleth-20, and fragrance.

Action and Uses: Diaparene Baby Wash Cloths contain lanolin and a mild cleansing solution to clean and condition baby's skin.

Administration and Dosage: Wipe baby's skin with solution-impregnated wash cloths as required.

How supplied: Canisters in sizes of 70 and 150 wash cloths.
Shown in Product Identification Section, page 410

MIDOL®

Composition: Each Caplet® contains Aspirin 454 mg (7 grains); Cinnamedrine Hydrochloride 14.9 mg; Caffeine 32.4 mg.

Action and Uses: Analgesic, smooth muscle relaxant. For fast relief of functional menstrual pain, cramps, irritability; headache, aches from swelling, and the irritability associated with premenstrual tension; headache, and low backache associated with menstruation.

Usage Adult Dosage: Two Caplets with water. Repeat two Caplets every four hours as needed, up to eight Caplets per day.

How Supplied: White, capsule-shaped Caplets.
NDC-12843-151-34, bottles of 12 Caplets
NDC 12843-151-02, sample size of 6 caplets
NDC-12843-151-36, bottles of 30 Caplets
NDC-12843-151-38, bottles of 60 Caplets

Samples Supplied: Available upon request.
Shown in Product Identification Section, page 410

MAXIMUM STRENGTH MIDOL® PMS

Composition: Each capsule contains: Acetaminophen 500 mg., Pamabrom 25 mg., Pyrilamine Maleate 15 mg.

Action and Uses: Relieves the symptoms of Premenstrual Syndrome. For fast relief from premenstrual tension, irritability, bloating, water-weight gain, cramps, backache and headache.

Usual Adult Dosage: Two capsules with water. Repeat two capsules every four hours as needed, up to eight capsules per day.

How Supplied: Red and white capsules.

NDC 12843-153-42 bottles of 8 capsules
NDC 12843-153-43 bottles of 16 capsules
NDC 12843-153-44 bottles of 32 capsules

Samples Supplied: Available upon request.

*Shown in Product Identification
Section, page 410*

MAXIMUM STRENGTH MIDOL® FOR CRAMPS

Composition: Each Caplet® Contains: Aspirin 500 mg., Cinnamedrine Hydrochloride 14.9 mg., Caffeine 32.4 mg.

Action and Uses: Analgesic, antispasmodic. For fast relief of cramps, functional menstrual pain, headache, backache, leg aches, aches from swelling. Inhibits the body's production of prostaglandins, known to be a major cause of menstrual cramps.

Usual Adult Dosage:
Two Caplets with water. Repeat two Caplets every four hours as needed, up to eight Caplets per day.

How Supplied: White capsule shaped Caplets
NDC 12843-152-48 bottles of 8 Caplets
NDC 12843-152-49 bottles of 16 Caplets
NDC 12843-152-50 bottles of 32 Caplets

Samples Supplied: Available upon request.

*Shown in Product Identification
Section, page 410*

CHILDREN'S PANADOL®
Acetaminophen Chewable Tablets, Liquid, Drops

Description: Each Children's PANADOL Chewable Tablet contains 80 mg. acetaminophen in a fruit flavored tablet. Children's PANADOL Acetaminophen Liquid is fruit flavored, red in color, and is both alcohol free and sugar free. Each ½ teaspoon contains 80 mg. of acetaminophen. Infant's PANADOL Drops are fruit flavored, red in color, and are both alcohol free and sugar free. Each 0.8 ml. (one calibrated dropper full) contains 80 mg. acetaminophen.

Actions and Indications: Acetaminophen, the active ingredient in PANADOL, is the analgesic/antipyretic most widely recommended by pediatricians for fast, effective relief of children's fevers. It also relieves the aches and pains of colds and flu, earaches, headaches, teething, immunizations, tonsillectomy, and childhood illnesses.

Precautions and Adverse Reactions: Children's PANADOL Tablets, Liquid, and Drops are aspirin free and contain no alcohol or sugar. The pleasant tasting formulations are not likely to upset ot irritate children's stomachs.

Usual Dosage: Dosing is based on single doses in the range of 10–15 mg/kg body weight. Doses may be repeated every four hours up to 4 or 5 times daily, but not to exceed 5 doses in 24 hours. The package labeling states that for children under 2 years to "consult a physician". Children's PANADOL Chewable Tablets: Children 2–3 years 2 tablets, 4–5 years 3 tablets, 6–8 years 4 tablets, 9–10 years 5 tablets, 11–12 years 6 tablets. For children under 2 consult your physician. Dosage may be repeated every four hours, no more than 5 times in 24 hours. Children's PANADOL Liquid: (a special 3 teaspoon cup for accurate measurement is provided) Under 2 years consult a physician, 2–3 years 1 teaspoon, 4–5 years 1½ teaspoons, 6–8 years 2 teaspoons, 9–10 years 2½ teaspoons, 11 years 3 teaspoons. Repeat every 4 hours up to 5 times in a 24 hour period. Children's PANADOL Liquid may be administered alone or mixed with formula, milk, juice, cereal, etc.
Infant's PANADOL Drops: Under 2 years consult a physician, 2–3 years 1.6 ml. (2 droppers filled to 0.8 mark), 4–5 years 2.4 ml. (3 droppers filled to 0.8 mark). May be repeated every 4 hours, up to 5 times in a 24 hour period.

Warning: Since Children's PANADOL Acetaminophen Chewable Tablets, Liquid, and Drops are available without a prescription as an analgesic/antipyretic, the following appears on the package labels: "WARNING: Do not take this product for more than 5 days. If symptoms persist or new ones occur, consult physician. Keep this and all medicines out of the reach of children. In case of accidental overdose, consult a physician immediately. As with any drug, if you are pregnant or nursing a baby, seek the advice of a health professional before using the product. High fever, severe or persistent sore throat, headache nausea, or vomiting may be serious; consult a physician."
Tamper Resistant: Children's PANADOL Acetaminophen Chewable Tablets, packaging provides tamper resistant features on both the outer carton and bottle. The following copy appears on the end flaps of this carton—"Purchase only if carton end flaps are sealed. Use only if printed neck seal over cap is intact." Children's PANADOL Liquid and Drops provide tamper resistant features on the bottle—"Use only if printed neck seal over cap is intact."

How Supplied: Chewable Tablets (colored pink and scored)—bottles of 30. Liquid (colored red)—bottles of 2 fl. oz. and 4 fl. oz. Drops (colored red)—bottles of ½ oz. (15 ml.).
All packages listed above have child resistant safety caps and tamper resistant features.

*Shown in Product Identification
Section, page 410*

Maximum Strength PANADOL®
Tablets and Capsules

Active Ingredient: Each Maximum Strength Panadol Tablet or Capsule contains 500 mg Acetaminophen.

Actions and Uses: Where regular strength analgesics and antipyretics are not sufficient, Maximum Strength Panadol Tablets and Capsules provide increased strength for effective relief of pain and reduction of fever. Maximum Strength Panadol provides relief from pain of headache, colds or "flu", menstrual cramps, dental pain, sinusitis, neuralgia, muscular backache, muscular aches from overexertion, minor arthritis aches.
Maximum Strength Panadol Tablets and Capsules are usually well tolerated in persons sensitive to aspirin.

Contraindications: Rare instances of hypersensitivity attributed to acetaminophen have been reported: in these instances, the drug should be stopped.

Precautions: Do not give to children under 6 or use for more than 10 days unless directed by a physician. Keep this and all medications out of the reach of children. In case of accidental overdose, contact a physician If pregnant or nursing, consult a physician before using this or any medication Store at room temperature.

Overdosage: Adverse effects are rare when acetaminophen is used as recommended. However, massive overdose of acetaminophen may result in hepatic toxicity in some patients. In case of overdose, contact a physician or your local poison control center immediately.

Dosage and Administration: Adults: Two tablets or capsules (1,000 mg) every 4 hours as needed, up to 8 tablets or capsules in a 24 hour period unless directed otherwise by a physician.

How Supplied: Tablets (colored white, imprinted "Panadol" and "500")—bottles of 10, 30, 60, and 100; capsules (colored white and imprinted Panadol 500 mg)—bottles of 10, 24, 50 and 75. All packages are tamper resistant.

*Shown in Product Identification
Section, page 410*

PHILLIPS' MILK OF MAGNESIA

Composition: A suspension of magnesium hydroxide, meeting all USP specifications.

Action and Uses: Phillips' Milk of Magnesia is a mild saline laxative and is indicated for the relief of constipation especially in patients with hemorrhoids, obstetric patients, cardiacs, and in geriatric patients where straining at stool is contraindicated. Phillips' also acts as an antacid, and is effective for the relief of symptoms associated with gastric hyperacidity.

Administration and Dosage: As a laxative, adults 2 to 4 tbsp. followed by a glass of water. Children—infants 1 tsp.; over one year ¼ to ½ adult dose, depending on age. As a antacid, 1 to 3 tsps. with a little water, up to four times a day. Children—1 to 12 years: ¼ to ½ adult dose up to four times a day.

Caution: Habitual use of laxatives may result in dependence upon them. If pregnant or nursing, consult physician.

Continued on next page

Glenbrook—Cont.

Contraindications: Abdominal pain, nausea, vomiting or other symptoms of appendicitis. This product is not to be used by persons with kidney disease, except under the advice and supervision of a physician.

How Supplied: Phillips' Milk of Magnesia is available in regular and mint in bottles of:

Regular
4 fl. oz.	NDC-12843-353-01
12 fl. oz.	NDC-12843-353-02
26 fl. oz.	NDC-12843-353-03

Mint
4 fl. oz.	NDC-12843-363-04
12 fl. oz.	NDC-12843-363-05
26 fl. oz.	NDC-12843-363-06

Also available in tablet form.
Shown in Product Identification Section, page 410

STRI–DEX® REGULAR STRENGTH PADS and STRI–DEX® MAXIMUM STRENGTH PADS

Active Ingredients:
Stri-Dex® Regular Strength: Salicylic Acid 0.5%, Alcohol 28% by volume.
Stri-Dex® Maximum Strength: Salicylic Acid 2.0%, SD Alcohol 40 44%.

Indications: Topical medication for the treatment of acne vulgaris. These products also clean the skin and help remove oil. They penetrate pores to clear most blackheads and acne pimples and they help prevent new acne pimples from forming.
They are more efficacious than benzoyl peroxide in the treatment of mild to moderate acne vulgaris.

Warning: For external use only. Keep away from eyes. If skin irritation develops, discontinue use and consult physician. Occasional signs of dryness and peeling is one indication that Stri-Dex is working.

Dosage and Administration: See labeling instructions for use.

How Supplied:
Stri-Dex Regular Strengths—Plastic Jar/42 Pads, Plastic Jar/75 Pads
Stri-Dex Maximum Strength—Plastic Jar/42 Pads

VANQUISH®

Composition: Each Caplet contains aspirin 227 mg., acetaminophen 194 mg., caffeine 33 mg., dried aluminum hydroxide gel 25 mg.; magnesium hydroxide 50 mg.

Action and Uses: A buffered analgesic, antipyretic for relief of headache; muscular aches and pains; neuralgia and neuritic pain; pain following dental procedures; for painful discomforts and fever of colds and flu; functional menstrual pain, headache and pain due to cramps; temporary relief from minor pains of arthritis, rheumatism, bursitis, lumbago, sciatica.

Usual Adult Dosage: Two caplets with water. May be repeated every four hours if necessary up to 12 tablets per day. Larger or more frequent doses may be prescribed by physician if necessary.

Contraindications: Hypersensitivity to salicylates.
(To be used with caution during anticoagulant therapy or in asthmatic patients.)

How Supplied: White, capsule-shaped Caplets in bottles of:
15 Caplets NDC 12843-171-42
30 Caplets NDC 12843-171-44
60 Caplets NDC 12843-171-46
100 Caplets NDC 12843-171-48
Shown in Product Identification Section, page 410

Goody's Manufacturing Corporation
P.O. BOX 10518
WINSTON-SALEM, NC 27108

GOODY'S HEADACHE POWDERS

Active Ingredient: 520 mg. Aspirin, 260 mg. Acetaminophen, 32.5 mg. Caffeine per powder

Indications: For relief of pain due to simple headache, muscular aches and pains, headaches accompanying head colds.

Actions: Combination of active ingredients have analgesic, antipyretic and anti-inflammatory activity.

Warnings: Do not take more than recommended dosage or take regularly for more than 10 days without consulting your physician. Keep out of reach of children. In case of accidental overdose, contact a physician immediately. As with any drug, if you are pregnant or nursing a baby seek the advice of a health professional before using this product.

Symptoms and Treatment of Oral Overdosage: Symptoms consist of dizziness, ringing in the ears, nausea, diarrhea, incoherent speech, and coma. Treatment varies but drinking two glasses of milk will dilute and slow absorption. Activated charcoal may be given orally in a 5 ml/kg dose. Emptying the stomach is advised.

Dosage and Administration: Adults: one powder with water or other liquid. May be repeated in 3 or 4 hours. Do not take more than 4 powders in any 24 hour period. For children under 12, only as directed by a physician.

How Supplied: Available in 2 dose envelope, 6 dose small box, 24 and 50 dose carton. All tamper resistant cellophane wrapped.
Shown in Product Identification Section, page 410

Hoechst-Roussel Pharmaceuticals Inc.
SOMERVILLE, NJ 08876

DOXIDAN®
Laxative with Stool Softener

Active Ingredients: Doxidan is a combination of 60 mg docusate calcium USP, 50 mg danthron USP and up to 1.5% alcohol (w/w).

Actions: Doxidan has a highly effective stool softener and a mild peristaltic stimulant that acts mainly in the lower bowel. Due to the effectiveness of the stool softening component, Doxidan produces soft, formed, easily evacuated stools, with the least possible disturbance of normal body physiology.

Indications: Doxidan is a safe, gentle laxative for the management of constipation. It has proved clinically effective in the management of constipation in geriatric or inactive patients, obstetric patients, and following surgery, particularly anorectal procedures. It may be used as a safe and effective evacuant prior to x-ray examination of the colon in preparing patients for barium enema.

Warnings: Do not use when abdominal pain, nausea, or vomiting is present. Frequent or prolonged use of this preparation may result in dependence on laxatives. A harmless pink or orange discoloration may appear in urine. In some patients occasional cramping may occur. As with any drug, if you are pregnant or nursing a baby, seek the advice of a health professional before using this product. Keep this and all medication out of the reach of children.

Dosage and Administration: Adults and children over 12—one or two capsules daily. Children 6 to 12—one capsule daily. Best given at bedtime, Doxidan will usually provide a gentle evacuation in 8 to 12 hours. Dosage should be maintained for 2 to 3 days or until bowel movements return to normal. For use in children under 6, consult a physician.

How Supplied: Maroon, soft gelatin capsules—packages of 10 and 30, bottles of 100 and 1000, and Unit Dose 100s (10 × 10 strips).
Shown in Product Identification Section, page 410

FESTAL® II
Digestive Aid

Composition: Each enteric-coated tablet contains the following: Lipase 6,000 USP units, Amylase 30,000 USP units and Protease 20,000 USP units.

Actions and Uses: Festal® II provides a high degree of protected digestive activity in a formula of standardized enzymes. Enteric coating of the tablet prevents release of ingredients in the stomach so that high enzymatic potency is delivered to the site in the intestinal tract where digestion normally takes place.

Festal® II is indicated in any condition where normal digestion is impaired by insufficiency of natural digestive enzymes, or when additional digestive enzymes may be beneficial. These conditions often manifest complaints of discomfort due to excess intestinal gas, such as bloating, cramps and flatulence. The following are conditions or situations where Festal® II may be helpful: pancreatic insufficiency, chronic pancreatitis, pancreatic necrosis, and removal of gas prior to x-ray examination.

Dosage: Usual adult dose is one or two tablets with each meal, or as directed by a physician.

Contraindications: Festal® II should not be given to patients sensitive to protein of porcine origin.

How Supplied: Bottles of 100 and 500 white, enteric-coated tablets for oral use.
Shown in Product Identification Section, page 411

SURFAK®
Stool Softener

Active Ingredient: Each 240 mg capsule contains 240 mg docusate calcium USP and up to 3% alcohol (w/w). Each 50 mg capsule contains 50 mg docusate calcium USP and up to 1.3% alcohol (w/w).

Actions: Surfak provides homogenization and formation of soft, easily evacuated stools without disturbance of body physiology, discomfort of bowel distention or oily leakage. Surfak is non-habit forming.

Indications: Surfak is indicated for the prevention and treatment of constipation in conditions in which hard stools may cause discomfort, or in those conditions where laxative therapy is undesirable or contraindicated. Surfak is useful in patients who require only stool softening without propulsive action to accomplish defecation. Surfak does not cause peristaltic stimulation, and because of its safety it may be effectively used in patients with heart conditions, anorectal conditions, obstetrical patients, following surgical procedures, ulcerative colitis, diverticulitis and bedridden patients.

Warnings: Surfak has no known side effects or disadvantages, except for the unusual occurrence of mild, transitory cramping pains. If cramping pain occurs, discontinue the medication. As with any drug, if you are pregnant or nursing a baby, seek the advice of a health professional before using this product. Keep this and all medication out of reach of children.

Overdosage: Overdosage does not lead to systemic toxicity.

Dosage and Administration: Adults—one red 240 mg capsule daily for several days or until bowel movements are normal. Children and adults with minimal needs—one to three orange 50 mg capsules daily. For use in children under 6, consult a physician.

How Supplied: 240 mg red, soft gelatin capsules—packages of 7 and 30, bottles of 100 and 500, and Unit Dose 100s (10 × 10 strips); 50 mg orange, soft gelatin capsules—bottles of 30 and 100.
Shown in Product Identification Section, page 411

Holland-Rantos Company, Inc.
P.O. BOX 385
865 CENTENNIAL AVE.
PISCATAWAY, NJ 08854
See YOUNGS DRUG PRODUCTS CORPORATION

Hynson, Westcott & Dunning
Division of Becton Dickinson and Co.
CHARLES & CHASE STS.
BALTIMORE, MD 21201

LACTINEX® TABLETS AND GRANULES

Composition: A viable mixed culture of *Lactobacillus acidophilus* and *L. bulgaricus* with the naturally occurring metabolic products that are produced by these organisms.

Action and Uses: Lactinex has been found to be useful in the treatment of uncomplicated diarrhea (including that due to antibiotic therapy) and acute fever blisters (cold sores).

Indications and Dosage: (for adults and children):
Gastrointestinal Disturbances—4 tablets or 1 packet of granules added to or taken with cereal, food, milk, fruit juice or water; three or four times a day.
Fever Blisters (Cold Sores)—4 tablets or 1 packet of granules chewed and swallowed three or four times a day. Each dose may be followed by a small amount of milk, fruit juice or water.

Lactinex Must Be Refrigerated
Individuals sensitive to milk products should not use Lactinex.

How Supplied: Tablets—bottles of fifty (NDC 0011-8368-50). Granules, boxes of twelve, 1 gram packets (unit dose dispensing), (NDC 0011-8367-12).

Literature Available: On request.
Shown in Product Identification Section, page 411

Products are cross-indexed
by product classifications
in the
BLUE SECTION

Jeffrey Martin, Inc.
410 CLERMONT TERRACE
UNION, NJ 07083

AYDS®
Appetite Suppressant Candy

Active Ingredient: Each candy contains 5 mg. Benzocaine.

Indications: Helps control appetite to aid weight reduction when used in conjunction with reduced caloric intake described in the accompanying diet plan.

Warnings: Do not take this product for periods exceeding 3 months. Do not give this product to children under 12 years of age. Do not take this product if allergic to benzocaine.

Dosage and Administration: Adults: Eat two candies 30 minutes before each meal. Do not exceed nine (9) candies a day.

How Supplied: Consumer packs of 12, 48, and 96 pieces. Available in Vanilla, Chocolate, Chocolate mint, Butterscotch, Caramel, and Peanut Butter chewy flavors.

BANTRON®
Smoking Deterrent Tablets

Active Ingredient: Lobeline Sulfate Alkaloids 2 mg; Tribasic Calcium Phosphate 130 mg; Magnesium Carbonate 130 mg.

Indications: A temporary aid to breaking the cigarette habit.

Actions: Decreases the physical craving for nicotine.

Warnings: Neither smoking nor the use of Bantron is recommended during pregnancy. Keep out of reach of children.

Dosage and Administration: 1 tablet after each meal with half a glass of water for up to 6 weeks.

How Supplied: Consumer packages of 18 and 36 blister packed tablets.

COMPOZ®
Nighttime Sleep Aid

Active Ingredient: Diphenhydramine HCl 50 mg.

Indications: For relief of occasional sleeplessness.

Warnings: Do not give to children under 12 years of age. If sleeplessness persists more than 2 weeks, consult your physician. Do not take this product if you have asthma, glaucoma, or enlargement of the prostate gland, except under the advice and supervision of a physician. Keep out of reach of children.
Take this product with caution if alcohol is being consumed.

Dosage and Administration: 1 tablet at bedtime, or as directed by a physician.

How Supplied: Consumer packs of 24 blister packed tablets.

Continued on next page

Jeffrey Martin—Cont.

CUTICURA®
Antibacterial Medicated Soap

Active Ingredient: Triclocarban 1%.

Indications: Antibacterial soap.

Actions: Cuticura Medicated Soap cleans deep to remove unwanted oil, dirt, makeup and impurities. It removes excess oil from oily areas but won't dry your skin because it contains emollients to help dry skin areas stay soft, supple and moisturized.

Warnings: Do not use this product on infants under 6 months of age. For external use only. Keep out of reach of children.

Dosage and Administration: At least twice daily, lather with Cuticura and warm water. Rinse thoroughly with cool water.

How Supplied: 3.25 oz. and 5 oz. individually packaged bars.

DOAN'S® Backache Spray

Active Ingredient: Methyl Salicylate 15%; Menthol 8.4%; Methyl Nicotinate 0.6%.

Indications: For temporary relief of minor aches and pains of muscles and joints such as simple backache, lumbago, arthritis, neuralgia, strains, bruises and strains.

Actions: Analgesic and provides soothing warmth to painful muscles and joints.

Warnings: For external use only. Avoid spraying in eyes, face, genital and anal area. If condition worsens or if symptoms persist for more than 7 days, discontinue use of this product and consult a physician. Do not apply to wounds or damaged skin. Do not bandage. Contents under pressure. Do not puncture or incinerate. Do not store at temperatures above 120°F. Keep out of reach of children.

Precaution: Flammable. Do not use near fire or flame. Avoid using while smoking. Use only as directed. Intentional misuse by deliberately concentrating and inhaling contents can be harmful or fatal.

Dosage and Administration: For adults and children over 2 years of age. Point valve opening toward area of pain. Even works if can is upside down. Hold 6 inches from skin. Spray painful area no more than 3 or 4 times per day. For children under 2 years of age, there is no recommended dosage, except under the advice and supervision of a physician.

How Supplied: Aerosol can, Net wt. 4 oz.

DOAN'S® Pills

Active Ingredient: Each tablet contains magnesium salicylate 325 mg.

Indications: For temporary relief of headache, occasional minor aches and pains including muscular backache pain.

Warnings: If pain persists for more than 10 days, discontinue use and consult a physician. Do not take this product except under the advice and supervision of a physician for arthritis, or if you have kidney disease, or if you are allergic to salicylates. Stop taking this product if ringing in the ears or other symptoms occur. Keep out of reach of children.

Precaution: Do not take this product except under the advice and supervision of a physician during the last 3 months of pregnancy, *or* if you have stomach distress, ulcers, bleeding problems, *or* if you are presently taking a prescription for anticoagulation (thinning the blood), diabetes, gout or arthritis.

Dosage and Administration: To be taken by adults only. Take 2 tablets with a full glass of water every 4 hours. Do not exceed 12 pills during a 24 hour period.

How Supplied: Consumer packs of 24 and 48 blister packed tablets.

PORCELANA®
Skin Bleaching Agent

Active Ingredient: Regular: Hydroquinone 2.0 percent; Porcelana with Sunscreen: Hydroquinone 2.0 percent, Octyl dimethyl PABA 2.5%.

Indications: 1) For the gradual fading of "age spots", "liver spots", freckles and melasma (the "mask of pregnancy", a condition of the skin that may also result from use of oral contraceptives). 2) Lightens dark pigment in the skin.

Warnings: Sun exposure should be avoided to prevent darkening from recurring. Avoid contact with eyes. If skin irritation develops, use of this product should be discontinued or a physician consulted. If no improvement is seen after 3 months of treatment, use of this product should be discontinued. Not for use by children under 12. Keep out of reach of children.

Dosage and Administration: Apply a thin film morning and night to discolored area. May be used under makeup.

How Supplied: 2 oz and 4 oz regular; 4 oz sunscreen.

PURSETTES®
Premenstrual Tablets

Active Ingredient: Each tablet contains acetaminophen 500 mg; pamabrom 25 mg; pyrilamine maleate 15 mg.

Indications: For relief of the following symptoms associated with the premenstrual period: emotional changes such as anxiety; nervous tension; irritability; pain of cramps; backache; temporary water weight gain; bloating.

Warnings: If pain persists for more than 10 days, discontinue use and consult your physician. Do not exceed the recommended dosage because severe liver damage may occur. This preparation may cause drowsiness. Do not drive or operate machinery while taking this medication. As with any drug, if pregnant or nursing an infant, do not use this product without consulting a health professional. Keep out of the reach of children.

Dosage and Administration: Take 2 tablets at the first sign of premenstrual distress, followed by 2 tablets every 6 hours while symptoms persist or as directed by a physician. Do not exceed 8 tablets in a 24-hour period.

How Supplied: Consumer packs of 24 blister packed tablets.

Johnson & Johnson
Baby Products Company
GRANDVIEW ROAD
SKILLMAN, NJ 08558

JOHNSON'S BABY CREAM
SKIN PROTECTANT

Active Ingredients: Dimethicone 2%.

Other Ingredients: Water, Mineral Oil, Lanolin, White Wax, Paraffin, Synthetic Beeswax, Glyceryl Stearate, Ceresin, Sodium Borate, Propylparaben, Fragrance.

Indications: Helps prevent diaper rash by providing protection for more than 8 continuous hours against irritating wetness. Provides soothing relief of diaper rash and minor irritations such as chafed, chapped, cracked, windburned and sunburned skin.
Moisturizes to provide soothing relief and long lasting protection from skin dryness and roughness.

Actions: Protects injured or exposed skin or mucous membrane surface from harmful or annoying stimuli.

Warnings: For external use only. If condition worsens or does not improve within 7 days, consult a doctor. Not to be applied over deep or punctured wounds, infections, or lacerations. Avoid contact with eyes.

Directions: Apply liberally as often as necessary.

How Supplied: Available in 2 oz. plastic tube and in 4 oz. and 6 oz. plastic jars.
Shown in Product Identification Section, page 411

SUNDOWN® SUNSCREENS
WATERPROOF
LOTIONS
Moderate Protection (SPF 4)
Extra Protection (SPF 6)
Maximal Protection (SPF 8)
Ultra Protection (SPF 15)
STICKS
Sunscreen Stick (SPF 8)
Sunblock Stick (SPF 15)

LOTIONS	SPF	*PADIMATE O	OXYBENZONE
Moderate	4	3.3%	—
Extra	6	3.3%	1.0%
Maximal	8	4.75%	1.75%
Ultra	15	6.5%	3.0%
STICKS			
Maximal	8	5.3%	1.75%
Ultra	15	7.0%	3.0%

*Octyl Dimethyl PABA

Active Ingredients:
[See table above].

Indications: Sunscreens to help prevent harmful effects from the sun. The SPF values designate that the products provide 4, 6, 8, and 15 times your natural sunburn protection, respectively. SPF 4 and 6 permit tanning, SPF 8 permits minimal tanning and SPF 15 permits no tanning. All formulas are waterproof providing protection for at least 80 minutes in water and resist removal by sweating. All formulas are ideal for both adults and children, especially those with very active lifestyles. Liberal and regular use may help reduce the chance of premature aging and wrinkling of the skin and skin cancer due to overexposure to the sun.

Actions: Screens out Ultraviolet rays.

Warnings: For external use only. Avoid contact with eyes. In cases of accidental ocular instillation, flush eye(s) with lukewarm water or normal saline. Discontinue use if signs of irritation or rash appear. Use on children under 6 months of age only with the advice of physician. Keep out of reach of children.

Symptoms and Treatment of Accidental Ingestion: Should ingestion of less than 30 ml (1 oz.) by an average weight one year old child be known or suspected, encourage fluid intake to dilute product. If a larger quantity is suspected, observe and treat symptomatically. Consideration may be given to gastric lavage or emesis induction.

Dosage and Administration:
Lotion: Shake well. Apply generously and evenly to all exposed areas.
Stick: For spot applications, apply generously and evenly to nose, lips, face, ears and shoulders.
All formulas are waterproof but should be reapplied after 80 minutes in water or after excessive perspiration.

How Supplied: Lotion in 4 fl. oz. plastic bottles; Stick in 0.35 oz. tube.
Shown in Product Identification Section, page 411

Johnson & Johnson Products, Inc.
501 GEORGE STREET
NEW BRUNSWICK, NJ 08903

ATHLETICARE™ Pretaping Underwrap
Description: The AthletiCare™ Pretaping Underwrap is a thin, lightweight, high quality foam underwrap which consists of a very fine polyurethane film.

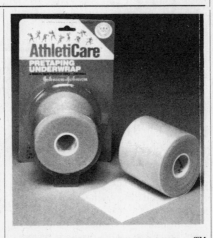

Actions and Uses: The AthletiCare™ Pretaping Underwrap is designed to assist in the application and removal of Sports Tape. It eliminates the need to shave before taping, allowing for painless removal of tape. It conforms easily to the skin, gives no restriction of motion, reduces friction and is easy to tear, apply and remove.

Directions: AthletiCare™ Pretaping Underwrap is applied directly to the skin. To remove, cut under tape and underwrap with scissors. The product must be used with tape.

How Supplied: The AthletiCare™ Pretaping Underwrap is sold in a roll that is 2¾ inches wide and 30 yards long. It is packaged in a blister-pack.

ATHLETICARE™ Sports Tape

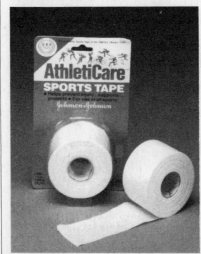

Description: Athleticare™ Sports Tape has a cloth backing and an adhesive that sticks firmly.

Actions and Uses: AthletiCare™ Sports Tape is indicated for use in wrapping hands, wrists, ankles, knees, fingers, etc. It is used to help prevent strains, sprains and fractures. It also helps speed recovery after injuries by providing support. Its porosity allows the skin to breath and moisture to escape. The tape has a number of secondary uses such as improving the grip on various sports equipment and securing protective padding, clothes and laces.

Precautions: Avoid ridges and lumps when tape is applied, to prevent irritation or blister formation. If a rash or irritation should occur, discontinue use of tape immediately. Tape applied too tightly can impede blood circulation.

Directions: Apply AthletiCare™ Sports Tape to skin that has been cleansed and is free from skin oil and hair. Tape directly from the roll. Apply smoothly and avoid excessive tightness. When used as a support, remove after each activity. The use of AthletiCare™ Pretaping Underwrap is recommended to assist in tape application and removal.

How Supplied: AthletiCare™ Sports Tape is sold in a roll that is 1½″ wide and 15 yards long. It is packaged in a blister-pack.

BIOCLUSIVE™
Transparent Dressing

Usage: For protection of post-surgical incisions, cuts, abrasions and blisters. Used in hospitals for prevention and treatment of pressure sores.
Provides an optimal wound healing environment.
- Breathes like skin.
- Waterproof barrier for protection of wound sites.
- Flexible to allow coverage of mobile body parts.
- Durable to protect against excessive friction.
- Hypo-Allergenic.
- For home and hospital use.

Precautions: Not to be used over dirty/contaminated wounds. Consult your physician if redness or inflammation occurs and also in cases of deep puncture wounds or serious burns.

Administration: Apply transparent dressing to clean, dry wound site.

Availability: 8—2 in. × 3 in. dressings per box; 2 six-packs per case.
Shown in Product Identification Section, page 411

Johnson & Johnson CLINICYDIN
Broad Spectrum Antibiotic Ointment

Each gram contains: Bacitracin, 400 units: Polymyxin B Sulfate, 5,000; Neomycin Sulfate (equiv. to 3.5 mg. Neomycin). 5mg.

Continued on next page

Johnson & Johnson—Cont.

Indications: Helps prevent infection and aids healing of minor cuts, scrapes and burns.

Warnings: For external use only. KEEP OUT OF REACH OF CHILDREN. In case of deep puncture wounds, serious burns, consult a physician.

Cautions: If redness, irritation, swelling or pain persists or increases or if infection occurs, discontinue use and consult a physician. Do not use in the eyes.

Directions: Apply to affected area 1–2 times daily and cover with a dry sterile dressing, if desired. Store at room temperature.

Shown in Product Identification Section, page 411

JOHNSON & JOHNSON FIRST AID CREAM
Skin Wound Protectant

Contains: Cetyl alcohol, Glyceryl stearate, Isopropyl palmitate, Stearyl alcohol, Synthetic beeswax as the skin wound protectants.

Indications: For minor cuts, scrapes and burns.

Actions: Helps protect minor skin wounds against contamination.

Cautions: Not for use on large, deep, or puncture wounds, serious burns or animal bites. If redness, irritation, swelling, or pain persists or increases, or if infection occurs, discontinue use and consult physician. Should not be used for more than ten days. If condition worsens or persists, see your physician. Not for use in eyes or on chronic skin conditions. KEEP OUT OF REACH OF CHILDREN.

Directions: For minor cuts and scrapes, first gently cleanse the area with mild soap and water, rinse and dry, and then smooth First Aid Cream gently over the affected area. Cover with a sterile dressing and tape securely.

Shown in Product Identification Section, page 411

K–Y® LUBRICATING JELLY
BACTERIOSTATIC K–Y® JELLY

Description: K-Y® Brand Lubricating Jelly is a greaseless, water-soluble jelly which is clear, spreads easily and is non-irritating.

Indications: K-Y® Jelly is indicated as a sexual lubricant which is safe and non-irritating for both men and women. It may also be used for easy insertion of rectal thermometers, tampons and other devices inserted into body cavities.

Actions: Helps lubricate body cavities for easier insertion. When used as a sexual lubricant, K-Y® Jelly helps overcome vaginal dryness caused by menopause, postnatal and psychological reasons.

Cautions: KEEP OUT OF EYES AND EARS. For external use only. Keep out of reach of children.

Directions: Apply to the area of insertion the desired amount of jelly and spread smoothly over the area. Repeat applications may be used.

How Supplied: Bacteriostatic K-Y® Jelly is available in 2 and 4 oz. tubes.
Shown in Product Identification Section, page 411

The Kendall Company
ONE FEDERAL STREET
BOSTON, MA 02101

DERMASSAGE® MEDICATED SKIN LOTION

Active Ingredient: 0.11% Menthol

Other Ingredient: Water, mineral oil, TEA-stearate, propylene glycol, stearic acid, diammonium phosphate, methylparaben, lanolin, triclosan, fragrance, urea, propylparaben.

Indications: Dermassage Medicated Skin Lotion is a rich, creamy formula that replaces lost moisture and helps soothe and smooth away rough, dry, chapped skin.

Actions: Dermassage Medicated Skin Lotion contains moisturizers and emollients that work deep into pores to soften the skin and prevent dryness from becoming soreness. The active ingredient (menthol) works as an anti-pruritic and a mild analgesic.

Contraindications: Sensitivity to any ingredient in this product.

Warnings: For External Use Only. Not for use on mucous membranes.

Dosage and Administration: Used daily Dermassage helps keep skin feeling soft and moist. Apply as desired to relieve the itching and irritation of dry, sore skin.

How Supplied:
6 oz.
10 oz.
15 oz.
Dermassage Medicated Skin Lotion is supplied in white opaque plastic bottles.

IDENTIFICATION PROBLEM?
Consult the
Product Identifcation Section
where you'll find
products pictured
in full color.

Kremers-Urban Company
See WILLIAM H. RORER, INC.

LactAid Inc.
600 FIRE ROAD
POST OFFICE BOX 111
PLEASANTVILLE, NJ
08232-0111

LACTAID®
LactAid liquid drops
and
LactAid Tablets
(lactase enzyme)

Description:
LIQUID: Each 5 drop dosage contains not less than 1000 NLU (Neutral Lactase Units) of Beta-D-galactosidase derived from Kluyveromyces lactis yeast. The enzyme is in a liquid carrier of glycerol (50%), water (30%), and inert yeast dry matter (20%). 4–5 drops hydrolyzes approximately 70% of the lactose in 1 quart of milk at refrigerator temperature, @ 42°F–6°C in 24 hours, or will do the same in 2 hours @ 85°F–30°C. Additional time and/or enzyme required for 100% lactose conversion. 1 U.S. quart of milk will contain approximately 50 gm lactose prior to lactose hydrolysis and will contain 15 gm or less, after 70% conversion.

Action: Hydrolysis converts the lactose into its simple sugar components: glucose and galactose.

Indications: Lactase insufficiency in the patient, suspected from g.i. disturbances after consumption of milk or milk content products: e.g., bloat, distension, flatulence, diarrhea; or identified by a lactose tolerance test.

Usage: Added to milk. 4–10 drops per quart of milk depending on level of lactose conversion desired.

Other Uses: In vivo activity has been demonstrated, indicating usage in tube feedings and other lactose-content solid and liquid foods, with addition at time of consumption.

How Supplied: Lactase enzyme in a stable liquid form, in sales units of 4, 12, 30 and 75 one-quart dosages at 5 drops per dose.
TABLETS: Each tablet contains not less than 3300 FCC lactase units of Beta-D-Galactosidase from Aspergillis oryzae. 1 to 2 tablets taken with a meal will normally handle a lactose challenge equal to 1 glass of milk. In severe cases, 3 tablets may be required.

How Supplied: In bottles of 100 and boxes of 12.

Toxicity: none.

Drug Interactions: none. Both liquid and tablets are classified as food, not drugs.

Precautions: Diabetics should be aware that the milk sugar will now be metabolically available and must be taken into account (25 gm glucose and 25 gm galactose per quart @ 100% hydrolysis). No reports received of any diabetics' reactions. Galactosemics may not have milk in any form, lactase enzyme modified or not.

Also in most areas of the U.S.: Fresh hydrolyzed lowfat milk from dairies, ready to drink, sold in food markets. Lactose hydrolysis level: 70%. If desired, further conversion of the dairy-treated milk can be done at home or institution with the LactAid liquid enzyme. Also in some areas: LactAid lactose reduced cottage cheese, American process cheese, ice cream.

Any person or institution unable to locate LactAid enzyme locally can order direct from LactAid Inc. retail or wholesale. Samples and full product information to doctors, institutions and nutritionists on request. Call toll-free 800-257-8650.

Shown in Product Identification Section, page 411

The Lannett Company, Inc.
9000 STATE ROAD
PHILADELPHIA, PA 19136

ACNEDERM™ LOTION

Composition: Grease-free, water-washable, non-staining suspension containing dispersible sulfur 5%, zinc sulfate 1% and zinc oxide 10% in a flesh-tinted powder foundation base. Isopropyl alcohol, 21% by volume.

Action and Uses: Medication of acne lesions. Combats oiliness of skin and excessive keratinization of sebaceous glands; promotes drying and peeling in acne, seborrheic dermatitis, rosacea, tinea corporis and tinea versicolor.

Administration and Dosage: Apply several times daily and at bedtime to affected areas, either with finger tips or sponge. Allow to dry and remove excess with powder puff or cleansing tissue.

Precautions: Discontinue treatment if excessive dryness or skin irritation occurs.

How Supplied: Bottles of 2 fl. oz.

Literature Available: Yes.

MAGNATRIL™ SUSPENSION AND TABLETS

Composition: Each tablet contains: Aluminum Hydroxide Gel (dried) 4 grs., Magnesium Trisilicate 7 grs., Magnesium Hydroxide 2 grs. Each teaspoonful of suspension contains: Colloidal suspension of Magnesium and Aluminum Hydroxides with 4 grs. Magnesium Trisilicate.

Action and Uses: Indicated to alleviate the symptoms of heartburn, sour stomach, and/or acid indigestion.

Drug Interaction Precautions: Do not take this product if you are presently taking a prescription of antibiotic drug containing any form of tetracycline.

Warning: Do not take more than 16 teaspoonsful in a 24 hour period, or use the maximum dosage of this product for more than 2 weeks, except under the advice and supervision of a physician. Do not use this product except under the advice and supervision of a physician if you have kidney disease.

Administration and Dosage: Tablets — Adults: 2 tablets well chewed, 1 or 2 hours following meals, or whenever symptoms are pronounced. Suspension —Adults, 1 to 4 teaspoonsful in water or milk four times a day, twenty minutes after meals and at bedtime, or as directed by a physician.

How Supplied: Tablets—Boxes of 50 and 100 cellophane-stripped tablets. Suspension—Bottles of 12 fl. oz.

Literature Available: Yes.

Lavoptik Company, Inc.
661 WESTERN AVENUE N.
ST. PAUL, MN 55103

LAVOPTIK® Eye Wash

Description: Isotonic LAVOPTIK Eye Wash is a buffered solution designed to help physically remove contaminants from the surface of the eye and lids. Formulated to buffer contaminants toward the safe range and help restore normal salts and water ratios in the tears.

Contents: Each 100 ml
Sodium Chloride	0.49 grams
Sodium Biphosphate	0.40 grams
Sodium Phosphate	0.45 grams
Preservative Agent	
Benzalkonium Chloride	0.005 grams

Precautions: If you experience severe eye pain, headache, rapid change in vision (side or straight ahead); sudden appearance of floating objects, acute redness of the eyes, pain on exposure to light or double vision consult a physician at once. If symptoms persist or worsen after use of this product, consult a physician. If solution changes color or becomes cloudy do not use. Keep this and all medicines out of reach of children. Keep container tightly closed. Do not use if safety seal is broken at time of purchase.

Administration: 6 ounce size with Eye Cup.
Rinse cup with clean water immediately before and after each use, avoid contamination of rim and inside surfaces of cup. Apply cup, half-filled with LAVOPTIK Eye Wash tightly to the eye. Tilt head backward. Open eyelids wide, rotate eyeball and blink several times to insure thorough washing. Discard washings. Repeat other eye. Tightly cap bottle. 32 ounce size.
Break seal as you remove cap and pour directly on contaminated area.

How Supplied: 6 ounce bottle with eyecup, NDC 10651-01040. 32 ounce bottle, NDC 10651-01019.

Lederle Laboratories
A Division of American Cyanamid Co.
WAYNE, NJ 07470

LEDERMARK®
Product Identification Code

Many Lederle tablets and capsules bear an identification code. A current listing appears in the Product Information Section of the 1985 PDR for Prescription Drugs.

CALTRATE™ 600
High Potency Calcium Supplement
Nature's Most Concentrated Form of Calcium™
No Sugar
No Salt
No Lactose
No Preservatives
Film-Coated for easy swallowing

ONE TABLET DAILY PROVIDES: 1500 mg CALCIUM CARBONATE which provides 600 mg elemental calcium
For Adults—
Percentage of U.S. Recommended Daily Allowance (U.S. RDA)
60%

Recommended Intake: One or two tablets daily or as directed by the physician.

Warnings: Keep this and all medications out of the reach of children.

How Supplied: Bottle of 60—NDC 0005-5510-19
Store at Controlled Room Temperature 15–30°C (59–86°F)
Shown in Product Identification Section, page 411

CALTRATE™ 600 + Vitamin D
High Potency Calcium Supplement
Nature's Most Concentrated Form of Calcium™
No Sugar
No Salt
No Lactose
No Preservatives
Film-Coated for easy swallowing

Active Ingredient: Calcium Carbonate–1500 mg

The information on each product appearing here is based on labelling effective in November, 1984 and is either the entire official brochure or an accurate condensation therefrom. Official brochures are enclosed in product packages. Information concerning all Lederle products may be obtained from the Professional Services Department, Lederle Laboratories, Pearl River, New York 10965.

Lederle—Cont.

Vitamin D–125 I.U.
ONE TABLET DAILY PROVIDES:

	Adults—U.S. RDA
1500 mg Calcium Carbonate which provides 600 mg elemental calcium	60%
Vitamin D 125 I.U.	31%

Recommended Intake: Minimum dosage one tablet daily, two or more as directed by the physician.
Keep out of the reach of children.
Store at Controlled Room Temperature 15-30° C (59-86° F).

How Supplied: Bottles of 60—
NDC-0005-5509-19
*Shown in Product Identification
Section, page 411*

CENTRUM®
High Potency
Multivitamin-Multimineral Formula,
Advanced Formula

Each tablet contains: For Adults

	Percentage of U.S. Recommended Daily Allowance (U.S. RDA)
Vitamin A (as Acetate)	5000 I.U. (100%)
Vitamin E (as dl-Alpha Tocopheryl Acetate)	30 I.U. (100%)
Vitamin C (as Ascorbic Acid)	90 mg (150%)
Folic Acid	400 mcg (100%)
Vitamin B_1 (as Thiamine Mononitrate)	2.25 mg (150%)
Vitamin B_2 (as Riboflavin)	2.6 mg (153%)
Niacinamide	20 mg (100%)
Vitamin B_6 (as Pyridoxine Hydrochloride)	3 mg (150%)
Vitamin B_{12} (as Cyanocobalamin)	9 mcg (150%)
Vitamin D	400 I.U. (100%)
Biotin	45 mcg (15%)
Pantothenic Acid (as Calcium Pantothenate)	10 mg (100%)
Calcium (as Tribasic Calcium Phosphate)	162 mg (16%)
Phosphorus (as Dibasic Calcium Phosphate)	125 mg (13%)
Iodine (as Potassium Iodide)	150 mcg (100%)
Iron (as Ferrous Fumarate)	27 mg (150%)
Magnesium (as Magnesium Oxide)	100 mg (25%)
Copper (as Cupric Oxide)	2 mg (100%)
Manganese (as Manganese Sulfate)	5 mg*
Potassium (as Potassium Chloride)	30 mg*
Chloride (as Potassium Chloride)	27.2 mg*
Chromium (as Chromium Chloride)	25 mcg*
Molybdenum (as Sodium Molybdate)	25 mcg*
Selenium (as Sodium Selenate)	25 mcg*
Zinc (as Zinc Sulfate)	15 mg (100%)

EACH TABLET CONTAINS:

VITAMINS	Quantity per tablet	Percentage of U.S. Recommended Daily Allowance (U.S. RDA) For Children 2 to 4 (½ tablet)	For Children Over 4 (1 tablet)
Vitamin A (as Acetate)	5,000 I.U.	(100%)	(100%)
Vitamin D	400 I.U.	(50%)	(100%)
Vitamin E (as Acetate)	30 I.U.	(150%)	(100%)
Vitamin C (as Ascorbic Acid and Sodium Ascorbate)	300 mg	(375%)	(500%)
Folic Acid	400 mcg	(100%)	(100%)
Biotin	45 mcg	(15%)	(15%)
Thiamine (as Thiamine Mononitrate)	1.5 mg	(107%)	(100%)
Pantothenic Acid (as Calcium Pantothenate)	10 mg	(100%)	(100%)
Riboflavin	1.7 mg	(107%)	(100%)
Niacinamide	20 mg	(111%)	(100%)
Vitamin B_6 (as Pyridoxine Hydrochloride)	2 mg	(143%)	(100%)
Vitamin B_{12} (as Cyanocobalamin)	6 mcg	(100%)	(100%)
Vitamin K_1 (as Phytonadione)	10 mcg*		
MINERALS			
Iron (as Ferrous Fumarate)	18 mg	(90%)	(100%)
Magnesium (as Magnesium Oxide)	40 mg	(10%)	(10%)
Iodine (as Potassium Iodide)	150 mcg	(107%)	(100%)
Copper (as Cupric Oxide)	2 mg	(100%)	(100%)
Phosphorous (as Tribasic Calcium Phosphate)	50 mg	(6.25%)	(5.0%)
Calcium (as Tribasic Calcium Phosphate)	108 mg	(13.5%)	(10.8%)
Zinc (as Zinc Oxide)	15 mg	(93%)	(100%)
Manganese (as Manganese Sulfate)	1 mg*		
Molybdenum (as Sodium Molybdate)	20 mcg*		
Chromium (as Chromium Chloride)	20 mcg*		

*Recognized as essential in human nutrition but no U.S. RDA established.

Vitamin K_1 25 mcg*
(as Phytonadione)
*Recognized as essential in human nutrition, but no U.S. RDA established.

Recommended Intake: Adults, 1 tablet daily.

How Supplied:
Capsule-shaped tablets, light peach, engraved LL—Embossed C1 Combopack*
NDC 0005-4239-30
*Bottles of 100 plus 30
Store at Controlled Room Temperature
15–30℃ (59–86°F)
*Shown in Product Identification
Section, page 411*

ADVANCED FORMULA
CENTRUM, Jr.®
CHILDREN'S CHEWABLE
Vitamin/Mineral Formula+EXTRA C

[See table below].

Warnings: CONTAINS IRON, WHICH CAN BE HARMFUL IN LARGE DOSES. CLOSE TIGHTLY AND KEEP OUT OF THE REACH OF CHILDREN. IN CASE OF ACCIDENTAL OVERDOSE, CONTACT A PHYSICIAN OR POISON CONTROL CENTER IMMEDIATELY.
Store at Controlled Room Temperature 15–30° C (59–86° F).

How Supplied: Bottle of 60
NDC 0005-4249-19
*Shown in Product Identification
Section, page 412*

CENTRUM Jr.®
Children's Chewable
Vitamin/Mineral Formula + Iron
Tablets

Each tablet contains:
[See table on next page].

Recommended Intake: 2 to 4 years of age: Chew one-half tablet daily. Over 4 years of age: Chew one tablet daily. CONTAINS IRON, WHICH CAN BE HARMFUL IN LARGE DOSES. CLOSE TIGHTLY AND KEEP OUT OF THE REACH OF CHILDREN. IN CASE OF ACCIDENTAL OVERDOSE, CONTACT A PHYSICIAN OR POISON CONTROL CENTER IMMEDIATELY.

How Supplied: Assorted Flavors —Uncoated Tablet—Partially Scored —Engraved Lederle C2 and CENTRUM, JR. Bottles of 60 NDC 0005-4234-19
*Shown in Product Identification
Section, page 411*

FERRO-SEQUELS®
sustained release iron
Capsules

Composition: Each capsule contains 150 mg. of ferrous fumarate equivalent to approximately 50 mg. of elemental iron, so prepared that it is released over a 5 to 6 hour period, and 100 mg. of docusate sodium (DSS) to counteract constipating effect of iron.

Indications: For the treatment of iron deficiency anemias.

	Quantity per tablet	Percentage of U.S. Recommended Daily Allowance (U.S. RDA)	
		For Children 2 to 4 (½ tablet)	For Children Over 4 (1 tablet)
VITAMINS			
Vitamin A (as Acetate)	5,000 I.U.	(100%)	(100%)
Vitamin D	400 I.U.	(50%)	(100%)
Vitamin E (as Acetate)	15 I.U.	(75%)	(50%)
Vitamin C (as Ascorbic Acid and Sodium Ascorbate)	60 mg	(75%)	(100%)
Folic Acid	400 mcg	(100%)	(100%)
Biotin	45 mcg	(15%)	(15%)
Thiamine (as Thiamine Mononitrate)	1.5 mg	(107%)	(100%)
Pantothenic Acid (as Calcium Pantothenate)	10 mg	(100%)	(100%)
Riboflavin	1.7 mg	(107%)	(100%)
Niacinamide	20 mg	(111%)	(100%)
Vitamin B_6 (as Pyridoxine Hydrochloride)	2 mg	(143%)	(100%)
Vitamin B_{12} (as Cyanocobalamin)	6 mcg	(100%)	(100%)
MINERALS			
Iron (as Ferrous Fumarate)	18 mg	(90%)	(100%)
Magnesium (as Magnesium Oxide)	25 mg	(6.25%)	(6.25%)
Iodine (as Potassium Iodide)	150 mcg	(107%)	(100%)
Copper (as Cupric Oxide)	2 mg	(100%)	(100%)
Zinc (as Zinc Oxide)	10 mg	(62%)	(67%)
Manganese (as Manganese Sulfate)	1 mg*		
Molybedenum (as Sodium Molybdate)	20 mcg*		
Chromium (as Chromium Chloride)	20 mcg*		

*Recognized as essential in human nutrition but no U.S. RDA established

Dosage: 1 capsule, once or twice daily or as prescribed by the physician.

Warning: As with any drug, if you are pregnant or nursing a baby, seek the advice of a health professional before using this product. Keep this and all medications out of the reach of children. In case of accidental overdose, seek professional assistance or contact a Poison Control Center immediately.

How Supplied: Capsules (green) printed Lederle and FERRO-SEQUELS® F2
Bottle of 30—NDC 0005-4612-13
Bottle of 100—NDC 0005-4612-23
Unit Dose Pkg., 10-10's—NDC 0005-4612-60
Bottle of 1,000—NDC 0005-4612-34
Store at Controlled Room Temperature 15–30° C (59–86° F)
Military and USPHS Depots:
NSN 6505-00-149-0103, 30's
NSN 6505-00-074-2981, 1000's
NSN 6505-00-131-8870, individually sealed 100's
Shown in product Identification Section, page 412

FILIBON®
prenatal tablets

Each tablet contains:

	For Pregnant or Lactating Women Percentage of U.S. Recommended Daily Allowance (U.S. RDA)
Vitamin A (as Acetate)	5000 I.U. (63%)
Vitamin D_2	400 I.U. (100%)
Vitamin E (as dl-Alpha Tocopheryl Acetate)	30 I.U. (100%)
Vitamin C (Ascorbic Acid)	60 mg (100%)
Folic Acid (Folacin)	0.4 mg (50%)
Vitamin B_1 (as Thiamine Mononitrate)	1.5 mg (88%)
Vitamin B_2 (as Riboflavin)	1.7 mg (85%)
Niacinamide	20 mg (100%)
Vitamin B_6 (as Pyridoxine Hydrochloride)	2 mg (80%)
Vitamin B_{12} (as Cyanocobalamin)	6 mcg (75%)
Calcium (as Calcium Carbonate)	125 mg (10%)
Iodine (as Potassium Iodide)	150 mcg (100%)
Iron (as Ferrous Fumarate)	18 mg (100%)
Magnesium (as Magnesium Oxide)	100 mg (22%)

A phosphorus-free vitamin and mineral dietary supplement for use in prenatal care and lactation.

Recommended Intake: 1 daily, or as prescribed by the physician.

How Supplied: Capsule-shaped tablets (film-coated, pink) engraved LL F4—bottles of 100 NDC-0005-4294-23

FOOTWORK™
Athlete's Foot Remedy

Indications: FOOTWORK™ Antifungal Remedy is clinically proven effective in the treatment and prevention of athlete's foot, jock itch, and ringworm. Soothing relief of itching, scaling, burning and discomfort that can accompany these conditions begins within 24 hours. FOOTWORK spray powder and powder also keep feet dry and comfortable with daily use.

Directions: Cleanse skin with soap and water and dry thoroughly.
Cream: Apply a thin layer over affected area morning and night or as directed by a doctor.
Powder: Sprinkle powder liberally over affected area morning and night or as directed by a doctor.
Solution: Apply two or three drops and massage gently to cover the affected area morning and night or as directed by a doctor.
Aerosol Powder: SHAKE WELL BEFORE USING. Cleanse skin with soap and water and dry thoroughly. Spray powder liberally over affected area morning and night or as directed by a doctor.

For athlete's foot, pay special attention to the spaces between the toes. Use FOOTWORK daily to prevent reinfection.

Warning: Do not use on children under two years of age except under the advice and supervision of a doctor. Children under 12 years of age should be supervised in the use of this product. For external use only. If irritation occurs or if there is no improvement within 4 weeks (for athlete's foot or ringworm) or within two weeks (for jock itch), discontinue use and consult a doctor or pharmacist. This product is not effective on the scalp or nails. Keep this and all drugs out of the reach of children. In case of accidental ingestion, seek professional assistance or contact a Poison Control Center immediately.

Caution: *Aerosol Powder:* FLAMMABLE. Avoid spraying into eyes. Contents under pressure. Do not puncture or incinerate or store at a temperature above 120° F (49° C). Use only as directed. Intentional misuse by deliberately concentrating and inhaling aerosol products can be harmful or fatal. Do not use near flame or spark or while smoking.

Continued on next page

Lederle—Cont.

DO NOT FREEZE. Store at Controlled Room Temperature 15–30° C (59–86° F).

Active Ingredient: Tolnaftate 1% Contains 15% alcohol.

How Supplied: Cream: 1.0 oz tube (28.5 g)
NDC 0005-2610-32
0.5 oz. tube (15 g)
NDC 0005-2610-09
Powder: 2.75 oz squeeze bottle (78 g)
NDC 0005-2614-70
Solution: $\frac{1}{3}$ oz bottle (10 ml)
NDC 0005-2611-34
Aerosol Powder: 3.5 oz. spray can (100 g)
NDC 0005-2613-69
Shown in Product Identification Section, page 412

GEVRABON®
vitamin-mineral supplement

Composition: Each fluid ounce (30 ml.) contains:

	For Adults Percentage of U.S. Recommended Daily Allowance (U.S. RDA)
Vitamin B₁ (as Thiamine Hydrochloride)	5 mg (333%)
Vitamin B₂ (as Riboflavin-5-Phosphate Sodium)	2.5 mg (147%)
Niacinamide	50 mg (250%)
Vitamin B₆ (Pyridoxine Hydrochloride)	1 mg (50%)
Vitamin B₁₂ (as Cyanocobalamin)	1 mcg (17%)
Pantothenic Acid (as D-Pantothenyl Alcohol)	10 mg (100%)
Iodine (as Potassium Iodide)	100 mcg (67%)
Iron (as Ferrous Gluconate)	15 mg (83%)
Magnesium (as Magnesium Chloride)	2 mg (0.5%)
Zinc (as Zinc Chloride)	2 mg (13%)
Inositol	100 mg*
Choline (as Tricholine Citrate)	100 mg.*
Manganese (as Manganese Chloride)	2 mg.*

Alcohol 18%
*Recognized as essential in human nutrition but no U.S. RDA established.

Indications: For use as a nutritional supplement.

Caution: If Pregnant Or Nursing, Consult Your Physician Or Pharmacist Before Taking This Or Any Medicine. Keep this preparation out of the reach of children.

Administration and Dosage: Adult: One ounce (30 ml.) daily or as prescribed by the physician as a nutritional supplement.

Important Note: In time a slight natural deposit, characteristic of the sherry wine base, may occur. This does not indicate in any way a loss of quality.

How Supplied: Syrup (sherry flavor) decanters of 16 fl. oz. NDC 0005-5110-35

Bottles of 1 Gallon—NDC 0005-5110-73
Keep Out of Direct Sunlight
Store at controlled room temperature 15–30°C (59–86°F)
DO NOT FREEZE
VA Depots:
NSN 6505-01-091-7541A

GEVRAL®
Multivitamin and Multimineral Supplement
TABLETS

Composition: Each tablet contains:

	For Adults Percentage of U.S. Recommended Daily Allowance (U.S. RDA)
Vitamin A (as Acetate)	5000 I.U. (100%)
Vitamin E (as *dl*-Alpha Tocopheryl Acetate)	30 I.U. (100%)
Vitamin C (as Ascorbic Acid)	60 mg (100%)
Folic Acid	0.4 mg (100%)
Vitamin B₁ (as Thiamine Mononitrate)	1.5 mg (100%)
Vitamin B₂ (as Riboflavin)	1.7 mg (100%)
Niacinaminde	20 mg (100%)
Vitamin B₆ (as Pyridoxine Hydrochloride)	2 mg (100%)
Vitamin B₁₂ (as Cyanocobalamin)	6 mcg (100%)
Calcium (as Dibasic Calcium Phosphate)	162 mg (16%)
Phosphorus (as Dibasic Calcium Phosphate)	125 mg (13%)
Iodine (as Potassium Iodide)	150 mcg (100%)
Iron (as Ferrous Fumarate)	18 mg (100%)
Magnesium (as Magnesium Oxide)	100 mg (25%)

Indications: Supplementation of the diet.

Administration and Dosage: One tablet daily or as prescribed by the physician.
Keep this and all medications out of the reach of children.

How Supplied: Tablets (film-coated, brown) engraved LL G1—bottle of 100
NDC 0005-4289-23
Store at Controlled Room Temperature 15–30°C (59–86°F)
A SPECTRUM® Product

GEVRAL® T
High Potency Multivitamin and Multimineral Supplement
TABLETS

Each tablet contains:

	Percentage of U.S. Recommended Daily Allowance (U.S. RDA)
Vitamin A (as Acetate)	5000 I.U. (100%)
Vitamin E (as *dl*-Alpha Tocopheryl Acetate)	45 I.U. (150%)
Vitamin C (as Ascorbic Acid)	90 mg (150%)
Folic Acid	0.4 mg (100%)
Vitamin B₁ (as Thiamine Mononitrate)	2.25 mg (150%)
Vitamin B₂ (as Riboflavin)	2.6 mg (153%)
Niacinamide	30 mg (150%)
Vitamin B₆ (as Pyridoxine Hydrochloride)	3 mg (150%)
Vitamin B₁₂ (as Cyanocobalamin)	9 mcg (150%)
Vitamin D₂	400 I.U. (100%)
Calcium (as Dibasic Calcium Phosphate)	162 mg (16%)
Phosphorus (as Dibasic Calcium Phosphate)	125 mg (13%)
Iodine (as Potassium Iodide)	225 mcg (150%)
Iron (as Ferrous Fumarate)	27 mg (150%)
Magnesium (as Magnesium Oxide)	100 mg (25%)
Copper (as Cupric oxide)	1.5 mg (75%)
Zinc (as Zinc Oxide)	22.5 mg (150%)

Indications: For the treatment of vitamin and mineral deficiencies.

Dosage: 1 tablet daily or as prescribed by physician.
Keep this and all medications out of the reach of children.

How Supplied: Tablets (film coated, maroon). Printed LL G2—bottle of 100
NDC 0005-4286-23
Store at Controlled Room Temperature 15–30°C (59–86°F)
A SPECTRUM® Product

INCREMIN®
WITH IRON SYRUP
Vitamins + Iron
DIETARY SUPPLEMENT
(Cherry Flavored)

Composition: Each teaspoonful (5 ml.) contains:

Elemental Iron (as Ferric Pyrophosphate)	30 mg
L-Lysine HCl	300 mg
Thiamine HCl (B₁)	10 mg
Pyridoxine HCl (B₆)	5 mg
Vitamin B₁₂ (Cyanocobalamin)	25 mcgm
Sorbitol	3.50 Gm
Alcohol	0.75%

Each teaspoonful (5 ml.) supplies the following Minimum Daily Requirements:

	Child under 6	Child over 6	Adult
Vitamin B₁	20 MDR	13⅓ MDR	10 MDR
Iron	4 MDR	3 MDR	3 MDR

Indications: For the prevention and treatment of iron deficiency anemia in children and adults.

Warning: As with any drug, if you are pregnant or nursing a baby, seek the advice of a health professional before using this product.
Keep this and all medications out of the reach of children.

Administration and Dosage: or as prescribed by a physician.

Children: One teaspoonful (5 ml) daily for the prevention of iron deficiency anemia.

Adults: One teaspoonful (5 ml) daily for the prevention of iron deficiency anemia.

Notice: To protect from light always dispense in this container or in an amber bottle.

Store at Controlled Room Temperature 15–30° C (59–86° F)

How Supplied: Syrup (cherry flavor)—bottles of 4 fl. oz.—NDC 0005-5604-58 and 16 fl. oz.—NDC 0005-5604-65
Store at Controlled Room Temperature 15–30°C (59–86°F)

LEDERPLEX®
Dietary Supplement of B-Complex Vitamins for Adults and Children 4 or More Years of Age
Capsules—Liquid

Each Capsule or Tablet Contains:
For Adults-
Percentage of U.S.
Recommended Daily
Allowance (U.S. RDA)

Vitamin B_1 (as Thiamine
  Hydrochloride) .... 2.25 mg (150%)
Vitamin B_2 (as
  Riboflavin) .... 2.6 mg (153%)
Niacinamide .... 30 mg (150%)
Vitamin B_6 (as Pyridoxine
  Hydrochloride) .... 3 mg (150%)
Vitamin B_{12} (as
  Cyanocobalamin) .... 9 mcg (150%)
Pantothenic Acid (as Cal-
  cium Pantothenate) ... 15 mg (150%)

Indications: For the prevention of Vitamin B complex deficiencies.

Dosage: *Children*—1 capsule daily.
Adults—1 or 2 capsules daily.

Each 10 ml (2 teaspoonfuls) contains:

Vitamin B_1 (as Thiamine
  Mononitrate) .... 2.25 mg (150%)
Vitamin B_2 (Riboflavin) 2.6 mg (153%)
Niacinamide .... 30 mg (150%)
Vitamin B_6 (as Pyridoxine
  Hydrochloride) .... 3 mg (150%)
Vitamin B_{12} (as
  Cobalamin) .... 9 mcg (150%)
Pantothenic Acid (as
  Panthenol) .... 15 mg (150%)

Indications: For the prevention of Vitamin B complex deficiencies:
KEEP COLD TO ENHANCE FLAVOR

Recommended intake:
Adults—10 ml. or 2 teaspoonfuls daily. Keep this and all medications out of the reach of children.

How Supplied: Capsules (hard shell, brown) L6—bottles of 100. NDC-0005-4280-23 Liquid (orange flavor)—bottles of 12 fl. oz. NDC 0005-4299-63
Store at Controlled Room Temperature 15–30°C (59–86°F)

NEOLOID®
emulsified castor oil

Composition: NEOLOID Emulsified Castor Oil USP 36.4% (w/w) with 0.1% (w/w) Sodium Benzoate and 0.2% (w/w)

Potassium Sorbate added as preservatives, emulsifying and flavoring agents in water. NEOLOID is an emulsion with an exceptionally bland, pleasant taste.

Indications: For the treatment of isolated bouts of constipation.
SHAKE WELL

Administration and Dosage:
Infants—½ to 1½ teaspoonfuls.
Children—Adjust between infant and adult dose.
Adult—Average dose, 2 to 4 tablespoonfuls.

Precautions: Not to be used when abdominal pain, nausea, vomiting, or other symptoms of appendicitis are present. Frequent or continued use of this preparation may result in dependence on laxatives. Do not use during pregnancy except on a physician's advice. Keep this and all drugs out of the reach of children.

Warning: As with any drug, if you are pregnant or nursing a baby, seek the advice of a health professional before using this product. In case of accidental overdose, seek professional assistance or contact a Poison Control Center immediately.

How Supplied: Bottles of 4 fl. oz. (peppermint flavor) NDC-0005-5442-58
Store at Controlled Room Temperature 15–30°C (59–86°F)
DO NOT FREEZE

PERITINIC®
hematinic with vitamins and fecal softener
Tablets

Each tablet contains:
Elemental Iron
  (as Ferrous Fumarate) ....100 mg.
Docusate Sodium U.S.P. (DSS)
  (to counteract the con-
  constipating effect of iron) ......100 mg.
Vitamin B_1
  (as Thiamine Mononitrate) ......7.5 mg.
  (7 ½ MDR)
Vitamin B_2 (Riboflavin) ....7.5 mg.
  (6¼ MDR)
Vitamin B_6
  (Pyridoxine Hydrochloride) ....7.5 mg.
Vitamin B_{12}
  (Cyanocobalamin) ....50 mcg.
Vitamin C (Ascorbic Acid) ....200 mg.
  (6⅔ MDR)
Niacinamide (3 MDR) ....30 mg.
Folic Acid ....0.05 mg.
Pantothenic Acid
  (as D-Pantothenyl Alcohol) ....15 mg.
MDR—Adult Minimum Daily Requirement

Warning: As with any drug, if you are pregnant or nursing a baby, seek the advice of a health professional before using this product. In case of accidental overdose, seek professional assistance or contact a Poison Control Center immediately. Keep out of the reach of children.

Action and Uses: In the prevention of nutritional anemias, certain vitamin deficiencies, and iron-deficiency anemias.

Administration and Dosage:
Adults: 1 or 2 tablets daily.

How Supplied: Tablets (maroon, capsule-shaped, film coated) P8—bottles of 60 NDC 0005-5124-19

SPARTUS®
High Potency Vitamins & Minerals plus Electrolytes

Each tablet contains:
For Adults
Percentage of U.S.
Recommended Daily
Allowance (U.S. RDA)

Vitamin A   5000 I.U. (100%)
  (as Acetate)
Vitamin E   30 I.U. (100%)
  (as *dl*-Alpha Tocopheryl Acetate)
Vitamin C   300 mg (500%)
  (as Ascorbic Acid)
Folic Acid   400 mcg (100%)
  (as Folacin)
Vitamin B_1 7.5 mg (500%)
  (as Thiamine Mononitrate)
Vitamin B_2 8.5 mg (500%)
  (as Riboflavin)
Niacinamide   100 mg (500%)
Vitamin B_6 10 mg (500%)
  (as Pyridoxine Hydrochloride)
Vitamin B_{12} 30 mcg (500%)
  (as Cyanocobalamin)
Vitamin D   400 I.U. (100%)
Biotin   45 mcg (15%)
Pantothenic Acid   25 mg (250%)
  (as Calcium Pantothenate)
Iodine   150 mcg (100%)
  (as Potassium Iodide)
Magnesium   100 mg (25%)
  (as Magnesium Oxide)
Copper   2 mg (100%)
  (as Cupric Oxide)
Chromium   25 mcg*
  (as Chromium Chloride)
Molybdenum   25 mcg*
  (as Sodium Molybdate)
Selenium   25 mcg*
  (as Sodium Selenate)
Manganese   5 mg*
  (as Manganese Sulfate)
Potassium   40 mg*
  (as Potassium Chloride)
Chloride   36.3 mg*
  (as Potassium Chloride)
Zinc   15 mg (100%)
  (as Zinc Oxide)
Calcium   162 mg (16%)
  (as Calcium Phosphate)
Phosphorus   75 mg (8%)
  (as Calcium Phosphate)

Continued on next page

The information on each product appearing here is based on labelling effective in November, 1984 and is either the entire official brochure or an accurate condensation therefrom. Official brochures are enclosed in product packages. Information concerning all Lederle products may be obtained from the Professional Services Department, Lederle Laboratories, Pearl River, New York 10965.

Lederle—Cont.

*Recognized as essential in human nutrition, but no U.S. RDA established.

Warnings: Keep this and all medications out of the reach of children.

Recommended Intake: Adults, 1 tablet daily or as directed by the physician.

How Supplied: Blue, oval, scored engraved LL and S22. Bottle of 60—NDC 0005-4129-19

Store at Controlled Room Temperature 15–30° C (59–86° F)

Shown in Product Identification Section, page 412

LEDERLE LABORATORIES DIVISION
American Cyanamid Company,
Pearl River, N.Y. 10965

SPARTUS® + IRON
High Potency Vitamins & Minerals plus Electrolytes

Each tablet contains:

	For Adults Percentage of U.S. Recommended Daily Allowance (U.S. RDA)
Vitamin A (as Acetate)	5000 I.U. (100%)
Vitamin E (as *dl*-Alpha Tocopheryl Acetate)	30 I.U. (100%)
Vitamin C (as Ascorbic Acid)	300 mg (500%)
Folic Acid (as Folacin)	400 mcg (100%)
Vitamin B₁ (as Thiamine Mononitrate)	7.5 mg (500%)
Vitamin B₂ (as Riboflavin)	8.5 mg (500%)
Niacinamide	100 mg (500%)
Vitamin B₆ (as Pyridoxine Hydrochloride)	10 mg (500%)
Vitamin B₁₂ (as Cyanocobalamin)	30 mcg (500%)
Vitamin D	400 I.U. (100%)
Biotin	45 mcg (15%)
Pantothenic Acid (as Calcium Pantothenate)	25 mg (250%)
Iodine (as Potassium Iodide)	150 mcg (100%)
Iron (as Ferrous Fumarate)	27 mg (150%)
Magnesium (as Magnesium Oxide)	100 mg (25%)
Copper (as Cupric Oxide)	2 mg (100%)
Chromium (as Chromium Chloride)	25 mcg*
Molybdenum (as Sodium Molybdate)	25 mcg*
Selenium (as Sodium Selenate)	25 mcg*
Manganese (as Manganese Sulfate)	5 mg*
Potassium (as Potassium Chloride)	40 mg*
Chloride (as Potassium Chloride)	36.3 mg*
Zinc (as Zinc Oxide)	15 mg (100%)
Calcium (as Calcium Phosphate)	162 mg (16%)
Phosphorus (as Calcium Phosphate)	75 mg (8%)

*Recognized as essential in human nutrition, but no U.S. RDA established.

Warnings: Keep this and all medications out of the reach of children.

Recommended Intake: Adults, 1 tablet daily or as directed by the physician.

How Supplied: Bottle of 60—NDC 0005-4130-19

Store at Controlled Room Temperature 15–30° C (59–86° F)

Shown in Product Identification Section, page 412

LEDERLE LABORATORIES DIVISION
American Cyanamid Company,
Pearl River, N.Y. 10965

STRESSCAPS®
Stress formula B+C vitamins

Each capsule contains:

	For Adults-Percentage of U.S. Recommended Daily Allowance (U.S. RDA)
Vitamin B₁ (as Thiamine Mononitrate)	10 mg (667%)
Vitamin B₂ (as Riboflavin)	10 mg (588%)
Vitamin B₆ (as Pyridoxine Hydrochloride)	2 mg (100%)
Vitamin B₁₂ (as Cyanocobalamin)	6 mcg (100%)
Vitamin C (as Ascorbic Acid)	300 mg (500%)
Niacinamide	100 mg (500%)
Pantothenic Acid (as Calcium Pantothenate)	20 mg (200%)

Indications: For the treatment of vitamin deficiencies.

Dosage and Administration: Adults, 1 capsule daily or as directed by the physician.

How Supplied: *Capsules* (hard shell, opaque brown) printed Lederle S5—Bottle of 30—NDC 0005-4205-13
Bottle of 100—NDC 0005-4205-23

STRESSTABS® 600 Advanced Formula
High Potency
Stress Formula Vitamins

Each tablet contains:

	For Adults-Percentage of U.S. Recommended Daily Allowance (U.S. RDA)
Vitamin E (as *dl*-Alpha Tocopheryl Acetate)	30 I.U. (100%)
Vitamin C (L-Ascorbic Acid)	600 mg (1000%)
B VITAMINS	
Folic Acid	400 mcg (100%)
Vitamin B₁ (as Thiamine Mononitrate)	15 mg (1000%)
Vitamin B₂ (as Riboflavin)	15 mg (882%)
Niacinamide	100 mg (500%)
Vitamin B₆ (as Pyridoxine Hydrochloride)	5 mg (250%)
Vitamin B₁₂ (as Cyanocobalamin)	12 mcg (200%)
Biotin	45 mcg (15%)
Pantothenic Acid (as Calcium Pantothenate USP)	20 mg (200%)

Recommended Intake: Adults, 1 tablet daily or as directed by physician.

Supplied:
Bottle of 30—NDC 0005-4124-13
Bottle of 60—NDC 0005-4124-19
Unit Dose 10 × 10's —NDC 0005-4124-60

Shown in Product Identification Section, page 412

STRESSTABS® 600 with IRON
Advanced Formula
High Potency
Stress Formula Vitamins

Each tablet contains:

	For Adults-Percentage of U.S. Recommended Daily Allowance (U.S. RDA)
Vitamin E (as *dl*-Alpha Tocopheryl Acetate)	30 I.U. (100%)
Vitamin C (L-Ascorbic Acid)	600 mg (1000%)
B VITAMINS	
Folic Acid	400 mcg (100%)
Vitamin B₁ (as Thiamine Mononitrate)	15 mg (1000%)
Vitamin B₂ (as Riboflavin)	15 mg (882%)
Niacinamide	100 mg (500%)
Vitamin B₆ (as Pyridoxine Hydrochloride)	5 mg (250%)
Vitamin B₁₂ (as Cyanocobalamin)	12 mcg (200%)
Biotin	45 mcg (15%)
Pantothenic Acid (as Calcium Pantothenate USP)	20 mg (200%)
Iron (as Ferrous Fumarate)	27 mg (150%)

Recommended Intake: Adults, 1 tablet daily or as directed by physician.

Supplied: Capsule-shaped tablets (film-coated, orange-red, scored) Engraved LL S2—
Bottle of 30—NDC 0005-4126-13
Bottle of 60—NDC 0005-4126-19

Shown in Product Identification Section, page 412

STRESSTABS® 600 with Zinc
Advanced Formula
High Potency
Stress Formula Vitamins

Each tablet contains:

	For Adults-Percentage of U.S. Recommended Daily Allowance (U.S. RDA)
Vitamin E (as *dl*-Alpha Tocopheryl Acetate)	30 I.U. (100%)
Vitamin C (L-Ascorbic Acid)	600 mg. (1000%)
B VITAMINS	
Folic Acid	400 mcg. (100%)
Vitamin B₁ (as Thiamine Mononitrate)	20 mg. (1333%)
Vitamin B₂ (as Riboflavin)	10 mg. (588%)
Niacinamide	100 mg. (500%)
Vitamin B₆ (as Pyridoxine Hydrochloride)	5 mg. (250%)

Vitamin B$_{12}$ (as Cyano-
Cobalamin)................12 mcg. (200%)
Biotin...............................45 mcg. (15%)
Pantothenic Acid (as Calcium
Pantothenate USP) 25 mg. (250%)
Copper (as Cupric
Oxide)...........................3 mg. (150%)
Zinc (as Zinc Sulfate)23.9 mg. (159%)

Recommended Intake: Adults, 1 tablet daily or as directed by the physician.

Supplied: Capsule-shaped Tablet (film coated, peach color) Engraved LL S3—
Bottle of 30—NDC 0005-4125-13
Bottle of 60—NDC 0005-4125-19
Store at Controlled Room Temperature 15–30°C (59–86°F)
*Shown in Product Identification
Section, page 412*

ZINCON® Improved Richer, Thicker Formula
Dandruff Shampoo

Contains: Pyrithione zinc (1%), water, sodium methyl cocoyl taurate, cocamide MEA, sodium chloride, magnesium aluminum silicate, sodium cocoyl isethionate, fragrance, glutaraldehyde, D&C green #5, citric acid or sodium hydroxide to adjust pH if necessary.

Indications: Relieves the itching and scalp flaking associated with dandruff. Relieves the itching, irritation, and skin flaking associated with seborrheic dermatitis of the scalp.

Directions: For best results use twice a week. Wet hair, apply to scalp and massage vigorously. Rinse and repeat.
SHAKE WELL BEFORE USING.

Warnings: Keep this and all drugs out of the reach of children. For external use only. Avoid contact with the eyes—if this happens, rinse thoroughly with water. If condition worsens or does not improve after regular use of this product as directed, consult a doctor. Do not use on children under 2 years of age except as directed by a doctor.

How Supplied:
4 oz. Bottle—NDC 0005-5455-58
8 oz. Bottle—NDC 0005-5455-61
*Shown in Product Identification
Section, page 412*

Leeming Division
Pfizer, Inc.
**100 JEFFERSON ROAD
PARSIPPANY, NJ 07054**

BEN–GAY® External Analgesic Products

Description: Ben-Gay is a combination of methyl salicylate and menthol in a suitable base for topical application. In addition to the Original Ointment (methyl salicylate, 18.3%; menthol, 16%), Ben-Gay is offered as a Greaseless/Stainless Ointment (methyl salicylate, 15%; menthol, 10%), an Extra Strength Balm (methyl salicylate, 30%; menthol, 8%), a Lotion and a Clear Gel (both of which contain methyl salicylate, 15%; menthol, 7%).

Action and Uses: Methyl salicylate and menthol are external analgesics which stimulate sensory receptors, including receptors of warmth and cold. This produces a counter-irritant response which alleviates the more severe pain in the joints and muscles where applied to provide transient, temporary symptomatic relief.

Several double blind clinical studies of Ben-Gay products have shown the effectiveness of the menthol-methyl salicylate combination in counteracting minor pain of skeletal muscle stress and arthritis.

Three studies involving a total of 102 normal subjects in which muscle soreness was experimentally induced showed statistically significant beneficial results from use of the active product vs. placebo for lowered Muscle Action Potential (spasms), greater rise in threshold of muscular pain and greater reduction in perceived muscular pain.

Six clinical studies of a total of 207 subjects suffering from minor pain and skeletal muscular spasms due to osteoarthritis and rheumatoid arthritis showed the active product to give statistically significant beneficial results vs. placebo for lowered Muscle Action Potential (spasm), greater relief of perceived pain, increased range of motion of the affected joints and increased digital dexterity.

In two studies designed to measure the effect of topically applied Ben-Gay vs. Placebo on muscular endurance, discomfort, onset of exercise pain and fatigue, and cardiovascular efficiency, 30 subjects performed a submaximal three-hour run and another 30 subjects performed a maximal treadmill run. Ben-Gay was found to significantly decrease the discomfort during the submaximal and maximal run, and increase the time before onset of fatigue during the maximal run. It did not improve cardiovascular function or affect recovery.

Directions: Rub generously into painful area, then massage gently until Ben-Gay disappears. Repeat as necessary.

Warning: Use only as directed. Keep away from children to avoid accidental poisoning. Do not swallow. If swallowed, induce vomiting, call a physician. Keep away from eyes, mucous membrane, broken or irritated skin. If skin irritation develops, pain lasts 10 days or more, redness is present, or with arthritis-like conditions in children under 12, call a physician.

DESITIN® OINTMENT

Description: Desitin Ointment is a combination of Zinc Oxide (40%), Cod Liver Oil (high in Vitamins A & D), and Talc in a petrolatum-lanolin base suitable for topical application.

Actions and Uses: Desitin Ointment is designed to provide relief of diaper rash, superficial wounds and burns, and other minor skin irritations. It helps prevent incidence of diaper rash, protects against urine and other irritants, soothes chafed skin and promotes healing.

Relief and protection is afforded by the combination of Zinc Oxide, Cod Liver Oil, Lanolin and Petrolatum. They provide a physical barrier by forming a protective coating over skin or mucous membrane which serves to reduce further effects of irritants on the affected area and relieves burning, pain or itch produced by them. In addition to its protective properties, Zinc Oxide acts as an astringent that helps heal local irritation and inflammation by lessening the flow of mucus and other secretions.

Several studies have shown the effectiveness of Desitin Ointment in the relief and prevention of diaper rash.

Two clinical studies involving 90 infants demonstrated the effectiveness of Desitin Ointment in curing diaper rash. The diaper rash area was treated with Desitin Ointment at each diaper change for a period of 24 hours, while the untreated site served as controls. A significant reduction was noted in the severity and area of diaper dermatitis on the treated area.

Ninety-seven (97) babies participated in a 12-week study to show that Desitin Ointment helps prevent diaper rash. Approximately half of the infants (49) were treated with Desitin Ointment on a regular daily basis. The other half (48) received the ointment as necessary to treat any diaper rash which occurred. The incidence as well as the severity of diaper rash was significantly less among the babies using the ointment on a regular daily basis.

In a comparative study of the efficacy of Desitin Ointment vs. a baby powder, forty-five babies were observed for a total of eight weeks. Results support the conclusion that Desitin Ointment is a better prophylactic against diaper rash than the baby powder.

In another study, Desitin was found to be dramatically more effective in reducing the severity of medically diagnosed diaper rash than a commercially available diaper rash product in which only anhydrous lanolin and petrolatum are listed as ingredients. Fifty infants participated in the study, half of whom were treated with Desitin and half with the other product. In the group (25) treated with Desitin, seventeen infants showed significant improvement within 10 hours which increased to twenty-three improved infants within 24 hours. Of the group (25) treated with the other product, only three showed improvement at ten hours with a total of four improved within twenty-four hours. These results are statistically valid to conclude that Desitin Ointment reduces severity of diaper rash within ten hours.

Several other studies show that Desitin Ointment helps relieve other skin disorders, such as contact dermatitis.

Directions: To prevent diaper rash, apply Desitin Ointment to the diaper area—especially at bedtime when exposure to wet diapers may be prolonged. If

Continued on next page

Leeming—Cont.

diaper rash is present, or at the first sign of redness, minor skin irritation or chafing, simply apply Desitin Ointment three or four times daily as needed. In superficial noninfected surface wounds and minor burns, apply a thin layer of Desitin Ointment, using a gauze dressing, if necessary. For external use only.

How Supplied: Desitin Ointment is available in 1 ounce (28g), 2 ounce (57g), 4 ounce (113g), 8 ounce (226g) tubes, and 1-lb. (452g) jar.

RHEABAN® TABLETS
(attapulgite)

Description: Rheaban is an anti-diarrheal medication containing activated attapulgite and is offered in tablet form. Each white Rheaban tablet contains 600 mg. of collodial activated attapulgite. Rheaban contains no narcotics, opiates or other habit-forming drugs.

Actions and Uses: Rheaban is indicated for relief of diarrhea and the cramps and pains associated with it. Attapulgite, which has been activated by thermal treatment, is a highly sorptive substance which absorbs nutrients and digestive enzymes as well as noxious gases, irritants, toxins and some bacteria and viruses that are common causes of diarrhea.

In clinical studies to show the effectiveness in relieving diarrhea and its symptoms, 100 subjects suffering from acute gastroenteritis with diarrhea participated in a double-blind comparison of Rheaban to a placebo. Patients treated with the attapulgite product showed significantly improved relief of diarrhea and its symptoms vs. the placebo.

Dosage and Administration:
TABLETS

Adults—2 tablets after initial bowel movement, 2 tablets after each subsequent bowel movement.

Children 6 to 12 years—1 tablet after initial bowel movement, 1 tablet after each subsequent bowel movement.

Warnings: Do not use for more than two days, or in the presence of high fever, Tablets should not be used for children under 6 years of age unless directed by physician. If diarrhea persists consult a physician.

How Supplied:
Tablets—Boxes of 12 tablets

UNISOM® NIGHTTIME SLEEP AID
(doxylamine succinate)

Description: Pale blue oval scored tablets containing 25 mg. of doxylamine succinate, 2-(α-(2-dimethylaminoethoxy)α-methylbenzyl) pyridine succinate.

Action and Uses: Doxylamine succinate is an antihistamine of the ethanolamine class, which characteristically shows a high incidence of sedation. In a comparative clinical study of over 20 antihistamines on more than 3000 subjects, doxyl-

amine succinate 25 mg. was one of the three most sedating antihistamines, producing a significantly reduced latency to end of wakefulness and comparing favorably with established hypnotic drugs such as secobarbital and pentobarbital in sedation activity. It was chosen as the antihistamine, based on dosage, causing the earliest onset of sleep. In another clinical study, doxylamine succinate 25 mg. scored better than secobarbital 100 mg. as a nighttime hypnotic. Two additional, identical clinical studies involving a total of 121 subjects demonstrated that doxylamine succinate 25 mg. reduced the sleep latency period by a third, compared to placebo. Duration of sleep was 26.6% longer with doxylamine succinate, and the quality of sleep was rated higher with the drug than with placebo. An EEG study of 6 subjects confirmed the results of these studies.

Administration and Dosage: One tablet 30 minutes before retiring. Not for children under 12 years of age.

Side Effects: Occasional anticholinergic effects may be seen.

Precautions: Unisom® should be taken only at bedtime.

Contraindications: Asthma, glaucoma, enlargement of the prostate gland. This product should not be taken by pregnant women, or those who are nursing a baby.

Warnings: Should be taken with caution if alcohol is being consumed. Product should not be taken if patient is concurrently on any other drug, without prior consultation with physician. Should not be taken for longer than two weeks unless approved by physician.

How Supplied: Boxes of 8, 16, 32 or 48 tablets.

VISINE® Eye Drops
(tetrahydrozoline hydrochloride)

Description: Visine is a sterile, isotonic, buffered ophthalmic solution containing tetrahydrozoline hydrochloride 0.05%, boric acid, sodium borate, sodium chloride and water. It is preserved with benzalkonium chloride 0.01% and edetate disodium 0.1%.

Indications: Visine is a decongestant ophthalmic solution designed to provide symptomatic relief of conjunctival edema and hyperemia secondary to ocular allergies, minor irritations, and so called non-specific or catarrhal conjunctivitis. Beneficial effects include amelioration of burning, irritation, pruritus, soreness, and excessive lacrimation. Relief is afforded by tetrahydrozoline hydrochloride, a sympathomimetic agent, which brings about decongestion by vasoconstriction. Reddened eyes are rapidly whitened by this effective vasoconstrictor, which limits the local vascular response by constricting the small blood vessels. The onset of vasoconstriction becomes apparent within minutes and the effect is prolonged. While some vasoconstrictors may produce a dilation of the pupil or cause rebound hyperemia,

there is no evidence that the use of Visine, with tetrahydrozoline hydrochloride, results in either condition.

The effectiveness of Visine in relieving conjunctival hyperemia and associated symptoms has been demonstrated by numerous clinicals, including several double blind studies, involving more than 2,000 subjects suffering from acute or chronic hyperemia induced by a variety of conditions. Visine was found to be efficacious in providing relief from conjunctival hyperemia and associated symptoms in over 90% of subjects.

Dosage and Administration: Place 1–2 drops in each eye two or three times a day or as directed by a physician. To avoid contamination of this product, do not touch tip of container to any other surface. Replace cap after using.

Warning: Visine should be used only for minor eye irritations. If relief is not obtained within 48 hours, or if irritation or redness persists or increases, discontinue use and consult your physician. In some instances irritation or redness is due to serious eye conditions such as infection, foreign body in the eye, or chemical corneal trauma requiring the attention of a physician. If you experience severe eye pain, headache, rapid change of vision, sudden appearance of floating spots, acute redness of the eyes, pain on exposure to light, or double vision, consult a physician at once. If you have glaucoma, do not use this product except under the advice and supervision of a physician. Remove contact lenses before using.

How Supplied: In 0.5 fl. oz., 0.75 fl. oz. and 1.0 fl. oz. plastic dispenser bottle and 0.5 fl. oz. plastic bottle with dropper.

VISINE® A.C. Eye Drops
(tetrahydrozoline hydrochloride and zinc sulfate)

Description: Visine A.C. is a sterile, isotonic, buffered ophthalmic solution containing tetrahydrozoline hydrochloride 0.05%, zinc sulfate 0.25%, boric acid, sodium citrate, sodium chloride, and water. It is preserved with benzalkonium chloride 0.01% and edetate disodium 0.1%.

Indications: Visine A.C. is an ophthalmic solution combining the effects of the decongestant tetrahydrozoline hydrochloride with the astringent effects of zinc sulfate. It is designed to provide symptomatic relief of conjunctival edema and hyperemia secondary to ocular allergies, minor irritation due to colds and other causes, as well as the so called non-specific or catarrhal conjunctivitis. Beneficial effects include amelioration of burning, irritation, pruritus, soreness, excessive lacrimation and removal of mucus from the eye. Relief is afforded by both ingredients, tetrahydrozoline hydrochloride and zinc sulfate. Tetrahydrozoline hydrochloride is a sympathomimetic agent, which brings about decongestion by vasoconstriction. Reddened eyes are rapidly whitened by this effective vasoconstrictor, which limits the local vascular response by constricting the small blood vessels. The onset of vasoconstriction becomes apparent within minutes and the effect is prolonged. While some vasoconstrictors produce a dilation of the pupil or cause rebound hyperemia, there is no evidence that the use of Visine, with tetrahydrozoline hydrochloride, results in either condition. Zinc sulfate is an ocular astringent which, by precipitating protein, helps to clear mucus from the outer surface of the eye.

The effectiveness of Visine A.C. in relieving conjunctival hyperemia and associated symptoms induced by cold and allergy has been clinically demonstrated. In one double blind study involving cold and allergy sufferers experiencing acute episodes of minor eye irritation, Visine A.C. produced statistically significant beneficial results versus a placebo of normal saline solution in relieving irritation of bulbar conjunctiva, irritation of palpebral conjunctiva, and mucous build-up. Treatment with Visine A.C. also significantly improved burning and itching symptoms.

Dosage and Administration: Place 1–2 drops in each eye two or three times a day or as directed by a physician. To avoid contamination of this product, do not touch tip of container to any other surface. Replace cap after using

Warning: Visine A.C. should be used only for minor eye irritations. If relief is not obtained within 72 hours, or if irritation or redness persists or increases, discontinue use and consult your physician. In some instances irritation or redness is due to serious eye conditions such as infection, foreign body in the eye, or other mechanical or chemical corneal trauma requiring the attention of a physician. If you experience severe eye pain, headache, rapid change in vision, sudden appearance of floating spots, acute redness of the eyes, pain on exposure to light, or double-vision consult a physician at once. If you have glaucoma, do not use this product except under the advice and supervision of a physician. Remove contact lenses before using.

How Supplied: In 0.5 fl. oz. and 1.0 fl. oz. plastic dispenser bottle.

Lemar Laboratories, Inc.
BUILDING B-200
10 PERIMETER WAY, N.W.
ATLANTA, GA 30339

HEALTHBREAK
Smoking Deterrent Gum and Lozenge

Active Ingredient: Silver Acetate 6 mg., Ammonium Chloride 10 mg., Cocarboxylase .025 mg.

Actions and Uses: Provides temporary aid in breaking the cigarette habit. Active ingredients react with tobacco smoke to produce a temporarily unpleasant taste in the mouth of the smoker. Unpleasant taste occurs only in the presence of tobacco smoke. Works on the principle of aversion therapy. Does not effect taste of food of beverage.

Warnings: It is not advisable to smoke or use a smoking deterrent during pregnancy. Discontinue use if prolonged nausea or allergic reaction occurs.

Dosage and Administration: Chew up to 6 gum tablets daily for 3 weeks (lozenge dissolve in mouth), one every 3 or 4 hours as needed. Chew gum tablets slowly for 20–30 minutes. If smoking has not been stopped or greatly reduced in 3 weeks time, discontinue treatment. After this period, may be used occasionally as needed—not more than 1 or 2 tablets per day—for up to 6 months, if helpful in continuing not smoking. Caution—excessive use may cause harmless skin discoloration.

How Supplied: Consumer package of 24 and 72 blister-packed gum tablets, 12 blister-packed lozenges.
Shown in Product Identification Section, page 412

Loma Linda Foods
11503 PIERCE STREET
RIVERSIDE, CA 92515

SOYALAC®   K PAREVE

Description: A milk free nutritionally balanced formula for infants. Liquid products are packed in solderless cans, eliminating lead from this source. Soyalac has a high polyunsaturated to saturated fatty acid ratio together with a liberal supply of Vitamin E. When prepared as directed, one quart of Soyalac daily contains essential nutrients in balanced combination and sufficient quantities to provide adequate nutrition for infants.

Action and Uses: Soyalac provides a highly satisfactory alternative or supplement for infants when breast milk is not available or the supply is inadequate. It is especially valuable for all infants, children, and adults - who may be sensitive to dairymilk, or who prefer a vegetarian diet. It may also be prescribed successfully for use in hypocholestrogenic diets; for pre-operative and post-operative diets; for fortifying any milk free diet; for geriatric cases, etc.

Preparation: Standard dilution is—
Ready to Serve—as canned
Concentrate—one part mixed with an equal part of water
Powder (can)—four scoops to one cup of water

Typical Analysis: Standard Dilution

SOYALAC

	NUTRIENTS PER 100 KILO-CALORIES	PER LITER
Protein (g)	3.1	21
Fat (g)	5.5	37
Carbohydrate (g)	9.8	66
Calories		680
Calories Per Fluid Ounce		20

Essential Fatty Acids (linoleate) (g)	2.8	19
Vitamins:		
A (IU)	310	2100
D (IU)	62	420
K (mcg)	7.8	53
E (IU)	2.3	16
C (ascorbic acid) (mg)	9.4	63
B$_1$ (thiamine) (mg)	0.078	0.53
B$_2$ (riboflavin) (mg)	0.093	0.63
B$_6$ (Pyridoxine) (mg)	0.062	0.42
B$_{12}$ (mcg)	0.31	2.1
Niacin (mg)	1.2	8.5
Folic acid (mcg)	15	106
Pantothenic acid (mg)	0.47	3.2
Biotin (mcg)	7.8	53
Choline (mg)	15	106
Inositol (mg)	15	106
Minerals:		
Calcium (mg)	93	630
Phosphorus (mg)	62	420
Magnesium (mg)	11	74
Iron (mg)	1.9	13
Iodine (mcg)	7	48
Zinc (mg)	0.78	5.3
Copper (mg)	0.078	0.53
Manganese (mg)	0.16	1.06
Sodium (mg)	51	350
Potassium (mg)	110	740
Chloride (mg)	58	390

Supply:
Soyalac Ready to Serve liquid:
 32 fl. oz. cans, 6 cans per case
Soyalac Double Strength Concentrate:
 13 fl. oz. cans, 12 cans per case
Soyalac Powder—Cans:
 14 oz. cans, 6 cans per case

I–SOYALAC   K PAREVE

Description: A corn free, milk free nutritionally balanced formula for infants. i-Soyalac contains a negligible amount of soy carbohydrates and has a high polyunsaturated to saturated fatty acid ratio together with a liberal supply of Vitamin E. In every respect except for the absence of corn derivatives and its negligible content of soy carbohydrates, i-Soyalac conforms to the description given on the page for Soyalac.

Action and Uses: Same as Soyalac, with the added advantage that it may be used with confidence by infants, children and adults who may be sensitive to corn and corn products.

Preparation: Standard dilution is—
Ready to Serve—as canned
Concentrate—one part mixed with an equal part water

Continued on next page

Loma Linda—Cont.

Supply:
i-Soyalac RTS liquid
   32 fl. oz. cans, 6 cans per case
i-Soyalac Double Strength Concentrate
   13 fl. oz. cans, 12 cans per case

Luyties Pharmacal Company
P.O. BOX 8080
ST. LOUIS, MO 63156

YELLOLAX

Description: YELLOLAX is a combination of time proven Yellow-phenolphthalein, and the Homeopathic ingredients, Bryonia and Hydrastis. Clinically YELLOLAX is an oral laxative. Each tablet contains two grains of yellow phenolphthalein and the Bryonia and Hydrastis approximately one fortieth grain each.

Action: Yellow-phenolphthalein is an effective and safe laxative, which is not contraindicated in pregnancy. Homeopathic Bryonia is used to treat constipation and the pain associated with constipation. Homeopathic Bryonia tends to increase mucous membrane moisture. Homeopathic Hydrastis is also included in the treatment of constipation because, the Homeopathic Hydrastis provides some relief of constipation and the associated pain and headaches by relaxing mucous membranes and encouraging their secretion. YELLOLAX has been safely used in pregnancy, children, and as conjunctive treatment with hemorrhoidal complications.

Indications: YELLOLAX is indicated in the management of simple constipation. YELLOLAX is also indicated in those conditions which require a gentle laxative.

Contraindications: YELLOLAX and all laxatives are contraindicated in appendicitis. All laxatives containing phenolphthalein are contraindicated in patients who have hypersensitivity to phenolphthalein.

Warnings: Do not use laxatives in cases of severe colic, nausea and other symptoms of appendicitis. Do not use laxatives habitually nor continually. If condition persists consult physician. Keep this and all medication out of the reach of children. DO NOT exceed the recommended dosage.

Caution: Frequent or prolonged use may result in laxative dependence. If skin rash appears, discontinue use.

Side Effects: The phenolphthalein may impart a red color to the urine, (phenolphthalein is also used as a pH indicator), this is normal.

Dosage: For adults one or two tablets chewed before retiring. For children over six a quarter tablet to half tablet before retiring. Tablets should be well chewed. For younger children consult physician.

Supplied: Compressed tablets packed in glass bottles of 36 (NDC 0618-0832-55) and 100 (NDC 0618-0832-12), and in repackers of 1000 tablets.

Homoeopathic
Luyties also manufactures a complete line of homoeopathic products. If more information is needed contact them direct.

3M Company
Personal Care Products
3M CENTER
ST. PAUL, MN 55144

DORBANE®
(brand of danthron)
Laxative

Dorbane promotes colonic peristalsis and is a superior laxative in the management and treatment of constipation.

Composition: Each tablet contains: Danthron 75 mg.

Warnings: Do not use when abdominal pain, nausea or vomiting are present. Frequent or prolonged use of this preparation may result in dependence on laxatives.

Dosage and Administration: 1 or 2 tablets once daily, 1 hour after the evening meal. As treatment progresses, dosage may be gradually decreased. May cause harmless discoloration of the urine.

Availability: Bottles of 100 (NDC 0089-0173-10) orange, scored tablets.

DORBANTYL® Laxative
Stool Softener

For relief of occasional constipation. May cause harmless discoloration of urine.

Composition: Each capsule contains: Danthron, 25 mg.; docusate sodium, 50 mg.

Warnings: Do not use when abdominal pain, nausea or vomiting are present. Frequent or prolonged use of this preparation may result in dependence on laxatives.
Keep this and all medications out of the reach of children.

Dosage and Administration: ADULTS: 2 capsules at bedtime; repeat following day if needed to cause bowel movement. CHILDREN: 6 to 12 years of age: 1 capsule taken as above. Under 6 years of age: use only on advice of physician. Contains color additives including FD&C Yellow No. 5 (tartrazine).

Availability: Bottles of 30 (NDC 0089-0174-03) and 100 (NDC 0089-0174-10) orange and black capsules.

DORBANTYL® FORTE
Laxative Stool Softener

For relief of occasional constipation. May cause harmless discoloration of urine.

Composition: Each capsule contains: Danthron, 50 mg.; docusate sodium, 100 mg.

Warnings: Do not use when abdominal pain, nausea or vomiting are present. Frequent or prolonged use of this preparation may result in dependence on laxatives. Keep this and all medication out of the reach of children.

Dosage and Administration: ADULTS: 1 capsule at bedtime; repeat following day if needed to cause bowel movement.
CHILDREN: Use regular Dorbantyl. Contains color additives including FD&C yellow No. 5 (tartrazine).

Note: 1 Dorbantyl Forte capsule is equivalent to 2 regular Dorbantyl capsules.

Availability: 30 (NDC 0089-0178-03) and 100 (NDC 0089-0178-10) orange and grey capsules.

TITRALAC® Tablets and Liquid
(calcium carbonate)

Description: Liquid: Each teaspoonful (5 ml.) of white, spearmint-flavored liquid contains calcium carbonate 1.0 gm. and glycine for a smooth, pleasant taste. One teaspoonful of liquid approximates two tablets.
Tablets: Each white, spearmint-flavored tablet contains calcium carbonate 0.42 gm. and glycine for a smooth, pleasant taste.

Indications: As an antacid for the relief of heartburn, sour stomach and/or acid indigestion and symptomatic relief of hyperacidity associated with the diagnosis of peptic ulcer, gastritis, peptic esophagitis, gastric hyperacidity, and hiatal hernia.

Warnings: Do not take more than 19 tablets or 8 teaspoonfuls in a 24-hour period or use maximum dosage for more than two weeks, except under the advice and supervision of a physician. Keep this and all medication out of the reach of children. In case of accidental overdose, seek professional assistance or contact your Poison Control Center immediately.

Dosage and Administration: One teaspoonful, or two tablets, taken one hour after meals or as directed by a physician. Tablets can be chewed, swallowed, or allowed to melt in the mouth.

Neutralizing Capacity: Titralac Liquid: 19 milliequivalents per 5 ml. Titralac Tablets: 15 milliequivalents per 2 tablets. These neutralization equivalents are expressed as milliequivalents of acid neutralized in 15 minutes when tested in accordance with USP antacid effectiveness test as prescribed in the code of Federal Regulations for OTC antacid products.
Sugar Free
Sodium Content:
Titralac Tablets: Not more than 0.3 mg (0.01 mEq.) sodium per tablet.
Titralac Liquid: Not more than 11 mg. (0.5 mEq.) sodium per teaspoon (5 ml.).

Availability:

Tablets: bottles of 40 (NDC 0089-0355-04), 100 (NDC 0089-0355-10) and 1000 (NDC 0089-0355-80), box of 50 individually film wrapped tablets (UPC 021200-18412)

Liquid: bottles of 12 fl. oz. (NDC 0089-0355-12)

Shown in Product Identification Section, page 412

Macsil, Inc.
1326 FRANKFORD AVENUE
PHILADELPHIA, PA 19125

BALMEX® BABY POWDER

Composition: Contains BALSAN® (specially purified balsam Peru), zinc oxide, talc, starch, calcium carbonate.

Action and Uses: Absorbent, emollient, soothing—for diaper irritation, intertrigo, and other common dermatological conditions. In acute, simple miliaria, itching ceases in minutes and lesions dry promptly. For routine use after bathing and each diaper change.

How Supplied: 4 oz. shaker top cans.

BALMEX® EMOLLIENT LOTION

Gentle and effective scientifically compounded infant's skin conditioner.

Composition: Contains a special lanolin oil (non-sensitizing, dewaxed, moisturizing fraction of lanolin), BALSAN® (specially purified balsam Peru) and silicone.

Action and Uses: The special Lanolin Oil aids nature lubricate baby's skin to keep it smooth and supple. Balmex Emollient Lotion is also highly effective as a physiologic conditioner on adult's skin.

How Supplied: Available in 6 oz. dispenser-top plastic bottles.

BALMEX® OINTMENT

Composition: Contains BALSAN® (specially purified balsam Peru), vitamins A and D, zinc oxide, and bismuth subnitrate in an ointment base containing silicone.

Action and Uses: Emollient, protective, anti-inflammatory, promotes healing—for diaper rash, minor burns, sunburn, and other simple skin conditions; also decubitus ulcers, skin irritations associated with ileostomy and colostomy drainage. Nonstaining, readily washes out of diapers and clothing.

How Supplied: 1, 2, 4 oz. tubes; 1 lb. plastic jars (½ oz. tubes for Hospitals only). Balmex Ointment-All Commercial Sizes-Safety Sealed.

A.G. Marin Pharmaceuticals
P.O. BOX 174
MIAMI, FL 33144

MAREPA
Marine Lipid Concentrate

Active Ingredients: Each 1200 mg capsule contains eicosapentaenoic acid (EPA) 216 mg and docosahexaenoic acid (DHA) 144 mg.

Indications: Provides a dietary source of OMEGA-3 fatty acids.

Dosage and Administration: 1 or 2 capsules three times daily with meals.

How Supplied: 1200 mg capsules available in bottles of 60. Store capsules in a dry place at a temperature of 59°–86°F.

Marion Laboratories, Inc.
Pharmaceutical Products Division
MARION INDUSTRIAL PARK
MARION PARK DRIVE
KANSAS CITY, MO 64137

AMBENYL®-D Decongestant Cough Formula
Antitussive, Expectorant, Nasal Decongestant

Two teaspoonfuls (10 ml) contain the following active ingredients:

Guaifenesin (glyceryl guaiacolate)	200 mg
Pseudoephedrine hydrochloride	60 mg
Dextromethorphan hydrobromide	30 mg

Also contains 9.5% alcohol.

Indications: AMBENYL®-D is for temporary relief of nasal congestion due to the common cold or associated with sinusitis, helps loosen phlegm, calms cough impulses without narcotics, and temporarily helps you cough less.

Directions for Use: Adult Dose (12 years and over)—Two teaspoonfuls every six hours. Child Dose (6 to 12 years)—One teaspoonful every six hours. (2 to 6 years)—One-half teaspoonful every six hours. No more than four doses per day.

Warnings: Do not give this product to children under 2 years, except under the advice and supervision of a physician. Do not take this product for persistent or chronic cough such as occurs with smoking, asthma, or emphysema, or where cough is accompanied by excessive secretions, except under the advice and supervision of a physician.
Do not exceed recommended dosage because at higher doses nervousness, dizziness, or sleeplessness may occur.

Caution: A persistent cough may be a sign of a serious condition. If cough persists for more than 1 week, tends to recur, or is accompanied by high fever, rash, or persistent headache, consult a physician.

If symptoms do not improve within seven days or are accompanied by high fever, consult a physician before continuing use. Do not take this product if you have high blood pressure, heart disease, diabetes, or thyroid disease, except under the advice and supervision of a physician.
If pregnant or nursing a baby, consult your physician or pharmacist before using this product.

Drug Interaction Precaution: Do not take this product if you are presently taking a prescription antihypertensive or antidepressant drug containing a monoamine oxidase inhibitor, except under the advice and supervision of a physician.
Store at a controlled room temperature (59°–86°F).
Keep this and all drugs out of reach of children.
In case of accidental overdose, seek professional assistance or contact a poison control center immediately.

How Supplied: Ambenyl-D Decongestant Cough Formula is supplied in a 4-fl-oz bottle.

Issued 5/84

Shown in Product Identification Section, page 412

DEBROX® Drops

Description: Carbamide peroxide 6.5% in a specially prepared anhydrous glycerol.

Actions: DEBROX® penetrates, softens, and facilitates removal of earwax. DEBROX Drops foams on contact with earwax due to the release of oxygen.

Indications: DEBROX Drops provides a safe, nonirritating method of softening and removing earwax.

Directions: Use directly from bottle. Tilt head sideways and squeeze bottle gently so that 5 to 10 drops flow into ear. Tip of bottle should not enter ear canal. Keep drops in ear for several minutes while head remains tilted or by inserting cotton. Repeat twice daily for up to four days if needed or as directed by physician. Any remaining wax may be removed by flushing with warm water, using a soft rubber bulb ear syringe. Avoid excessive pressure.

Warnings: Do not use if you have ear drainage or discharge, ear pain, irritation or rash in the ear, or are dizzy, unless directed by a physician. Do not use if you have an injury or perforation (hole) of the eardrum or after ear surgery, unless directed by a physician. Do not use for more than four consecutive days. If excessive earwax remains after use of this product, consult a physician. Consult a physician prior to use in children under 12.

Cautions: Avoid exposing bottle to excessive heat and direct sunlight. Keep color tip on bottle when not in use. **AVOID CONTACT WITH EYES. KEEP THIS AND ALL DRUGS OUT**

Continued on next page

Marion—Cont.

OF THE REACH OF CHILDREN. IN CASE OF ACCIDENTAL INGESTION, SEEK PROFESSIONAL ASSISTANCE OR CONTACT A POISON CONTROL CENTER IMMEDIATELY.

How Supplied: DEBROX Drops in ½- or 1-fl-oz plastic squeeze bottles with applicator spouts. Issued 8/83

Shown in Product Identification Section, page 412

GAVISCON® Antacid Tablets

Composition: Each chewable tablet contains the following active ingredients:
Aluminum hydroxide dried gel... 80 mg
Magnesium trisilicate .... 20 mg
and the following inactive ingredients: sucrose, alginic acid, sodium bicarbonate, starch, calcium stearate, and flavoring.

Actions: Unique formulation produces soothing foam which floats on stomach contents. Foam containing antacid precedes stomach contents into the esophagus when reflux occurs to help protect the sensitive mucosa from further irritation. GAVISCON acts locally without neutralizing entire stomach contents to help maintain integrity of the digestive process. Endoscopic studies indicate that GAVISCON® Antacid Tablets are equally as effective in the erect or supine patient.

Indications: GAVISCON is specifically formulated for the temporary relief of heartburn (acid indigestion) due to acid reflux. GAVISCON is not indicated for the treatment of peptic ulcers.

Directions: Chew two to four tablets four times a day or as directed by a physician. Tablets should be taken after meals and at bedtime or as needed. For best results follow by a half glass of water or other liquid. DO NOT SWALLOW WHOLE.

Warnings: Do not take more than 16 tablets in a 24-hour period or 16 tablets daily for more than 2 weeks, except under the advice and supervision of a physician. Do not use this product except under the advice and supervision of a physician if you are on a sodium-restricted diet. Each GAVISCON Tablet contains approximately 0.8 mEq sodium.

Drug Interaction Precautions: Do not take this product if you are presently taking a prescription antibiotic drug containing any form of tetracycline.
Store at a controlled room temperature in a dry place.
Keep this and all drugs out of the reach of children. In case of accidental overdose, seek professional assistance or contact a poison control center immediately.

How Supplied: Available in bottle of 100 tablets and in foil-wrapped 2's in box of 30 tablets. Issued 12/83
Shown in Product Identification Section, page 412

GAVISCON® Liquid Antacid

Each tablespoonful (15 ml) contains the following active ingredients:
Aluminum hydroxide .... 95 mg
Magnesium carbonate .... 412 mg
and the following inactive ingredients: water, sorbitol solution, glycerin, sodium alginate, xanthan gum, edetate disodium, preservatives, flavorings, and colors.

Indications: For the relief of heartburn, sour stomach, and/or acid indigestion, and upset stomach associated with heartburn, sour stomach, and/or acid indigestion.

Directions: Shake well before using. Take 1 or 2 tablespoonfuls four times a day or as directed by a physician. GAVISCON® Liquid should be taken after meals and at bedtime, followed by half a glass of water.

Warnings: Except under the advice and supervision of a physician, do not take more than 8 tablespoonfuls in a 24-hour period or 8 tablespoonfuls daily for more than 2 weeks. May have laxative effect. Do not use this product if you have a kidney disease; do not use this product if you are on a sodium-restricted diet. Each tablespoonful of GAVISCON Liquid contains approximately 1.7 mEq sodium.

Drug Interaction Precautions: Do not take this product if you are presently taking a prescription antibiotic drug containing any form of tetracycline.
Keep tightly closed. Avoid freezing. Store at a controlled room temperature.
Keep this and all drugs out of the reach of children.
In case of accidental overdose, seek professional assistance or contact a poison control center immediately.

How Supplied: GAVISCON® Liquid Antacid is available in 12-fl-oz (355-ml) and 6-fl-oz (177-ml) bottles.
Issued 5/84
Shown in Product Identification Section, page 412

GAVISCON®-2 Antacid Tablets

Composition: Each chewable tablet contains the following active ingredients:
Aluminum hydroxide dried gel 160 mg
Magnesium trisilicate .... 40 mg
and the following inactive ingredients: sucrose, alginic acid, sodium bicarbonate, starch, calcium stearate, and flavoring.

Indications: GAVISCON® is specifically formulated for the temporary relief of heartburn (acid indigestion) due to acid reflux. GAVISCON is not indicated for the treatment of peptic ulcers.

Directions: Chew one to two tablets four times a day or as directed by a physician. Tablets should be taken after meals and at bedtime or as needed. For best results follow by a half glass of water or other liquid. DO NOT SWALLOW WHOLE.

Warnings: Do not take more than eight tablets in a 24-hour period or eight tablets daily for more than 2 weeks, except under the advice and supervision of a physician. Do not use this product except under the advice and supervision of a physician if you are on a sodium-restricted diet. Each GAVISCON-2 Tablet contains approximately 1.6 mEq sodium.

Drug Interaction Precautions: Do not take this product if you are presently taking a prescription antibiotic drug containing any form of tetracycline.
Store at a controlled room temperature in a dry place.
Keep this and all drugs out of the reach of children. In case of accidental overdose, seek professional assistance or contact a poison control center immediately.

How Supplied: Box of 48 foil-wrapped tablets.
Issued 12/83
Shown in Product Identification Section, page 412

GLY-OXIDE® Liquid

Description: Carbamide peroxide 10% in specially prepared anhydrous glycerol. Artificial flavor added.

Actions: GLY-OXIDE® is a safe, stabilized oxygenating agent. Specifically formulated for topical oral administration, it provides unique chemomechanical cleansing and debriding action which allows normal healing to occur.

Indications: Local treatment and hygienic prevention (as an aid to professional care) of minor oral inflammation such as canker sores, denture irritation, and postdental procedure irritation. GLY-OXIDE Liquid provides effective aid to oral hygiene when normal cleansing measures are inadequate or impossible (eg, total-care geriatric patients). As an adjunct to oral hygiene (orthodontics, dental appliances) after regular brushing.

Precautions: Severe or persistent oral inflammation or denture irritation may be serious. If these or unexpected effects occur, consult physician or dentist promptly.

Dosage and Administration: DO NOT DILUTE—use directly from the bottle. Apply four times daily after meals and at bedtime, or as directed by a dentist or physician. Place several drops on affected area; expectorate after two to three minutes; or place 10 drops onto tongue, mix with saliva, swish for several minutes, expectorate. Do not rinse. Foams on contact with saliva.
Avoid contact with eyes. Protect from heat and direct sunlight. Keep this and all drugs out of the reach of children. In case of accidental ingestion, seek professional assistance or contact a poison control center immediately.

How Supplied: GLY-OXIDE Liquid in ½-fl-oz and 2-fl-oz nonspill plastic squeeze bottles with applicator spouts.

Issued 3/84

Shown in Product Identification Section, page 413

OS–CAL® 250 Tablets
(calcium supplement with vitamin D added)

Each Tablet Contains: 625 mg of calcium carbonate from oyster shell, an organic calcium source.
Elemental calcium .... 250 mg
Vitamin D .... 125 USP Units

Directions: One tablet three times a day with meals, or as recommended by your physician.

Three Tablets Provide:

	% U.S. RDA for Adults
Calcium .... 750 mg	75%
Vitamin D ..... 375 Units	94%

Store at room temperature. Keep out of reach of children.

How Supplied: OS-CAL® 250 is available in bottles of 100, 240, 500, and 1000 tablets.

Issued 11/83

Shown in Product Identification Section, page 413

OS–CAL® 500 Tablets
(calcium supplement)

Each Tablet Contains: 1250 mg of calcium carbonate from oyster shell, an organic calcium source.
Elemental calcium ....500 mg

Directions: One tablet two to three times a day with meals, or as recommended by your physician.

Two Tablets Provide: 1000 mg calcium, 100% of U.S. RDA for adults and children 12 or more years of age.

Three Tablets Provide: 1500 mg calcium, 115% of U.S. RDA for pregnant and lactating women.

Store at room temperature. Keep out of reach of children.

How Supplied: OS-CAL® 500 is available in bottles of 60 and 120 tablets.

Issued 5/84

Shown in Product Identification Section, page 413

OS–CAL FORTE®Tablets
(multivitamin and mineral supplement)

Each Tablet Contains:
Vitamin A (palmitate) 1668 USP Units
Vitamin D .... 125 USP Units
Thiamine mononitrate
  (vitamin B₁).................... 1.7 mg
Riboflavin (vitamin B₂)................ 1.7 mg
Pyridoxine hydrochloride
  (vitamin B₆)..................... 2.0 mg
Cyanocobalamin (vitamin B₁₂) 1.6 mcg
Ascorbic acid (vitamin C)............. 50 mg
dl-alpha-tocopherol acetate
  (vitamin E)................................. 0.8 IU

Niacinamide .... 15 mg
Calcium (from oyster shell*)...... 250 mg
Iron (as ferrous fumarate).............. 5 mg
Copper (as sulfate)........................ 0.3 mg
Iodine (as potassium iodide)...... 0.05 mg
Magnesium (as oxide)................... 1.6 mg
Manganese (as sulfate)................. 0.3 mg
Zinc (as sulfate)............................ 0.5 mg
*Trace minerals from oyster shell: copper, iron, magnesium, manganese, silica, and zinc.

Indication: Multivitamin and mineral supplement.

Dosage: One tablet three times daily or as directed by physician.

How Supplied: Bottles of 100 tablets. Keep this and all drugs out of reach of children. In case of accidental overdose, seek professional assistance or contact a poison control center immediately. Store at room temperature.

Issued 11/83

OS–CAL–GESIC® Tablets
(antiarthritic)

Each Tablet Contains:
Salicylamide .... 400 mg
Calcium (from oyster shell) .... 100 mg
Vitamin D ....50 USP Units

Indication: For temporary relief of symptoms associated with arthritis.

Dosage: Initially—2 tablets hourly for 3 or 4 doses. Maintenance—1 or 2 tablets 4 times daily.

How Supplied: OS-CAL-GESIC® is available in bottles of 100 tablets. Keep this and all drugs out of reach of children. In case of accidental overdose, seek professional assistance or contact a poison control center immediately. Store at room temperature.

Issued 11/83

OS–CAL® Plus Tablets
(multivitamin and multimineral supplement)

Each Tablet Contains:
Calcium (from oyster shell) .... 250 mg
Vitamin D .... 125 USP Units

Plus:
Vitamin A (palmitate) 1666 USP Units
Vitamin C (ascorbic acid).......... 33.0 mg
Vitamin B₂ (riboflavin).............. 0.66 mg
Vitamin B₁ (thiamine
  mononitrate)........................... 0.5 mg
Vitamin B₆ (pyridoxine HCl)...... 0.5 mg
Niacinamide................................ 3.33 mg
Iron (as ferrous fumarate) .... 16.6 mg
Zinc (as the sulfate).................... 0.75 mg
Manganese (as the sulfate)....... 0.75 mg
Copper (as the sulfate)............. 0.036 mg
Iodine (as potassium iodide) ... 0.036 mg

Indications: As a multivitamin and multimineral supplement.

Dosage: One tablet three times a day before meals or as directed by a physician. For children under 4 years of age, consult a physician.

How Supplied: Bottles of 100 tablets. Store at room temperature. Keep this and all drugs out of reach of children. In case of accidental overdose, seek professional assistance or contact a poison control center immediately.

Issued 11/83

THROAT DISCS® Throat Lozenges

Description: Each lozenge contains capsicum, peppermint, anise, cubeb, glycyrrhiza extract (licorice), and linseed.

Indications: Effective for soothing, temporary relief of minor throat irritations from hoarseness and coughs due to colds.

Precautions: For severe or persistent cough or sore throat, or sore throat accompanied by high fever, headache, nausea, and vomiting, consult physician promptly. Not recommended for children under 3 years of age.

Directions: Allow lozenge to dissolve slowly in mouth. One or two should give the desired relief. Do not use more than four lozenges per hour.

How Supplied: Box of 60 lozenges.

Issued 2/83

Shown in Product Identification Section, page 413

Marlyn Co., Inc.
350 PAUMA PLACE
ESCONDIDO, CA 92025

MARLYN PMS™
**Nutritional Supplement For Women
Multi-Vitamin Mineral Pak
Five tablets/capsules per pak**

Each Pak Contains			*%USRDA
VITAMIN A, D, & E CAPSULE			
Vitamin A	5000	I.U.	100
(Fish Liver Oil)			
Vitamin D	400	I.U.	100
(Fish Liver Oil)			
Vitamin E	200	I.U.	333
(d-Alpha Tocopherol)			
In a base of safflower oil containing:			
Linoleic Acid 113.07 mg			
Linolenic Acid 0.754 mg.			
VITAMIN B COMPLEX, SUSTAINED RELEASE W/PANCREATIN			
Vitamin B₁	25	mg.	1666
(Thiamine)			
Vitamin B₂	25	mg.	1470
(Riboflavin)			
Niacinamide	25	mg.	80
Vitamin B₆	125	mg.	6250
(Pyridoxine)			
Vitamin B₁₂	50	mcg.	833
(Cobalamin Conc.)			
Biotin	25	mcg.	8.3
Pantothenic Acid	25	mg.	250
(d-Cal. Panto.)			
Folic Acid	200	mcg.	50
Choline	50	mg.	**
(Bitartrate)			
Inositol	50	mg.	**
Paraminobenzoic	50	mg.	**
Acid			

Continued on next page

Marlyn—Cont.

In a base containing pancreatin
VITAMIN C COMPLEX, SUSTAINED
RELEASE

Vitamin C	500 mg.	833
(Ascorbic Acid)		
Lemon Bioflavonoids	100 mg.	**
Hesperidin	100 mg.	**

MULTI-MINERALS, AMINO ACID
CHELATED

Iron	9 mg.	50
(Chelated Gluconate)		
Calcium	200 mg.	20
(Dicalcium Phosphate & Bone Meal)		
Phosphorus	155 mg.	15
(Dicalcium Phosphate & Bone Meal)		
Iodine (Kelp)	75 mcg.	50
Zinc	7.5 mg.	50
(Chelated Gluconate)		
Copper	1 mg.	50
(Chelated Gluconate)		
Manganese	5 mg.	**
(Chelated Gluconate)		
Potassium	25 mg.	**
(Amino Acid Complex)		
Chromium	1 mcg.	**
(Organically Bound Yeast)		
Selenium	50 mcg.	**
(Organically Bound Yeast)		

MAGNESIUM TABLET, AMINO ACID
CHELATED

Magnesium	250 mg.	62

*United States Recommended Daily
Allowance
**USRDA not established

Gelatin Capsules & Tablets contain no
artificial preseratives, coloring or flavoring. Tablets are also free of sugar and
starch.

Suggested Use: Two paks daily, preferably morning and evening after meals.

How Supplied: Boxes of 60 paks each.
*Shown in Product Identification
Section, page 413*

SOFT STRESS
**Multi-Vitamin/Mineral Stress
Formula in Easy to Swallow, Soft
Gelatin Capsules**

Each four gelatin capsules contain:

		%USRDA
Beta Carotene	15 mg.	500
(Equivalent to 25,000 I.U. Vit.A)		
Vitamin D	400 I.U.	100
(Cholicalciferol)		
Vitamin E	200 I.U.	666
(Mixed Tocopherols)		
Vitamin C	500 mg.	833
(Vegetable)		
Folic Acid	200 mcg.	50
(Whole Rice, Folic Acid)		
Vitamin B$_1$	25 mg.	1666
(Whole Rice, Thiamine)		
Vitamin B$_2$	25 mg.	1470
(Whole Rice, Riboflavin)		
Niacinamide	25 mg.	125
(Whole Rice, Niacinamide)		
Vitamin B$_6$	25 mg.	1250
(Whole Rice, Pyridoxine)		
Vitamin B$_{12}$	25 mcg.	416
(Cobalamin)		
Biotin	25 mcg.	8333
(Whole Rice, Biotin)		

Pantothenic Acid	25 mg.	250
(Whole Rice, Calcium Pantothenate)		
Calcium	200 mg.	20
(Dicalcium Phosphate)		
Phosphorus	152 mg.	15
(Dicalcium Phosphate)		
Iron	18 mg.	100
(Iron Sulphate)		
Magnesium	50 mg.	12
(Magnesium Oxide)		
Copper	0.5 mg.	25
(Copper Sulphate)		
Zinc	15 mg.	100
(Zinc Oxide)		
Potassium	30 mg.	**
(Potassium Sulphate)		
Choline Bitartrate	25 mg.	**
(Whole Rice, Choline Bitartrate)		
Inositol	25 mg.	**
(Whole Rice, Inositol)		
Paraminobenzoic Acid	25 mg.	**
(Whole Rice, PABA)		
Chromium	7.5 mcg.	**
(Yeast)		
Selenium	12.5 mcg.	**
(Yeast)		
Octacosanol	375 mcg.	**

In natural vegetable oils; soybean and
lecithin
**USRDA not established
Preservative Free. No artificial color or
flavors.

Suggested Use: One pak daily.

Max Factor & Co.
**1655 N. McCADDEN PLACE
HOLLYWOOD, CA 90028**

ERACE ACNE CONTROL COVER–UP
with 5% Benzoyl Peroxide

Active Ingredient: Benzoyl Peroxide
5% in a skin-tinted stick containing Mineral Oil, Cyclomethicone, Ozokerite, Fragrance, Titanium Dioxide and Iron Oxides.

Indications: For the topical treatment
of Acne Vulgaris.

Actions: ERACE Acne Control Cover-
Up is a safe and effective medicated antibacterial acne control stick containing
5% benzoyl peroxide which:
(1) Dries and clears acne pimples as it
helps prevent new lesions from forming by killing the acne causing bacteria Propionbacterium acnes.
(2) Cosmetically conceals while treating
acne lesions. Available in an easy to
use stick in four skin-matched tones.
Application is precise and controlled
without unsightly blotches or a
"masky-medicine" look.

Warnings: For external use only.
Other topical acne medications should
not be used concurrently. Persons with
very sensitive skin or a sensitivity to benzoyl peroxide should not use this medication. If excessive dryness or uncomfortable irritation occur, reduce frequency of
use. If symptoms persist, discontinue use
and/or consult a physician promptly.
Keep away from eyes, lips, mouth and
sensitive areas of the neck. The product
may bleach hair or dyed fabrics. Keep

this and all medicines out of the reach of
children.

Directions for Use: Wash and dry
skin thoroughly. Swivel up stick and apply directly to affected areas. Using fingertips, blend with skin. Because excessive drying of the skin may occur, do not
apply more than 2 to 3 times a day.

How Supplied: Self-service/blister card
package holds swivel-up stick containing
.09oz of ERACE Acne Control Cover-Up
in 1 of 4 skin-matching shades.
*Shown in Product Identification
Section, page 413*

FOR YOUR EYES ONLY™ Mascara

Description: A safe and gentle, hypo-
allergenic formula mascara especially
for sensitive eyes. Also, formulated for
contact lens wearers.

Action: Lengthens and separates as it
colors the lashes. Flakeproof. Resists
smudging and smearing. Dermatologist
tested. Ophthalmologist tested on contact lens wearers. Available in velvet
black, black, black/brown. Removes easily with soap and water or any Max Factor Eye Make-Up Remover.

How Supplied: Self-service/blister
card package holds tube containing .45 fl.
oz. mascara with brush wand.
*Shown in Product Identification
Section, page 413*

SKIN PRINCIPLE™

SKIN PRINCIPLE Skin Support System
is a serious line of hypo-allergenic skin
care formulated to help skin breathe. It
consists of cleansing, clarifying and moisturizing products especially formulated
for Oily/Partly Oily, Normal, Dry/-
Partly Dry skin types.
All products are hypo-allergenic, fragrance free, dermatologist tested and
clinically tested.
*Shown in Product Identification
Section, page 413*

SKIN PRINCIPLE™
Purifying Cleansing Lotion

Composition: Water, Mineral Oil, Iso-
propyl Palmitate, Butylene Glycol, PEG-
100 Stearate, Glyceryl Stearate, Isocetyl
Stearate, Sorbitan Stearate, Urea, Mat-
ricaria Oil, Allantoin, Benzophenone-11,
Carbomer 941, Triethanolamine, Gly-
cine, Potassium and Ammonium PCA,
Leucine, Glucose Glutamate, Serine,
Proline, Collagen Amino Acids, Tyro-
sine, Tryptophan, Aspartic Acid, Valine,
Alanine, Isoleucine, Sodium Lactate,
Ethylparaben, Methylparaben, Propyl-
paraben, Imidazolidinyl Urea, BHA,
D&C Green No. 5, FD&C Red No. 4,
FD&C Yellow No. 5.

Actions: Cleanses and helps skin
breathe by gently removing make-up,
dirt, grime and skin-dulling dead cells.
Recommended for: Dry/Partly Dry and
Normal Skin.

Administration: Twice daily, morning
and night.

How Supplied: 8.3 fl. oz. lotion (plastic bottle).

Shown in Product Identification Section, page 413

SKIN PRINCIPLE™
Basic Clarifying Lotion

Composition: Water, SD Alcohol 40, Propyene Glycol, Horse Chestnut Extract, Butylene Glycol, Alcloxa, Matricaria Oil, Polysorbate 20, Benzophenone-4, Glycine, Potassium and Ammonium PCA, Leucine, Glucose Glutamate, Serine, Proline, Collagen Amino Acids, Tyrosine, Tryptophan, Aspartic Acid, Valine, Alanine, Isoleucine, Sodium Lactate, Lactic Acid, Methylparaben, Propylparaben, Imidazolidinyl Urea, FD&C Red. No. 40, FD&C Yellow No. 5.

Actions: Removes final traces of cleanser. Works with body chemistry to tone, refine and normalize pH balance. Prepares skin for moisturizing benefits. Recommended for: Oily/Partly Oily, Normal, Dry/Partly Dry Skin.

Caution: For dry skin, dampen cotton ball with water before use.

Administration: Twice daily, morning and night after cleansing. Oily skin types may reapply throughout day as needed.

How Supplied: 8.3 fl. oz. liquid (plastic bottle).

Shown in Product Identification Section, page 413

SKIN PRINCIPLE™
Daily Light Moisture Lotion

Composition: Water, Butylene Glycol, Soluble Collagen Complex, Octyl Palmitate, Glyceryl Stearate, Myristyl Myristate, Sorbitan Stearate, PEG-100 Stearate, Squalane, Urea, Sesame Oil, Matricaria Oil, Collagen, Hydrogenated Cottonseed Glyceride, Caprylic/Capric Triglyceride, Sodium Ribonucleate, Benzophenone-11, Cetearyl Alcohol, Leteareth-20, Polysorbate 60, Dimethicone, Carbomer 941, Triethanolamine, Glycine, Potassium and Ammonium PCA, Leucine, Glucose Glutamate, Serine, Proline, Collagen Amino Acids, Tyrosine, Tryptophan, Aspartic Acid, Valine, Alanine, Isoleucine, Sodium Lactate, Ethylparaben, Methylparaben, Propylparaben, Imidazolidinyl Urea, BHA, D&C Green No. 5, FD&C Red No. 4, FD&C Yellow No. 5.

Actions: Non-occlusive formula provides moisture where needed. Helps combat drying effects of the environment. Softens and smoothes skin. Suitable for under make-up. Recommended for: Partly Oily and Normal Skin.

Caution: Avoid oily T-zone.

Administration: Twice daily, morning and night.

How Supplied: 4.2 fl. oz. lotion (bottle).

Shown in Product Identification Section, page 413

SKIN PRINCIPLE™
Daily Rich Moisture Lotion

Composition: Water, Soluble Collagen Complex, Butylene Glycol, Octyl Palmitate, Glyceryl Stearate, PEG-100 Stearate, Myristyl Myristate, Sorbitan Stearate, Squalane, Urea, Hybrid Safflower Oil, Sesame Oil, Sunflower Seed Oil, Matricaria Oil, Collagen, Caprylic/Capric Triglyceride, Sodium Ribonucleate, Benzophenone-11, Cetearyl Alcohol, Ceteareth-20, Polysorbate 60, Dimethicone, Carbomer 941, Triethanolamine, Glycine, Potassium and Ammonium PCA, Leucine, Glucose Glutamate, Serine, Proline, Collagen Amino Acids, Tyrosine, Tryptophan, Aspartic Acid, Valine, Alanine, Isoleucine, Sodium Lactate, Ethylparaben, Methylparaben, Propylparaben, Imidazolidinyl Urea, BHA, D&C Green No. 5, FD&C Red No. 4, FD&C Yellow No. 5.

Actions: Non-occlusive moisture lotion works with body chemistry to renew and rebalance moisture reserves. Enhances elasticity to instantly soften and smoothe skin. Suitable for under make-up. Recommended for: Dry/Partly Dry Skin.

Administration: Twice daily, morning and night.

How Supplied: 4.2 fl. oz. lotion (bottle).

Shown in Product Identification Section, page 413

SKIN PRINCIPLE™
Serious Moisture Supplement

Composition: Water, Soluble Collagen Complex, Isostearyl Neopentanoate, Isocetyl Stearate, Hybrid Safflower Oil, Sesame Oil, Sunflower Seed Oil, Butylene Glycol, Sorbitan Stearate, Glyceryl Stearate, PEG-100 Stearate, Squalane, Caprylic/Capric Triglyceride, Matricaria Oil, Urea, Ceteareth-20, Cetearyl Alcohol, Cetyl Alcohol, Elastin, Sodium Ribonucleate, Ascorbic Acid, Tocopherol, Sodium Citrate, Benzophenone-11, Dimethicone, Glycine, Potassium and Ammonium PCA, Leucine, Glucose Glutamate, Serine, Proline, Collagen Amino Acids, Tyrosine, Trypotophan, Aspartic Acid, Valine, Alanine, Isoleucine, Xanthan Gum, Sodium Lactate, Ethylparaben, Methylparaben, Propylparaben, Imidazolidinyl Urea, BHA, Trisodium EDTA, D&C Green No. 5, FD&C Red No. 4, D&C Red No. 33.

Actions: Non-occlusive moisture concentrate. Minimizes dry skin lines to help skin appear younger and fresher looking. Suitable for use under make-up by extra dry skin types. Recommended for: Dry/Partly Dry Skin or a mature complexion.

Administration: Once nightly. Extra-dry skin types may also use in the morning under make-up if desired.

How Supplied: 2 oz. cream (glass jar).

Shown in Product Identification Section, page 413

Mayrand, Inc.
P.O. BOX 8869
FOUR DUNDAS CIRCLE
GREENSBORO, NC 27419-0869

ELDERTONIC
Vitamin-Mineral Supplement

Description: Each 45 ml. (3 tablespoonfuls) contains:

	For Adults Percentage of U.S. RDA
Thiamine HCl. (B_1)	1.5 mg.
Riboflavin (B_2)	1.7 mg.
Niacinamide	20 mg.
Dexpanthenol	10 mg.
Pyridoxine HCl. (B_6)	2 mg.
Cyancobalamin (B_{12})	6 mcg.
Zinc (Elemental) (as Zinc Sulfate)	15 mg.
Manganese (as Manganese Sulfate)	2 mg.
Magnesium (as Magnesium Sulfate)	*2 mg.
Alcohol	13.5%

*Minimum concentration as added magnesium

Action: ELDERTONIC is a highly palatable elixir prepared in a special sherry wine base, with essential B-complex vitamins and minerals to help maintain nutritional status. ELDERTONIC is especially useful for elderly patients requiring appetite stimulation and nutritional support.

The extremely palatable elixir increases patient acceptance and, therefore, compliance. This helps to preclude skipped doses which interfere with the effectiveness of the regimen. Chilling prior to administration will enhance the flavor of this fine sherry wine vehicle.

Indications: ELDERTONIC is indicated for nutritional support for those requiring dietary supplementation of minerals and vitamins.

THIS PRODUCT PROVIDES 100% OF THE ESTABLISHED RDA OF THE LISTED VITAMINS PER 45 ml. IT ALSO PROVIDES 100% OF THE ESTABLISHED RDA FOR ZINC, 50% OF RDA FOR MANGANESE, AND 0.5% (minimum) OF RDA FOR MAGNESIUM.

Dosage and Administration: Adult: One tablespoon three times daily, with or before meals.

How Supplied: ELDERTONIC is supplied in 8 oz, NDC 0259-0351-08; pints, NDC 0259-0351-16; and gallons, NDC 0259-0351-28.

GLYTUSS TABS
Expectorant Tablets

Composition: Each tablet contains:
Guaifenesin .... 200 mg.

Actions and Use: Guaifenesin is an expectorant that enhances the output of respiratory tract fluid by reducing the

Continued on next page

Mayrand—Cont.

viscosity of the fluid. This results in a less dry, more productive cough.

Indications: Glytuss is useful in the treatment of dry, unproductive coughing associated with the common cold, influenza and bronchitis.

Warning: Persons with high fever, or persistent cough that recurs should consult a physician since one or more of these symptoms may indicate a serious condition. Glytuss should not be taken for persistent coughs associated with smoking, asthma or emphysema, or coughs associated with excessive secretions, except under supervision of a physician.

Caution: Safe use of this product in pregnancy has not been established.

How Supplied: Bottles of 100 tablets, NDC 0259-0288-01. Tablets are imprinted Mayrand.

NU–IRON 150 Caps
NU–IRON Elixir
(polysaccharide-iron complex)
Iron Supplement

Composition: NU-IRON is a highly water soluble complex of iron and a low molecular weight polysaccharide. Each NU-IRON 150 Capsule contains 150 mg. elemental iron. Each 5 ml. (teaspoonful) of NU-IRON Elixir contains 100 mg. elemental iron, alcohol 10% (Sugar free).

Action and Uses: NU-IRON is a non-ionic, easily assimilated, relatively non-toxic form of iron. Full therapeutic doses may be achieved with virtually no gastrointestinal side effects. There is no metallic aftertaste and no staining of teeth.

Indications: For treatment of uncomplicated iron deficiency anemia.

Contraindications: Hemochromatosis, hemosiderosis or a known hypersensitivity to any of the ingredients.

Usual Dosage: ADULTS; One or two NU-IRON 150 Caps daily, or one to two teaspoonfuls NU-IRON Elixir daily. CHILDREN; 6 to 12 years old; one teaspoonful NU-IRON Elixir daily; 2 to 6 years old: ½ teaspoonful daily; under 2 years: ¼ teaspoonful daily.

How Supplied: NU-IRON 150 Caps in bottles of 100. NU-IRON Elixir in 8 fl. oz. bottles.

Products are cross-indexed by
generic and chemical names
in the
YELLOW SECTION

McNeil Consumer Products Company
McNEILAB, INC.
FORT WASHINGTON, PA 19034

COTYLENOL® Cold Medication Tablets and Capsules

Description: Each CoTYLENOL Tablet or Capsule contains acetaminophen 325 mg., chlorpheniramine maleate 2 mg., pseudoephedrine hydrochloride 30 mg. and dextromethorphan hydrobromide 15 mg.

Actions: CoTYLENOL Cold Medication Tablets and Capsules contain a clinically proven analgesic-antipyretic, decongestant, cough suppressant and antihistamine. Acetaminophen produces analgesia by elevation of the pain threshold and antipyresis through action on the hypothalamic heat-regulating center. Pseudoephedrine hydrochloride is a sympathomimetic amine which provides temporary relief of nasal congestion. Dextromethorphan is a cough suppressant which provides temporary relief of coughs due to throat irritations that may occur with the common cold. Chlorpheniramine is an antihistamine which helps provide temporary relief of runny nose and sneezing due to the common cold.

Indications: CoTYLENOL provides effective symptomatic relief of fever, aches, pains and general discomfort associated with colds and other upper respiratory infections.

Adverse Reactions: While the acetaminophen component is equal to aspirin in analgesic and antipyretic effectiveness, it is unlikely to produce many of the side effects associated with aspirin and aspirin-containing products. Although pseudoephedrine is virtually without pressor effect in normotensive patients, it should be used with caution in hypertensives.

Usual Dosage: Adults: Two tablets or capsules every 6 hours, not to exceed 8 tablets or capsules in 24 hours. Children (6–12 years): One tablet or capsule every 6 hours, not to exceed 4 tablets or capsules in 24 hours.

Note: Since CoTYLENOL Cold Medication Tablets and Capsules are available without prescription, the following appears on the package label: "WARNING: Do not administer to children under 6 or exceed the recommended dosage because nervousness, dizziness or sleeplessness may result. Do not take if you have asthma, glaucoma, high blood pressure, heart disease, diabetes, thyroid disease, enlargement of the prostate gland, persistent cough due to smoking or emphysema, or are presently taking a prescription drug for the treatment of high blood pressure or emotional disorders, without the advice and supervision of a doctor. This product may cause drowsiness. Do not drive, operate machinery or drink alcoholic beverages while taking. Persistent cough may indicate a serious condition. Consult a doctor after 3 days if fever persists, or after 7 days if symptoms do not improve or cough persists, tends to recur or is accompanied by high fever, rash, or persistent headaches. Do not use if carton is opened, or if printed green neck wrap or printed foil inner seal is broken (for Capsules). Do not use if carton is opened or printed foil seal is broken (for Tablets). Keep this and all medication out of the reach of children. As with any drug, if you are pregnant or nursing a baby, seek the advice of a health professional before using this product. In case of accidental overdosage, contact a physician or poison control center immediately."

Overdosage: Acetaminophen in massive overdosage may cause hepatic toxicity in some patients. In all cases of suspected overdose, immediately call your regional poison center or the Rocky Mountain Poison Center's toll-free number (800-525-6115) for assistance in diagnosis and for directions in the use of N-acetylcysteine as an antidote, a use currently restricted to investigational status. In adults, hepatic toxicity has rarely been reported with acute overdoses of less than 10 grams and fatalities with less than 15 grams. Importantly, young children seem to be more resistant than adults to the hepatotoxic effect of an acetaminophen overdose. Despite this, the measures outlined below should be initiated in any adult or child suspected of having ingested an acetaminophen overdose.

Early symptoms following a potentially hepatotoxic overdose may include: nausea, vomiting, diaphoresis and general malaise. Clinical and laboratory evidence of hepatic toxicity may not be apparent until 48 to 72 hours postingestion. The stomach should be emptied promptly by lavage or by induction of emesis with syrup of ipecac. Patients' estimates of the quantity of a drug ingested are notoriously unreliable. Therefore, if an acetaminophen overdose is suspected, a serum acetaminophen assay should be obtained as early as possible, but no sooner than four hours following ingestion. Liver function studies should be obtained initially and repeated at 24 hour intervals. The antidote, N-acetylcysteine, should be administered as early as possible, and within 16 hours of the overdose ingestion for optimal results. Following recovery, there are no residual, structural or functional hepatic abnormalities.

Chlorpheniramine toxicity should be treated as you would an antihistamine/anticholinergic overdose and is likely to be present within a few hours after acute ingestion.

Symptoms from pseudoephedrine overdose consist most often of mild anexiety, tachycardia and/or mild hypertension. Symptoms usually appear within 4 to 8 hours of ingestion and are transient, usually requiring no treatment.

Acute dextromethorphan overdose usually does not result in serious signs and symptoms unless massive amounts have been ingested. Signs and symptoms of a substantial overdose may include nausea and vomiting, visual disturbances, CNS disturbances, and urinary retention.

How Supplied: Tablets (colored yellow, imprinted "CoTYLENOL") — blister packs of 24, tamper-resistant bottles of 50 and 100. Capsules (colored dark green and light yellow, imprinted "CoTYLENOL")—blister packs of 20 and tamper-resistant bottles of 40.

Shown in Product Identification Section, page 414

CoTYLENOL® Cold Medicine Liquid

Description: Each 30 ml (1 fl. oz.) contains acetaminophen 650 mg., chlorpheniramine maleate 4 mg., pseudoephedrine hydrochloride 60 mg., and dextromethorphan hydrobromide 30 mg. (alcohol 7.5%).

Actions: CoTYLENOL Liquid Cold Medication contains a clinically proven analgesic-antipyretic, decongestant, cough suppressant and antihistamine. Acetaminophen produces analgesia by elevation of the pain threshold and antipyresis through action on the hypothalamic heat-regulating center. Pseudoephedrine hydrochloride is a sympathomimetic amine which provides temporary relief of nasal congestion. Dextromethorphan is a cough suppressant which provides temporary relief of coughs due to throat irritations that may occur with the common cold. Chlorpheniramine is an antihistamine which helps provide temporary relief of runny nose and sneezing due to the common cold.

Indications: CoTYLENOL provides effective symptomatic relief of fever, aches, pains and general discomfort associated with colds and other upper respiratory infections.

Adverse Reactions: While the acetaminophen component is equal to aspirin in analgesic and antipyretic effectiveness, it is unlikely to produce many of the side effects associated with aspirin and aspirin-containing products. Although pseudoephedrine is virtually without pressor effect in normotensive patients, it should be used with caution in hypertensives.

Usual Dosage: Measuring cup is provided and marked for accurate dosing. Adults: 1 fluid ounce (2 tbsp.) every 6 hours as needed, not to exceed 4 doses in 24 hours. Children (6–12 yrs): ½ the adult dose (1 tbsp.) as indicated on the measuring cup provided, not to exceed 4 doses in 24 hours.
Note: Since CoTYLENOL Liquid Cold Medication is available without a prescription, the following appears on the package label: "WARNING: Do not administer to children under 6 or exceed the recommended dosage because nervousness, dizziness or sleeplessness may result. Do not take if you have asthma, glaucoma, high blood pressure, heart disease, diabetes, thyroid disease, enlargement of the prostate gland, persistant cough due to smoking or emphysema, or are presently taking a prescription drug

for the treatment of high blood pressure or emotional disorders, without advice and supervision of a doctor. This product may cause drowsiness. Do not drive, operate machinery or drink alcoholic beverages while taking. Persistent cough may indicate a serious condition. Consult a doctor after 3 days if fever persists, or after 7 days if symptoms do not improve or cough persists, tends to recur or is accompanied by high fever, rash, or persistent headaches. **Do not use if carton is opened, or if printed plastic overwrap or printed foil inner seal is broken. Keep this and all medication out of the reach of children. As with any drug, if you are pregnant or nursing a baby, seek the advice of a health professional before using this product. In case of accidental overdosage, contact a physician or poison control center immediately."**

Overdosage: Acetaminophen in massive overdosage may cause hepatic toxicity in some patients. In all cases of suspected overdose, immediately call your regional poison center or the Rocky Mountain Poison Center's toll-free number (800-525-6115) for assistance in diagnosis and for directions in the use of N-acetylcysteine as an antidote, a use currently restricted to investigational status. In adults, hepatic toxicity has rarely been reported with acute overdoses of less than 10 grams and fatalities with less than 15 grams. Importantly, young children seem to be more resistant than adults to the hepatotoxic effect of an acetaminophen overdose. Despite this, the measures outlined below should be initiated in any adult or child suspected of having ingested an acetaminophen overdose.
Early symptoms following a potentially hepatotoxic overdose may include: nausea, vomiting, diaphoresis and general malaise. Clinical and laboratory evidence of hepatic toxicity may not be apparent until 48 to 72 hours postingestion. The stomach should be emptied promptly by lavage or by induction of emesis with syrup of ipecac. Patients' estimates of the quantity of a drug ingested are notoriously unreliable. Therefore, if an acetaminophen overdose is suspected, a serum acetaminophen assay should be obtained as early as possible, but no sooner than four hours following ingestion. Liver function studies should be obtained initially and repeated at 24-hour intervals. The antidote, N-acetylcysteine, should be administered as early as possible, and within 16 hours of the overdose ingestion for optimal results. Following recovery, there are no residual, structural or functional hepatic abnormalities.
Chlorpheniramine toxicity should be treated as you would an antihistamine/anticholinergic overdose and is likely to be present within a few hours after acute ingestion.
Symptoms from pseudoephedrine overdose consist most often of mild anxiety, tachycardia and/or mild hypertension. Symptoms usually appear within 4 to 8

hours of ingestion and are transient, usually requiring no treatment.
Acute dextromethorphan overdose usually does not result in serious signs and symptoms unless massive amounts have been ingested. Signs and symptoms of a substantial overdose may include nausea and vomiting, visual disturbances, CNS disturbances, and urinary retention.

How Supplied: Cherry/mint mentholated flavored (colored amber) in 5 oz. bottles with child-resistant safety cap, special dosage cup graded in ounces and tablespoons, and tamper-resistant packaging.

Children's CoTYLENOL® Chewable Cold Tablets and Liquid Cold Formula

Description: Each Children's CoTYLENOL Chewable Cold Tablet contains acetaminophen 80 mg, chlorpheniramine maleate 0.5 mg, and phenylpropanolamine hydrochloride 3.125 mg. Children's CoTYLENOL Liquid Cold Formula is stable, cherry-flavored, red in color and contains 8.5% alcohol. Each teaspoon (5 ml) contains acetaminophen 160 mg, chlorpheniramine maleate 1 mg, and phenylpropanolamine hydrochloride 6.25 mg.

Actions and Indications: Children's CoTYLENOL Chewable Cold Tablets and Liquid Cold Formula combine the nonsalicylate analgesic-antipyretic acetaminophen with the decongestant phenylpropanolamine hydrochloride and the antihistamine chlorpheniramine maleate to help relieve nasal congestion, dry runny noses and prevent sneezing as well as to relieve the fever, aches, pains and general discomfort associated with colds and upper respiratory infections.
While the acetaminophen component is equal to aspirin in analgesic and antipyretic effectiveness, it is unlikely to produce the following side effects often associated with aspirin or aspirin-containing products: allergic reactions, even in aspirin-sensitive children or those with a history of allergy in general; "therapeutic toxicity" in feverish children, since electrolyte imbalance and acid-base changes are not likely to occur; and gastric irritation even in children with an already upset stomach.

Dosage: Children's CoTYLENOL Chewable Cold Tablets: 2–5 years—2 tablets, 6–11 years—4 tablets.
Children's CoTYLENOL Liquid Cold Formula: Measuring Cup is provided and marked for accurate dosing. 2–5 years—1 teaspoonful; 6–11 years—2 teaspoonsful. Doses may be repeated every 4 hours as needed, not to exceed 5 doses in 24 hours.
Note: Since Children's CoTYLENOL Chewable Cold Tablets and Liquid Cold Formula are available without prescription, the following information appears on the package labels: "WARNING: Do not exceed the recommended dosage. Reduce dosage if nervousness, restlessness or sleeplessness occurs. Do not use if

Continued on next page

McNeil Consumer—Cont.

glaucoma, high blood pressure, heart disease, diabetes, or thyroid disease is present. This preparation may cause drowsiness, or in some instances, excitability. If presently taking a prescription drug for the treatment of high blood pressure or emotional disorders, or if you have asthma, do not use except under advice and supervision of a physician. Do not drive or operate machinery while taking this medication. If symptoms do not improve within seven days, or are accompanied by high fever or persistent cough, consult a physician before continuing use.

Do not use if carton is opened, or if printed plastic bottle wrap or printed foil inner seal is broken. Keep this and all medicine out of the reach of children. In case of accidental overdosage, contact a physician or poison control center immediately.

Overdosage: Acetaminophen in massive overdosage may cause hepatic toxicity in some patients. In all cases of suspected overdose, immediately call your regional poison center or the Rocky Mountain Poison Center's toll-free number (800-525-6115) for assistance in diagnosis and for directions in the use of N-acetylcysteine as an antidote, a use currently restricted to investigational status.

The occurence of acetaminophen overdose toxicity is uncommon in the pediatric age group. Even with large overdoses, children appear to be less vulnerable than adults to developing hepatotoxicity. This may be due to age-related differences that have been demonstrated in the metabolism of acetaminophen. Despite these differences, the measures outlined below should be immediately initiated in any child suspected of having ingested an acetaminophen overdose.

Early symptoms following a potentially hepatotoxic overdose may include: nausea, vomiting, diaphoresis and general malaise. Clinical and laboratory evidence of hepatic toxicity may not be apparent until 48 to 72 hours post-ingestion.

The stomach should be emptied promptly by lavage or by induction of emesis with syrup of ipecac. If an acute dose of 150 mg/kg body weight or greater was ingested, or if the dose cannot be accurately determined, a serum acetaminophen assay should be obtained as early as possible, but no sooner than four hours following ingestion. If in the toxic range, liver function studies should be obtained at 24-hour intervals. The antidote, N-acetylcysteine, should be administered as early as possible, and within 16 hours of the overdose ingestion for optimal results. Following recovery, there are no residual, structural or functional hepatic abnormalities.

Chlorpheniramine toxicity should be treated as you would an antihistamine/anticholinergic overdose and is likely to be present within a few hours after acute ingestion.

Phenylpropanolamine may produce central nervous system stimulation and sympathomimetic effects on the cardiovascular system which are likely to be manifested within a few hours following ingestion. Hypertension is the most likely manifestation.

How Supplied: Chewable Tablets (colored orange, scored, imprinted "CoTYLENOL")—bottles of 24. Cold Formula—bottles (colored red) of 4 fl. oz.

Shown in Product Identification Section, page 414

PEDIACARE™ 1 Children's Cough Relief Liquid
PEDIACARE™ 2 Children's Cold Relief Liquid
PEDIACARE™ 3 Children's Cold Relief Liquid and Chewable Tablets

Description: Each 5 ml (teaspoon) of PediaCare 1 Children's Cough Relief Liquid contains dextromethorphan hydrobromide 5 mg.

Each 5 ml of PediaCare 2 Children's Cold Relief Liquid contains pseudoephedrine hydrochloride 15 mg and chlorpheniramine maleate 1 mg.

Each 5 ml of PediaCare 3 Children's Cold Relief Liquid contains pseudoephedrine hydrochloride 15 mg, chlorpheniramine maleate 1 mg and dextromethorphan hydrobromide 5 mg.

Each PediaCare 3 Cold Relief Chewable Tablet contains pseudoephedrine hydrochloride 7.5 mg, chlorpheniramine maleate 0.5 mg and dextromethorphan hydrobromide 2.5 mg.

PediaCare Liquid Products are stable, cherry flavored and red in color.

PediaCare 3 Chewable Tablets are fruit-flavored and pink in color.

Actions and Indications: PediaCare Cold Products are available in three different formulas, allowing you to select the ideal cold product to temporarily relieve the patient's particular cold symptoms.

PediaCare 1 Liquid contains a cough suppressant, dextromethorphan hydrobromide, to provide temporary relief of coughs due to minor throat irritations that may occur with the common cold.

PediaCare 2 Liquid contains a decongestant, pseudoephedrine hydrochloride, and an antihistamine, chlorpheniramine maleate, to provide temporary relief of nasal congestion, runny nose and sneezing due to the common cold, hay fever or other upper respiratory allergies.

PediaCare 3 Liquid and Chewable Tablets contain all three of the above ingredients to provide temporary relief of nasal congestion, runny nose, sneezing and coughing due to the common cold, hay fever or other upper respiratory allergies.

Professional Dosage: A calibrated dosage cup is provided for accurate dosing of the PediaCare Liquid formulas. All PediaCare 1 Liquid doses may be repeated every 4 hours, not to exceed 6 doses in 24 hours. All doses of PediaCare 2 Liquid and PediaCare 3 Liquid and Chewable Tablets may be repeated every 4–6 hours, not to exceed 4 doses in 24 hours.

[See table below].

Note: Since PediaCare cold products are available without prescription, the following information appears on the package labels: "WARNINGS: Do not use if carton is opened, or if printed plastic bottle wrap or foil inner seal is broken. Keep this and all medication out of the reach of children. In case of accidental overdosage, contact a physician or poison control center immediately."

The following information appears on the appropriate package labels:

PediaCare 1 Children's Cough Relief Liquid: "Do not take for persistent or chronic cough such as occurs with asthma or where cough is accompanied by excessive mucus except under the advice and supervision of a physician. A persistent cough may be a sign of a serious condition. If cough persists for more than seven days, tends to recur or is accompanied by a high fever, rash or persistent headache, consult a physician".

PediaCare 2 Children's Cold Relief Liquid: "Do not exceed the recommended dosage because nervousness, dizziness or sleeplessness may occur. If symptoms do not improve within seven days or are accompanied by a high fever, consult a physician before continuing use. This preparation may cause drowsiness, or in some cases, excitability. Do not drive or operate heavy machinery while taking this medication. Do not take if you have high blood pressure, heart disease, diabetes, thyroid disease, glaucoma or asthma, or are taking a prescription antihypertensive or antidepressant drug, except under the advice and supervision of a physician".

PediaCare 3 Children's Cold Relief Liquid and Chewable Tablets: "Do not exceed the recommended dosage because nervousness, dizziness or sleeplessness may occur. A persistent cough may be a sign of a serious condition. If symptoms do not improve within seven days or are accompanied by a high fever, rash, excessive mucus, persistent cough or headache, consult a physician before continuing use. This preparation may cause drowsiness or, in some cases,

Age Group (yrs)	2–3	4–5	6–8	9–10	11	Dosage
Weight (lbs)	24–35	36–47	48–59	60–71	72–95	
PediaCare 1 Liquid	1 tsp	1½ tsp	2 tsp	2½ tsp	3 tsp	q4h
PediaCare 2 Liquid	1 tsp	1½ tsp	2 tsp	2½ tsp	3 tsp	q4–6h
PediaCare 3 Liquid	1 tsp	1½ tsp	2 tsp	2½ tsp	3 tsp	q4–6h
Chewable Tablets	2 tabs	3 tabs	4 tabs	5 tabs	6 tabs	q4–6h

excitability. Do not drive or operate machinery while taking this medication. Do not take if you have high blood pressure, heart disease, diabetes, thyroid disease, glaucoma or asthma, or are taking a prescription antihypertensive or antidepressant drug, except under the advice and supervision of a physician." PediaCare 3 Chewable Tablets also contain the warning, "Phenylketonurics: contains phenylalanine."

Overdosage: Acute dextromethorphan overdose usually does not result in serious signs and symptoms unless massive amounts have been ingested. Signs and symptoms of a substantial overdose may include nausea and vomiting, visual disturbances, CNS disturbances, and urinary retention.

Symptoms from pseudoephedrine overdose consist most often of mild anxiety, tachycardia and/or mild hypertension. Symptoms usually appear within 4 to 8 hours of ingestion and are transient, usually requiring no treatment.

Chlorpheniramine toxicity should be treated as you would an antihistamine/anticholinergic overdose and is likely to be present within a few hours after acute ingestion.

How Supplied: PediaCare Liquid products (colored red)—bottles of 4 fl. oz. with child-resistant safety cap and calibrated dosage cup. PediaCare 3 Chewable Tablets (pink, scored)—bottles of 24 with child-resistant safety cap.

Show in Product Identification Section, page 413

SINE–AID®
Sinus Headache Tablets

Description: Each SINE-AID® Tablet contains acetaminophen 325 mg and pseudoephedrine hydrochloride 30 mg.

Actions: SINE-AID® Tablets contain a clinically proven analgesic-antipyretic and a decongestant. Acetaminophen produces analgesia by elevation of the pain threshold and antipyresis through action on the hypothalamic heat-regulating center. Pseudoephedrine hydrochloride is a sympathomimetic amine which promotes proper sinus cavity drainage by reducing nasopharyngeal mucosal congestion.

Indications: SINE-AID® Tablets provide effective symptomatic relief from sinus headache pain and pressure caused by sinusitis.

Adverse Reactions: While the acetaminophen component is equal to aspirin in analgesic and antipyretic effectiveness, it is unlikely to produce many of the side effects associated with aspirin and aspirin-containing products. Since the product contains no antihistamine, SINE-AID® Tablets will not produce the drowsiness that may interfere with work, driving an automobile or operating dangerous machinery. SINE-AID® is particularly well-suited in patients with aspirin allergy, hemostatic disturbances (including anticoagulant therapy), and bleeding diatheses (e.g. hemophilia) and

upper gastrointestinal disease (e.g. ulcer, gastritis, hiatus hernia). If a rare sensitivity occurs, the drug should be discontinued. Although pseudoephedrine is virtually without pressor effect in normotensive patients, it should be used with caution in hypertensives.

Usual Dosage: Adult dosage: Two tablets every four to six hours. Do not exceed eight tablets in any 24 hour period. Note: Since SINE-AID® Tablets are available without a prescription, the following appears on the package labels: "WARNING: Do not exceed the recommended dosage or administer to children under 12. Reduce dosage if nervousness or sleeplessness occurs. If you have high blood pressure, heart disease, diabetes, or thyroid disease or are presently taking a prescription drug for the treatment of high blood pressure or emotional disorders, do not take except under the advice and supervision of a physician. If symptoms persist for 7 days or are accompanied by high fever, consult a physician. **Do not use if carton is opened, or printed foil inner seal is broken. Keep this and all medication out of the reach of children. As with any drug, if you are pregnant or nursing a baby, seek the advice of a health professional before using this product. In case of accidental overdosage, contact a physician or poison control center.**

Overdosage: Acetaminophen in massive overdosage may cause hepatic toxicity in some patients. In all cases of suspected overdose, immediately call your regional poison center or the Rocky Mountain Poison Center's toll-free number (800-525-6115) for assistance in diagnosis and for directions in the use of N-acetylcysteine as an antidote, a use currently restricted to investigational status. In adults hepatic toxicity has rarely been reported with acute overdoses of less than 10 grams and fatalities with less than 15 grams. Importantly, young children seem to be more resistant than adults to the hepatotoxic effect of an acetaminophen overdose. Despite this, the measures outlined below should be initiated in any adult or child suspected of having ingested an acetaminophen overdose.

Early symptoms following a potentially hepatotoxic overdose may include: nausea, vomiting, diaphoresis and general malaise. Clinical and laboratory evidence of hepatic toxicity may not be apparent until 48 to 72 hours postingestion. The stomach should be emptied promptly by lavage or by induction of emesis with syrup of ipecac. Patients' estimates of the quantity of a drug ingested are notoriously unreliable. Therefore, if an acetaminophen overdose is suspected, a serum acetaminophen assay should be obtained as early as possible, but no sooner than four hours following ingestion. Liver function studies should be obtained initially and repeated at 24-hour intervals. The antidote, N-acetylcysteine, should be administered as early as possible, and within 16 hours of the

overdose ingestion for optimal results. Following recovery, there are no residual structural or functional hepatic abnormalities.

Symptoms from pseudoephedrine overdose consist most often of mild anxiety, tachycardia and/or mild hypertension. Symptoms usually appear within 4 to 8 hours of ingestion and are transient, usually requiring no treatment.

How Supplied: Tablets (colored white, imprinted "SINE-AID®")—tamper-resistant bottles of 24, 50 and 100.
Shown in Product Identification Section, page 414

EXTRA–STRENGTH SINE–AID®
Sinus Headache Capsules

Description: Each EXTRA-STRENGTH SINE-AID® Capsule contains acetaminophen 500 mg and pseudoephedrine hydrochloride 30 mg.

Actions: EXTRA-STRENGTH SINE-AID® Capsules contain a clinically proven analgesic-antipyretic and a decongestant. Maximum allowable nonprescription levels of acetaminophen and pseudoephedrine provide temporary relief of sinus congestion and pain. Acetaminophen produces analgesia by elevation of the pain threshold and antipyresis through action on the hypothalamic heat-regulating center. Pseudoephedrine hydrochloride is a sympathomimetic amine which promotes proper sinus cavity drainage by reducing nasopharyngeal mucosal congestion.

Indications: EXTRA-STRENGTH SINE-AID® Capsules provide effective symptomatic relief from sinus headache pain and pressure caused by sinusitis.

Adverse Reactions: While the acetaminophen component is equal to aspirin in analgesic and antipyretic effectiveness, it is unlikely to produce many of the side effects associated with aspirin and aspirin-containing products. Since the product contains no antihistamine, EXTRA-STRENGTH SINE-AID® Capsules will not produce the drowsiness that may interfere with work, driving an automobile or operating dangerous machinery. SINE-AID® is particularly well-suited in patients with aspirin allergy, hemostatic disturbances (including anticoagulant therapy), and bleeding diatheses (e.g. hemophilia) and upper gastrointestinal disease (e.g. ulcer, gastritis, hiatus hernia). If a rare sensitivity occurs, the drug should be discontinued. Although pseudoephedrine is virtually without pressor effect in normotensive patients, it should be used with caution in hypertensives.

Usual Dosage: Adult dosage: Two capsules every four to six hours. Do not exceed eight capsules in any 24 hour period. **Note:** Since EXTRA-STRENGTH SINE-AID® Capsules are available without a prescription, the following appears on the package labels: "WARNING: Do not exceed the recommended dosage or

Continued on next page

McNeil Consumer—Cont.

administer to children under 12. Reduce dosage if nervousness or sleeplessness occurs. If you have high blood pressure, heart disease, diabetes, or thyroid disease or are presently taking a prescription drug for the treatment of high blood pressure or emotional disorders, do not take except under the advice and supervision of a physician. If symptoms persist for 7 days or are accompanied by high fever, consult a physician. **Do not use if carton is opened, or if printed redneck wrap or printed foil inner seal is broken. Keep this and all medication out of the reach of children. As with any drug, if you are pregnant or nursing a baby, seek the advice of a health professional before using this product. In case of accidental overdosage, contact a physician or poison control center.**

Overdosage: Acetaminophen in massive overdosage may cause hepatic toxicity in some patients. In all cases of suspected overdose, immediately call your regional poison center or the Rocky Mountain Center's toll-free number (800-525-6115) for assistance in diagnosis and for directions in the use of N-acetylcysteine as an antidote, a use currently restricted to investigational status. In adults hepatic toxicity has rarely been reported with acute overdoses of less than 10 grams and fatalities with less than 15 grams. Importantly, young children seem to be more resistant than adults to the hepatotoxic effect of an acetaminophen overdose. Despite this, the measures outlined below should be initiated in any adult or child suspected of having ingested an acetaminophen overdose.

Early symptoms following a potentially hepatotoxic overdose may include: nausea, vomiting, diaphoresis and general malaise. Clinical and laboratory evidence of hepatic toxicity may not be apparent until 48 to 72 hours postingestion. The stomach should be emptied promptly by lavage or by induction of emesis with syrup of ipecac. Patients' estimates of the quantity of a drug ingested are notoriously unreliable. Therefore, if an acetaminophen overdose is suspected, a serum acetaminophen assay should be obtained as early as possible, but no sooner than four hours following ingestion. Liver function studies should be obtained initially and repeated at 24-hour intervals. The antidote, N-acetylcysteine, should be administered as early as possible, and within 16 hours of the overdose ingestion for optimal results. Following recovery, there are no residual structural or functional hepatic abnormalities.

Symptoms from pseudoephedrine overdose consist most often of mild anxiety, tachycardia and/or mild hypertension. Symptoms usually appear within 4 to 8 hours of ingestion and are transient, usually requiring no treatment.

How Supplied: Capsules (colored yellow and white imprinted "EXTRA-

STRENGTH SINE-AID®")—tamper-resistant bottles of 20.

Shown in Product Identification Section, page 414

Children's TYLENOL®
acetaminophen
Chewable Tablets, Elixir, Drops

Description: Each Children's TYLENOL Chewable Tablet contains 80 mg. acetaminophen in a fruit flavored tablet. Children's TYLENOL acetaminophen Elixir is stable, cherry flavored, red in color and is alcohol free. Infants' TYLENOL Drops are stable, fruit flavored, orange in color and are alcohol free. Children's TYLENOL Elixir: Each 5 ml. contains 160 mg. acetaminophen. Infant's TYLENOL Drops: Each 0.8 ml. (one calibrated dropperful) contains 80 mg. acetaminophen.

Actions: TYLENOL acetaminophen is an effective antipyretic/analgesic. It produces antipyresis through action on the hypothalamic heat-regulating center and analgesia by elevation of the pain threshold.

Indications: Children's TYLENOL Chewable Tablets, Elixir and Drops are designed for treatment of infants and children with conditions requiring reduction of fever or relief of pain—such as mild upper respiratory infections (tonsillitis, common cold, "grippe"), headache, myalgia, post-immunization reactions, post-tonsillectomy discomfort and gastroenteritis. TYLENOL acetaminophen is useful as an analgesic and antipyretic in many bacterial or viral infections, such as bronchitis, pharyngitis, tracheobronchitis, sinusitis, pneumonia, otitis media, and cervical adenitis.

Precautions and Adverse Reactions: TYLENOL acetaminophen has rarely been found to produce any side effects. If a rare sensitivity reaction occurs, the drug should be stopped. It is usually well tolerated by aspirin-sensitive patients.

Usual Dosage: Doses may be repeated 4 or 5 times daily, but not to exceed 5 doses in 24 hours.
Children's TYLENOL Chewable Tablets: 1–2 years: one and one half tablets. 2–3 years: two tablets. 4–5 years: three tablets. 6–8 years: four tablets. 9–10 years: five tablets. 11–12 years: six tablets.
Children's TYLENOL Elixir: (special cup for measuring dosage is provided) 4–11 months: one-half teaspoon. 12–23 months: three-quarters teaspoon. 2–3 years: one teaspoon. 4–5 years: one and one-half teaspoons. 6–8 years: 2 teaspoons. 9–10 years: two and one-half teaspoons. 11–12 years: three teaspoons.
Infants' TYLENOL Drops: 0–3 months: 0.4 ml. 4–11 months: 0.8 ml. 12–23 months: 1.2 ml. 2–3 years: 1.6 ml. 4–5 years: 2.4 ml.
Note: Since Children's TYLENOL acetaminophen Chewable Tablets, Elixir and Drops are available without prescription as an analgesic, the following appears on the package labels: "WARNING: Consult your physician if fever persists for more

than three days or if pain continues for more than five days. **Do not use if safety seals are broken. Keep this and all medication out of the reach of children. In case of accidental overdosage, contact a physician or poison control center immediately.**"

Overdosage: Acetaminophen in massive overdosage may cause hepatic toxicity in some patients. In all cases of suspected overdose, immediately call your regional poison center or the Rocky Mountain Poison Center's toll-free number (800-525-6115) for assistance in diagnosis and for directions in the use of N-acetylcysteine as an antidote, a use currently restricted to investigational status. The occurence of acetaminophen overdose toxicity is uncommon in the pediatric age group. Even with large overdoses, children appear to be less vulnerable than adults to developing hepatotoxicity. This may be due to age-related differences that have been demonstrated in the metabolism of acetaminophen. Despite these differences, the measures outlined below should be immediately initiated in any child suspected of having ingested an overdose of acetaminophen.

Early symptoms following a potentially hepatotoxic overdose may include: nausea, vomiting, diaphoresis and general malaise. Clinical and laboratory evidence of hepatic toxicity may not be apparent until 48 to 72 hours post-ingestion. The stomach should be emptied promptly by lavage or by induction of emesis with syrup of ipecac. If an acute dose of 150 mg/kg body weight or greated was ingested, or if the dose cannot be accurately determined, a serum acetaminophen assay should be obtained as early as possible, but no sooner than four hours post-ingestion. If in the toxic range, liver function studies should be obtained and repeated at 24-hour intervals. The antidote N-acetylcysteine should be administered as early as possible, and within 16 hours of the overdose ingestion for optimal results. Following recovery there are no residual, structural or functional hepatic abnormalities.

How Supplied: Chewable Tablets (colored pink, scored, imprinted "TYLENOL")—Bottles of 30. Elixir (colored red)—bottles of 2 and 4 fl. oz. Drops (colored orange)—bottles of ½ oz. (15 ml.) with calibrated plastic dropper.
All packages listed above have child-resistant safety caps.

Shown in Product Identification Section, page 414

Junior Strength TYLENOL®
acetaminophen
Swallowable Tablets

Description: Each Junior Strength Swallowable Tablet contains 160mg acetaminophen in a small, coated, capsule shaped tablet.

Actions: TYLENOL acetaminophen is an effective antipyretic/analgesic. It produces antipyresis through action on the hypothalmic heat-regulating center and analgesia by elevation of the pain threshold.

Indications: Junior Strength TYLENOL Swallowable Tablets are designed for older children and young adults with conditions requiring reduction of fever or relief of pain—such as mild upper respiratory infections (tonsillitis, common cold, "grippe"), headache, myalgia, post-immunization reactions, post-tonsillectomy discomfort and gastroenteritis. TYLENOL acetaminophen is useful as an analgesic and antipryetic in many bacterial or viral infections, such as bronchitis, pharyngitis, tracheobronchitis, sinusitis, pneumonia, otitis media and cervical adenitis.

Precautions and Adverse Reactions: TYLENOL acetaminophen has rarely been found to produce any side effects. If a rare sensitivity reaction occurs, the drug should be stopped. It is usually well tolerated by aspirin-sensitive patients.

Usual Dosage: Doses may be repeated 4 or 5 times daily, but not to exceed 5 doses in 24 hours each. For ages: 6–8 years: two tablets, 9–10 years: two and one-half tablets, 11 years: three tablets, 12–14 years: four tablets.
Note: Since Junior Strength TYLENOL acetaminophen Swallowable Tablets are available without a prescription as an analgesic, the following appears on the package labels:
Warnings: Do not use if carton is opened or if a blister unit is broken. Keep this and all medications out of the reach of children. In case of accidental overdosage, contact a physician or poison control center immediately. Consult your physician if fever persists for more than three days or if pain continues for more than five days. As with any drugs, if you are pregnant or nursing a baby, seek the advise of a health professional before using this product. Not for children who have difficulty swallowing tablets.

Overdosage: Acetaminophen in massive overdosage may cause hepatic toxicity in some patients. In all cases of suspected overdose, immediately call your regional poison control center or the Rocky Mountain Poison Center's toll-free number (800-525-6115) for assistance in diagnosis and for directions in the use of N-acetylcysteine as an antidote, a use currently restricted to investigational status. The occurence of acetaminophen overdose toxicity is uncommon in the pediatric age group. Even with large overdoses, children appear to be less vulnerable than adults to developing hepatotoxicity. This may be due to age-related differences that have been demonstrated in the metabolism of acetaminophen. Despite these differences, the measures outlined below should be immediately initiated in any child suspected of having ingested an overdose of acetaminophen.
Early symptoms following a potentially hepatotoxic overdose may include: nausea, vomiting, diaphoresis and general malaise. Clinical and laboratory evidence of hepatic toxicity may not be apparent until 48 to 72 hours post-ingestion. The stomach should be emptied promptly by lavage or by induction of emesis with syrup of ipecac. If an acute dose of 150mg/kg body weight or greater was ingested, or if the dose cannot be accurately determined, a serum acetaminophen assay should be obtained as early as possible, but no sooner than four hours following ingestion. If in the toxic range, liver function studies should be obtained and repeated at 24-hour intervals. The antidote N-acetylsteine, should be administered as early as possible, and within 16 hours of the overdose ingestion for optimal results. Following recovery there are no residual, structual or functional hepatic abnormalities.

How Supplied: Swallowable Tablets, (colored white, coated, scored, imprinted "TYLENOL"). Package of 30. All packages are safety sealed and use child resistant blister packaging.
Shown in Product Identification Section, page 414

Regular Strength
TYLENOL® acetaminophen
Tablets and Capsules

Description: Each Regular Strength TYLENOL Tablet or Capsule contains acetaminophen 325 mg.

Actions: TYLENOL acetaminophen is a clinically proven analgesic and antipyretic. TYLENOL acetaminophen produces analgesia by elevation of the pain threshold and antipyresis through action on the hypothalamic heat-regulating center.

Indications: TYLENOL acetaminophen provides effective analgesia in a wide variety of arthritic and rheumatic conditions involving musculoskeletal pain, as well as in other painful disorders such as headache, dysmenorrhea, myalgias and neuralgias. In addition, TYLENOL acetaminophen is indicated as an analgesic and antipyretic in diseases accompanied by discomfort and fever, such as the common cold and other viral infections. TYLENOL acetaminophen is particularly well-suited as an analgesic-antipyretic in the presence of aspirin allergy, hemostatic disturbances (including anticoagulant therapy), and bleeding diatheses (e.g. hemophilia) and upper gastrointestinal disorders (e.g., ulcer, gastritis, hiatus hernia).

Precautions and Adverse Reactions: If a rare sensitivity reaction occurs, the drug should be stopped. TYLENOL acetaminophen has rarely been found to produce any side effects. It is usually well-tolerated by aspirin-sensitive patients.

Usual Dosage: *Adults:* One to two tablets or capsules every 4–6 hours. Not to exceed 12 tablets or capsules per day. *Children (6 to 12):* One-half to one tablet 3 or 4 times daily. (TYLENOL acetaminophen Junior Strength Swallowable Tablets, Chewable Tablets, Elixir and Drops are available for greater convenience in younger patients.)

Note: Since TYLENOL acetaminophen tablets and capsules are available without prescription as an analgesic, the following appears on the package labels: "Consult a physician for use by children under 6 or for use longer than 10 days. WARNING: **Do not use if printed red neck wrap or printed foil inner seal is broken.** Keep this and all medication out of the reach of children. As with any drug, if you are pregnant or nursing a baby, seek the advice of a health professional before using this product. In case of accidental overdosage, contact a physician or poison control center immediately." In connection with its use for temporary relief of minor aches and pains of arthritis and rheumatism: "Caution: If pain persists for more than 10 days, or redness is present, or in arthritic or rheumatic conditions affecting children under 12 years, consult a physician immediately."

Overdosage: Acetaminophen in massive overdosage may cause hepatic toxicity in some patients. In all cases of suspected overdose, immediately call your regional poison center or the Rocky Mountain Poison Center's toll-free number (800-525-6115) for assistance in diagnosis and for directions in the use of N-acetylcysteine as an antidote, a use currently restricted to investigational status. In adults, hepatic toxicity has rarely been reported with acute overdoses of less than 10 grams and fatalities with less than 15 grams. Importantly, young children seem to be more resistant than adults to the hepatotoxic effect of an acetaminophen overdose. Despite this, the measures outlined below should be initiated in any adult or child suspected of having ingested an acetaminophen overdose.
Early symptoms following a potentially hepatotoxic overdose may include: nausea, vomiting, diaphoresis and general malaise. Clinical and laboratory evidence of hepatic toxicity may not be apparent until 48 to 72 hours postingestion. The stomach should be emptied promptly by lavage or by induction of emesis with syrup of ipecac. Patients' estimates of the quantity of a drug ingested are notoriously unreliable. Therefore, if an acetaminophen overdose is suspected, a serum acetaminophen assay should be obtained as early as possible, but no sooner than four hours following ingestion. Liver function studies should be obtained initally and repeated at 24-hour intervals. The anitdote, N-acetylcysteine, should be administered as early as possible, and within 16 hours of the overdose ingestion for optimal results. Following recovery, there are no residual, structural or functional hepatic abnormalities.

How Supplied: Tablets (colored white, scored, imprinted "TYLENOL" and "325")—tamper-resistant tins and vials of 12 and bottles of 24, 50, 100 and 200. Capsules (colored gray and white, imprinted "TYLENOL 325 mg")—tamper-resistant bottles of 24, 50 and 100.

Continued on next page

McNeil Consumer—Cont.

Also available: Extra-Strength TYLE-NOL® Tablets, Capsules and Caplets, 500 mg. and Extra-Strength TYLENOL® Adult Liquid Pain Reliever (colored green; 1 fl. oz. = 1000 mg.).

Shown in Product Identification Section, page 413

Extra-Strength TYLENOL® acetaminophen Tablets, Capsules and Caplets

Description: Each Extra-Strength TYLE-NOL Tablet, Capsule and Caplet contains acetaminophen 500 mg.

Actions: TYLENOL acetaminophen is a clinically proven analgesic and antipyretic. Acetaminophen produces analgesia by elevation of the pain threshold and antipyresis through action on the hypothalamic heat-regulating center.

Indications: For relief of pain and fever. Extra-Strength TYLENOL Tablets, Capsules and Caplets provide increased analgesic strength for minor conditions when the usual doses of mild analgesics are insufficient.

Precautions and Adverse Reactions: If a rare sensitivity reaction occurs, the drug should be stopped. TYLENOL acetaminophen has rarely been found to produce any side effects. It is usually well-tolerated by aspirin-sensitive patients.

Usual Dosage: Adults: Two tablets, capsules or caplets 3 or 4 times daily. No more than a total of eight tablets, capsules or caplets in any 24-hour period. *Note:*Since Extra-Strength TYLENOL Tablets, Capsules and Caplets are available without a prescription, the following appears on the package labels: "Severe or recurrent pain or high or continued fever may be indicative of serious illness. Under these conditions, consult a physician. WARNING: **Do not use if printed red neck wrap or printed foil inner seal is broken.** Keep this and all medication out of the reach of children. As with any drug, if you are pregnant or nursing a baby, seek the advice of a health professional before using this product. In case of accidental overdosage, contact a physician or poison control center immediately."

Overdosage: Acetaminophen in massive overdosage may cause hepatic toxicity in some patients. In all cases of suspected overdose, immediately call your regional poison center or the Rocky Mountain Poison Center's toll-free number (800-525-6115) for assistance in diagnosis and for directions in the use of N-acetylcysteine as an antidote, a use currently restricted to investigational status. In adults, hepatic toxicity has rarely been reported with acute overdoses of less than 10 grams and fatalities with less than 15 grams. Importantly, young children seem to be more resistant than adults to the hepatotoxic effect of an acetaminophen overdose. Despite this, the measures outlined below should be initi-ated in any adult or child suspected of having ingested an acetaminophen overdose.

Early symptoms following a potentially hepatotoxic overdose may include: nausea, vomiting, diaphoresis and general malaise. Clinical and laboratory evidence of hepatic toxicity may not be apparent until 48 to 72 hours postingestion. The stomach should be emptied promptly by lavage or by induction of emesis with syrup of ipecac. Patients' estimates of the quantity of a drug ingested are notoriously unreliable. Therefore, if an acetaminophen overdose is suspected, a serum acetaminophen assay should be obtained as early as possible, but no sooner than four hours following ingestion. Liver function studies should be obtained initially and repeated at 24-hour intervals. The antidote, N-acetylcysteine, should be administered as early as possible, and within 16 hours of the overdose ingestion for optimal results. Following recovery, there are no residual, structural or functional hepatic abnormalities.

How Supplied: Tablets (colored white, imprinted "TYLENOL" and "500")—tamper-resistant vials of 10 and bottles of 30, 60, 100 and 200, Capsules (colored red and white, imprinted "TYLENOL 500 mg.")—tamper-resistant vials of 8 and bottles of 24, 50, 100 and 165, Caplets (colored white, imprinted "TYLENOL 500 mg.")—tamper-resistant bottles of 24, 50 and 100.

Also Available: For adults who prefer liquids or can't swallow solid medication, Extra-Strength TYLENOL® Adult Liquid Pain Reliever (1 fl. oz. = 1000 mg.).

Shown in Product Identification Section, page 413

Extra-Strength TYLENOL® acetaminophen Adult Liquid Pain Reliever

Description: Each 15 ml. (½ fl. oz. or one tablespoonful) contains 500 mg. acetaminophen (alcohol 8½%).

Actions: TYLENOL acetaminophen is a clinically proven analgesic and antipyretic. Acetaminophen produces analgesia by elevation of the pain threshold and antipyresis through action on the hypothalamic heat-regulating center.

Indications: TYLENOL acetaminophen provides fast, effective relief of pain and/or fever for adults who prefer liquids or can't swallow solid medication, e.g., the tablets, capsules or caplets.

Precautions and Adverse Reactions: If a rare sensitivity reaction occurs, the drug should be stopped. TYLENOL acetaminophen has rarely been found to produce any side effects. It is usually well-tolerated by aspirin-sensitive patients.

Usual Dosage: Extra-Strength TYLENOL Adult Liquid is an adult preparation. Not for use in children under 12. Measuring cup is marked for accurate dosage. Extra-Strength Dose—1 fl. oz. (30 ml or 2 tablespoonsful, 1000 mg) which is equiva-lent to two 500 mg Extra-Strength TYLE-NOL Tablets, Capsules or Caplets. Take every 4 to 6 hours, no more than 4 doses in any 24 hour period.

Note: Since Extra-Strength TYLENOL Adult Liquid Pain Reliever is available without a prescription, the following appears on the package labels: "Severe or recurrent pain or high or continued fever may be indicative of serious illness. Under these conditions, consult a physician. WARNING: **Do not use if printed plastic overwrap or printed foil seal is broken.** Keep this and all medication out of the reach of children. As with any drug, if you are pregnant or nursing a baby, seek the advice of a health professional before using this product. In case of accidental overdosage, contact a physician or poison control center immediately."

Overdosage: Acetaminophen in massive overdosage may cause hepatic toxicity in some patients. In all cases of suspected overdose, immediately call your regional poison center or the Rocky Mountain Poison Center's toll-free number (800-525-6115) for assistance in diagnosis and for directions in the use of N-acetylcysteine as an antidote, a use currently restricted to investigational status. In adults, hepatic toxicity has rarely been reported with acute overdoses of less than 10 grams and fatalities with less than 15 grams. Importantly, young children seem to be more resistant than adults to the hepatotoxic effect of an acetaminophen overdose. Despite this, the measures outlined below should be initiated in any adult or child suspected of having ingested an acetaminophen overdose.

Early symptoms following a potentially hepatotoxic overdose may include: nausea, vomiting, diaphoresis and general malaise. Clinical and laboratory evidence of hepatic toxicity may not be apparent until 48 to 72 hours post-ingestion. The stomach should be emptied promptly by lavage or by induction of emesis with syrup of ipecac. Patients' estimates of a drug ingested are notoriously unreliable. Therefore, if an acetaminophen overdose is suspected, a serum acetaminophen assay should be obtained as early as possible, but no sooner than four hours following ingestion. Liver function studies should be obtained initially and at 24-hour intervals. The antidote, N-acetylcysteine, should be administered as early as possible, and within 16 hours of the overdose ingestion for optimal results. Following recovery, there are no residual, structural or functional hepatic abnormalities.

How Supplied: Mint-flavored liquid (colored green), 8 fl. oz. tamper-resistant bottle, with child resistent safety cap and special dosage cup.

Maximum-Strength TYLENOL® Sinus Medication Tablets and Capsules

Description: Each Maximum-Strength TYLENOL® Sinus Medication tablet or capsule contains acetaminophen 500 mg.

and pseudoephedrine hydrochloride 30 mg.

Actions: TYLENOL Sinus Medication contains a clinically proven analgesic-antipyretic and a decongestant. Maximum allowable non-prescription levels of acetaminophen and pseudoephedrine provide temporary relief of sinus congestion and pain.
TYLENOL® Acetaminophen produces analgesia by elevation of the pain threshold and antipyresis through action on the hypothalamic heat-regulating center. Pseudoephedrine hydrochloride is a sympathomimetic amine which promotes proper sinus cavity drainage by reducing nasopharyngeal mucosal congestion.

Indications: Maximum-Strength TYLENOL Sinus Medication provides effective syptomatic relief from sinus headache pain and pressure caused by sinusitus.

Adverse Reactions: While Maximum-Strength TYLENOL Sinus Medication's acetaminophen component is equal to aspirin in analgesic and antipyretic effectiveness, it is unlikely to produce many of the side effects associated with aspirin and aspirin-containing products. Since it contains no antihistamine, TYLENOL Sinus Medication will not produce the drowsiness that may interfere with work, driving an automobile or operating dangerous machinery. Maximum-Strength TYLENOL Sinus Medication is particularly well-suited in patients with aspirin allergy, hemostatic disturbances (including anticoagulant therapy), and bleeding diatheses (e.g. hemophilia) and upper gastrointestinal disease (e.g. ulcer, gastritis, hiatus hernia). If a rare sensitivity occurs, the drug should be discontinued. Although pseudoephedrine is virtually without pressor effect in normotensive patients, it should be used with caution in hypertensives.

Usual Dosage: Adult dosage: Two tablets or capsules every four to six hours. Do not exceed eight tablets or capsules in any 24 hour period. **Note:** Since TYLENOL Sinus Medication tablets and capsules are available without a prescription, the following appears on the package labels: "WARNING: Do not exceed the recommended dosage or administer to children under 12. Reduce dosage if nervousness or sleeplessness occurs. If you have high blood pressure, heart disease, diabetes, or thyroid disease, or are presently taking a prescription drug for the treatment of high blood pressure or emotional disorders, do not take except under the advice and supervision of a physician. If symptoms persist for 7 days or are accompanied by high fever, consult a physician." **Do not use tablets or capsules if carton is open or if printed foil inner seal is broken. Do not use capsules if carton is opened or if printed green neck wrap or printed foil inner seal is broken. Keep this and all medication out of the reach of children. As with any drug, if you are pregnant or nusing a baby, seek the advice of a health professional before using this prod-**uct. **In case of accidental overdosage, contact a physician or poison control center.**

Overdosage: Acetaminophen in massive overdosage may cause hepatic toxicity in some patients. In all cases of suspected overdose, immediately call your regional poison center or the Rocky Mountain Center's toll-free number (800-525-6115) for assistance in diagnosis and for directions in the use of N-acetylcysteine as an antidote, a use currently restricted to investigational status. In adults hepatic toxicity has rarely been reported with acute overdoses of less than 10 grams and fatalities with less than 15 grams. Importantly, young children seem to be more resistant than adults to the hepatotoxic effect of an a-cetaminophen overdose. Despite this, the measures outlined below should be initiated in any adult or child suspected of having ingested an acetaminophen overdose.
Early symptons following a potentially hepatotoxic overdose may include: nausea, vomiting, diaphoresis and general malaise. Clinical and laboratory evidence of hepatic toxicity may not be apparent until 48 to 72 hours postingestion. The stomach should be emptied promptly by lavage or by induction of emesis with syrup of ipecac. Patients' estimates of the quanitity of a drug ingested are notoriously unreliable. Therefore, if an acetaminophen overdose is suspected, a serum acetaminophen assay should be obtained as early as possible, but no sooner than four hours following ingestion. Liver function studies should be obtained initially and repeated at 24-hour intervals. The antidote, N-acetylcysteine, should be administered as early as possible, and within 16 hours of the overdose ingestion for optimal results. Following recovery, there are no residual structural or functional hepatic abnormalities.
Symptoms from pseudoephedrine overdose consist most often of mild anxiety, tachycardia and/or mild hypertension. Symptoms usually appear within 4 to 8 hours of ingestion and are transient, usually requiring no treatment.

How Supplied: Tablets (colored light green, imprinted "Maximum-Strength TYLENOL Sinus")—tamper-resistant bottles of 24 and 50. Capsules (colored green and white, imprinted "Maximum-Strength TYLENOL Sinus")—tamper-resistant bottles of 20 and 40.
Shown in Product Identification Section, page 414

Products are
indexed alphabetically
in the
PINK SECTION

Mead Johnson
Nutritional Division
Mead Johnson & Company
2404 W. PENNSYLVANIA ST.
EVANSVILLE, IN 47721

CASEC® powder
Calcium caseinate

Composition: Consists of dried, soluble calcium caseinate (88% protein) derived from skim milk curd and lime water (calcium carbonate) by a special process. Contains only 43 mg sodium per 6 packed level tbsp (1 ounce).

Action and Uses: Supplementing diets of children and adults, including sodium restricted diets and diets low in fat or cholesterol.

Precautions: When Casec is used to modify tube feedings, water intake should be monitored to assure the patient's daily water requirement is met. This is particularly important for comatose or semicomatose patients.

Preparation: Casec powder may be mixed with cereals, vegetables, meat dishes, or blended into milk drinks. For protein supplementation—give as needed.

How Supplied: Casec® powder
NDC 0087-0390-02   Cans of 3⅓ oz (94.5 g)

CE-VI-SOL®
Vitamin C supplement drops
For infants

Composition: Each 0.6 ml supplies 35 mg ascorbic acid. Contains 5% alcohol.

Action and Uses: Dietary supplement of vitamin C for infants.

Administration and Dosage: 0.6 ml (35 mg) or as indicated. Dropper calibrated for doses of 0.6 and 0.3 ml (35 and 17.5 mg ascorbic acid).

How Supplied: Ce-Vi-Sol® drops (with calibrated dropper)
NDC 0087-0400-01 Bottles of 1⅔ fl oz (50 ml)
Shown in Product Identification Section, page 414

CRITICARE HN®
Ready-to-use high nitrogen elemental diet

Composition: Water, maltodextrin, enzymatically hydrolyzed casein, modified corn starch, safflower oil, potassium citrate, calcium gluconate, calcium glycerophosphate, magnesium chloride, choline bitartrate, L-methionine, carrageenan, L-tyrosine, diacetyl tartaric acid esters of mono- and diglycerides, magnesium oxide, L-tryptophan, vitamins (vitamin A palmitate, cholecalciferol, dl-alpha-tocopheryl acetate, sodium ascorbate, folic acid, thiamine hydrochloride, riboflavin, niacinamide, pyridoxine hydrochloride, cyanocobalamin, biotin, cal-

Continued on next page

Mead Johnson Nutr.—Cont.

cium pantothenate and phytonadione) and minerals (potassium iodide, ferrous gluconate, copper gluconate, zinc gluconate and manganese gluconate).

Criticare HN provides 14% of the calories as protein, 3% as fat and 83% as carbohydrate.

Actions and Uses: Criticare HN is the first complete, high nitrogen, elemental nutrition in a commercially sterile, ready-to-use liquid form for patients with impaired digestion and absorption. Under physician supervision, it is intended for use in patients with inflammatory bowel disease, chronic pancreatitis, short gut syndrome, cystic fibrosis, non-specific malabsorption/maldigestion states, and transitions from TPN to enteral nutrition.

Criticare HN contains at least 100% of the U.S. RDA's for all vitamins and minerals in 2000 Calories with extra amounts of vitamin C and B-complex vitamins to meet the increased requirements for these vitamins in the critically ill patient.

Criticare HN is lactose-free and has a moderate osmolality (650 mOsm/kg H_2O) to assure rapid patient adaptation and good patient tolerance.

Preparation: It is recommended that Criticare HN be tube fed and that tube feeding be initiated as follows:

Day 1—1:1 dilution of Criticare HN with water at 50 ml/hour (or full strength at 25 ml/hr).

Day 2—full strength at 50 ml/hour.

Day 3—full strength up to 100–125 ml/hour.

Opened bottles of unused Criticare HN should be covered, kept refrigerated and used within 48 hours of opening. Do not freeze or refrigerate unopened bottles of Criticare HN.

If used with an oral feeding, it is advisable to counsel patients that the flavor of Criticare HN differs significantly from other liquid diets because of the special characteristics of the protein.

Tube Feeding Precaution: Additional water should be given as needed to meet the patient's requirements. Particular attention should be given to water supply for comatose and unconscious patients and others who cannot express the usual sensation of thirst.

Additional water is important also when renal concentrating ability is impaired, when there is extensive breakdown of tissue protein, or when water requirements are high, as in fever, burns or under dry atmospheric conditions.

Criticare HN provides 830 ml of water per 1000 ml of formula.

How Supplied: Criticare HN® liquid NDC 0087-0563-41 Bottles of 8 fl oz

ENFAMIL®
Concentrated liquid • powder
Infant formula

Composition: A whey-predominant infant formula that is nutritionally closer to breast milk than casein-predominant formulas. Caloric distribution: 9% from protein, 50% from fat, 41% from carbohydrate.

Each quart of Enfamil formula (normal dilution, 20 kcal/fl oz) supplies 640 kilocalories, 14.4 g protein, 36 g fat, 66 g carbohydrate, 50 mg taurine and the following:

Vitamin A, IU	2000
Vitamin D, IU	400
Vitamin E, IU	20
Vitamin C, mg	52
Folic acid, mcg	100
Thiamine, mcg	500
Riboflavin, mg	1
Niacin, mg	8
Vitamin B_6, mcg	400
Vitamin B_{12}, mcg	1.5
Biotin, mcg	15
Pantothenic acid, mg	3
Vitamin K_1, mcg	55
Choline, mg	100
Inositol, mg	30
Calcium, mg	440
Phosphorus, mg	300
Iodine, mcg	65
Iron, mg	1

A minimum of 5.4 mg iron per quart should be supplied from other sources.

Magnesium, mg	50
Copper, mcg	600
Zinc, mg	5
Manganese, mcg	100
Chloride, mg	400
Potassium, mg	650
Sodium, mg	200

NOTE: Fer-In-Sol® iron supplement drops are a convenient source of added iron.

Action and Uses: For feeding of full term and premature infants during the first twelve months of life and a supplementary formula for breast-fed babies.

Preparation: For 20 kcal/fl oz: With concentrated liquid—1 part to 1 part water. With powder—1 level scoop to each 2 fl oz water; or 1 level cup to water sufficient to make a quart of formula.

Formula prepared from Enfamil concentrated liquid and opened cans of this liquid should be refrigerated and used within 48 hours. Formula prepared from Enfamil powder should be refrigerated and used within 24 hours. Opened cans of powder should be kept in a cool, dry place and used within 30 days.

How Supplied: Powder, 16-oz (1-lb) cans with measuring scoop. Concentrated liquid, 40 kcal/fl oz 13-fl oz cans.

Also available, Enfamil concentrated liquid or powder with iron; 12 mg iron per quart at 20 kcal/fl oz concentrated liquid, 13-fl oz cans. Powder, 16-oz (1-lb) cans with scoop.

Shown in Product Identification Section, page 414

ENFAMIL® with Iron
Concentrated liquid •powder
Infant formula

Composition: A whey-predominant infant formula which is nutritionally closer to breast milk than casein-predominant formulas, with added iron (12 mg/qt). Caloric distribution: 9% from protein, 50% from fat, 41% from carbohydrate. Except for the higher iron content, the normal dilution (20 kcal/fl oz) has the same vitamin and mineral content as Enfamil (see Enfamil).

Action and Uses: Enfamil with Iron supplies a daily intake of iron for full term and premature infants during the first twelve months of life. Feeding of infants with special needs for exogenous iron, such as: premature infants, offspring of anemic mothers, infants of multiple births, infants with low birth weights and those who grow rapidly, infants who have minor losses of blood at birth or in surgery. As a supplementary formula for breast-fed infants. For older infants the formula provides an easily digestible "beverage milk" plus a supplement of iron. One quart (32 fl oz) of formula supplies 12 mg of iron.

Preparation: See Enfamil section.

Precautions: If therapeutic or larger supplementary amounts of iron are indicated, the iron content of the formula should be taken into account (12 mg iron per qt) in calculating the total iron dosage.

How Supplied: Liquid—13-fl oz cans. Powder—16-oz (1-lb) cans.

Shown in Product Identification Section, page 414

ENFAMIL NURSETTE®
Infant formula

Composition: Glass formula bottle filled with ready-to-feed Enfamil® infant formula (20 kcal/fl oz) (See Enfamil concentrated liquid and powder for nutrient values.) A whey-predominant infant formula which is nutritionally closer to breast milk than casein-predominant formulas.

Action and Uses: A very convenient form of Enfamil for routine formula feeding for the first twelve months of life. Especially useful for feeding for first weeks at home, infants of working mothers, infant travel, emergency feedings, or as a supplementary formula for breast-fed babies.

Preparation: Remove cap, attach any standard sterilized nipple unit and feed baby. The Nursette bottle needs no refrigeration until opened and can be fed at room temperature. Interchangeable with Enfamil Ready-To-Use liquid in cans and formulas in normal dilution (20 kcal/fl oz) prepared from Enfamil concentrated liquid or powder.

Note: Contents remaining in bottle after feeding should be discarded. Nipples and collar rings should be washed, rinsed and sterilized before reuse; bottle not for reuse.

How Supplied: Available in convenient 4 fl oz, 6 fl oz, and 8 fl oz Nursette® bottles, packed four bottles to a sealed carton, six 4-packs per case.

Enfamil Nursette with Iron also available in 6-fl oz bottles.

ENFAMIL® ready-to-use Infant formula

Composition: Filled cans of ready-to-feed Enfamil infant formula 20 kcal/fl oz (see Enfamil concentrated liquid and powder for nutrient values). A whey-predominant infant formula which is nutritionally closer to breast milk than casein-predominant formulas.

Action and Uses: A very convenient form of Enfamil for routine formula feeding during the first twelve months of life. Especially useful for feeding infants of working mothers, infant travel, emergency feedings, as a supplementary formula for breast-fed babies.

Preparation: Pour liquid into sterilized nursing bottle without diluting. No refrigeration is necessary for the unopened cans. The formula need not be heated before feeding baby. Interchangeable with formulas in normal dilution (20 kcal/fl oz) prepared from Enfamil concentrated liquid or powder and Enfamil Nursette® in filled formula bottles.

Precautions: Opened cans of Enfamil ready-to-use formula should be stored in refrigerator and used within 48 hours.

How Supplied: 8-fl oz cans, in an easy to carry handy six-can pack, 4 packs per case, and 32-fl oz (1-qt) cans, six cans per case.

ENFAMIL® with Iron ready-to-use Infant formula

Composition: Filled cans of ready-to-feed Enfamil with Iron infant formula 20 kcal/fl oz (see Enfamil with Iron concentrated liquid & powder for nutrient values). A whey-predominant infant formula which is nutritionally closer to breast milk than casein-predominant formulas.
One quart (32 fl oz) of Enfamil with Iron ready-to-use infant formula supplies 12 mg of iron.

Action and Uses: A very convenient form of Enfamil with Iron for routine formula feeding during the first twelve months of life, especially useful for routine feeding during first weeks at home, infants of working mothers, infant travel, emergency feedings, as a supplementary formula for breast-fed babies.

Preparation: Pour desired amount of liquid into sterilized nursing bottle without diluting. No refrigeration is necessary for unopened cans. The formula need not be heated before feeding baby. Interchangeable with formulas in normal dilution (20 kcal/fl oz) prepared from Enfamil with Iron concentrated liquid or powder.

Precautions: If therapeutic or larger supplementary amounts of iron are indicated, the iron content of the formula should be taken into account (12 mg per qt) in calculating the total iron dosage. Opened cans of Enfamil with Iron ready-to-use formula should be stored in the refrigerator and used within 48 hours.

How Supplied: 8-fl oz cans, in an easy to carry handy six-can pack, 4 packs per case, and 32-fl oz (1-qt) cans, six cans per case.

FER-IN-SOL®
Iron supplement
- drops
- syrup
- capsules

Ferrous sulfate, Mead Johnson

Composition:

Fer-In-Sol	Ferrous Sulfate mg	As Elemental Iron mg	Alcohol %
Drops (per 0.6 ml dose)	75	15	.02
Syrup (per 5 ml teaspoonful)	90	18	5
Capsule (1 capsule)	190 (dried)	60	—

Action and Uses: Source of supplemental iron.

Administration and Dosage:
drops
0.6 ml daily supplies 15 mg of elemental iron, 100% of the U.S. RDA for infants and 150% of the U.S. RDA for children under 4 years of age.
Give in water or in fruit or vegetable juice.
Fer-In-Sol should be given immediately after meals. When an infant or child is taking iron, stools may appear darker in color. This is to be expected and should be no cause for concern. When drops containing iron are given to young babies, some darkening of the membrane covering the baby's teeth may occur. This is not serious or permanent. The enamel of the teeth is not affected. Should this darkening or staining occur, it may be removed by rubbing the baby's teeth with a little baking soda on a small cloth once a week.
syrup
1 teaspoon (5 ml) daily supplies 18 mg of elemental iron, 100% of the U.S. RDA for adults and children 4 or more years of age.
capsules
One capsule daily supplies 60 mg of elemental iron, 333% of the U.S. RDA for pregnant or lactating women.

How Supplied: Fer-In-Sol® drops (with calibrated 'Safti-Dropper')
NDC 0087-0740-02 Bottles of 1-⅔ fl oz (50 ml)
6505-00-664-0856 (1-⅔ fl oz, 50 ml) Defense
Fer-In-Sol® syrup
NDC 0087-0741-01 Bottles of 16 fl oz
Fer-In-Sol® capsules
NDC 0087-0742-01 Bottles of 100

ISOCAL®
Complete liquid diet

Composition: Water, maltodextrin, soy oil, calcium caseinate, sodium caseinate, medium chain triglycerides (fractionated coconut oil), soy protein isolate, potassium citrate, lecithin, calcium citrate, magnesium chloride, calcium chloride, dibasic calcium phosphate, dibasic magnesium phosphate, sodium citrate, carrageenan, potassium chloride, vitamins (vitamin A palmitate, cholecalciferol, dl-alpha-tocopheryl acetate, sodium ascorbate, folic acid, thiamine hydrochloride, riboflavin, niacinamide, pyridoxine hydrochloride, cyanocobalamin, biotin, calcium pantothenate, phytonadione, and choline chloride) and minerals (potassium iodide, ferrous sulfate, cupric sulfate, zinc sulfate and manganese sulfate).
Isocal provides 13% of the calories as protein, 37% as fat and 50% as carbohydrate.

Actions and Uses: Isocal is a complete liquid diet specifically formulated to provide well-balanced nutrition for tube-fed patients when used as the sole source of nourishment. Isocal is lactose-free, has an osmolality of 300 mOsm/kg water and provides at least 100% of the U.S. RDA for vitamins and minerals in 2000 Calories.

Preparation and Administration: Isocal is ready to feed and requires no additional water; shake well before opening. Unopened Isocal should be stored at room temperature. After opening, Isocal should be covered and refrigerated if not used immediately.
Nasogastric tube feedings with Isocal, Complete Liquid Diet, may be given using a standard tube feeding set, or the Isocal Tube Feeding Set. Feedings may be given by continuous drip or at intervals. The rate should be adjusted for the best comfort and needs of the individual patient. When initiating feedings it is recommended that the volume given be no more than 8 fluid ounces. This amount should be administered over a period of about 30 minutes.
Isocal has a bland, unsweetened taste because it is specifically formulated for tube feedings. However, patients on long-term oral diet may prefer the taste of Isocal to the sweet taste of some oral liquid nutritional supplements.

Precautions: Additional water may be needed to meet the patient's requirements. Particular attention should be given to water needs of comatose and unconscious patients and others who cannot express the usual sensations of thirst. Additional water is important also when renal-concentrating ability is impaired, when there is extensive breakdown of tissue protein, or when water requirements are high, as in fever. Isocal provides 843 ml of water per 1000 ml.
Tube feeding preparations should be at room temperature during administration.

Continued on next page

Mead Johnson Nutr.—Cont.

How Supplied: Isocal® Complete Liquid Diet
NDC 0087-0355-01 Cans of 8 fl oz
NDC 0087-0355-02 Cans of 12 fl oz
NDC 0087-0355-44 Cans of 32 fl oz (1 quart)
NDC 0087-0356-01 Bottles of 8 fl oz
VA 8940-00-609-2636 (8-fl-oz bottles)

Also Available:
NDC 0087-0357-01 Isocal Tube Feeding Set
Shown in Product Identification Section, page 415

ISOCAL® HCN
High calorie and nitrogen nutritionally complete liquid tube-feeding formula

Composition: Water, corn syrup, soybean oil, calcium caseinate, medium chain triglycerides (fractionated coconut oil), sodium caseinate, lecithin, potassium citrate, magnesium chloride, potassium carbonate, magnesium phosphate, salt, calcium phosphate, carrageenan, potassium chloride, vitamins (vitamin A palmitate, cholecalciferol, dl-alpha-tocopheryl acetate, sodium ascorbate, folic acid, thiamine hydrochloride, riboflavin, niacinamide, pyridoxine hydrochloride, cyanocobalamin, biotin, calcium pantothenate, phytonadione and choline bitartrate) and minerals (potassium iodide, ferrous gluconate, cupric sulfate, zinc sulfate and manganese sulfate).

Indication: Isocal HCN is a complete, concentrated liquid tube feeding diet specifically formulated to provide patients with generous calorie (2.0 Cal/ml) and protein levels (75 g protein/1000 ml). Isocal HCN provides 15% of the calories as protein, 45% as fat, 40% as carbohydrate and 100% of the U.S. RDA of all essential vitamins and minerals in 1000 ml. This lactose-free formulation has an osmolality of 690 mOsm/kg water.

Actions and Uses: Isocal HCN is of particular value to patients who are fluid-restricted (neurosurgery, congestive heart failure, etc.) or are volume-restricted (cardiac or cancer cachexia, chronic obstructive lung disease) and require tube feeding.
Isocal HCN may be used as a nutritional supplement in situations: where taste perceptions have been altered by therapy and illness; where variety is indicated during long-term full liquid diet use; during the transition from tube feedings to conventional supplements and normal diets. Flavorings may be added to Isocal HCN to suit individual preferences.

Preparation: Isocal HCN is ready to feed; shake well before opening. Unopened Isocal HCN should be stored at room temperature. Unused Isocal HCN should be covered, kept refrigerated and used within 48 hours of opening.
It is recommended that Isocal HCN be tube fed and that tube feeding be initiated as follows:

Day 1—1:1 dilution of Isocal HCN to water at 50 ml/hour (or full strength at 25 ml/hr).
Day 2—full strength at 50 ml/hour.
Day 3—full strength up to 100–125 ml/hour.
Administration via infusion pump is recommended.

Precaution: Additional water may be given as needed to meet the patient's requirements. Particular attention should be given to water needs of comatose and unconscious patients, those who cannot express the usual sensation of thirst and patients with impaired renal concentrating capacity, extensive breakdown of tissue protein, or when water requirements are high, e.g. fever, burns, and dry atmospheric conditions. Isocal HCN provides 700 ml of water per 1000 ml of formula.

How Supplied: Isocal® HCN liquid
NDC 0087-0462-42 Cans of 8 fl oz
VA 8940-01-124-7909 (8-fl-oz cans)

LOFENALAC® powder
Low phenylalanine food

Composition: 49.2% corn syrup solids, 18.7% specially processed casein hydrolysate (an enzymic digest of casein containing amino acids and small peptides, processed to remove most of the phenylalanine), 18% corn oil, 9.57% modified tapioca starch, 1.45% calcium citrate, 0.8% L-tyrosine, 0.76% dibasic calcium phosphate, 0.58% dibasic potassium phosphate, 0.2% L-tryptophan, 0.18% L-histidine hydrochloride monohydrate, 0.12% potassium citrate, 0.1% magnesium oxide, 0.1% L-methionine, 0.04% calcium hydroxide, taurine (50 mg/qt normal dilution), vitamins (vitamin A palmitate, cholecalciferol, dl-alpha-tocopheryl acetate, sodium ascorbate, folic acid, thiamine hydrochloride, riboflavin, niacinamide, pyridoxine hydrochloride, cyanocobalamin, biotin, calcium pantothenate, phytonadione, choline chloride and inositol), and minerals (ferrous sulfate, cupric sulfate, zinc sulfate, manganese sulfate, and sodium iodide). *Proximate analysis* (powder): protein equivalent (N × 6.25) 15%, fat 18%, carbohydrate 60%, minerals (ash) 3.6%, moisture 3.8%. Phenylalanine content of Lofenalac powder is approximately 0.08% (not more than 0.1% nor less than 0.06%). Each 100 g of powder supplies about 460 kilocalories and 80 mg phenylalanine. One packed level scoop contains 9.5 g. Each quart of formula in normal dilution supplies the following:

	Per Qt.
Protein, equivalent (N × 6.25) g	21+
Vitamin A, IU	1600
Vitamin D, IU	400
Vitamin E, IU	10
Vitamin C, mg	52
Folic acid, mcg	100
Thiamine, mg	0.5
Riboflavin, mg	0.6
Niacin, mg	8
Vitamin B$_6$, mg	0.4
Vitamin B$_{12}$, mcg	2
Biotin, mcg	50
Pantothenic acid, mg	3
Vitamin K$_1$, mcg	100
Choline, mg	85
Inositol, mg	30
Calcium, mg	600
Phosphorus, mg	450
Iodine, mcg	45
Iron, mg	12
Magnesium, mg	70
Copper, mg	0.6
Zinc, mg	4
Manganese, mg	1
Chloride, mg	450
Potassium, mg	650
Sodium, mg	300

+The protein is incomplete since it contains an inadequate amount of the essential amino acid, phenylalanine, for normal growth. With added phenylalanine, the PER is greater than that of casein.

Action and Uses: For use as basic food in low phenylalanine dietary management of infants and children with phenylketonuria. Provides essential nutrients without the high phenylalanine content (approx. 5%) present in natural food proteins. Except for its low and carefully limited phenylalanine content, Lofenalac is nutritionally complete.

Preparation: 20 kcal/fl oz Formula for Infants: To make a quart of formula, add one packed level cup (139 g) of Lofenalac powder to 29 fl oz water. For smaller amounts of formula, add 1 packed level measuring scoop (9.5 g) of powder to each 2 fluid ounces of water.
To prepare as a beverage (about 30 kcal/fl oz) for older children and adults, add one packed level cup (139 g) of powder to 20 fl oz of warm water; mix with beater until smooth, then store in refrigerator. Prescribe a specific amount of this mixture daily, and carefully add specific amounts of other foods to the diet. Lofenalac contains approximately 110 mg of phenylalanine per quart of formula (17 mg/100 kcal). This low level does not provide sufficient phenylalanine to meet total daily requirements of the growing infant. Other foods should be given as required to bring phenylalanine intake to adequate, but not excessive, level. The diet and the phenylalanine intake must be adapted to individual needs.
Store bottled formula in refrigerator and use within 24 hours.

Contraindications: Lofenalac (low phenylalanine food) should not be used for normal infants and children, but should be used only as part of the diet of patients with phenylketonuria. Continued usage must be carefully and frequently supervised by the physician and the diet periodically adjusted on the basis of frequent tests of urine and blood.

How Supplied: Lofenalac® powder
NDC 0087-0340-01 Cans of 40 oz (2½ lb). List # 340-26
Consult PKU—A Guide for Dietary Management for details.

LONALAC® powder
Low sodium, high protein beverage mix

Composition: Lactose, casein, coconut oil, calcium phosphate, potassium carbonate, calcium citrate, potassium citrate, calcium hydroxide, calcium chloride, potassium chloride, magnesium oxide, calcium carbonate, vitamin A palmitate, thiamine hydrochloride, riboflavin, niacinamide, artificial color and flavor. Each 100 g of Lonalac powder supplies 27 g protein, 28 g fat and 38 g carbohydrate. Each quart (30 Cal/fl oz) contains the following:

Vitamin A, IU	1440
Thiamine, mg	0.6
Riboflavin, mg	2.6
Niacin, mg	1.2
Calcium, mg	1690
Phosphorus, mg	1500
Magnesium, mg	135
Chloride, mg	750
Potassium, mg	1800
Sodium, mg	38

It contains only 38 mg sodium per quart of normal dilution, in contrast to 480 mg per quart of milk.

Action and Uses: A substitute for milk when dietary sodium restriction is prescribed, as in congestive heart failure, hypertension, nephrosis, acute nephritis, toxemia of pregnancy, hepatic cirrhosis with ascites, and therapy with certain drugs.

Preparation: For 30 Cal/fl oz: add 1½ cups (188 g) Lonalac powder to 27 fl oz of water. Concentrated preparation: ½ cup Lonalac powder to 1 cup water.
Store bottled formula in refrigerator and use within 24 hours.

Precautions: Care should be taken to avoid additional sodium intake from other dietary or non-dietary sources. Subjects receiving low sodium diets must be observed for signs of sodium deprivation such as weakness, exhaustion and abdominal cramps. In long term management (using Lonalac), additional sources of sodium must be given since Lonalac is almost void of the essential nutrient sodium.

How Supplied: Lonalac® powder
NDC 0087-0391-01 Cans of 16 oz (1 lb)
VA 8940-00-191-6565 (1 lb can)

LYTREN®
Oral electrolyte solution

Lytren provides important electrolytes plus carbohydrate in a balanced formulation. It is designed for oral administration when food intake is discontinued.

Composition: Water, dextrose, potassium citrate, salt (sodium chloride), sodium citrate, citric acid.

Concentrations of Electrolytes:

Electrolyte	mEq/L
Sodium	50
Chloride	45
Citrate	30
Potassium	25
Total*	150

*NOTE: Lytren oral electrolyte solution has an osmolality of approximately 220 mOsm per kilogram of water.

Indications: When intake of the usual foods and liquids is discontinued, oral feedings of Lytren solution may be used:
- To supply water and electrolytes for maintenance.
- To replace mild to moderate fluid losses.

Such oral electrolyte feedings have particular application in mild and moderate diarrheas, to forestall dehydration,[1–6] and in postoperative states.

Intake and Administration: Feed by nursing bottle, glass or straw.
Administration of Lytren solution should be begun as soon as intake of usual foods and liquids is discontinued, and before serious fluid losses or deficits develop.
Intake of Lytren solution should approximate the patient's calculated daily water requirements, for maintenance and for replacement of losses. The prescribed quantity may be divided and used throughout the day as desired or appropriate. (Note: No more than this amount of Lytren should be given. Additional liquid to satisfy thirst should be water or other non-electrolyte-containing fluids.)
- **For infants and young children.** The water requirement should be calculated on the basis of body surface area. Estimated daily water requirements such as the following may be used as a general guide:
    For maintenance in illness—1500 ml (50 fl oz) per square meter.[7]
    For maintenance plus replacement of moderate losses (as in diarrhea or vomiting)—2400 ml (80 fl oz) per square meter.[7]
Daily amount of Lytren solution based on these estimated requirements is shown in the Intake Guide table. Intake should be adjusted according to the size of the individual patient and the clinical conditions.
- **For older children and adults.** When fluid losses are mild to moderate, amounts such as the following may be given daily: Children 5 to 10 years—1 to

LYTREN INTAKE GUIDE
for infants and young children
(Adjust to meet individual needs)

	Body Weight		Average Surface Area	Maintenance Approx.	Maintenance plus Replacement of Moderate Losses Approx.
*Averages of Benedict-Talbot estimated surface areas for boys and girls.[8]	Kg	Lb	Sq Meter*	Fl Oz†	Fl Oz‡
†Based on water requirement of 1500 ml (50 fl oz) per sq meter.[7]	3	6–7	0.2	10	16
	5	11	0.29	15	23
	7	15	0.38	19	30
‡Based on water requirement of 2400 ml (80 fl oz) per sq meter.[7]	10	22	0.49	25	40
	12	26	0.55	28	44
	15	33	0.64	32	51
	18	40	0.76	38	61

LYTREN SOLUTION DAILY INTAKE

2 quarts. Older children and adults—2 to 3 quarts.[7]
Intake should be adjusted on the basis of clinical indications, amount of fluid loss, patient's usual water intake and other relevant factors.
[See table above].
- Lytren in conjunction with other fluids. When severe fluid losses or accumulated deficits require parenteral fluid therapy, Lytren solution by mouth <u>may be</u> given simultaneously to supply <u>part</u> of the estimated fluid requirement. After emergency needs have been met, Lytren solution alone may be used.

Contraindications:
Lytren should not be used:
- In the presence of severe, continuing diarrhea or other critical fluid losses requiring parenteral fluid therapy.
- In intractable vomiting, adynamic ileus, intestinal obstruction or perforated bowel.
- When renal function is depressed (anuria, oliguria) or homeostatic mechanisms are impaired.

Precautions: Lytren oral electrolyte solution should only be used in the recommended volume intakes in order to avoid excessive electrolyte ingestion. Do not mix with, or give with, other electrolyte-containing liquids, such as milk or fruit juices.
Urgent needs in severe fluid imbalances must be met parenterally. When Lytren solution by mouth is used in addition to parenteral fluids, do not exceed total water and electrolyte requirements.
Intake of Lytren should be discontinued upon reintroduction of other electrolyte-containing foods into the diet. Should be administered on physician's orders only.

How Supplied:
Lytren—8 fl oz, Ready to Use. List # 294-02
Lytren is also available in the hospital in an 8-fl oz Nursette® Disposable Bottle. List # 292-04

References:
1. Darrow DC: Pediatrics *9*:519–533 (May) 1952. 2. Harrison HE: Pediat Clin North America, (May) 1954. pp 335–348. 3. Vaughan VC, III, in Nelson WE: Text-

Continued on next page

Mead Johnson Nutr.—Cont.

book of Pediatrics, ed 7, Philadelphia, WB Saunders Company, 1959, pp 187–189. 4. Brooke CE, Anast CS: JAMA *179*:148–153 (March) 1962. 5. Darrow DC, Welsh JS: J Pediat *56*:204–210 (Feb) 1960. 6. Cooke RE: JAMA *167*:1243–1246 (July 5) 1958. 7. Worthen HG, Raile RB: Minnesota Med *37*:558–564 (Aug) 1954. 8. McLester JS, Darby WJ: Nutrition and Diet in Health and Disease, ed 6, Philadelphia, WB Saunders Company, 1952, pp 32–34.

MCT Oil
Medium chain triglycerides oil

Composition: MCT Oil contains triglycerides of medium chain fatty acids which are more easily digested and absorbed than conventional food fat.
MCT Oil is bland tasting and light yellow in color. It provides 8.3 Cal/g. One tablespoon (15 ml) weighs 14 g and contains 115 Cal. It is a lipid fraction of coconut oil and consists primarily of the triglycerides of C_8 and C_{10} saturated fatty acids. MCT Oil does not provide essential fatty acids.
Approximate percentages are:

Fatty Acid	%
Shorter than C_8	<6
C_8 (Octanoic)	67
C_{10} (Decanoic)	23
Longer than C_{10}	<4

Actions and Uses: MCT Oil is a special dietary supplement for use in the nutritional management of children and adults who cannot efficiently digest and absorb conventional long chain food fats. One tablespoonful 3 to 4 times per day or as recommended by the physician. MCT Oil should be mixed with fruit juices, used on salads and vegetables, incorporated into sauces for use on fish, chicken, or lean meat, or used in cooking or baking. Recipes or professional literature available upon request.

Precaution: In persons with advanced cirrhosis of the liver, large amounts of medium chain triglycerides in the diet may result in elevated blood and spinal fluid levels of medium chain fatty acids (MCFA), due to impaired hepatic clearance of these fatty acids, which are rapidly absorbed via the portal vein. These elevated levels have been reported to be associated with reversible coma and precoma in certain subjects with advanced cirrhosis, particularly with portacaval shunts. Therefore, diets containing high levels of medium chain triglyceride fat should be used with caution in persons with hepatic cirrhosis and complications thereof, such as portacaval shunts or tendency to encephalopathy.
Use of MCT Oil-containing products in abetalipoproteinemia is not indicated.

How Supplied: MCT Oil
NDC 0087-0365-03 Bottles of 1 quart

NATURACIL®
Natural-fiber laxative

Description: Naturacil is a chewable bulk-forming laxative product providing natural fiber in a soft, chewable form for gentle relief from constipation. It contains psyllium seed husks, an excellent source of dietary fiber derived from **Plantago ovata**. Each adult dose (two pieces) contains 3.4 grams of psyllium seed husks and also contains artificial chocolate flavor and color, corn syrup, glycerin, nonfat milk, partially hydrogenated vegetable oil (soybean and cottonseed oil), sugar, 0.011 grams (11 mg) of sodium, 54 Calories, and 9.6 grams of available carbohydrate.

Indications: Naturacil is indicated for the relief and prevention of simple constipation in patients with the following diagnosis:
1. Women during pregnancy or the puerperal period.
2. Geriatric patients with poor eating habits whose abdominal and perineal muscles have lost their tone.
3. Children with functional chronic constipation.
4. Patients whose bowel motility has been altered through use of anticholinergic drugs or narcotics.
5. Patients with an episiotomy wound, painful thrombosed hemorrhoids or anal fissures.
6. Patients with irritable bowel syndrome.
7. Patients with diverticulosis.
Naturacil is non habit-forming and may be used when long-term therapy is necessary.

Actions: Although many factors may be involved in the causation of constipation, one of the most important is the amount of fiber in the diet. The psyllium seed husks in Naturacil, when taken with adequate fluids, provide a source of dietary fiber which promotes evacuation of the bowels by increasing bulk volume and water content of stools.

Warnings: Laxatives should not be used when abdominal pain, nausea, or vomiting are present.

Dosage and Administration: The usual adult dosage is two pieces (one piece for children 6–12) one to three times per day. A full glass (8 fl oz) of liquid should be taken with each dose. Results usually occur within 24 hours, although continued use for two or three days may be needed for optimal benefit.

Contraindications: Intestinal obstruction, fecal impaction.

How Supplied: Naturacil® Natural fiber laxative
NDC 0087-0444-01 Carton of 24 pieces (12 adult doses)
NDC 0087-0444-02 Carton of 40 pieces (20 adult doses)
No ℞ required.

Shown in Product Identification Section, page 414

NUTRAMIGEN® powder
Protein hydrolysate formula

Composition: 43.3% sugar (sucrose), 19.2% casein enzymically hydrolyzed and charcoal-treated to reduce allergenicity, 18% corn oil, 16.5% modified tapioca starch, 1.12% dibasic calcium phosphate, 0.91% potassium citrate, 0.34% calcium citrate, 0.3% calcium hydroxide, 0.1% magnesium oxide, 0.057% potassium chloride, taurine (50 mg/qt normal dilution), vitamins (vitamin A palmitate, cholecalciferol, dl-alpha-tocopheryl acetate, sodium ascorbate, folic acid, thiamine hydrochloride, riboflavin, niacinamide, pyridoxine hydrochloride, cyanocobalamin, biotin, calcium pantothenate, phytonadione, choline chloride and inositol), and minerals (ferrous sulfate, manganese sulfate, cupric sulfate, zinc sulfate, and sodium iodide).
One quart of Nutramigen formula (4.9 oz Nutramigen powder) supplies 640 kilocalories and the following:

Vitamin A, IU	1600
Vitamin D, IU	400
Vitamin E, IU	10
Vitamin C, mg	52
Folic acid, mcg	100
Thiamine, mg	0.5
Riboflavin, mg	0.6
Niacin, mg	8
Vitamin B_6, mg	0.4
Vitamin B_{12}, mcg	2
Biotin, mcg	50
Pantothenic acid, mg	3
Vitamin K_1, mcg	100
Choline, mg	85
Inositol, mg	30
Calcium, mg	600
Phosphorus, mg	450
Iodine, mcg	45
Iron, mg	12
Magnesium, mg	70
Copper, mg	0.6
Zinc, mg	4
Manganese, mcg	200
Chloride, mg	450
Potassium, mg	650
Sodium, mg	300

Action and Uses: Feeding of infants and children allergic or intolerant to intact proteins of cow's milk and other foods. Provides a formula with predigested protein for infants with diarrhea, colic or other gastrointestinal disturbances. Provides lactose-free feedings in galactosemia.

Precautions: Initial feedings of Nutramigen should be diluted to 10 kcal/fl oz and gradually increased to 20 kcal/fl oz over a period of 3 to 5 days. Nutramigen is not recommended for routine use in highly stressed low birthweight infants. Some of these infants may be at increased risk of developing gastrointestinal complications.

Preparation: For 10 kcal/fl oz: 1 packed level scoop to 4 fl oz water, or ½ cup, packed level, to water sufficient to make a quart of formula. For 20 kcal/fl oz: 1 packed level scoop powder (9.5 g) to 2 fl oz water, or 1 level cup (139 g) to water sufficient to make a quart of formula.

Store bottled formula in refrigerator and use within 24 hours.

How Supplied: Nutramigen® powder NDC 0087-0338-01 Cans of 16 oz (1 lb), with scoop. List # 338-21

POLY-VI-SOL®
Vitamin drops • chewable tablets

Composition: Usual daily doses supply: [See table above].

Action and Uses: Daily vitamin supplementation for infants and children. Chewable tablets useful also for adults.

Administration and Dosage: Usual doses as above, or as indicated.

How Supplied: Poly-Vi-Sol® vitamin drops: (with 'Safti-Dropper' marked to deliver 1.0 ml)
NDC 0087-0402-02 Bottles of 1 fl oz (30 ml)
NDC 0087-0402-03 Bottles of 1⅔ fl oz (50 ml)
6505-00-104-8433 (50 ml) (Defense)
Poly-Vi-Sol® chewable vitamins tablets:
NDC 0087-0412-03 Bottles of 100
Poly-Vi-Sol® chewable vitamins tablets in Circus Shapes:
NDC 0087-0414-02 Bottles of 100
Shown in Product Identification Section, page 414

POLY-VI-SOL® with Iron
Vitamin and Iron drops

Composition: Each 1.0 ml supplies:

		% U.S. RDA Infants
Vitamin A, IU	1500	100
Vitamin D, IU	400	100
Vitamin E, IU	5	100
Vitamin C, mg	35	100
Thiamine, mg	0.5	100
Riboflavin, mg	0.6	100
Niacin, mg	8	100
Vitamin B_6, mg	0.4	100
Iron, mg	10	67

Action and Uses: Daily vitamin and iron supplement for infants.

Administration and Dosage: Drop into mouth with 'Safti-Dropper.' Dose: 1.0 ml daily, or as indicated.
When an infant or child is taking iron, stools may appear darker in color. This is to be expected and should be no cause for concern. When drops containing iron are given to infants or young children, some darkening of the plaque on the teeth may occur. This is not serious or permanent as it does not affect the enamel. The stains can be removed or prevented by rubbing the teeth with a little baking soda or powder on a toothbrush or small cloth once or twice a week.

How Supplied: Poly-Vi-Sol® vitamin and iron drops (with dropper marked to deliver 1 ml)
NDC 0087-0405-01 Bottles of 1⅔ fl oz (50 ml)
Shown in Product Identification Section, page 414

	Drops 1.0 ml	% U.S. RDA for Infants	Chewable Tablets 1 tablet	% U.S. RDA	
				Children under 4	Adults and Children 4 or more
Vitamin A, IU	1500	100	2500	100	50
Vitamin D, IU	400	100	400	100	100
Vitamin E, IU	5	100	15	150	50
Vitamin C, mg	35	100	60	150	100
Folic acid, mg	—	—	0.3	150	75
Thiamine, mg	0.5	100	1.05	150	70
Riboflavin, mg	0.6	100	1.2	150	70
Niacin, mg	8	100	13.5	150	68
Vitamin B_6, mg	0.4	100	1.05	150	53
Vitamin B_{12}, mcg	2	100	4.5	150	75

POLY-VI-SOL® with Iron and Zinc
Chewable vitamins with Iron and Zinc

Composition: Each tablet supplies same vitamins as Poly-Vi-Sol tablets (see above) plus 12 mg iron and 8 mg zinc.

Action and Uses: Daily vitamin and mineral supplement for adults and children.

Administration and Dosage: 1 tablet daily.

How Supplied: Poly-Vi-Sol® chewable vitamins with Iron and Zinc tablets.
NDC 0087-0455-02 Bottles of 100
Poly-Vi-Sol® chewable vitamins with Iron and Zinc tablets in Circus Shapes.
NDC 0087-0456-02 Bottles of 100
Shown in Product Identification Section, page 414

PORTAGEN®
Nutritionally complete dietary with Medium Chain Triglycerides
U.S. Patent No. 3,450,819

Composition: Corn syrup solids, medium chain triglycerides (fractionated coconut oil), sodium caseinate, sugar (sucrose), corn oil, calcium citrate, potassium chloride, dibasic magnesium phosphate, dicalcium phosphate, potassium citrate, lecithin, vitamins (vitamin A palmitate, cholecalciferol, dl-alpha-tocopheryl acetate, sodium ascorbate, folic acid, thiamine hydrochloride, riboflavin, niacinamide, pyridoxine hydrochloride, cyanocobalamin, biotin, calcium pantothenate, phytonadione, and choline chloride), and minerals (ferrous sulfate, cupric sulfate, zinc sulfate, manganese sulfate, and sodium iodide).
Portagen powder provides 14% of the calories as protein, 41% as fat (87% of the fat is Medium Chain Triglycerides) and 45% as carbohydrate. One quart of prepared Portagen at 20 Cal/fl oz supplies 640 Calories; one quart at 30 Cal/fl oz supplies 960 Calories; one quart at 60 Cal/fl oz supplies 1920 Calories.

Action and Uses: A nutritionally complete dietary is prepared by adding Portagen powder to water. Portagen may be used where conventional food fats are not well digested or absorbed such as in patients with cystic fibrosis, pancreatic or hepatic disease, lymphatic system disorders and in some patients with "fat storage" disorders.

This dietary may be used, according to physician recommendation, as the major or sole constituent of the diet. Or, it may be used as a beverage to be consumed with each meal, or it may be incorporated in various recipes. Recipes or professional literature available upon request.

Preparation: *To Prepare as a Beverage (30 kilocalories per fluid ounce):* Add 1½ packed level cups of Portagen powder (203 g) to 3 cups of water. Mix with electric mixer, egg beater or fork until smooth. Then stir in enough water to make 1 quart of beverage.
To Prepare as an Infant Formula (in normal dilution of 20 kilocalories per fluid ounce): Add 1 packed level cup (136 g) of Portagen powder to 3 cups of water. Mix with electric mixer, egg beater or fork until smooth. Then stir in enough water to make 1 quart of formula.
Store bottled formula in refrigerator and use within 24 hours.

Precautions: Recent studies indicate that, contrary to earlier recommendations, Portagen should not be used in cases of abetalipoproteinemia (faulty chylomicron formation). The usual intake of water should be maintained when Portagen beverage is used as the sole article or major part of the diet.

How Supplied: Portagen® powder
NDC 0087-0387-01 Cans of 16 oz (1 lb)

PREGESTIMIL®
Protein hydrolysate formula with medium chain triglycerides and added amino acids

Composition: 52.4% corn syrup solids, 15.5% casein enzymatically hydrolyzed and charcoal-treated to reduce allergenicity, 10.5% corn oil, 10.3% modified tapioca starch, 7.7% medium chain triglycerides (fractionated coconut oil), 1.1% calcium citrate, 0.88% potassium citrate, 0.79% calcium phosphate, 0.18% soy lecithin, 0.16% potassium chloride, 0.15% L-cystine, 0.15% L-tyrosine, 0.08% magnesium oxide, 0.06% L-tryptophan, taurine (50 mg/qt normal dilution), vitamins (vitamin A palmitate, cholecalciferol, dl-alpha-tocopheryl acetate, sodium ascorbate, folic acid, thiamine hydrochloride, riboflavin, niacinamide, pyridoxine hydrochloride, cyanocobalamin, biotin, calcium pantothenate, phytonadione, choline chloride, and ino-

Continued on next page

Mead Johnson Nutr.—Cont.

sitol) and minerals (ferrous sulfate, cupric sulfate, zinc sulfate, manganese sulfate and sodium iodide).

One quart of Pregestimil formula (20 kcal/fl oz) supplies 18 g protein equivalent, 26 g fat, 86 g carbohydrate and the following:

		% U. S. RDA Children 1–4
Vitamin A, IU	2000	80
Vitamin D, IU	400	100
Vitamin E, IU	15	150
Vitamin C, mg	52	130
Folic acid, mcg	100	50
Thiamine, mg	0.5	71
Riboflavin, mg	0.6	75
Niacin, mg	8	89
Vitamin B_6, mg	0.4	57
Vitamin B_{12}, mcg	2	67
Biotin, mcg	50	33
Pantothenic acid, mg	3	60
Vitamin K_1, mcg	100	*
Choline, mg	85	*
Inositol, mg	30	*
Calcium, mg	600	75
Phosphorus, mg	400	50
Iodine, mcg	45	64
Iron, mg	12	120
Magnesium, mg	70	35
Copper, mg	0.6	60
Zinc, mg	4	50
Manganese, mg	0.2	*
Chloride, mg	550	*
Potassium, mg	700	*
Sodium, mg	300	*

*U.S. Recommended Daily Allowance (U.S. RDA) has not been established.

Action and Uses: Provides very easily digestible and assimilable fat, carbohydrate, and protein for feeding of infants and children with severe problems of diarrhea, dietary intolerance, disaccharidase deficiency, or malabsorption. For the nutritional management of infants with cow's milk-protein allergy, colic, following intestinal resection where temporary deficiency of intestinal enzymes may be found, or in infants with cystic fibrosis. In infants with severe malabsorption problems of non-specific etiologies, such as chronic diarrhea, nutritional maintenance with Pregestimil permits trial of specific disaccharides, milk protein or regular dietary fats to determine if the dietary intolerance is due to a component of conventional feedings.

Precautions: Initial feedings of Pregestimil should be diluted to 10 kcal/fl oz or less and gradually increased to 20 kcal/fl oz over a period of 3 to 5 days. This product is not recommended for routine use in highly stressed low birthweight infants. Some of these infants may be at increased risk of developing gastrointestinal complications.

Preparation: For 10 kcal/fl oz: add one packed level scoop (enclosed) (9.7 g) of Pregestimil powder to each 4 fl oz (120 ml) of water. Always add powder to water. To make a quart of 10 kcal/fl oz formula, add 1/2 packed level cup (71 g) of powder to 29 fl oz (858 ml) of water. For 20 kcal/fl oz: add one packed level scoop (9.7 g) of Pregestimil powder to each 2 fl oz (60 ml) of water. To make a quart of 20 kcal/fl oz formula, add one packed level cup (141 g) of powder to 29 fl oz (858 ml) of water.

Caution: Store remaining liquid formula in refrigerator in a covered container and use within 24 hours after mixing.

How Supplied: Pregestimil® powder NDC 0087-0367-01 Cans of 16 oz (1 lb) with measuring scoop. List # 367-21

PROSOBEE® concentrated liquid • ready-to-use liquid • powder
Milk-free formula with soy protein isolate

ProSobee Concentrated Liquid

Composition: 74.9% water, 13.2% corn syrup solids, 4.1% soy protein isolate, 3.6% coconut oil, 3% soy oil, and less than 1% of each of the following: tribasic calcium phosphate, tribasic potassium citrate, soy lecithin, mono- and diglycerides, salt, magnesium chloride, L-methionine, carrageenan, vitamins (vitamin A palmitate, cholecalciferol, dl-alpha-tocopheryl acetate, sodium ascorbate, folic acid, thiamine hydrochloride, riboflavin, niacinamide, pyridoxine hydrochloride, cyanocobalamin, biotin, calcium pantothenate, phytonadione, choline chloride and inositol), taurine (50 mg/qt normal dilution), and minerals (potassium iodide, ferrous sulfate, cupric sulfate and zinc sulfate).

ProSobee Ready-To-Use

Composition: 87.1% water, 6.8% corn syrup solids, 2.1% soy protein isolate, 1.9% coconut oil, 1.5% soy oil, and less than 1% of each of the following: tribasic calcium phosphate, tribasic potassium citrate, soy lecithin, mono- and diglycerides, salt, magnesium chloride, L-methionine, carrageenan, vitamins (vitamin A palmitate, cholecalciferol, dl-alpha-tocopheryl acetate, sodium ascorbate, folic acid, thiamine hydrochloride, riboflavin, niacinamide, pyridoxine hydrochloride, cyanocobalamin, biotin, calcium pantothenate, phytonadione, choline chloride and inositol), taurine (50 mg/qt), and minerals (potassium iodide, ferrous sulfate, cupric sulfate and zinc sulfate).

ProSobee Powder

Composition: 51% corn syrup solids, 17.4% soy protein isolate, 15.3% coconut oil, 12.5% corn oil, and less than 2% of each of the following: calcium phosphate, potassium chloride, potassium citrate, magnesium phosphate, sodium citrate, calcium carbonate, L-methionine, taurine (50 mg/qt normal dilution), vitamins (vitamins A palmitate, cholecalciferol, dl-alpha-tocopheryl acetate, sodium ascorbate, folic acid, thiamine hydrochloride, riboflavin, niacinamide, pyridoxine hydrochloride, cyanocobalamin, biotin, calcium pantothenate, phytonadione, choline chloride and inositol) and minerals (sodium iodide, ferrous sulfate, cupric sulfate and zinc sulfate).

One quart of ProSobee formula, normal dilution (20 kcal/fl oz) supplies 640 kilocalories and the following:

Vitamin A, IU	2000
Vitamin D, IU	400
Vitamin E, IU	20
Vitamin C, mg	52
Folic acid, mcg	100
Thiamine, mcg	500
Riboflavin, mcg	600
Niacin, mg	8
Vitamin B_6, mcg	400
Vitamin B_{12}, mcg	2
Biotin, mcg	50
Pantothenic acid, mg	3
Vitamin K_1, mcg	100
Choline, mg	50
Inositol, mg	30
Calcium, mg	600
Phosphorus, mg	475
Iodine, mcg	65
Iron, mg	12
Magnesium, mg	70
Copper, mcg	600
Zinc, mg	5
Manganese, mcg	200
Chloride, mg	520
Potassium, mg	740
Sodium, mg	275

Action and Uses: Milk-free, lactose-free and sucrose-free formula with soy protein for infants with common feeding problems associated with milk sensitivity, such as: mild diarrhea, fussiness, spitting up, rash and eczema. ProSobee should be considered for infants sensitive to milk, with lactose or sucrose intolerance, or with galactosemia. As a milk substitute for children and adults with poor tolerance to milk.

Preparation: *Concentrated liquid:* For 20 kcal/fl oz, 1 part ProSobee concentrated liquid to 1 part water. ProSobee may be used to replace milk as a beverage or in cooking. A pleasant-tasting beverage is made with two parts ProSobee concentrated liquid to one part water. An opened can of ProSobee liquid should be covered, refrigerated and used within 48 hours.
Powder: To make a quart of formula, add 1 unpacked level cup of powder to 29 fl oz of water; for single bottle feeding, add 1 level scoop of powder to each 2 fl oz of water. Mix vigorously. Reconstituted powder should be covered, kept refrigerated and used within 24 hours. ProSobee powder needs no refrigeration.

How Supplied: ProSobee®
List 308-01 Cans of 13 fl oz concentrated liquid (40 kcal/fl oz)
List 309-01 Cans of 32 fl oz (1 qt) ready-to-use (20 kcal/fl oz)
List 309-42 Cans of 8 fl oz ready-to-use (20 kcal/fl oz)
List 3101-21 Cans of 14 oz powder

SMURF™
chewable vitamins

Composition: Usual daily doses supply:
[See table on next page].

Action and Uses: Daily vitamin supplementation for children and adults.

Administration and Dosage: 1 tablet daily.

How Supplied: Smurf™ chewable vitamins:

NDC 0087-0484-01 Bottles of 60
Shown in Product Identification Section, page 415

SMURF™
chewable vitamins with Iron and Zinc

Composition: Each tablet supplies same vitamins as Smurf™ chewable vitamins (see above) plus 12 mg iron and 8 mg zinc.

Action and Uses: Daily vitamin and mineral supplement for children and adults.

Administration and Dosage: 1 tablet daily.

How Supplied: Smurf™ chewable vitamins with Iron and Zinc:

NDC 0087-0485-01 Bottles of 60
Shown in Product Identification Section, page 415

SUSTACAL®
- liquid (ready to use)
- powder (mix with milk)
- pudding (ready-to-eat)

Nutritionally complete food

Composition: (Vanilla Liquid)
Water, sugar (sucrose), corn syrup, calcium caseinate, partially hydrogenated soy oil, soy protein isolate, sodium caseinate, potassium citrate, artificial flavor, dibasic magnesium phosphate, salt (sodium chloride), potassium chloride, calcium carbonate, dibasic calcium phosphate, sodium citrate, lecithin, carrageenan, vitamins (vitamin A palmitate, cholecalciferol, dl-alpha-tocopheryl acetate, sodium ascorbate, folic acid, thiamine hydrochloride, riboflavin, niacinamide, pyridoxine hydrochloride, cyanocobalamin, biotin, calcium pantothenate, phytonadione and choline bitartrate) and minerals (sodium iodide, ferric pyrophosphate, ferrous sulfate, cupric sulfate, zinc sulfate and manganese sulfate). (In addition to the above, Chocolate liquid contains Dutch process cocoa [alkalized], and artificial color.) Eggnog flavored liquid contains artificial color.

Each 12-fl-oz can of Sustacal supplies 21.7 g protein, 8.3 g fat, 49.6 g carbohydrate, 360 Calories (1 Calorie per ml) and 33% of the U.S. RDA for all essential vitamins and minerals. Sustacal liquid is lactose free.

Vanilla Powder—Nonfat milk, sugar, corn syrup solids, artificial flavor, dibasic magnesium phosphate, vitamins (vitamin A palmitate, cholecalciferol, dl-alpha-tocopheryl acetate, sodium ascorbate, folic acid, thiamine hydrochloride, niacinamide, pyridoxine hydrochloride, cyanocobalamin, biotin and calcium pantothenate) and minerals (ferrous sulfate, cupric carbonate, zinc sulfate, and manganese sulfate). (In addition to the above, Chocolate Powder contains Dutch process cocoa [alkalized], and lecithin.)

| | | Percentage of U.S. Recommended Daily Allowance | |
		Children 2–4 Years	Adults & Children 4 or More
Vitamin A, IU	2500	100	50
Vitamin D, IU	400	100	100
Vitamin E, IU	15	150	50
Vitamin C, mg	60	150	100
Folic acid, mg	0.3	150	75
Thiamine, mg	1.05	150	70
Riboflavin, mg	1.2	150	70
Niacin, mg	13.5	150	68
Vitamin B$_6$, mg	1.05	150	53
Vitamin B$_{12}$, mcg	4.5	150	75
Iron, mg	12	120	67
Zinc, mg	8	100	53

With the exception of lactose, one pouch of Sustacal powder mixed with 8-fl oz whole milk provides essentially the same nutritional value as a 12 fl oz can of Sustacal.

Vanilla Pudding—Water, nonfat milk, sugar, partially hydrogenated soy oil, modified food starch, dibasic magnesium phosphate, sodium stearoyl lactylate, dibasic sodium phosphate, natural and artificial flavor, carrageenan, artificial color (includes FD&C Yellow No. 5), and vitamins and minerals (vitamin A palmitate, sodium ascorbate, thiamine hydrochloride, riboflavin, niacinamide, ferric pyrophosphate, cholecalciferol, dl-alpha-tocopheryl acetate, pyridoxine hydrochloride, folic acid, cyanocobalamin, zinc sulfate, cupric sulfate, biotin and calcium pantothenate).

In addition to the above, Chocolate contains Dutch process cocoa (alkalized) but no FD&C Yellow No. 5. Butterscotch does not contain FD&C Yellow No. 5. Sustacal Pudding provides 11% of Calories as protein, 36% as fat, 53% as carbohydrate and 15% of the U.S. RDA for all essential vitamins and minerals in a 5 oz serving.

Action and Uses: Sustacal liquid and powder are ideally formulated to provide for the nutritional needs of the broad range of patients requiring an oral supplement or high protein diet (21.7 g protein in one 12 fl oz serving).

Sustacal liquid is of particular value to patients who require a supplement and can be used effectively for anorectic cancer patients, hypermetabolic patients (as in burn or multiple trauma patients) and elderly patients. It is also recommended to be used as the sole source of diet in the above mentioned patients and in those patients who require less than 1500 Cal per day (Sustacal liquid is designed to provide 100% of the daily nutrient needs in less than 1500 Cal.)

Sustacal Pudding is a convenient and well-accepted means of providing supplemental nutrition and is especially appropriate to help avoid taste fatigue and monotony associated with liquid supplements.

Preparation: Liquid: ready to serve in 30 Cal/fl oz dilution (one Cal per milliliter). Powder: mix contents of one packet with 8-fl oz whole milk to prepare a 40 Calorie per fluid ounce dilution. To prepare powder in 30 Calorie per fluid ounce dilution, add 90 ml (3 fl oz) of water to the above mixture to yield approximately 12 fl oz. Both forms may be used orally or by tube. Vanilla flavor is recommended for tube feeding if chocolate allergy is suspected.

In initiating tube feeding, particularly for malnourished patients, feedings should be diluted to half-strength on Day 1; increase volume and concentration gradually over a period of several days.

Precautions: When Sustacal liquid is used as the sole food, give additional water as needed for adequate daily intake. This is particularly important for unconscious or semiconscious patients. Do not begin postoperative tube feedings until peristalsis is reestablished. Electrolyte content of Sustacal should be considered for cardiac patients and others who tend to have edema. Sustacal liquid supplies 840 ml of water per 1000 ml.

Store bottled formula in refrigerator and use within 48 hours.

How Supplied: Sustacal® Vanilla liquid and powder.
NDC 0087-0351-42 Cans of 8 fl oz
NDC 0087-0351-01 Cans of 12 fl oz
NDC 0087-0351-44 Cans of 32 fl oz (1 quart)
NDC 0087-0353-01 Packets of 1.9 oz, 4 packets per carton
NDC 0087-0353-43 Cans of 3.8 lb
VA 8940-01-024-6421 (8 fl oz, van.)
Sustacal® Chocolate liquid and powder.
NDC 0087-0350-42 Cans of 8 fl oz
NDC 0087-0350-01 Cans of 12 fl oz
NDC 0087-0350-44 Cans of 32 fl oz (1 quart)
NDC 0087-0352-01 Packets of 1.9 oz, 4 packets per carton
VA 8940-01-048-3360 (8 fl oz, choc.)
Sustacal® Eggnog liquid.
NDC 0087-0457-42 Cans of 8 fl oz, 12 cans per case
NDC 0087-0457-44 Cans of 32 fl oz, 6 cans per case
VA 8940-01-087-2875 (8 fl oz, eggnog)
Sustacal® Pudding
NDC 0087-0409-41 Vanilla, 5 oz cans, 4 cans per carton, 12 cartons per case
NDC 0087-0410-41 Chocolate, 5 oz cans, 4 cans per carton, 12 cartons per case

Continued on next page

Mead Johnson Nutr.—Cont.

NDC 0087-0415-41 Butterscotch, 5 oz cans, 4 cans per carton, 12 cartons per case

VA8940-01-074-3125 (Vanilla, 5 oz cans)

VA8940-01-074-3124 (Chocolate, 5 oz cans)

VA8940-01-074-3123 (Butterscotch, 5 oz cans)

Shown in Product Identification Section, page 415

SUSTACAL® HC
High calorie nutritionally complete food

Composition: (Vanilla Flavored Liquid) Water, corn syrup solids, corn oil, sugar, calcium caseinate, sodium caseinate, lecithin, potassium chloride, dibasic magnesium phosphate, calcium carbonate, artificial flavor, sodium citrate, carrageenan, potassium citrate, vitamins (vitamin A palmitate, cholecalciferol, dl-alpha-tocopheryl acetate, sodium ascorbate, folic acid, thiamine hydrochloride, riboflavin, niacinamide, pyridoxine hydrochloride, cyanocobalamin, biotin, calcium pantothenate, phytonadione and choline bitartrate) and minerals (sodium iodide, ferric pyrophosphate, ferrous sulfate, cupric sulfate, zinc sulfate and manganese sulfate).

Sustacal HC is available in vanilla, chocolate, and eggnog flavors. (In addition to the above, chocolate flavored liquid contains Dutch process cocoa [alkalized], and artificial color. Eggnog flavored liquid also contains artificial color.)

Each 8-fl oz can of Sustacal HC supplies 14.4 g protein, 13.6 g fat, 45 g carbohydrate, 360 Calories (1.5 Cal/ml) and at least 20% of the U.S. RDA for all essential vitamins and minerals.

Actions and Uses: Sustacal HC liquid is formulated to meet the supplemental or total nutritional needs of patients requiring generous calorie and protein intake (1.5 Cal/ml; 14.4 g protein/8 fl oz) while limiting total fluid volume. Sustacal HC is of particular value to patients in these situations: hypermetabolic states (burn, major trauma, thyrotoxicosis, etc.); fluid restrictions (neurosurgery, congestive heart failure, etc.); volume restrictions (cardiac or cancer cachexia, chronic obstructive lung disease); and lactose intolerance.

Preparation: Sustacal HC is ready to drink. Shake well before opening. Unopened Sustacal HC should be stored at room temperature. Refrigerate unused Sustacal HC and use within 48 hours. Acceptance by some patients is enhanced if Sustacal HC liquid is chilled before serving. Very ill patients should be directed to sip the liquid slowly.

Preparation for Tube Feeding: If Sustacal HC is used for this purpose, initial feedings should be diluted to half strength (0.75 Cal/ml) on the first day and three-fourths strength (1.12 Cal/ml) on the second day. This will allow the body to adjust to the osmolality of Sustacal HC Liquid. As tolerance is established, Sustacal HC Liquid can be fed full strength—1.5 Cal/ml.

Tube Feeding Precaution: Additional water should be given as needed to meet the patient's requirements. Particular attention should be given to water supply for comatose and unconscious patients and others who cannot express the usual sensation of thirst. Additional water is important also when renal concentrating ability is impaired, when there is extensive breakdown of tissue protein, or when water requirements are high, as in fever, burns or under dry atmospheric conditions. Sustacal HC provides 775 ml of water per 1000 ml of formula.

How Supplied: Sustacal® HC vanilla flavored liquid.
   NDC 0087-0460-42 Cans of 8 fl oz
Sustacal HC chocolate flavored liquid
   NDC 0087-0466-42 Cans of 8 fl oz
Sustacal HC eggnog flavored liquid
   NDC 0087-0461-42 Cans of 8 fl oz

SUSTAGEN® powder
Nutritional supplement

Composition: Corn syrup solids, nonfat milk, powdered whole milk, calcium caseinate, dextrose, artificial vanilla flavor, vitamins (vitamin A palmitate, cholecalciferol, dl-alpha-tocopheryl acetate, ascorbic acid, folic acid, thiamine hydrochloride, riboflavin, niacinamide, pyridoxine hydrochloride, cyanocobalamin, biotin, calcium pantothenate, phytonadione, and choline bitartrate), and minerals (ferrous sulfate, dibasic magnesium phosphate, cupric carbonate, zinc sulfate, and manganese sulfate).

Chocolate-flavored Sustagen also contains sugar and cocoa. High in protein, low in fat; generous in vitamins, calcium and iron. Easily mixed with water to make a pleasant-tasting beverage or a feeding via nasogastric tube.

One quart of prepared Sustagen supplies 107 g protein, 300 g carbohydrate, 15.9 g fat and at least 100% of the U.S. RDA for all essential vitamins and minerals:

Actions and Uses: Orally or by tube, provides extra nutritional support for ill, injured, surgical, and convalescent patients and those with impediments to eating or swallowing. Useful in peptic ulcer for buffering effect plus nutrition.

Preparation: Oral dilution: Mix equal parts (by volume) of Sustagen powder and water. This yields about 50 Cal/fl oz. One pound (3 packed level cups) Sustagen powder and 3 cups water make about a quart. ⅔ packed level cup Sustagen powder and ⅔ cup water make a single serving.

Refrigerate reconstituted Sustagen and use within 24 hours.

Tube-feeding dilution: Use 400 g Sustagen powder to 800 ml water for 1 liter. This mixture yields about 45 Cal/fl oz. More dilute mixtures may be utilized if desired. **In initiating tube feeding,** particularly for malnourished patients, feedings should be diluted to half strength on Day 1; increase volume and concentration gradually over a period of several days. Vanilla flavor is recommended for tube feeding if chocolate allergy is suspected.

Precautions: When Sustagen is used as the sole food, give additional water as needed for adequate daily intake. This is particularly important for unconscious or semiconscious patients. Do not begin post-operative tube feedings until peristalsis is reestablished. Electrolyte content of Sustagen should be considered for cardiac patients and others who tend to have edema.

How Supplied: Sustagen® vanilla
   NDC 0087-0393-21 Cans of 16 oz (1 lb)
   NDC 0087-0393-76 Cans of 5 lb
Sustagen chocolate
   NDC 0087-0394-21 Cans of 16 oz (1 lb)

TEMPRA®
Acetaminophen
Drops • syrup • chewable tablets
For infants and children

Composition: Tempra is acetaminophen, a safe and effective analgesic-antipyretic. It is not a salicylate. It contains no phenacetin or caffeine. It has no effect on prothrombin time. Tempra offers prompt, non-irritating therapy. Because it provides significant freedom from side effects, it is particularly valuable for patients who do not tolerate aspirin well. Tempra drops contain 10% alcohol. Tempra syrup contains no alcohol. Tempra chewable tablets are sugar-free.

Action and Uses: Tempra drops, syrup and chewable tablets are useful for reducing fever and for the temporary relief of minor aches, pains and discomfort associated with the common cold or "flu," inoculations or vaccination. Tempra syrup is valuable in reducing pain following tonsillectomy and adenoidectomy. When Tempra is used by pregnant or nursing women, there are no known adverse effects upon fetal development or nursing infants.

Administration and Dosage:
Every 4 hours as needed but not more than 5 times daily.
[See table on next page].
Drops given with calibrated 'Safti-Dropper' or mixed with water or fruit juices. Syrup given by teaspoon.

Precaution: Acetaminophen has been reported to potentiate the effect of orally administered anticoagulants.

Side Effects: Infrequent, nonspecific side effects have been reported with the therapeutic use of acetaminophen.

Overdosage: Acetaminophen in massive overdosage may cause hepatic toxicity in some patients. In all cases of suspected overdose, **immediately** contact a Poison Control Center for assistance in diagnosis and for information on the antidotes used to treat acetaminophen overdosage. The Rocky Mountain Poison Center toll-free number is (800) 525-6115. Following the ingestion of a large quantity of acetaminophen, patients may be asymptomatic for several days. Likewise, clinical laboratory evidence of hepatotoxicity may be delayed for up to a week. Parents' estimates of the quantity of a drug ingested are often also unreliable. Therefore, any report of the ingestion of an overdose should be corroborated by assaying for the acetaminophen plasma concentration. Since plasma levels at specific time points following an overdose correlate closely with the potential occurrence and probable severity of hepatotoxicity, it is important to accurately determine the elapsed time from ingestion of an overdose to the time of plasma acetaminophen determination.

Close clinical monitoring and serial hepatic enzyme studies are recommended for patients who delay presentation until several days following a reported acetaminophen overdose.

Note: A prescription is not required for Tempra drops, syrup or tablets as an analgesic. To prevent its misuse by the layman, the following information appears on the package label:

Warning: If fever persists for more than 3 days (72 hours) or if pain continues for more than 5 days, consult your physician.

As with any drug, if you are pregnant or nursing a baby, seek the advice of a health professional before using this product.

Phenylketonurics: Tablets contain phenylalanine.

How Supplied: Tempra® (acetaminophen) drops: (with calibrated 'Safti-Dropper') cherry-flavored

  NDC 0087-0730-01 Bottles of 15 ml
Tempra® (acetaminophen) syrup: cherry-flavored

  NDC 0087-0733-04 Bottles of 4 fl oz
  NDC 0087-0733-03 Bottles of 16 fl oz
Tempra chewables: grape-flavored, no sucrose

  NDC 0087-0738-01 Bottles of 30 tablets
No ℞ required.

Shown in Product Identification Section, page 415

TRAUMACAL™
High nitrogen and high calorie nutritionally complete formula for traumatized patients
Liquid (ready to use)

Composition: Water, corn syrup, calcium caseinate, soybean oil, sodium caseinate, sugar, medium chain triglycerides (fractionated coconut oil), lecithin, potassium citrate, magnesium chloride, salt, artificial flavor, potassium chloride, calcium carbonate, carrageenan, vitamins (vitamin A palmitate, cholecalciferol, dl-alpha-tocopheryl acetate, sodium ascorbate, folic acid, thiamine hydrochloride, riboflavin, niacinamide, pyridoxine hydrochloride, cyanocobalamin, biotin, calcium pantothenate, phytonadione and choline bitartrate) and minerals (potassium iodide, ferrous sulfate, cupric sulfate, zinc sulfate and manganese sulfate).

Age	Approximate Weight Range*	Dosage		
		Drops	Syrup	Chewables
Under 3 mo	Under 13 lb	½ dropper	¼ tsp	—
3 to 9 mo	13–20 lb	1 dropper	½ tsp	—
10 to 24 mo	21–26 lb	1½ dropper	¾ tsp	—
2 to 3 yr	27–35 lb	2 droppers	1 tsp	2 tablets
4 to 5 yr	36–43 lb	3 droppers	1½ tsp	3 tablets
6 to 8 yr	44–62 lb	—	2 tsp	4 tablets
9 to 10 yr	63–79 lb	—	2½ tsp	5 tablets
11 yr	80–89 lb	—	3 tsp	6 tablets
12 yr and older	90 lb & over	—	3–4 tsp	6–8 tablets

Dosage may be given every 4 hours as needed but not more than 5 times daily.
HOW SUPPLIED:
DROPS: Each 0.8 ml dropper contains 80 mg (1.23 grains) acetaminophen.
SYRUP: Each 5 ml teaspoon contains 160 mg (2.46 grains) acetaminophen.
CHEWABLES: Each tablet contains 80 mg (1.23 grains) acetaminophen.
*If child is significantly under- or overweight, dosage may need to be adjusted accordingly.

Indication: TraumaCal is a nutritionally complete ready-to-use liquid specifically formulated for patients requiring high nitrogen and calorie intake in limited volume (multiple trauma, moderate to severe burns). This formula may be fed orally or as a tube-feeding.

Actions: TraumaCal provides 22% of the total calories as protein, 40% as fat and 38% as carbohydrate in a 1.5 Cal/ml formula. TraumaCal is lactose-free with an osmolality of 490 mOsm/kg water.

Preparation: TraumaCal liquid is ready to feed; shake well before opening. Unused TraumaCal should be covered, refrigerated and used within 48 hours of opening.

It is recommended that TraumaCal be tube fed and that tube feeding be initiated as follows: Day 1—1:1 dilution of TraumaCal to water at 50 ml/hour (or full strength at 25 ml/hour). Day 2—full strength at 50 ml/hour. Day 3—full strength up to 100–125 ml/hour. Administration via infusion pump is recommended. If gravity feeding is utilized, larger diameter indwelling tubes are recommended to facilitate flow rate (12 French or larger.)

Precaution: Additional water should be given as needed to meet the patient's requirements. Particular attention should be given to water supply for comatose and unconscious patients and others who cannot express the usual sensation of thirst. Additional water is important also when renal concentrating ability is impaired, when there is extensive breakdown of tissue protein, or when water requirements are high, as in fever, burns or under dry atmospheric conditions. TraumaCal provides 780 ml of water per 1000 ml of formula.

How Supplied: TraumaCal liquid
NDC 0087-0464-42 Cans of 8 fl oz

TRIND® liquid
Antihistamine • nasal decongestant
Sugar-free

Composition: per 5 ml teaspoonful
Phenylpropanolamine
  hydrochloride .... 12.5 mg
Chlorpheniramine
  maleate .... 2.0 mg
  Contains 5% alcohol

Action and Uses: Trind contains two active ingredients to effectively relieve cold symptoms for children and adults. Pleasant tasting, orange-flavored liquid clears nasal passages, dries runny nose, relieves itchy, watery eyes and helps stop sneezing. When Trind is used by pregnant or nursing women according to the recommended dosage schedule, there are no known adverse effects upon fetal development or nursing infants.

Dosage: One dose every 4 hours as needed but not more than 6 times daily. Use enclosed dosage cup to measure correct dosage.

Age	Approximate Weight Range*	Dosage
Under 3 months	Under 11 lb	As directed by physician
3–9 months	12–18 lb	⅛ tsp
10–24 months	19–24 lb	¼ tsp
2–5	25–52 lb	½ tsp
6–12	53–99 lb	1 tsp
Adult	100 lb and over	2 tsp

*If child is significantly under or overweight, consult a physician for appropriate dosage.

Continued on next page

Mead Johnson Nutr.—Cont.

Warning: If symptoms do not improve within 3-5 days, or are accompanied by fever, consult a physician before continuing use. Do not take this product except under the advice and supervision of a physician if you have asthma, glaucoma, high blood pressure, heart disease, diabetes, thyroid disease, or difficulty in urination due to enlargement of the prostate. May cause excitability in children. Do not exceed recommended dosage because at higher doses nervousness, dizziness, or sleeplessness may occur. Caution: May cause marked drowsiness. Avoid alcoholic beverages, driving a motor vehicle or operating machinery.

As with any drug, if you are pregnant or nursing a baby, seek the advice of a health professional before using this product.

How Supplied: Trind® liquid (available without prescription)
NDC 0087-0750-44 Bottles of 5 fl oz

TRIND-DM® liquid
Cough suppressant • antihistamine • nasal decongestant
Sugar-free

Composition: per 5 ml
                                                teaspoonful
Phenylpropanolamine
   hydrochloride .... 12.5 mg
Dextromethorphan
   hydrobromide .... 7.5 mg
Chlorpheniramine
   maleate .... 2.0 mg
   Contains 5% alcohol

Action and Uses: Trind-DM contains three active ingredients to effectively relieve cough and cold symptoms for children and adults. When Trind-DM is used by pregnant or nursing women according to the recommended dosage schedule, there are no known adverse effects on fetal development or nursing infants. Pleasant tasting, fruit-flavored liquid suppresses cough, clears nasal passages, dries runny nose, relieves itchy, watery eyes and helps stop sneezing.

Dosage: One dose every 4 hours as needed but not more than 6 times daily. Use enclosed dosage cup to measure correct dosage.

	Approximate	
Age	Weight Range*	Dosage
Under 3 months	Under 11 lb	As directed by physician
3–9 months	12–18 lb	⅛ tsp
10–24 months	19–24 lb	¼ tsp
2–5	25–52 lb	½ tsp
6–12	53–99 lb	1 tsp
Adult	100 lb and over	2 tsp

*If child is significantly under or overweight, consult a physician for appropriate dosage.

Warning: If symptoms do not improve within 3–5 days, or are accompanied by fever, consult a physician before continuing use. Do not take this product except

under the advice and supervision of a physician if you have asthma, glaucoma, high blood pressure, heart disease, diabetes, thyroid disease, or difficulty in urination due to enlargement of the prostate. May cause excitability in children. Do not exceed recommended dosage because at higher doses nervousness, dizziness, or sleeplessness may occur. Caution: A persistent cough may be a sign of a serious condition. If cough persists, tends to recur, is accompanied by fever, rash, persistent headache, or if symptoms do not improve within 3–5 days, consult a physician before continuing use. May cause marked drowsiness. Avoid alcoholic beverages, driving a motor vehicle or operating machinery.

As with any drug, if you are pregnant or nursing a baby, seek the advice of a health professional before using this product.

How Supplied: Trind-DM® liquid: (Available without prescription.)
NDC 0087-0753-44 Bottles of 5 fl oz

TRI-VI-SOL®
Vitamins A, D and C drops

	Drops 1.0 ml	% U.S. RDA for Infants
Vitamin A, IU	1500	100
Vitamin D, IU	400	100
Vitamin C, mg	35	100

Action and Uses: Tri-Vi-Sol drops provide vitamins A, D and C.

How Supplied: Tri-Vi-Sol® drops: (with 'Safti-Dropper' marked to deliver 1 ml)
NDC 0087-0403-02 Bottles of 1 fl oz (30 ml)
NDC 0087-0403-03 Bottles of 1⅔ fl oz (50 ml)
Shown in Product Identification Section, page 415

TRI-VI-SOL® with Iron
Vitamins A, D, C and Iron drops

Composition: Each 1.0 ml supplies same vitamins as in Tri-Vi-Sol® vitamin drops (see above) plus 10 mg iron.

Action and Uses: Tri-Vi-Sol with Iron vitamins A, D, C and Iron for infants and children.

Administration and Dosage: Drop into mouth with 'Safti-Dropper'. Dose: 1.0 ml daily, or as indicated.

How Supplied: Tri-Vi-Sol® vitamin drops with Iron (with dropper marked to deliver 1 ml)
NDC 0087-0453-03 Bottles of 1⅔ fl oz (50 ml)
Shown in Product Identification Section, page 415

Products are cross-indexed by generic and chemical names in the
YELLOW SECTION

Mead Johnson
Pharmaceutical Division
Mead Johnson & Company
2404 W. PENNSYLVANIA ST.
EVANSVILLE, INDIANA 47721

COLACE®
Docusate sodium, Mead Johnson capsules • syrup • liquid (drops)

Description: Colace (Docusate sodium) is a stool softener.

Actions and Uses: Colace, a surface active agent, helps to keep stools soft for easy, natural passage. Not a laxative, thus not habit forming. Useful in constipation due to hard stools, in painful anorectal conditions, in cardiac and other conditions in which maximum ease of passage is desirable to avoid difficult or painful defecation, and when peristaltic stimulants are contraindicated. *Note.* When peristaltic stimulation is needed due to inadequate bowel motility, see Peri-Colace® (laxative and stool softener).

Contraindications: There are no known contraindications to Colace.

Side Effects: The incidence of side effects—none of a serious nature—is exceedingly small. Bitter taste, throat irritation, and nausea (primarily associated with the use of the syrup and liquid) are the main side effects reported. Rash has occurred.

Administration and Dosage: *Orally*—Suggested daily Dosage: *Adults and older children:* 50 to 200 mg. *Children 6 to 12:* 40 to 120 mg. *Children 3 to 6:* 20 to 60 mg. *Infants and children under 3:* 10 to 40 mg. The higher doses are recommended for initial therapy. Dosage should be adjusted to individual response. The effect on stools is usually apparent one to three days after the first dose. Give Colace liquid in half a glass of milk or fruit juice or in infant formula, to mask bitter taste. *In enemas*—Add 50 to 100 mg. Colace (5 to 10 ml. Colace liquid) to a retention or flushing enema.

Warning: As with any drug, if you are pregnant or nursing a baby, seek the advice of a health professional before using this product.

How Supplied: Colace® capsules, 50 mg.
NDC 0087-0713-01 Bottles of 30
NDC 0087-0713-02 Bottles of 60
NDC 0087-0713-03 Bottles of 250
NDC 0087-0713-05 Bottles of 1000
NDC 0087-0713-07 Cartons of 100 single unit packs
Colace® capsules, 100 mg.
NDC 0087-0714-43 Cartons of 10 single unit packs
NDC 0087-0714-01 Bottles of 30
NDC 0087-0714-02 Bottles of 60
NDC 0087-0714-03 Bottles of 250
NDC 0087-0714-05 Bottles of 1000
NDC 0087-0714-07 Cartons of 100 single unit packs

Note: Colace capsules should be stored at controlled room temperature (59°–86°F. or 15°–30°C.)

Colace® liquid, 1% solution; 10 mg./ml. with calibrated dropper)

NDC 0087-0717-04 Bottles of 16 fl. oz.
NDC 0087-0717-02 Bottles of 30 ml.
6505-00-045-7786 (Bottle of 30 ml) Defense

Colace® syrup, 20 mg./5-ml. teaspoon; contains not more than 1% alcohol

NDC 0087-0720-01 Bottles of 8 fl. oz.
NDC 0087-0720-02 Bottles of 16 fl. oz.

Shown in Product Identification Section, page 415

PERI-COLACE® capsules • syrup
Casanthranol and docusate sodium

Description: Peri-Colace is a combination of the mild stimulant laxative Peristim (casanthranol, Mead Johnson) and the stool-softener Colace® (docusate sodium, Mead Johnson). Each capsule contains 30 mg of Peristim and 100 mg of Colace; the syrup contains 30 mg of Peristim and 60 mg of Colace per 15-ml tablespoon (10 mg of Peristim and 20 mg of Colace per 5-ml teaspoon) and 10% alcohol.

Action and Uses: Peri-Colace provides gentle peristaltic stimulation and helps to keep stools soft for easier passage. Bowel movement is induced gently—usually overnight or in 8 to 12 hours. Nausea, griping, abnormally loose stools, and constipation rebound are minimized. Useful in management of chronic or temporary constipation.

Note: To prevent hard stools when laxative stimulation is not needed or undesirable, see Colace (stool softener).

Side Effects: The incidence of side effects—none of a serious nature—is exceedingly small. Nausea, abdominal cramping or discomfort, diarrhea, and rash are the main side effects reported.

Administration and Dosage:
Adults—1 or 2 capsules, or 1 or 2 tablespoons syrup at bedtime, or as indicated. In severe cases, dosage may be increased to 2 capsules or 2 tablespoons twice daily, or 3 capsules at bedtime. *Children*—1 to 3 teaspoons of syrup at bedtime, or as indicated.

Warnings: Do not use when abdominal pain, nausea, or vomiting are present. Frequent or prolonged use of this preparation may result in dependence on laxatives. As with any drug, if you are pregnant or nursing a baby, seek the advice of a health professional before using this product.

Overdosage: In addition to symptomatic treatment, gastric lavage, if timely, is recommended in cases of large overdosage.

How Supplied: Peri-Colace® Capsules
NDC 0087-0715-43 Cartons of 10 single unit pack

NDC 0087-0715-01 Bottles of 30
NDC 0087-0715-02 Bottles of 60
NDC 0087-0715-03 Bottles of 250
NDC 0087-0715-05 Bottles of 1000
NDC 0087-0715-07 Cartons of 100 single unit packs

Note: Peri-Colace capsules should be stored at controlled room temperatures (59°–86°F or 15°–30°C).

Peri-Colace® Syrup
NDC 0087-0721-01 Bottles of 8 fl. oz.
NDC 0087-0721-02 Bottles of 16 fl. oz.

Shown in Product Identification Section, page 415

Medicone Company
225 VARICK ST.
NEW YORK, NY 10014

DERMA MEDICONE® Ointment

Composition: Each gram contains:
Benzocaine.................................. 20.0 mg.
8-Hydroxyquinoline sulfate...... 10.5 mg.
Menthol....................................... 4.8 mg.
Ichthammol................................. 10.0 mg.
Zinc oxide....................................137.3 mg.
Petrolatum, Lanolin, perfume............q.s.

Action and Uses: For prompt, temporary relief of intolerable itching, burning and pain associated with minor skin irritations. A bland, non-toxic, well balanced formula in a non-drying base which will not disintegrate or liquefy at body temperature and is not washed away by urine, perspiration or exudate. Exerts a soothing, cooling influence on irritated skin surfaces by affording mild anesthesia to control the scratch reflex, promotes healing of the affected area and checks the spread of infection. Useful for symptomatic relief in a wide variety of pruritic skin irritations resulting from insect bites, prickly heat, eczema, chafed and raw skin surfaces, sunburn, fungus infections, plant poisoning, pruritus ani and pruritus vulvae—mouth sores, cracked lips, under dentures.

Administration and Dosage: Apply liberally directly to site of irritation and gently rub into affected area for better penetration and absorption. Cover area with gauze if necessary.

Precautions: Do not use in the eyes. If the condition for which this preparation is used persists, or if rash or irritation develops, discontinue use and consult physician.

How Supplied: 1 ounce tubes.

MEDICONE® DRESSING Cream

Composition: Each gram contains:
Benzocaine.................................... 5.0 mg.
8-Hydroxyquinoline sulfate...... 0.5 mg.
Cod liver oil ....125.0 mg.
Zinc oxide....................................125.0 mg.
Menthol.. 1.8 mg.
Petrolatum, Lanolin, talcum,
paraffin & perfume...........................q.s.

Action and Uses: Meets the first requisite in the treatment of minor burns, wounds and other denuded skin lesions by exerting mild, cooling anesthetic action for the prompt temporary relief of pain, burning and itching. A stable, nontoxic anesthetic dressing which does not liquefy or wash off at body temperature, nor is it decomposed by exudate, urine or perspiration. Promotes granulation and aids epithelization of affected tissue. The anesthetic, antipruritic, antibacterial properties make Medicone Dressing ideal for the treatment of 1st and 2nd degree burns, minor wounds, abrasions, diaper rashes and a wide variety of pruritic skin irritations.

Administration and Dosage: The smooth, specially formulated consistency allows comfortable application directly to the painful, irritated affected area. It may be spread on gauze before application or covered with gauze as desired.

Precautions: Do not use in the eyes. If the condition for which this preparation is used persists or if a rash or irritation develops, discontinue use and consult physician.

How Supplied: Tubes of 1 ounce.

MEDICONET®
(medicated rectal wipes)

Composition: Each cloth wipe medicated with Benzalkonium chloride, 0.02%; Ethoxylated lanolin, 0.5%; Methylparaben, 0.15%; Hamamelis water, 50%; Glycerin, 10%; Purified water, USP and Perfume, q.s.

Action and Uses: Soft disposable cloth wipes which fulfill the important requisite in treating anal discomfort by providing the facility for gently and thoroughly cleansing the affected area. For the temporary relief of intolerable pain, itching and burning in minor external hemorrhoidal, anal and outer vaginal discomfort. Lanolized, delicately scented, durable and delightfully soft. Antiseptic, antipruritic, astringent. Useful as a substitute for harsh, dry toilet tissue. May also be used as a compress in the pre- and post-operative management of anorectal discomfort. The hygienic Mediconet pad is generally useful in relieving pain, burning and itching in diaper rash, sunburn, heat rash, minor burns and insect bites.

How Supplied: Boxes of 20 individually packaged, pre-moistened cleansing cloths.

RECTAL MEDICONE®
SUPPOSITORIES

Composition: Each suppository contains:
Benzocaine .... 2 gr.
8-Hydroxyquinoline sulfate..............¼ gr.
Zinc oxide... 3 gr.
Menthol...⅐ gr.
Balsam Peru .... 1 gr.

Continued on next page

Medicone—Cont.

Cocoa butter—vegetable & petroleum oil base; Certified color added ....q.s.

Action and Uses: A soothing, non-toxic, comprehensive formula carefully designed to meet the therapeutic requirements in adequately treating simple hemorrhoids and minor anorectal disorders. Performs the primary function of promptly alleviating pain, burning and itching temporarily by exerting satisfactory local anesthesia. The muscle spasm, present in many cases of painful anal and rectal conditions, is controlled and together with the emollients provided, helps the patient to evacuate the bowel comfortably and normally. The active ingredients reduce congestion and afford antisepsis, accelerating the normal healing process. Used pre- and post-surgically in hemorrhoidectomy, in prenatal and postpartum care and whenever surgery is contraindicated for the comfort and well-being of the patient during treatment of an underlying cause.

Administration and Dosage: One suppository in the morning and one at night and after each stool, or as directed. Use of the suppositories should be continued for 10 to 15 days after cessation of discomfort to help protect against recurrence of symptoms. See Rectal Medicone Unguent for concurrent internal-external use.

Precautions: If a rash or irritation develops, or bleeding from the rectum occurs, discontinue use and consult physician.

How Supplied: Boxes of 12 and 24 individually foil-wrapped green suppositories.

RECTAL MEDICONE® UNGUENT

Composition: Each gram contains:

Benzocaine	20	mg.
8-Hydroxyquinoline sulfate	5	mg.
Menthol	4	mg.
Zinc oxide	100	mg.
Balsam Peru	12.5	mg.
Petrolatum	625	mg.
Lanolin	210	mg.

Certified color added

Action and Uses: A soothing, effective formulation which affords prompt, temporary relief of pain, burning and itching by exerting surface anesthetic action on the affected area in minor internal-external hemorrhoids and anorectal disorders. The active ingredients promote healing and protect against irritation, aiding inflamed tissue to retrogress to normal. The emollient petrolatum-lanolin base provides lubrication making bowel movements easier and more comfortable. Accelerates the normal healing process. Non-toxic. Rectal Medicone Unguent and Rectal Medicone Suppositories are excellent for concurrent management of internal-external irritations.

Administration and Dosage: For internal use—attach pliable applicator and lubricate tip with a small amount of Un-

guent to ease insertion. Apply liberally into affected area morning and night and after each stool or as directed. When used externally, cover area with gauze. When used with Rectal Medicone Suppositories, insert a small amount of Unguent into the rectum before inserting suppository.

Precautions: If a rash or irritation develops or rectal bleeding occurs, discontinue use and consult physician.

How Supplied: 1½ ounce tubes with pliable rectal applicator.

Medtech Laboratories, Inc.
P.O. BOX 2930
1501 STAMPEDE AVENUE
CODY, WY 82414-2930

IODEX™ Regular
Anti-infective

Description: Iodex contains 4.7% iodine in organic combination with oleic acid. The iodine is loosely combined with a fatty acid carrier and suspended in a neutral petrolatum base. As long as Iodex remains in contact with body tissues in minor cuts, wounds and abrasions, the iodine gradually separates from the molecule of the carrier and inhibits the growth and action of bacteria and promotes healing.

Directions: Apply and rub until color disappears. If area is too tender, apply freely and cover with a light loose bandage.

Caution: Do not use tight or air-excluding bandage. Consult a physician in the following cases: deep or puncture wounds, serious burns; or if redness, irritation, swelling or pain persists or increases; or if infection occurs.

How Supplied: Iodex Regular is available in 1 oz. and 14.5 oz.

IODEX™ with Methyl Salicylate
Counter Irritant

Description: Iodex contains 4.7% iodine in organic combination with oleic acid and 4.8% oil of wintergreen (synthetic). The iodine is loosely combined with a fatty acid carrier and suspended in a natural petrolatum base. Iodex with Methyl Salicylate will relieve local congestion moderating the symptoms: local aches and pains, soreness and stiffness of muscles. Iodex is also useful in giving relief to ordinary muscle strains and sprains.

Directions: Apply and rub until color disappears. If area is too tender, apply freely and cover with a light loose bandage.

Caution: Do not use tight or heavy air-excluding bandage. Discontinue use if excessive irritation of the skin develops. Avoid getting into eyes or mucous membrane.

How Supplied: Iodex with Methyl Salicylate is available in 1 oz. and 14.5 oz.

Menley & James Laboratories
a SmithKline Beckman company
ONE FRANKLIN PLAZA
P. O. BOX 8082
PHILADELPHIA, PA 19101

A.R.M.® Allergy Relief Medicine
Maximum Strength

Product Infromation: A.R.M. combines two important medicines in one safe fast-acting tablet:

- The highest level of antihistamine available without prescription-for better relief of sneezing, runny nose and itchy, weepy eyes.
- A clinically-proven sinus decongestant to help ease breathing and drain sinus congestion for hours.

Dosage: One tablet every 4 hours, not to exceed 4 tablets daily. Children (6–12 years): one-half the adult dose. Children under 6 years use only as directed by physician.

Warning: Do not exceed recommended dosage. If symptoms do not improve within 7 days, or are accompanied by high fever, consult a physician before continuing use. Stop use if dizziness, sleeplessness or nervousness occurs. If you have or are being treated for depression, high blood pressure, glaucoma, diabetes, asthma, difficulty in urination due to enlarged prostate, heart disease or thyroid disease, use only as directed by physician. As with any drug, if you are pregnant or nursing a baby, seek the advice of a health professional before using this product. Do not take this product if you are taking another medication containing phenylpropanolamine.

Avoid alcoholic beverages while taking this product. Do not drive or operate heavy machinery as this preparation may cause drowsiness.

May cause excitability, especially in children. Keep this and all medicines out of reach of children. In case of accidental overdose, consult physician or poison control center immediately. Store at controlled room temperature (59°–86°F).

TAMPER-RESISTANT PACKAGE FEATURE: Each tablet in sealed unit; do not use if broken.

Formula: Each A.R.M. tablet contains chlorpheniramine maleate, 4.0 mg. phenylpropanolamine HCl, 25 mg.

How Supplied: Consumer packages of 20 and 40 tablets.

Shown in Product Identification Section, page 415

ACNOMEL® CREAM
acne therapy

Description: *Cream*—sulfur, 8%; resorcinol, 2%; alcohol, 11% (w/w); non-greasy, dries oily skin, easy to apply.

Directions: Wash and dry affected areas thoroughly. Apply a thin coating of Acnomel Cream once or twice daily, making sure it does not get into the eyes or on eyelids. Do not rub in. If a marked chapping effect occurs, discontinue use temporarily.

Warning: Acnomel should not be applied to acutely inflamed area. If undue skin irritation develops or increases, discontinue use and consult physician. Keep this and all medicines out of reach of children. In case of accidental ingestion, contact a physician or poison control center immediately. Keep tube tightly closed to prevent drying. Store at controlled room temperature (59° to 86°F).

How Supplied: *Cream*—in specially lined 1 oz. tubes.
Shown in Product Identification Section, page 415

BENZEDREX® INHALER
nasal decongestant

For temporary relief of nasal congestion in colds and hayfever; also for ear block and pressure pain during air travel.

Composition: Each inhaler packed with propylhexedrine, 250 mg. Inactive ingredients: Lavender Oil, Menthol.

Directions: Insert in nostril. Close other nostril. Inhale twice. Treat other nostril the same way. Avoid excessive use. Inhaler loses potency after 2 or 3 months' use but some aroma may linger.

Warning: Ill effects may result if taken internally. In the case of accidental overdose or ingestion of contents, seek professional assistance or contact a poison control center immediately. Keep this and all drugs out of reach of children.
TAMPER-RESISTANT PACKAGE FEATURE: Inhaler sealed with imprinted cellophane. Do not use if broken.

How Supplied: In single plastic tubes.
in Product Identification Section, page 415

CONGESTAC™
Congestion Relief Medicine
Decongestant/Expectorant

Helps you breathe easier by temporarily relieving nasal congestion associated with the common cold, sinusitis, hay fever and allergies. Also helps relieve chest congestion by loosening phlegm and clearing bronchial passages of excess mucus. Contains no antihistamines which may overdry or make you drowsy.

Dosage: One tablet every 4 hours, not to exceed 4 tablets in 24 hours. Children (6 to 12 years): one-half the adult dose (break tablet in half). Children under 6 years use only as directed by physician.
TAMPER-RESISTANT PACKAGE FEATURE: EACH TABLET IN SEALED UNIT: DO NOT USE IF BROKEN.

Warning: Do not exceed recommended dosage. If symptoms do not improve within 7 days or are accompanied by high

fever, rash, shortness of breath or persistent headache, consult a physician before continuing use. Do not use if you have high blood pressure, heart disease, diabetes, thyroid disease or persistent or chronic cough, except under the advice and supervision of a physician. Keep this and all medicines out of reach of children. In case of accidental overdosage, contact a physician or poison control center immediately. As with any drug, if you are pregnant or nursing a baby, seek the advice of a health professional before using this product.

Drug Interaction Precaution: Do not take this product if you are presently taking a prescription antihypertensive or antidepressant drug containing a monoamine oxidase inhibitor except under the advice and supervision of a physician.

Formula: Each tablet contains pseudoephedrine hydrochloride 60 mg., guaifenesin 400 mg.
Store at controlled room temperature (59°–86°F.).

How Supplied: Available in packages of 24 and 50 tablets.
Shown in Product Identification Section, page 415

CONTAC®
Continuous Action Nasal
Decongestant/Antihistamine
Capsules

Composition:
(See table next page)

Product Information: Contac provides an increased amount of decongestant and antihistamine to give prolonged, round-the-clock relief from nasal congestion due to the common cold, hay fever and sinusitis. With just one capsule in the morning and one at bedtime, you feel better all day, sleep better all night, to awake refreshed, breathing freely without congestion.

Product Benefits: Each Contac continuous action capsule contains over 600 "tiny time pills". Some go to work right away for fast relief. The rest are scientifically timed to dissolve slowly, to give up to 12 hours of prolonged relief. Contac provides increased amounts of:
- A DECONGESTANT to help clear nasal and sinus passages and to reduce swollen nasal and sinus tissues.
- AN ANTIHISTAMINE to help relieve itchy, watery eyes; sneezing, running nose and postnasal drip.

Dosage: One capsule every 12 hours.

Warnings: Children under 12 should use only as directed by physician. Do not exceed recommended dosage. If symptoms do not improve within 7 days, or are accompanied by high fever, consult a physician before continuing use. Stop use if dizziness, sleeplessness or nervousness occurs.
Individuals with high blood pressure, glaucoma, diabetes, asthma, difficulty in urination due to enlarged prostate, heart disease or thyroid disease should use

only as directed by physician. Do not take this product if you are taking another medication containing phenylpropanolamine.
Avoid alcoholic beverages while taking this product. Do not drive or operate heavy machinery as this preparation may cause drowsiness.
May cause excitability, especially in children. Keep this and all medicines out of reach of children. In case of accidental overdose, consult physician or poison control center immediately. Store at controlled room temperature (59°–86°F.).
As with any drug, if you are pregnant or nursing a baby, seek the advice of a health professional before using this product.

Drug Interaction Precaution: Do not take if you are presently taking a prescription antihypertensive or antidepressant drug containing a monoamine oxidase inhibitor except under the advice and supervision of a physician.

Formula: Each capsule contains phenylpropanolamine hydrochloride 75.0 mg.; chlorpheniramine maleate 8.0 mg.
TAMPER-RESISTANT PACKAGE FEATURE: 40's—Bottle has seal under cap; do no use if broken. 10's, 20's & 30's—Each capsule in sealed unit; Do not use if broken.

How Supplied: Consumer packages of 10, 20, 30 and 40 capsules. Also, Industrial Dispensary Package of 200 capsules (2's in strip dispenser) for industrial dispensaries only.
Shown in Product Identification Section, page 415

CONTAC® Cough Capsules

Composition:
[See table on next page].

Product Information: Contac Cough Capsules provide strong and effective cough relief—all the relief of cough syrups concentrated in a capsule. Each capsule delivers maximum strength ingredients for temporary relief from coughing and nasal congestion due to the common cold.
New Contac Cough Capsules—concentrated to control your cough for hours.

Product Benefits:
- Effective cough relief
- Easy-to-swallow capsule form
- Concentrated cough relief in a capsule
- Convenient to carry
- Maximum Strength cough suppressant/decongestant

SAFETY SEALED PACKAGE FEATURE: EACH CAPSULE IN SEALED UNIT; DO NOT USE IF BROKEN.

Warning: Do not exceed recommended dosage. Do not give this product to children under 12 years except under the advice of a physician.

Caution: A persistent cough may be a sign of a serious condition. If cough persists for more than 1 week, tends to recur or is accompanied by high fever, fever

Continued on next page

Menley & James—Cont.

lasting more than 3 days, rash, persistent headache, shortness of breath or chest pain when breathing, consult a physician. As with any drug, if you are pregnant or nursing a baby, seek the advice of a health professional before using this product.

Stop use if dizziness, sleeplessness, or nervousness occurs. If you have or are being treated for depression, high blood pressure, diabetes, heart disease or thyroid disease, use only as directed by a physician.

Keep this and all medicines out of reach of children. In case of accidental overdose, consult a physician or poison control center immediately.

Store at controlled room temperature (59°–86°F.).

Dosage: One capsule every 6 hours, not to exceed 4 capsules daily. Children under 12 should use only as directed by a physician.

Formula: Each capsule contains Dextromethorphan Hydrobromide 30 mg. (cough suppressant) and Pseudoephedrine Hydrochloride 60 mg. (decongestant).

How Supplied: In consumer packages of 10's and 20's.

Shown in Product Identification Section, page 415

CONTAC®
Severe Cold Formula
Maximum Strength Capsules

Composition: [See table below].

Product Information: Two capsules every 6 hours help relieve discomforts of the severe cold (colds with flu-like symptoms such as fever, coughing, aches and pains).

Product Benefits: Contac Severe Cold Formula contains a non-aspirin analgesic, a cough suppressant, a decongestant and an antihistamine. These safe and effective ingredients provide temporary relief from these major cold symptoms: fever, coughing, body aches and pain, minor sore throat pain, headache, running nose, postnasal drip, sneezing, watery eyes and nasal congestion, sinus pressure, sinus congestion.

Dosage: Two capsules every 6 hours, not to exceed 8 capsules daily. Children

under 12 should use only as directed by physician.

Warnings: Do not exceed recommended dosage. If symptoms do not improve within 7 days, or worsen, or are accompanied by high fever, or difficulty in breathing, consult a physician before continuing use. Persistent cough may indicate the presence of a serious condition. Stop use if dizziness, sleeplessness, or nervousness occurs. Individuals with high blood pressure, glaucoma, diabetes, asthma, difficulty in urination due to enlarged prostate, heart disease or thyroid disease should use only as directed by physician. Avoid alcoholic beverages while taking this product. Do not drive or operate heavy machinery as this preparation may cause drowsiness. May cause excitability especially in children. Keep this and all medicines out of reach of children. In case of accidental overdose, consult physician or poison control center immediately. As with any drug, if you are pregnant or nursing a baby, seek the advice of a health professional before using this product. Store at controlled room temperature (59°–86°F.).

TAMPER-RESISTANT PACKAGE FEATURE: Each capsule in sealed unit; Do not use if broken.

Formula: Each capsule contains Pseudoephedrine Hydrochloride 30 mg.; Acetaminophen 500 mg. (500 mg. is a nonstandard dose of acetaminophen, as compared to the standard of 325 mg.); Dextromethorphan Hydrobromide 15 mg.; Chlorpheniramine Maleate 2 mg.

How Supplied: Consumer packages of 10 and 20 capsules.

Also Available: Contac Severe Cold Formula Night Strength Liquid—5 oz.

Shown in Product Identification Section, page 415

CONTAC®
Severe Cold Formula
Night Strength™

Composition: [See table below].

Product Information: Contac Severe Cold Formula Night Strength provides maximum strength relief from the discomforts of the severe cold (colds with flu-like symptoms such a fever, coughing, aches and pains).

Dosage: AT BEDTIME: take 1 fluid ounce in medicine cup provided. IF CONFINED TO BED OR AT HOME: take 1 fluid ounce every 6 hours as needed, not

to exceed 4 fluid ounces in 24 hours. Children under 12 should use only as directed by physician.

SAFETY SEALED PACKAGE FEATURE: IMPRINTED SEAL AROUND BOTTLE CAP; DO NOT USE IF SEAL IS BROKEN.

Warning: Do not exceed recommended dosage. If symptoms do not improve within 7 days, or worsen, or are accompanied by high fever, or difficulty in breathing, consult a physician before continuing use. A persistent cough may be a sign of a serious condition. If cough persists for more than 1 week, tends to recur or is accompanied by a high fever, fever lasting more than 3 days, rash, persistent headache, shortness of breath or chest pain when breathing, consult a physician. Stop use if dizziness, sleeplessness or nervousness occurs. Individuals who have been or are being treated for depression, high blood pressure, glaucoma, diabetes, asthma, difficulty in urination due to enlarged prostate, heart disease or thyroid disease should use only as directed by a physician. Avoid alcoholic beverages while taking this product. Do not drive or operate heavy machinery as this preparation may cause marked drowsiness. May cause excitability, especially in children. This package is child safe; however, keep this and all medicines out of reach of children. In case of accidental overdose, consult a physician or poison control center immediately. As with any drug, if you are pregnant or nursing a baby, seek the advice of a health professional before using this product.

Formula: Each fluid ounce (2 tablespoons) contains: acetaminophen 1000 mg. (1000 mg. is a non-standard dose of acetaminophen, as compared to the standard of 325 mg.) dextromethorphan hydrobromide 30 mg., pseudoephedrine hydrochloride 60 mg., doxylamine succinate 7.5 mg. Alcohol 25%.

Store at controlled room temperature (59°–86°F.).

How Supplied: Amber liquid in 5 oz. bottle.

Also Available: Contac Severe Cold Formula Capsules 10's and 20's.

Shown in Product Identification Section, page 415

CONTAC	Contac Continuous Action Decongestant Capsules	Contac Severe Cold Formula Capsules	Contac Severe Cold Formula Night Strength Liq. (each fluid ounce)	Contac Cough Capsules	Contac Jr. (each 5cc)
Phenylpropanolamine HCl	75.0 mg	—	—	—	9.375 mg
Chlorpheniramine maleate	8.0 mg	2.0 mg	—	—	—
Pseudoephedrine Hydrochloride	—	30.0 mg	60.0 mg	60.0 mg	—
Acetaminophen	—	500.0 mg	1000.0 mg	—	162.5 mg
Dextromethorphan Hydrobromide	—	15.0 mg	30.0 mg	30.0 mg	5.0 mg
Doxylamine succinate	—	—	7.5 mg	—	—
Alcohol	—	—	25%	—	10% by volume

CONTAC JR.®
The Complete Cold Medicine For Children

Composition:
[See table on preceding page]

Product Information: For congestion, coughing, body aches and fever due to colds. Relieves symptoms with these reliable medicines:

gentle decongestant. For temporary relief of nasal congestion. Helps your child breathe more freely. A safe, sensible, non-narcotic cough quieter. Calms worrisome coughs due to colds.

trusted, aspirin-free pain reliever and fever reducer. Provides temporary relief of muscular aches and pains, headaches, discomforts of fever due to colds and flu."

Product Benefits: The good medicines in Contac Jr. were specially chosen to help relieve your child's congestion, coughing, body aches and fever due to colds-without harsh drugs. Medical authorities know that for children, dose by weight-not age-means the dose you give is right for consistent controlled relief. Use the enclosed Contac Jr. Accu-Measure® Cup to select the right dose for your child's body weight.

Dosage: One dose every four hours, not to exceed 6 times daily. Use the enclosed Contac Jr. Accu-Measure® Cup to measure the right dose for your child. For dose by teaspoon see bottle label.

Caution: Do not exceed recommended dosage for your child's body weight. For children under 31 lbs. or under 3 years of age, consult a physician.

Warning: If symptoms persist for 7 days or are accompanied by high fever, severe or recurrent pain, or if child is being treated for depression, high blood pressure, diabetes, heart disease or thyroid disease, consult your physician. Stop use if dizziness, sleeplessness or nervousness occurs. Do not use if your child is taking another medication containing phenylpropanolamine. Keep this and all medicines out of children's reach. In case of accidental overdose, contact a physician immediately. Store at controlled room temperature 59°–86°F).

TAMPER-RESISTANT PACKAGE FEATURE: Imprinted seal around bottle cap; do not use if broken.

Formula: Each 5 cc (average teaspoon) contains: phenylpropanolamine HCl .375 mg.; acetaminophen 162.5 mg.; dextromethorphan hydrobromide 5.0 mg.; alcohol 10% by volume.

How Supplied: A clear red liquid in 4 oz. size bottle.
Shown in Product Identification Section, page 415

DIETAC™
Maximum Strength
Once-A-Day Diet Aid Capsules

Product Benefits:
- Caffeine free
- No stronger, longer-lasting appetite suppressant available without a prescription
- Timed-release—Just one capsule controls your appetite for 12 hours
- Contains the ingredient clinically proven safe and effective for weight loss

Dosage: Take one capsule each morning. This product's effectiveness is directly related to the degree to which you reduce your daily food intake.

Warning: Do not exceed recommended dosage. Do not take this product for periods exceeding three months. Do not give this product to children under 12 years. Do not take this product if you are taking another medication containing phenylpropanolamine. If you have or are being treated for high blood pressure, heart disease, diabetes, thyroid disease or depression, take this product only under the supervision of a physician. If you become nervous, sleepless or dizzy, stop the medication.
Keep this and all medicines out of reach of children. In case of accidental overdose, contact a physician or poison control center immediately.
As with any drug, if you are pregnant or nursing a baby, seek the advice of a health professional before using this product.

TAMPER-RESISTANT PACKAGE FEATURE: Each capsule in sealed unit; Do not use if broken.

Formula: Each capsule contains phenylpropanolamine HCl 75 mg. (appetite suppressant)

How Supplied: Consumer packages of 20 and 40 capsules
Shown in Product Identification Section, page 415

ECOTRIN®
Safety Coated Aspirin for Arthritis Pain

Product Information: This medication provides temporary relief of minor aches and pains of arthritis and rheumatism.

Usual Dosage: Adults, 1 or 2 tablets every 4 hours as necessary with water or fruit juice. Do not exceed 12 tablets in 24 hours unless directed by a physician. Children—as recommended by physician

Warning: If under medical care, do not use without physician's approval. If pain persists more than 10 days or redness is present, or in arthritic or rheumatic conditions affecting children under 12, consult a physician immediately. Discontinue use if dizziness, ringing in ears or impaired hearing occurs. If you experience persistent or unexplained stomach upset, consult a physician.

Keep this and all medicines out of reach of children. In case of accidental overdose contact a physician or poison control center immediately. As with any drug, if you are pregnant or nursing a baby, seek the advice of a health professional before using this product.

TAMPER-RESISTANT PACKAGE FEATURE: Bottle has imprinted seal under cap; do not use if broken.

Formula: Each Ecotrin tablet contains 325 mg. (5 gr.) aspirin.

How Supplied: Five grain tablets in bottles of 36, 100, 250 and 1000.
Shown in Product Identification Section, page 416

Maximum Strength
ECOTRIN® CAPSULES

Product Information: This maximum strength medication provides temporary relief of minor aches and pains of arthritis and rheumatism.

Usual Dosage: Adults, 2 capsules every 6 hours, with water or fruit juice. Do not exceed 8 capsules in 24 hours unless directed by a physician. Children—As recommended by a physician.

Formula: Each capsule contains 500 mg. (7.7 gr.) aspirin. (500 mg. is a nonstandard, maximum strength dosage of aspirin, as compared to the standard of 325 mg).

TAMPER RESISTANT PACKAGE FEATURE: BOTTLE HAS IMPRINTED SEAL UNDER CAP; DO NOT USE IF BROKEN.

Warning: If under medical care, do not use without your physician's approval. If pain persists for more than 10 days, or if redness is present, or in arthritic or rheumatic conditions affecting children under 12, consult a physician immediately. Discontinue use if dizziness, ringing in ears, or impaired hearing occurs. If you experience persistent or unexplained stomach upset, consult a physician. Keep this and all medicines out of children's reach. In case of accidental overdose, consult a physician or poison control center immediately. As with any medicine, if you are pregnant or nursing a baby, seek the advice of a health professional before using this product.
Store at controlled room temperature (59°–86°F.).

How Supplied: 500 mg. (7.7 grain) capsules, in bottles of 50 and 100.
Shown in Product Identification Section, page 416

Maximum Strength
ECOTRIN® TABLETS
Safety Coated Aspirin for Arthritis Pain

Product Information: This maximum strength medication provides temporary relief of minor aches and pains of arthritis and rheumatism.

Continued on next page

Menley & James—Cont.

Usual Dosage: Adults, 2 tablets every 6 hours as needed, with water or fruit juice. Do not exceed 8 tablets in 24 hours unless directed by a physician. Children —As recommended by physician.

Formula: Each tablet contains 500 mg. (7.7 gr.) aspirin. *(500 mg. is a non-standard, maximum-strength dosage of aspirin, as compared to the standard of 325 mg.)*

TAMPER-RESISTANT PACKAGE FEATURE: BOTTLE HAS IMPRINTED SEAL UNDER CAP; DO NOT USE IF BROKEN.

Warning: If under medical care, do not use without your physician's approval. If pain persists more than 10 days, or redness is present, or in arthritic or rheumatic conditions affecting children under 12, consult a physician immediately. Discontinue use if dizziness, ringing in ears or impaired hearing occurs. If you experience persistent or unexplained stomach upset, consult a physician. Keep this and all medicines out of children's reach. In case of accidental overdose, consult a physician or poison control center immediately. As with any medicine, if you are pregnant or nursing a baby, seek the advice of a health professional before using this product.
Store at controlled room temperature (59°–86°F.).

How Supplied: 500 mg. (7.7 grain) tablets, in bottles of 24, 60 and 150.
Shown in Product Identification Section, page 416

Regular Strength
ECOTRIN® CAPSULES

Product Information: This medication provides temporary relief of minor aches and pains of arthritis and rheumatism.

Usual Dosage: Adults, 1 or 2 capsules every 4 hours, as needed, with water or fruit juice. Do not exceed 12 capsules in 24 hours unless directed by a physician. Children—As recommended by physician.

Formula: Each capsule contains 325 mg. (5 gr.) aspirin.

TAMPER-RESISTANT PACKAGE FEATURE: BOTTLE HAS IMPRINTED SEAL UNDER CAP; DO NOT USE IF BROKEN.

Warning: If under medical care, do not use without your physician's approval. If pain persists for more than 10 days, or if redness is present, or in arthritic or rheumatic conditions affecting children under 12, consult a physician immediately. Discontinue use if dizziness, ringing in ears, or impaired hearing occurs. If you experience persistent or unexplained stomach upset, consult a physician. Keep this and all medicines out of children's reach. In case of accidental overdose, consult a physician or poison control center

immediately. As with any medicine, if you are pregnant or nursing a baby, seek the advice of a health professional before using this product.
Store at controlled room temperature (59°–86°F.).

How Supplied: 5 grain tablets in bottles of 70 and 140 shown in product identification section.
Shown in Product Identification Section, page 416

FEOSOL® ELIXIR
Hematinic

Description: Feosol Elixir, an unusually palatable iron elixir, provides the body with ferrous sulfate—iron in its most efficient form. The standard elixir for simple iron deficiency and iron-deficiency anemia when the need for such therapy has been determined by a physician.
Each 5 ml. (1 teaspoonful) contains ferrous sulfate USP, 220 mg. (44 mg. of elemental iron); alcohol, 5%.

Usual Dosage: *Adults*—1 to 2 teaspoonfuls three times daily. *Children*—½ to 1 teaspoonful three times daily preferably between meals. *Infants*—as directed by physician. Mix with water or fruit juice to avoid temporary staining of teeth; do not mix with milk or wine-based vehicles.

TAMPER-RESISTANT PACKAGE FEATURE: Imprinted seal around bottle cap; do not use if broken.

Warning: The treatment of any anemic condition should be under the advice and supervision of a physician. Since oral iron products interfere with absorption of oral tetracycline antibiotics, these products should not be taken within two hours of each other. Occasional gastrointestinal discomfort (such as nausea) may be minimized by taking with meals and by beginning with one teaspoonful the first day, two the second, etc. until the recommended dosage is reached. Iron-containing medication may occasionally cause constipation or diarrhea, and liquids may cause temporary staining of the teeth (this is less likely when diluted). Keep this and all medicines out of reach of children. In case of accidental overdose, contact a physician or poison control center immediately.
Caution: As with any drug, if you are pregnant or nursing a baby, seek the advice of a health professional before using this product.

How Supplied: A clear orange liquid in 16 fl. oz. bottles.

Also Available: Feosol® Tablets, Feosol® Capsules.
Shown in Product Identification Section, page 416

FEOSOL® CAPSULES
Hematinic

Description: Feosol capsules provide the body with ferrous sulfate—iron in its most efficient form—for simple iron deficiency and iron-deficiency anemia.

The special targeted-release capsule formulation—ferrous sulfate in pellets—reduces stomach upset, a common problem with iron.

Formula: Each capsule contains 16[?] mg. of dried ferrous sulfate USP (50 mg of elemental iron), equivalent to 250 mg of ferrous sulfate USP.

Dosage: Do not exceed recommended dosage. Adults: 1 or 2 capsules as directed by a physician. Children: As directed by a physician.

TAMPER-RESISTANT PACKAGE FEATURE: Each capsule in sealed unit; do not use if broken (30's). Bottle has imprinted seal under cap; do not use if broken (100's and 500's).

Warnings: The treatment of any anemic condition should be under the advice and supervision of a physician. Since oral iron products interfere with absorption of oral tetracycline antibiotics, these products should not be taken within two hours of each other. Keep this and all medicines out of reach of children. In case of accidental overdose, contact a physician or poison control center immediately. Iron-containing medicine may occasionally cause constipation or diarrhea.
Caution: As with any drug, if you are pregnant or nursing a baby, seek the advice of a health professional before using this product.

How Supplied: Bottles of 30, 100 and 500 capsules; in Single Unit Packages of 100 capsules (intended for institutional use only).
Also available in Tablets and Elixir.
Shown in Product Identification Section, page 416

FEOSOL® TABLETS
Hematinic

Product Information: Feosol Tablets provide the body with ferrous sulfate iron in its most efficient form, for iron deficiency and iron-deficiency anemia when the need for such therapy has been determined by a physician. The distinctive triangular-shaped tablet has a coating to prevent oxidation and improve palatability.

Formula: Each tablet contains 200 mg of dried ferrous sulfate USP (65 mg. of elemental iron), equivalent to 325 mg. (5 grains) of ferrous sulfate USP.

Usual Dosage: *Adults*—one tablet to 4 times daily, after meals and upon retiring. *Children 6 to 12 years*—one tablet three times a day after meals. *Children under 6 years and infants*—use Feosol® Elixir.

TAMPER-RESISTANT PACKAGE FEATURE: Bottle has imprinted seal under cap. Do not use if broken.

Warnings: Do not exceed recommended dosage. The treatment of an anemic condition should be under the advice and supervision of a physician. Since oral iron products interfere with absorption of oral tetracycline antibiotics

ics, these products should not be taken within two hours of each other.

Occasional gastrointestinal discomfort (such as nausea) may be minimized by taking with meals and by beginning with one tablet the first day, two the second, etc. until the recommended dosage is reached. Iron-containing medication may occasionally cause constipation or diarrhea.

Keep this and all medicines out of reach of children. In case of accidental overdose, contact a physician or poison control center immediately.

Caution: As with any drug, if you are pregnant or nursing a baby, seek the advice of a health professional before using this product.

How Supplied: Bottles of 100 and 1000 tablets; in Single Unit Packages of 100 tablets (intended for institutional use only).
Also available in Capsules and Elixir.
Shown in Product Identification Section, page 416

FEOSOL PLUS®
Iron plus vitamins

Description: For use in iron deficiency and iron-deficiency anemia where additional vitamins are indicated.

Formula: Each Feosol Plus capsule contains:
Dried ferrous sulfate ....200 mg.
  (equivalent to 325 mg. ferrous sulfate USP; 65 mg. of elemental iron)
Folic acid ....0.2 mg.
Ascorbic acid
  (Vitamin C) ....50 mg.
Thiamine HCl
  (Vitamin B$_1$) ....2 mg.
Riboflavin
  (Vitamin B$_2$) ....2 mg.
Pyridoxine HCl
  (Vitamin B$_6$) ....2 mg.
Vitamin B$_{12}$
  (activity equivalent) ....5 mcg.
  (derived from streptomyces fermentation)
Nicotinic acid (niacin) ....20 mg.

Usual Dosage: *Adults and Children (over 3 yrs.)*One capsule twice daily or as directed by physician.

TAMPER-RESISTANT PACKAGE FEATURE: Bottle has imprinted seal under cap; do not use if broken.

Warning: The treatment of any anemic condition should be under the advice and supervision of a physician.

Since oral iron products tend to interfere with absorption of oral tetracycline antibiotics, these products should not be taken within two hours of each other. Keep this and all medicines out of reach of children. In case of accidental overdose, contact a physician or poison control center immediately. Iron-containing medication may occasionally cause constipation or diarrhea.

Caution: As with any drug, if you are pregnant or nursing a baby, seek the advice of a health professional before using this product.

How Supplied: Bottles of 100 capsules.
Shown in Product Identification Section, page 416

ORNACOL®
Cough & Cold Capsules

Product Information: For temporary relief from coughing and nasal congestion due to common cold and sinusitis. NO ANTIHISTAMINE DROWSINESS/ ASPIRIN-FREE—especially suited for working people.

Dosage: Adults and children over 12—ONE CAPSULE four times a day.

TAMPER-RESISTANT PACKAGE FEATURE: EACH CAPSULE IN SEALED UNIT; DO NOT USE IF BROKEN.

Warning: Do not exceed recommended dosage. Persistent cough may indicate the presence of a serious condition. Persons with a high fever or persistent cough should not use this preparation unless directed by a physician. If you have or are being treated for depression, high blood pressure, diabetes, heart disease or thyroid disease, use only as directed by a physician. Stop use if dizziness, sleeplessness or nervousness occurs. If relief does not occur within three days, discontinue use and consult a physician. Do not take this product if you are taking another product containing phenylpropanolamine. Keep this and all medicines out of reach of children. In case of accidental overdose, contact a physician or poison control center immediately. As with any drug, if you are pregnant or nursing a baby, seek the advice of a health professional before using this product.

Formula: Each capsule contains 30 mg. dextromethorphan HBr, 25 mg. phenylpropanolamine HCl.
Store at controlled room temperature (59°–86°F.).

Supplied: Ornacol Cough & Cold Capsules in packages of 20.
Shown in Product Identification Section, page 416

ORNEX®
decongestant/analgesic

Composition: Each capsule contains: 12.5 mg. phenylpropanolamine hydrochloride; 325 mg. acetaminophen.

Action: For temporary relief of nasal congestion, headache, aches, pains and fever due to colds, sinusitis and flu. No antihistamine drowsiness.

Dosage: Adults—Two capsules every 4 hours. Do not exceed 8 capsules in 24 hours. Children (6 to 12 years)—One capsule every 4 hours. Do not exceed 4 capsules in 24 hours.

Warning: Do not exceed recommended dosage. Do not give to children under 6 or use for more than 10 days, unless directed by physician. If you have or are being treated for depression, high blood pressure, diabetes, heart disease or thyroid disease, use only as directed by physician. Stop use if dizziness, sleeplessness or nervousness occurs. Do not take this product if you are taking another medication containing phenylpropanolamine. This package is for households with young children. Keep this and all medicines out of reach of children. In case of accidental overdose, contact a physician or poison control center immediately. As with any drug, if you are pregnant or nursing a baby, seek the advice of a health professional before using this product.

TAMPER-RESISTANT PACKAGE FEATURE: Each capsule in sealed unit; do not use if broken.

Supplied: In consumer packages of 24 and 48 capsules, in bottles of 100 capsules. Also, Dispensary Packages of 800 capsules for industrial dispensaries and student health clinics only.
Shown in Product Identification Section, page 416

PRAGMATAR® OINTMENT

Description: Cetyl alcohol-coal tar distillate, 4%; precipitated sulfur, 3%; salicylic acid, 3%.

Action and Uses: Highly effective in common skin disorders in both adults and children: dandruff, cradle cap, dermatitis, eczema, itchy scaly skin, athlete's foot. Consult your physician for use in other conditions.

Directions: On the scalp: Part hair and massage into small areas at bedtime. Apply sparingly but thoroughly to entire scalp. Remove with a light shampoo the following morning. Use no more often than every other day. On other areas: Use small quantities, confining application to affected surfaces. Apply no more than once daily. Keep tube tightly closed to prevent drying. Store at controlled room temperature (59°–85°F).

Warning: Keep out of eyes and off eyelids. Use with care near the groin or on acutely inflamed areas. Do not use on blistered surfaces. If rash or irritation develops, discontinue use. Keep this and all medicines out of reach of children. In case of accidental ingestion, contact a physician or poison control center immediately.

How Supplied: 1 oz. tubes.
Shown in Product Identification Section, page 416

SINE–OFF® Extra Strength
Sinus Medicine
Aspirin-Free Capsules
Relieves headache and congestion

Composition:
[See table on next page].

Product Information: Sine-Off Extra Strength Capsules provide extra strength relief from headache and sinus pain. Relieves pressure and congestion

Continued on next page

Menley & James—Cont.

due to sinusitis, allergic sinusitis or the common cold. This formula contains acetaminophen, a pain reliever that is unlikely to cause gastric irritation or allergic reactions often associated with aspirin-containing products.

Product Benefits: Eases headache pain and pressure ● promotes sinus drainage ● shrinks swollen membranes to relieve congestion ● relieves postnasal drip.

Dosage: Adults and children over 12 years of age: 2 capsules every 6 hours, not to exceed 8 capsules in any 24-hour period. Children under 12 should use only as directed by physician.

Warnings: Do not exceed recommended dosage. If symptoms do not improve within 7 days, consult a physician before continuing use. Individuals being treated for depression, high blood pressure, asthma, heart disease, diabetes, thyroid disease, glaucoma or enlarged prostate should use only as directed by a physician.
Avoid alcoholic beverages while taking this product. Do not drive or operate heavy machinery as this preparation may cause drowsiness.
Stop use if dizziness, sleeplessness or nervousness occurs.
May cause excitability, especially in children. This package is child-safe; however, keep this and all medicines out of reach of children. In case of accidental overdose, contact a physician immediately.
As with any drug if pregnant or nursing, consult your physician before taking this or any medicine. Do not take this medication if you are taking another product containing phenylpropanolamine.

TAMPER-RESISTANT PACKAGE FEATURE: Each capsule in sealed unit; do not use if broken.

Formula: Each capsule contains: Chlorpheniramine maleate, 2.0 mg.; phenylpropanolamine HCl, 30 mg.; acetaminophen, 500 mg. **(500 mg. is a non-standard dosage of acetaminophen, as compared to the standard of 325 mg.).**

How Supplied: Consumer packages of 20 capsules.

Also Available: Sine-Off® Extra Strength Sinus Medicine Aspirin-Free Tablets 20's. Sine-Off® Sinus Medicine Tablets with Aspirin in 24's, 48's, 100's. Sine-Off® Extra Strength No Drowsiness Formula 20's

Shown in Product Identification Section, page 416

SINE–OFF® Extra Strength Sinus Medicine Aspirin-Free Tablets
Relieves sinus headache and congestion

Composition: [See table below].

Product Information: Sine-Off Extra Strength Tablets provide extra strength relief from headache and sinus pain. Relieves pressure and congestion due to sinusitis, allergic sinusitis or the common cold. This formula contains acetaminophen, a pain reliever that is unlikely to cause gastric irritation or allergic reactions often associated with aspirin-containing products.

Product Benefits: Eases headache, pain and pressure; promotes sinus drainage; shrinks swollen membranes to relieve congestion; relieves postnasal drip.

Dosage: Adults and children over 12 years of age: 2 tablets every 6 hours, not to exceed 8 tablets in any 24-hour period. Children under 12 should use only as directed by physician.

Warnings: Do not exceed recommended dosage. If symptoms do not improve within 7 days, consult a physician before continuing use. Individuals being treated for depression, high blood pressure, asthma, heart disease, diabetes, thyroid disease, glaucoma or enlarged prostrate should use only as directed by a physician. Do not take this product if you are taking another medication containing phenylpropanolamine.
Avoid alcoholic beverages while taking this product. Do not drive or operate heavy machinery as this preparation may cause drowsiness.
Stop use if dizziness, sleeplessness or nervousness occurs.
May cause excitability, especially in children. **This package is child-safe;** however, keep this and all medicines out of reach of children. In case of accidental overdose, contact a physician immediately. As with any drug, if you are pregnant or nursing a baby, seek the advice of a health professional before using this product.
Store at controlled room temperature (59°–86°F.).

TAMPER-RESISTANT PACKAGE FEATURE: Each tablet in sealed unit; do not use if broken.

Formula: Each tablet contains chlorpheniramine, 2.0 mg.; phenylpropanolamine HCl, 18.75 mg.; acetaminophen 500 mg. (500 mg. is a non-standard extra strength dosage of acetaminophen, as compared to the standard of 325 mg.).

How Supplied: Consumer packages of 20 tablets.

Also Available: Sine-Off® Tablets with Aspirin in 24's, 48's, 100's. Sine-Off® Extra Strength Aspirin-Free Capsules 20's. Sine-Off® Extra Strength No Drowsiness Formula 20's.

Shown in Product Identification Section, page 416

SINE–OFF® Extra Strength No Drowsiness Formula

Composition: [See table below].

Product Information: No Drowsiness Formula Sine-Off Extra Strength Capsules provide extra strength relief from headache and sinus pain. Relieves pressure and congestion due to sinusitis, allergic sinusitis or the common cold. This formula contains acetaminophen, a pain reliever that is unlikely to cause gastric irritation or allergic reactions often associated with aspirin-containing products.

Product Benefits: Eases headache, pain and pressure. Promotes sinus drainage ● shrinks swollen membranes to relieve congestion ● does not cause drowsiness.

Dosage: Adults and children over 12 years of age: 2 capsules every 6 hours, not to exceed 8 capsules in any 24-hour period. Children under 12 should use only as directed by physician.

Warnings: Do not exceed recommended dosage. If symptoms do not improve within 7 days, consult a physician before continuing use. Individuals being treated for depression, high blood pressure, heart disease, diabetes, thyroid disease should use only as directed by a physician. Do not take this product if you are taking another medication containing phenylpropanolamine.
Stop use if dizziness, sleeplessness or nervousness occurs. This package is child-safe; however, keep this and all medicines out of reach of children. In case of accidental overdose, contact a physician immediately. Store at controlled room temperature (59°–86°F.).
As with any drug, if you are pregnant or nursing a baby, seek the advice of a health professional before using this product.

TAMPER-RESISTANT PACKAGE FEATURE: Each capsule in sealed unit; do not use if broken.

Each tablet/ capsule contains:	Sine-Off Tablets-Aspirin Formula	Sine-Off Extra Strength Aspirin-Free Capsules	Sine-Off Extra Strength Aspirin-Free Tablets	Sine-Off Extra Strength No Drowsiness Formula Capsules
Chlorpheniramine maleate	2.0 mg	2.0 mg	2.0 mg	—
Phenylpropanolamine HCl	12.5 mg	30.0 mg	18.75 mg	—
Aspirin	325.0 mg	—	—	—
Acetaminophen	—	500.0 mg	500.0 mg	500.0 mg
Pseudoephedrine HCl	—	—	—	30.0 mg

Formula: Each capsule contains: 30 mg. pseudoephedrine hydrochloride, 500 mg. acetaminophen (500 mg. is a nonstandard dosage of acetaminophen, as compared to the standard of 325 mg.).

How Supplied: Consumer packages of 20 capsules.

Also Available:
Sine-Off® Tablets with Aspirin
Sine-Off® Extra Strength Tablets—aspirin-free
Sine-Off® Extra Strength Capsules—aspirin-free

Shown in Product Identification Section, page 416

SINE-OFF® Sinus Medicine Tablets–Aspirin Formula
Relieves sinus headache and congestion.

Composition:
[See table on preceding page].

Product Information: Sine-Off relieves headache, pain, pressure and congestion due to sinusitis, allergic sinusitis, or the common cold.

Product Benefits: Eases headache, pain and pressure; promotes sinus drainage; shrinks swollen membranes to relieve congestion; relieves postnasal drip.

Dosage: Adults: 2 tablets every 4 hours, not to exceed 8 tablets in any 24-hour period. Children (6–12) one-half the adult dosage. Children under 6 years should use only as directed by a physician.

Warning: Do not exceed recommended dosage. If symptoms do not improve within 7 days, consult a physician before continuing use. Individuals being treated for depression, high blood pressure, asthma, heart disease, diabetes, thyroid disease, glaucoma or enlarged prostate should use only as directed by a physician. Do not take this product if you are taking another medication containing phenylpropanolamine. □ Avoid alcoholic beverages while taking this product. Do not drive or operate heavy machinery as this preparation may cause drowsiness. □ Stop use if dizziness, sleeplessness or nervousness occurs. □ May cause excitability, especially in children. Keep this and all medicines out of reach of children. In case of accidental overdose, contact a physician immediately. As with any drug, if you are pregnant or nursing a baby, seek the advice of a health professional before using this product. Store at controlled room temperature (59°–86°F.).

TAMPER-RESISTANT PACKAGE FEATURE: Each tablet in sealed unit; do not use if broken.

Formula: Chlorpheniramine maleate 2.0 mg.; phenylpropanolamine HCl 12.5 mg. aspirin 325.0 mg.

How Supplied: Consumer packages of 24, 48 and 100 tablets

Also Available: Sine-Off® Extra Strength Aspirin-Free Capsules 20's, and Extra Strength Aspirin-Free Tablets 20's. Sine-Off® Extra Strength No Drowsiness 20's.
Shown in Product Identification Section, page 416

TELDRIN®
Chlorpheniramine maleate
Timed-Release Allergy Capsules, 8 mg. and Maximum Strength 12 mg.

Formula: Each capsule contains chlorpheniramine maleate 8 mg. or Maximum Strength 12 mg.

Description: Each Teldrin Timed-Release capsule contains chlorpheniramine maleate, 8 mg. or Maximum Strength 12 mg., so formulated that a portion of the antihistamine dose is released initially, and the remaining medication is released gradually over a prolonged period.

Indications for Use: Hay fever and allergies are caused by grass and tree pollen, dust and pollution. Teldrin provides up to 12 hours of relief from hay fever/upper respiratory allergy symptoms; sneezing; running nose; itchy, watery eyes. Teldrin is formulated to release some medication initially and the rest gradually over a prolonged period.

Dosage: Adults and children over 12 years of age: Just one capsule in the morning, and one in the evening. Do not give to children under 12 without the advice and consent of a physician. Not to exceed 24 mg. (3 capsules of 8 mg.; 2 capsules of 12 mg.) in 24 hours.

TAMPER-RESISTANT PACKAGE FEATURE: Packages of 12's and 24's—each capsule in sealed unit; do not use if broken.
Bottles of 50's and 500's—bottle has imprinted seal under cap; do not use if broken.

Warning: Do not take this product if you have asthma, glaucoma, or difficulty in urination due to enlargement of the prostate gland, except under the advice and supervision of a physician.
Do not drive or operate heavy machinery as this preparation may cause drowsiness. Avoid alcoholic beverages while taking this product. May cause excitability, especially in children. Keep this and all medicines out of the reach of children. In case of accidental overdose, contact a physician or poison control center immediately.
As with any drug, if you are pregnant or nursing a baby, seek the advice of a health professional before using this product.

How Supplied: 8 mg. and Maximum Strength 12 mg. Timed-Release capsules in packages of 12 and 24 capsules, in bottles of 50 and 500; in Single Unit Packages of 100 (intended for institutional use only).
Shown in Product Identification Section, page 416

TELDRIN®
Multi–Symptom Allergy Reliever

Product Information: Two capsules every 6 hours help relieve the discomforts of hay fever, allergies and sinusitis, caused by grass and tree pollen, dust and pollution.

Product Benefits: Teldrin Multi-Symptom Allergy Reliever contains an antihistamine, a decongestant, and an aspirin-free analgesic. These safe and effective ingredients provide fast and temporary relief from the following major hay fever/upper respiratory allergy symptoms: sneezing, itchy eyes, watery eyes, running nose, postnasal drip, nasal and sinus congestion, sinus pressure, headache and facial pain.

Dosage: Adults and children over 12: Two capsules every 6 hours, not to exceed 8 capsules in any 24-hour period. Children under 12 should use only as directed by a physician.

Warnings: Do not exceed recommended dosage. If symptoms do not improve within 7 days consult a physician before continuing use. Individuals being treated for depression, high blood pressure, asthma, heart disease, diabetes, thyroid disease, glaucoma or enlarged prostate should use only as directed by a physician. Avoid alcoholic beverages while taking this product. Do not drive or operate heavy machinery as this preparation may cause drowsiness. Stop use if dizziness, sleeplessness or nervousness occurs. May cause excitability, especially in children. This package is child-safe; however, keep this and all medicines out of reach of children. In case of accidental overdose, contact a physician or poison control center immediately.
As with any drug, if you are pregnant or nursing a baby, seek the advice of a health professional before using this product. Store at controlled room temperature (59°–86°F).

TAMPER RESISTANT PACKAGE FEATURE: Each capsule in sealed unit; do not use if broken.

Formula: Each capsule contains chlorpheniramine maleate, 2 mg.; acetaminophen, 325 mg.; pseudoephedrine HCl, 30 mg.

How Supplied: Consumer packages of 20 and 40 capsules.
Shown in Product Identification Section, page 416

TROPH–IRON®
Vitamins B₁, B₁₂ and Iron

Description: Each 5 ml. (1 teaspoonful) contains thiamine hydrochloride (vitamin B_1), 10 mg.; cyanocobalamin (vitamin B_{12}), 25 mcg.; iron, 20 mg., present as soluble ferric pyrophosphate.

Indications: For deficiencies of vitamins B_1, B_{12} and iron.

Dosage: Liquid—One teaspoonful daily, or as directed by physician. While its ef-

Continued on next page

Menley & James—Cont.

fectiveness is in no way affected, Troph-Iron Liquid may darken as it ages.

Warning: The treatment of any anemic condition should be under the advice and supervision of a physician. Since oral iron products interfere with absorption of oral tetracycline antibiotics, these products should not be taken within two hours of each other.

Iron-containing medications may occasionally cause gastrointestinal discomfort, such as nausea, constipation or diarrhea.

Keep this and all medicines out of reach of children. In case of accidental overdose, contact a physician or poison control center immediately.

As with any drug, if you are pregnant or nursing a baby, seek the advice of a health professional before using this product.

Store at room temperature (59°–86°F).

TAMPER-RESISTANT PACKAGE FEATURE: Sealed, imprinted bottle cap; do not use if broken.

How Supplied: Liquid—in 4 fl. oz. (118 ml) bottles.

Shown in Product Identification Section, page 416

TROPHITE®
Vitamins B₁ and B₁₂

Description: Each 5 ml (1 teaspoonful) and each tablet contains thiamine hydrochloride (vitamin B_1), 10 mg.; and cyanocobalamin (vitamin B_{12}), 25 mcg.

Indications: For deficiencies of vitamins B_1 and B_{12}.

Dosage and Administration: One 5 ml. teaspoonful or one tablet daily—or as directed by physician.

Important: Dispense liquid only in original bottle or an amber bottle. This product is light-sensitive. Never dispense in a flint, green, or blue bottle.

Trophite Liquid may be mixed with water, milk, or fruit or vegetable juices immediately before taking.

Store at controlled room temperature (59°–86°F).

Warning: Keep this and all medicines out of reach of children. In case of accidental overdose, contact a physician or poison control center immediately.

As with any drug, if you are pregnant or nursing a baby, seek the advice of a health professional before using this product.

TAMPER-RESISTANT PACKAGE FEATURE: Liquid—Sealed, imprinted bottle cap; do not use if broken. Tablets—Bottle has imprinted seal under cap; do not use if broken.

How Supplied: Liquid—4 fl. oz. (118 ml.) bottles. Tablets—bottles of 50.

Shown in Product Identification Section, page 416

The Mentholatum Company
1360 NIAGARA STREET BUFFALO, NY 14213

CALMOL 4® SUPPOSITORIES

Active Ingredient: Cocoa Butter 54.5%, Zinc Oxide 15.0%, also contains Cod Liver Oil.

Indications: For the temporary relief of itching associated with hemorrhoids, inflamed hemorrhoidal tissue or other anorectal disorders.

Actions: Cocoa butter and zinc oxide are protectants which act to prevent irritation of the anorectal area and water loss from the stratum corneum skin layer by forming a barrier on the skin. Protection of the perianal area from irritants such as fecal matter and air leads to a reduction in irritation and concomitant itching.

Warnings: If symptoms do not improve, do not use this product for more than 7 days and consult a physician. Do not exceed the recommended daily dosage except under the advice and supervision of a physician. If itching persists for more than 7 days, consult a physician. In case of bleeding consult a physician promptly. Keep this and all drugs out of the reach of children. In case of accidental ingestion, seek professional assistance or contact a Poison Control Center immediately.

Dosage and Administration: Adult dosage—insert one suppository after each bowel movement but do not exceed six applications in a 24 hour period, unless directed otherwise by physician. When practical to do so, wash the anorectal area with mild soap and warm water and rinse off all soap before application of this product. Remove Calmol 4 suppository from foil wrapper before inserting into rectum. Insert with gentle pressure, rounded end first.

How Supplied: Individually foil wrapped in boxes of 12 and 24.

FLETCHER'S CASTORIA FOR CHILDREN

Active Ingredients: Senna—equivalent to 6½% Alcohol—3½%

Indications: A natural vegetable laxative especially made for children. Mild, dependable, for use with children of all ages.

Warnings: Not to be used when abdominal pain, nausea, vomiting, or other symptoms of appendicitis are present. Habitual use of laxatives may result in dependence upon them. Keep this and all other medicine out of children's reach.

Directions: Shake well before using.

1–6 months	¼–½ Teaspoonful
7–12 months	½–1 Teaspoonful
1–5 years	1–2 Teaspoonfuls
6–12 years	2–3 Teaspoonfuls

How Supplied: 2½, 5 Oz. bottles

MEDI-QUIK AEROSOL SPRAY

Active Ingredients: Benzalkonium Chloride—0.13% w/w Lidocaine—2.0% w/w Camphor—0.2% w/w

Indications: Effective antiseptic/pain relieving skin wound cleanser. Helps prevent infection, and temporarily relieves pain and itching due to minor cuts, scrapes, scratches, sunburn, insect bites and minor burns.

Warnings: For external use only. Avoid spraying in eyes, mouth, and other sensitive areas. Not for use on wild or domestic animal bites. If you have animal bites consult your physician immediately. Puncture wounds should also be attended to by a physician. Do not use this product for more than seven days. If condition worsens or persists, see a physician. Do not bandage tightly. Do not use in large quantities, particularly over raw or blistered areas. Do not use on child under 2 yrs of age except under supervision of physician. Keep this and all drugs out of the reach of children. In case of accidental ingestion seek professional assistance or contact a poison center. Do not puncture or incinerate. Contents under pressure. Do not store at temperatures above 120°F. Use only as directed. Intentional misuse by deliberately concentrating and inhaling contents may be harmful or fatal.

Directions: Shake well. For adults and children 2 years of age and over: Apply to affected areas not more than four times daily. To spray or flush wound hold can upright 2–3 inches from surface and spray across wound. To aid in removing foreign particles dab wound with clean gauze saturated with product.

How Supplied: Aerosol 3-oz. can.

MENTHOLATUM DEEP HEATING® LOTION
Topical Analgesic

Active Ingredient: Methylsalicylate 20%, Menthol 6%.

Indications: For the temporary relief of minor arthritic and rheumatic pain. Also helps relieve muscle soreness and stiffness. Also for muscle tightness due to chest colds.

Actions: Acts as a counterirritant by stimulating cutaneous sensory receptors.

Warnings: For external use only. Keep this and all drugs out of the reach of children. In case of accidental ingestion, seek professional assistance or contact a Poison Control Center immediately. Use only as directed. If pain persists for more than 10 days, or redness is present, or in conditions affecting children under 12 years of age, consult a physician immediately. Discontinue use if excessive irritation of the skin develops. Avoid getting into the eyes or on mucous membranes.

Dosage and Administration: Massage on affected area until it is absorbed into the skin. Repeat as necessary.

Professional Labeling: Same as those under indications.

How Supplied: 2 oz. (safety cap) and 4 oz. bottles.

MENTHOLATUM DEEP HEATING® RUB
Topical Analgesic

Active Ingredient: Methylsalicylate 12.7%, Menthol 5.8%.

Indications: For the temporary relief of minor arthritic and rheumatic pain. Also helps relieve muscle soreness and stiffness. Also for muscle tightness due to chest colds.

Actions: Acts as a counterirritant by stimulating cutaneous sensory receptors.

Warnings: For external use only. Keep this and all drugs out of the reach of children. In case of accidental ingestion, seek professional assistance or contact a Poison Control Center immediately. Use only as directed. If pain persists for more than 10 days, or redness is present, or in conditions affecting children under 12 years of age, consult a physician immediately. Discontinue use if excessive irritation of the skin develops. Avoid getting into the eyes or on mucous membranes.

Dosage and Administration: Massage on affected area until it is absorbed into the skin. Repeat as necessary.

Professional Labeling: Same as those under indications.

How Supplied: 1¼, 3⅓ and 5 oz. aluminum tubes.

MENTHOLATUM® LIPBALM with SUNSCREEN
Lipbalm with sunscreen

Active Ingredient: Octyldimethyl PABA 8% in a petrolatum base. SPF 14.8.

Indications: Aids in the prevention and healing of winter chapped lips. Also prevents sunburned lips. Over exposure to sun may lead to lip cancer. Liberal and regular use over the years may reduce the sun's harmful effects.

Actions: Octyldimethyl paba is an effective sunscreen agent. Petrolatum is an effective skin moisturizing agent.

Warnings: For external use only. Avoid contact with the eyes. Discontinue use if signs of irritation or rash appear.

Dosage and Administration: For dry, chapped lips apply as needed. To help prevent dry, chapped sun or windburned lips, apply to lips before, during or following exposure to sun, wind, water and cold weather.

How Supplied: 4.5 gm. Lipsticks in regular, or Cherry, Strawberry and Lemon Ice flavors.

MENTHOLATUM® OINTMENT
Topical Analgesic, Skin protectant

Active Ingredient: Menthol 1.35%, Camphor 9% in a petrolatum base.

Indications: For the symptomatic relief of nasal congestion, bronchial mucous congestion, coughs, muscular tightness and muscular aches and pains due to cold. Also for chapped irritated skin, sunburn, scalds and insect bites.

Actions: Menthol and camphor are cutaneous sensory receptor depressants and thus produce a local analgesia. Petrolatum is an effective skin moisturizing agent.

Warnings: For conditions that persist or are accompanied by fever, see your doctor. For external use only. Do not place in mouth or nostrils. Keep this and all medicines out of the reach of children. In case of accidental ingestion, seek professional assistance or contact a poison control center immediately.

Dosage and Administration: To help relieve discomforts of head colds, chest colds, congestion, coughs, sore throat and that all-over "achy" feeling-rub Mentholatum Ointment on chest, throat and back. For most effective results, cover these areas with a warm cloth. Repeat as often as necessary. To help ease stuffy nose, place a dab of Mentholatum Ointment below each nostril. For skin soreness due to colds, sneezing or runny nose, spread a thin layer over irritated areas, lips and outside of nostrils. Also recommended for: chapped skin, sunburn, scalds, insect bites.

How Supplied: 1 and 3 oz. plastic jars and 1 oz. & ⅖ oz. tubes.

NYTILAX® TABLETS
(sennosides A and B)

Description: Each blue Nytilax Tablet contains 12 mg. of crystalline Sennosides A and B calcium salts (not U.S.P.), the most highly purified form available for these glycosides, derived from the Cassia Acutifolia plant and standardized by chemical rather than biological assay.

Actions and Uses: Indicated for relief of chronic or occasional functional constipation. Recent additional support has been given to the current theory that upon ingestion, the sugar glycosides Sennosides A and B are transported without chemical change through the alimentary canal to the colon, where they are hydrolyzed to their aglycone derivatives by the colonic flora leading to localized nerve plexus stimulation and peristalsis-induced defecation. The effect is gentle and predictable, with well-formed stools being produced, usualy within 8–10 hours. The high chemical purity of the Sennoside A and B calcium salts facilitates individualized dosage regulation and further minimizes the possibility of rare adverse reactions such as loose stools or abdominal discomfort. Sennosides A and B, as contained in Nytilax Tablets, have been found in numerous clinical studies to be highly effective for varieties of functional constipation: chronic, geriatric, drug-induced, pediatric and surgical-related, and in lower bowel x-ray preparative procedures.

Dosage and Administration:
Adults—Swallow 2 tablets with water at bedtime. In order to meet individual requirements, increase dose by 1 tablet or decrease by 1 tablet. Maximum dosage 3 tablets.
Children—Consult a physician.

Warnings: Do not take any laxative when abdominal pain, nausea or vomiting are present. Frequent or prolonged use of laxatives may result in dependence. As with any drug, if you are pregnant or nursing a baby, seek professional advice before using this product. Keep this and all drugs out of the reach of children. In case of accidental overdose seek professional assistance or contact a poison control center immediately.

How Supplied: Boxes of 12, 24 or 48 tablets. Each tablet is individually film wrapped.

RED CROSS TOOTHACHE MEDICATION
Toothache Drops

Active Ingredient: Eugenol 85%.

Indications: For the temporary relief of discomfort of a tooth with throbbing, persistent pain until a dentist can be seen.

Actions: Eugenol is an effective dental analgesic acting on tooth nerve endings to eliminate pain.

Warnings: Avoid touching tissue other than the tooth cavity. Keep this and all drugs out of reach of children.

Dosage and Administration: Rinse with water to remove food particles. Use tweezers to moisten pellet and place in cavity.

How Supplied: As a kit containing ⅛ fl. oz. (3.7 ml) bottle of drops, a pair of tweezers and a box of cotton pellets.

RESICORT® CREAM
Hydrocortisone Cream

Active Ingredient: Hydrocortisone acetate 0.5% in a cream base.

Indications: For the temporary relief of minor skin irritations, itching and rashes due to eczema, dermatitis, insect bites, poison ivy, poison oak, poison sumac, soaps, detergents, cosmetics, jewelry, and itchy genital and anal areas.

Actions: Hydrocortisone acetate is a topical anti-inflamatory and an antipruritic.

Warnings: For external use only. Avoid contact with eyes. If condition worsens or if symptoms persist more than 7 days discontinue use and consult a physician. Do not use on children under 2 years except under the advice of a physi-

Continued on next page

Mentholatum—Cont.

cian. Keep this and all drugs out of the reach of children.

Dosage and Administration: For adults and children 2 years and older, apply to affected area 3 to 4 times daily.

How Supplied: ½ oz. tubes.

Mericon Industries, Inc.
8819 N. PIONEER RD.
PEORIA, IL 61615

DELACORT
(hydrocortisone USP ½%)

Active Ingredient: Hydrocortisone USP ½%.

Indications: For the temporary relief of minor skin irritations, itching and rashes due to eczema, dermatitis, insect bites, poison ivy, poison oak, poison sumac, soaps; detergents, cosmetics, and jewelry, and for itchy genital and anal areas.

Warnings: For external use only. Avoid contact with the eyes. If condition worsens, or if symptoms persist for more than 7 days discontinue use (of this product) and consult a physician. Do not use on children 2 years of age except under the advice and supervision of a physician.

Precaution: KEEP OUT OF REACH OF CHILDREN.

Dosage and Administration: For adults and children 2 years of age and older: Apply to affected area 3 or 4 times daily.

How Supplied: 2 oz. and 4 oz. squeeze bottle.

ORAZINC®
(zinc sulfate)

Active Ingredient: Zinc Sulfate U.S.P. 220 mg. and 110 mg. Capsules.

Indications: A Dietary Supplement containing Zinc.

Warnings: Should be taken with milk or meals to alleviate possible gastric distress.

Symptoms and Treatment of Oral Overdosage: Nausea, mild diarrhea or rash—to control, reduce dosage or discontinue.

Dosage and Administration: One capsule daily or as recommended by physician.

How Supplied: Bottles of 100 and 1000 Capsules each.

ORAZINC® LOZENGES
(zinc gluconate)

Active Ingredient: Zinc (Zinc Gluconate) 10 mg. Contains no starch, no artificial colors, flavors or preservatives. Sweetened with sorbitol and fructose.

Directions: As a dietary supplement, slowly dissolve one or two lozenges in mouth. To alleviate possible gastric distress, do not take on empty stomach.

Warnings: Keep this and all medications out of the reach of children.

How Supplied: Bottles of 100 Lozenges (NDC 0394-0495-02).

Merrell Dow Pharmaceuticals Inc.
Subsidiary of The Dow Chemical Company
10123 ALLIANCE ROAD
CINCINNATI, OH 45242-9553

CĒPACOL® Mouthwash/Gargle

Description:
Ceepryn® (cetylpyridinium
chloride)... 1:2000
Alcohol 14%
Phosphate buffers and aromatics
Also contains FD&C Yellow No. 5 (tartrazine) as a color additive.
Cēpacol is a soothing, pleasant tasting mouthwash/gargle. It has a low surface tension, approximately ½ that of water. This property is the basis of the spreading action in the oral cavity as well as its foaming action. Cēpacol leaves the mouth feeling fresh and clean and helps provide soothing, temporary relief of dryness and minor irritations.

Uses: Recommended as a mouthwash and gargle for daily oral care; as an aromatic mouth freshener to provide a clean feeling in the mouth; as a soothing, foaming rinse to freshen the mouth.
Used routinely before dental procedures, helps give patient confidence of not offending with mouth odor. Often employed as a foaming and refreshing rinse before, during, and after instrumentation and dental prophylaxis. Convenient as a mouth-freshening agent after taking dental impressions. Helpful in reducing the unpleasant taste and odor in the mouth following gingivectomy.
Used in hospitals as a mouthwash and gargle for daily oral care. Also used to refresh and soothe the mouth following emesis, inhalation therapy, and intubations, and for swabbing the mouths of patients incapable of personal care.

Warning: Keep out of reach of children.

Instructions For Use: Rinse vigorously after brushing or any time to freshen the mouth. Particularly useful after meals or before social engagements. Aromatic Cēpacol leaves the mouth feeling refreshingly clean.
Use full strength every two or three hours as a soothing, foaming gargle, or as directed by a physician or dentist. May also be mixed with warm water.

How Supplied:
12 oz, 18 oz, 24 oz, and 32 oz
4 oz Hospital Bedside Bottles (not for retail sale)

CĒPACOL® Throat Lozenges

Description:
Ceepryn® (cetylpyridinium
chloride)..1:1500
Benzyl alcohol 0.3%
Aromatics
Yellow mint-flavored hard candy base
Also contains FD&C Yellow No. 5 (tartrazine) as a color additive.
Cetylpyridinium chloride (Ceepryn) is a cationic quaternary ammonium compound. This is a surface-active agent which in aqueous solution has a surface tension lower than that of water.
Cetylpyridinium chloride in the concentration used in Cēpacol is non-irritating to tissues.

Indications: Cēpacol Lozenges stimulate salivation to help provide soothing temporary relief of dryness and minor irritation of mouth and throat and resulting cough.

Warning: Severe sore throat or sore throat accompanied by high fever or headache or nausea and vomiting, or any sore throat persisting more than two days may be serious. Consult a physician promptly. Persons with a high fever or persistent cough should not use this preparation unless directed by physician. Do not administer to children under 3 years of age unless directed by physician. Keep this and all medication out of children's reach. As with any drug, if you are pregnant or nursing a baby, seek the advice of a health professional before using this product.

Instructions For Use: May be used as needed. Allow to dissolve slowly in the mouth.

How Supplied:
Trade Package: 18 lozenges in 2 pocket packs of 9 each.
Professional Package: 648 lozenges in 72 blisters of 9 each.

CĒPACOL® Anesthetic Lozenges (Troches)

Description:
Ceepryn® (cetylpyridinium chloride)... 1:1500
Benzocaine
Aromatics
Green citrus-flavored hard candy base
Also contains FD&C Yellow No. 5 (tartrazine) as a color additive.
Cetylpyridinium chloride (Ceepryn) is a cationic quaternary ammonium compound, which is a surface-active agent. Aqueous solutions of cetylpyridinium chloride have a surface tension lower than that of water.
Cetylpyridinium chloride in the concentration used in Cēpacol is non-irritating to tissues.

Actions:
Anesthetic effect for pain relief
Stimulates salivation—Relieves dryness

Indications: *Sore Throat:* For fast, temporary relief of pain and discomfort due to minor sore throat. For temporary relief of pain and discomfort associated with tonsillitis and pharyngitis. *Mouth*

Irritations: For fast, temporary relief of pain and discomfort due to minor mouth irritations. For temporary relief of discomfort associated with stomatitis. For adjunctive, temporary relief of pain and discomfort following periodontal procedures and minor surgery of the mouth.

Warning: Severe sore throat or sore throat accompanied by high fever or headache or nausea and vomiting, or any sore throat persisting more than two days may be serious. Consult a physician promptly. Do not administer to children under 3 years of age unless directed by physician. Keep this and all medication out of children's reach. As with any drug, if you are pregnant or nursing a baby, seek the advice of a health professional before using this product.

Instructions For Use: May be used as needed. Allow to dissolve slowly in the mouth.

How Supplied:
Trade Package: 18 troches in 2 pocket packs of 9 each.
Professional Package: 324 troches in 36 blisters of 9 each.

CEPASTAT®
sore throat lozenges

Description:
Lozenges–cherry flavor
Cherry-flavored, sugar-free lozenges containing phenol 0.73% and menthol 0.12% in a sorbitol base.
Lozenges–regular flavor
Cooling sugar-free lozenges containing phenol (1.45%) and menthol (0.12%) in a sorbitol base flavored with eucalyptus oil.

Indications:
1. Sore throat:
   For prompt temporary relief of minor pain or discomfort associated with pharyngitis or tonsillitis or following tonsillectomy.
2. Sore mouth or gums:
   For prompt temporary relief of minor pain or discomfort associated with pericoronitis or periodontitis or with dental procedures such as extractions, gingivectomies, and other minor oral surgery.

Action:
Phenol is a recognized topical anesthetic. Menthol provides a cooling sensation to aid in symptomatic relief and adds to the lozenge effect in stimulating salivary flow.

Warning*:
Do not exceed recommended dosage. If soreness is severe, persists for more than 2 days, or is accompanied by high fever, headache, nausea or vomiting, consult your physician or dentist promptly. Do not give to children under 6 years unless directed by physician or dentist. Do not use for more than 10 days at a time. As with any drug, if you are pregnant or nursing a baby, seek the advice of a health professional before using this product.

KEEP OUT OF REACH OF CHILDREN.
Note to Diabetics*: Each lozenge contains approximately 2 grams of carbohydrate as sorbitol.

Instructions for Use:
Lozenges–cherry flavor
Adults and Children over 12:
   Dissolve 1 lozenge, followed by another if needed, every 2 hours. Do not exceed 18 lozenges per day.
Children 6 to 12 years of age:
   Dissolve (do not chew) 1 lozenge, followed by another if needed, every 3 hours. Do not exceed 10 lozenges per day.
Lozenges–regular flavor
Adults:
   Dissolve 1 lozenge in mouth every 2 hours. Do not exceed 9 lozenges per day.
Children 6 to 12 years of age:
   Dissolve 1 lozenge in mouth every 3 hours. Do not exceed 4 lozenges per day.

How Supplied:
Lozenges–cherry flavor
   Boxes of 18 lozenges as 2 pocket packs of 9 lozenges each. 648 lozenges in 72 blisters of 9 each.
Lozenges–regular flavor
   300 lozenges in 100 strips of 3 each
   Boxes of 18 lozenges as 2 pocket packs of 9 lozenges each. 648 lozenges in 72 blisters of 9 each.

*This section appears on the label for the consumer.

DELCID®

Description: Each teaspoonful (5 ml) contains a balanced combination of 600 mg aluminum hydroxide [Al (OH)$_3$] and 665 mg magnesium hydroxide [Mg (OH)$_2$]. The sodium content is not more than 15 mg per teaspoonful.

Actions: The balanced ratio of antacids provides reduction of gastric acidity and gives symptomatic comfort to the patient. The acid neutralizing capacity is 42 mEq for each 5 ml.

Indications: Delcid is used to relieve the symptoms of hyperacidity associated with peptic ulcer, gastritis, peptic esophagitis, gastric hyperacidity, and hiatal hernia, and to relieve the following symptoms: heartburn, sour stomach, or acid indigestion.

Warnings*: Do not take more than 6 teaspoonfuls in a 24-hour period or use the maximum dosage of this product for more than 2 weeks, except under the advice and supervision of a physician. May have laxative effect. Do not use this product except under the advice and supervision of a physician if you have kidney disease. As with any drug, if you are pregnant or nursing a baby, seek the advice of a health professional before using this product. Keep this and all drugs out of the reach of children. In case of accidental overdose, seek professional assistance or contact a poison control center immediately.

Drug Interaction Precautions*: Do not take this product if you are presently taking a prescription antibiotic drug containing any form of tetracycline.

Adverse Reactions: Miscellaneous reports include diarrhea, nausea, and vomiting.

Dosage and Administration: 1 teaspoonful, ½ to 1 hour after meals and at bedtime or as directed.
Directions*: Take as needed to alleviate symptoms: 1 teaspoonful every 4 hours, or as directed by a physician.

How Supplied: 8 fl oz plastic bottles

---

*This section appears on the label for the consumer.

KOLANTYL®

Description: Each teaspoonful (5 ml) of Kolantyl Gel contains:
   Aluminum hydroxide
   [Al (OH)$_3$] .... 150 mg
   Magnesium hydroxide
   [Mg(OH)$_2$] .... 150 mg
Each Kolantyl Wafer contains:
   Aluminum hydroxide .... 180 mg
   (supplied as dried aluminum hydroxide gel)
   Magnesium hydroxide .... 170 mg

Actions: The balanced ratio of antacids provides reduction of gastric acidity and gives symptomatic comfort to the patient. The acid neutralizing capacity is 10.5 mEq for each 5 ml of gel and 10.8 mEq for each wafer.

Indications: Kolantyl is used to relieve the symptoms of hyperacidity associated with peptic ulcer, gastritis, peptic esophagitis, gastric hyperacidity, and hiatal hernia, and to relieve the following symptoms: heartburn, sour stomach, or acid indigestion.

Warnings*: Do not take more than 12 teaspoonfuls of gel or 12 wafers in a 24-hour period or use the maximum dosage of this product for more than 2 weeks, except under the advice and supervision of a physician. May have laxative effect. Do not use this product except under the advice and supervision of a physician if you have kidney disease. As with any drug, if you are pregnant or nursing a baby, seek the advice of a health professional before using this product. Keep this and all drugs out of the reach of children. In case of accidental overdose, seek professional assistance or contact a poison control center immediately.

Drug Interaction Precautions*: Do not take this product if you are presently taking a prescription antibiotic drug containing any form of tetracycline.

Adverse Reactions: Miscellaneous reports include nausea and vomiting, abdominal discomfort, stomatitis, rash, dizziness, and diarrhea.

Continued on next page

Merrell Dow—Cont.

Dosage and Administration:
Kolantyl Gel: 1 to 4 teaspoonfuls ½ to 1 hour after meals and at bedtime or as directed. May be taken undiluted or mixed with milk or water, particularly if the patient is on a regular milk regimen. Kolantyl Wafers: 1 to 4 wafers ½ to 1 hour after meals and at bedtime or as directed. Wafers may be chewed or allowed to dissolve in the mouth.

Directions*:
Kolantyl Gel—Take as needed to alleviate symptoms: 1 to 4 teaspoonfuls every 4 hours, or as directed by a physician.
Kolantyl Wafers—Take as needed to alleviate symptoms: 1 to 4 wafers every 4 hours, or as directed by a physician. Wafers may be chewed or allowed to dissolve in the mouth.

How Supplied:
Kolantyl Gel: 12 oz bottles
Kolantyl Wafers: boxes of 36 wafers, sealed in 6 blister packs of 6 wafers each.

*This section appears on the label for the consumer.

NOVAHISTINE® COUGH & COLD FORMULA
Antitussive-Decongestant-
Antihistamine
Liquid

Description: Each 5 ml. teaspoonful of NOVAHISTINE COUGH & COLD FORMULA contains dextromethorphan hydrobromide, 10 mg., pseudoephedrine hydrochloride, 30 mg., and chlorpheniramine maleate, 2 mg. The formulation also contains alcohol, 5%.

Actions: Dextromethorphan suppresses the cough reflex by a direct effect on the cough center in the medulla of the brain. Although it is chemically related to morphine, it produces no analgesia or addiction. Its antitussive activity is about equal to that of codeine.
Pseudoephedrine is an orally effective nasal decongestant. Pseudoephedrine is a sympathomimetic amine with peripheral effects similar to epinephrine and central effects similar to, but less intense than, amphetamines. It has the potential for excitatory side-effects. At the recommended oral dosage, pseudoephedrine has little or no pressor effect in normotensive adults. Patients have not been reported to experience the rebound congestion sometimes experienced with frequent, repeated use of topical decongestants.
Chlorpheniramine is an antihistaminic drug which possesses anticholinergic and sedative effects. It is considered one of the most effective and least toxic of the histamine antagonists. Chlorpheniramine antagonizes many of the pharmacologic actions of histamine. It prevents released histamine from dilating capillaries and causing edema of the respiratory mucosa.

Indications: For the relief of exhausting, nonproductive cough and nasal congestion associated, for example, with the common cold, acute upper respiratory infections, sinusitis, and hay fever or upper respiratory allergies.

Contraindications: NOVAHISTINE COUGH & COLD FORMULA is contraindicated in persistent or chronic cough such as occurs with smoking, asthma, or emphysema, or when cough is accompanied by excessive secretions, except on advice of a physician. It is also contraindicated in patients with narrow-angle glaucoma, urinary retention, peptic ulcer, or during an asthmatic attack, patients with severe hypertension, severe coronary artery disease, and patients on MAO inhibitor therapy.

Nursing Mothers: Pseudoephedrine is contraindicated in nursing mothers because of the higher than usual risk for infants from sympathomimetic amines.

Hypersensitivity: This drug is contraindicated in patients with hypersensitivity or idiosyncrasy to antitussives, sympathomimetic amines or antihistamines. Patient idiosyncrasy to adrenergic agents may be manifested by insomnia, dizziness, weakness, tremor or arrhythmias.

Warnings: Use judiciously and sparingly in patients with hypertension, diabetes mellitus, ischemic heart disease, increased intraocular pressure, hyperthyroidism, or prostatic hypertrophy. Sympathomimetics may produce central nervous system stimulation and convulsions or cardiovascular collapse with accompanying hypotension.
Do not exceed recommended dosage.
Use in Pregnancy: The safety of pseudoephedrine for use during pregnancy has not been established.
Use in Elderly: The elderly (60 years and older) are more likely to have adverse reactions to sympathomimetics. Overdosage of sympathomimetics in this age group may cause hallucinations, convulsions, CNS depression, and death. Antihistamines may cause excitability, especially in children. If cough persists for more than 1 week, tends to recur, or is accompanied by high fever, rash or persistent headache, consult a physician.

Precautions: Drugs containing pseudoephedrine should be used with caution in patients with diabetes, hypertension, cardiovascular disease and hyperreactivity to ephedrine. The antihistamine agent may cause drowsiness and ambulatory patients who operate machinery or motor vehicles should be cautioned accordingly.

Adverse Reactions: These occur infrequently with usual doses. When they occur, adverse reactions may include nausea and dizziness, gastrointestinal upset or vomiting.
Because of the pseudoephedrine in NOVAHISTINE COUGH & COLD FORMULA, hyperreactive individuals may display ephedrine-like reactions such as tachycardia, palpitations, headache, dizziness or nausea. Sympathomimetic drugs have been associated with certain untoward reactions including fear, anxiety, tenseness, restlessness, tremor, weakness, pallor, respiratory difficulty, dysuria, insomnia, hallucinations, convulsions, CNS depression, arrhythmias and cardiovascular collapse with hypotension.
Patients may experience mild sedation. Possible side effects from the antihistamine may include dry mouth, dizziness, weakness, anorexia, nausea, vomiting, headache, nervousness, polyuria, heartburn, diplopia, dysuria and, very rarely, dermatitis.

Drug Interactions: MAO inhibitors and beta adrenergic blockers increase the effects of pseudoephedrine (sympathomimetics). Sympathomimetics may reduce the antihypertensive effects of methyldopa, mecamylamine, reserpine and veratrum alkaloids.
Antihistamines have been shown to enhance one or more of the effects of tricyclic antidepressants, barbiturates, alcohol and other central nervous system depressants.

Dosage and Administration: Adults and children 12 years or older, 2 teaspoonfuls every 4 to 6 hours. Children 6 to under 12 years, 1 teaspoonful every 4 to 6 hours. Children 2 to under 6 years, ½ teaspoonful every 4 to 6 hours. Not more than 4 doses in 24 hours. For children under 2 years of age, at the discretion of the physician.

Note: NOVAHISTINE COUGH & COLD FORMULA does not require a prescription. The package label has dosage instructions as follows: Adults and children 12 years or older, 2 teaspoonfuls every 4 to 6 hours. Children 6 to under 12 years, 1 teaspoonful every 4 to 6 hours. Not more than 4 doses in 24 hours. For children under 6 years of age give only as directed by a physician.

How Supplied: In 4 fluid ounce bottles and 8 fluid ounce bottles.

NOVAHISTINE® DMX
Cough/Cold Formula &
Decongestant

Description: Each 5 ml teaspoonful of NOVAHISTINE DMX contains: dextromethorphan hydrobromide, 10 mg, pseudoephedrine hydrochloride, 30 mg, and guaifenesin, 100 mg. Dextromethorphan, a synthetic non-narcotic antitussive, is the dextrorotatory isomer of 3-methoxy-N-methylmorphinan. Pseudoephedrine hydrochloride is the salt of a pharmacologically active stereoisomer of ephedrine (1-phenyl-2-methylamino-1-propanol). The formulation also contains alcohol, 10%.

Actions: Dextromethorphan suppresses the cough reflex by a direct effect on the cough center in the medulla of the brain. Although it is chemically related to morphine, it produces no analgesia or addiction. Its antitussive activity is about equal to that of codeine.
Pseudoephedrine hydrochloride is an orally effective nasal decongestant. Pseudoephedrine is a sympathomimetic amine with peripheral effects similar to

epinephrine and central effects similar to, but less intense than, amphetamines. Therefore, it has the potential for excitatory side effects. Pseudoephedrine at the recommended oral dosage has little or no pressor effect in normotensive adults. Patients taking pseudoephedrine orally have not been reported to experience the rebound congestion sometimes experienced with frequent, repeated use of topical decongestants. Pseudoephedrine is not known to produce drowsiness.

Guaifenesin acts as an expectorant by increasing respiratory tract fluid which reduces the viscosity of tenacious secretions, thus making expectoration easier.

Indications: NOVAHISTINE DMX is indicated when exhausting, nonproductive cough accompanies respiratory tract congestion. It is useful in the symptomatic relief of upper respiratory congestion associated with the common cold, influenza, bronchitis, and sinusitis.

Contraindications: Sympathomimetic amines are contraindicated in patients with severe hypertension, severe coronary artery disease, and in patients on MAO inhibitor therapy. Patient idiosyncrasy to adrenergic agents may be manifested by insomnia, dizziness, weakness, tremor or arrhythmias.

Nursing mothers: Pseudoephedrine is contraindicated in nursing mothers because of the higher than usual risk for infants from sympathomimetic amines.

Hypersensitivity: This drug is contraindicated in patients with hypersensitivity or idiosyncrasy to sympathomimetic amines, dextromethorphan, or to other formula ingredients.

Warnings: Sympathomimetic amines should be used judiciously and sparingly in patients with hypertension, diabetes mellitus, ischemic heart disease, increased intraocular pressure, hyperthyroidism and prostatic hypertrophy. Sympathomimetics may produce central nervous system stimulation with convulsions or cardiovascular collapse with accompanying hypotension. See, however, Contraindications.

Use in pregnancy: The safety of pseudoephedrine for use during pregnancy has not been established.

Use in elderly: The elderly (60 years and older) are more likely to have adverse reactions to sympathomimetics. Overdosage of sympathomimetics in this age group may cause hallucinations, convulsions, CNS depression, and death.

Precautions: Pseudoephedrine should be used with caution in patients with diabetes, hypertension, cardiovascular disease and hyperreactivity to ephedrine. See, however, Contraindications.

Adverse Reactions: Adverse reactions occur infrequently with usual oral doses of NOVAHISTINE DMX. When they occur, adverse reactions may include gastrointestinal upset and nausea. Because of the pseudoephedrine in NOVAHISTINE DMX, hyperreactive individuals may display ephedrine-like

reactions such as tachycardia, palpitations, headache, dizziness or nausea. Sympathomimetic drugs have been associated with certain untoward reactions including fear, anxiety, tenseness, restlessness, tremor, weakness, pallor, respiratory difficulty, dysuria, insomnia, hallucinations, convulsions, CNS depression, arrhythmias, and cardiovascular collapse with hypotension.

Note: Guaifenesin interferes with the colorimetric determination of 5-hydroxyindoleacetic acid (5-HIAA) and vanillylmandelic acid (VMA).

Drug Interactions: MAO inhibitors and beta adrenergic blockers increase the effects of pseudoephedrine (sympathomimetics). Sympathomimetics may reduce the antihypertensive effects of methyldopa, mecamylamine, reserpine, and veratrum alkaloids.

Dosage: Adults and older children, two teaspoonfuls, 3 to 4 times a day. Children 6 to 12 years of age, one teaspoonful, 3 to 4 times a day. Children 2 to 5 years of age, one-half teaspoonful, 3 to 4 times a day. May be given to children under 2 at the discretion of the physician.

Note: NOVAHISTINE DMX does not require a prescription. The package label has dosage instructions as follows:

Adults, and children over 12 years of age, two teaspoonfuls, every 4 to 6 hours. Children 6 to 12 years of age, one teaspoonful, every 4 to 6 hours. Children 2 to 5 years of age, one-half teaspoonful, every 4 to 6 hours. Not more than four doses every 24 hours. For children under 2 years of age, give only as directed by a physician.

How Supplied: As a red syrup in 4 fluid ounce bottles and 8 fluid ounce bottles.

NOVAHISTINE® Elixir
Cold & Hay Fever Formula

Description: Each 5 ml teaspoonful of elixir contains: phenylephrine hydrochloride, 5 mg, chlorpheniramine maleate, 2 mg, and alcohol, 5%. Although considered sugar-free, each 5 ml contains 2.6 grams of carbohydrates.

Actions: Phenylephrine is a nasal decongestant. Its effects are similar to epinephrine, but it is less potent on a weight basis, and has a longer duration of action. Phenylephrine produces peripheral effects similar to epinephrine, but has little or no central nervous system stimulation. After oral administration, nasal decongestion may occur within 15 or 20 minutes and persist for 2 to 4 hours.

Chlorpheniramine maleate, an antihistaminic effective for the symptomatic relief of allergic rhinitis, possesses mild anticholinergic and sedative effects. Chlorpheniramine antagonizes many of the pharmacologic actions of histamine. It prevents released histamine from dilating capillaries and causing edema of the respiratory mucosa.

Indications: For the temporary relief of nasal congestion and eustachian tube

congestion associated with the common cold, sinusitis, and hay fever (allergic rhinitis). Also provides temporary relief of runny nose, sneezing, itching of nose or throat, and itchy and watery eyes as may occur in hay fever (allergic rhinitis). May be given concomitantly, when indicated, with analgesics and antibiotics.

Contraindications: Sympathomimetic amines are contraindicated in patients with severe hypertension, severe coronary artery disease, in patients on MAO inhibitor therapy, and in nursing mothers.

Antihistamines are contraindicated in patients with narrow-angle glaucoma, urinary retention, peptic ulcer, during an asthmatic attack, and in patients receiving MAO inhibitors.

NOVAHISTINE Elixir is also contraindicated in patients with hypersensitivity or idiosyncrasy to sympathomimetic amines or antihistamines.

Warnings: If sympathomimetic amines are used in patients with hypertension, diabetes mellitus, ischemic heart disease, increased intraocular pressure, hyperthyroidism, or prostatic hypertrophy, judicious caution should be exercised. The elderly (60 years and older) are more likely to have adverse reactions to sympathomimetics. Safety for use during pregnancy has not been established. Antihistamines may cause excitability, especially in children.

At dosages higher than the recommended dose, nervousness, dizziness, or sleeplessness may occur.

Precautions: Caution should be exercised if used in patients with high blood pressure, heart disease, diabetes or thyroid disease. The antihistamine may cause drowsiness, and ambulatory patients who operate machinery or motor vehicles should be cautioned accordingly.

Adverse Reactions: Drugs containing sympathomimetic amines have been associated with certain untoward reactions, including fear, anxiety, tenseness, restlessness, tremor, weakness, pallor, respiratory difficulty, dysuria, insomnia, hallucinations, convulsions, CNS depression, arrhythmias, and cardiovascular collapse with hypotension. Individuals hyperreactive to phenylephrine may display ephedrine-like reactions such as tachycardia, palpitation, headache, dizziness, or nausea.

Phenylephrine is considered safe and relatively free of unpleasant side effects when taken at recommended dosage. Patients sensitive to antihistamine drugs may experience mild sedation. Other side effects from antihistamines may include dry mouth, dizziness, weakness, anorexia, nausea, vomiting, headache, nervousness, polyuria, heartburn, diplopia, dysuria, and, very rarely, dermatitis.

Drug Interactions: MAO inhibitors and beta adrenergic blockers increase the effects of sympathomimetics. Sympathomimetics may reduce the antihyper-

Continued on next page

Merrell Dow—Cont.

tensive effects of methyldopa, mecamylamine, reserpine and veratrum alkaloids. Antihistamines have been shown to enhance one or more of the effects of tricyclic antidepressants, barbiturates, alcohol, and other central nervous system depressants.

Dosage: Adults, 2 teaspoonfuls every 4 hours; children 6 to 12 years, 1 teaspoonful every 4 hours; children 2 to 5 years, ½ teaspoonful every 4 hours.
For children under 2 years, at the discretion of the physician.

Note: NOVAHISTINE Elixir does not require a prescription. The package label has dosage instructions as follows:
Adults, 2 teaspoonfuls every 4 hours; children 6 to 12 years, 1 teaspoonful every 4 hours. Not more than 6 doses in 24 hours. For children under 6 years, consult a physician.

How Supplied: NOVAHISTINE Elixir, as a green liquid in 4 fluid ounce bottles and 8 fluid ounce bottles.
Product Information as of August, 1983

SIMRON™

Description:
Each maroon, soft-gelatin Simron capsule contains:
Elemental iron ....10 mg
(supplied by 86 mg ferrous gluconate USP)
Sacagen™ (polysorbate 20)......400 mg

Actions: Ferrous gluconate provides a source of elemental iron that will prevent and correct iron deficiency and iron-deficiency anemia. Sacagen (polysorbate 20) is polyoxyethylene 20 sorbitan monolaurate. It is an amber-colored liquid intended to enhance iron absorption and, as a surfactant, aids in the prevention of constipation.

Indications: For the prevention and treatment of iron deficiency and iron-deficiency anemia.
Simron is unusually well tolerated in patients who cannot tolerate other oral iron preparations and in patients with gastrointestinal disease, including peptic ulcer and ulcerative colitis.
Simron is indicated in the treatment of iron-deficiency anemia of patients with a potential for upper gastrointestinal bleeding because it rarely produces black stools, which could mask evidence of bleeding. Simron is indicated in the treatment of iron-deficiency anemia of patients with ulcerative colitis because only small amounts of unabsorbed irritant iron salts are present in the stool. Simron is indicated in the prevention and treatment of iron deficiency and iron-deficiency anemia of pregnancy.

Contraindications: Simron is contraindicated in the treatment of patients with disease associated with increased iron storage (hemochromatosis).

Warnings: Simron should be stored out of the reach of children because of the possibility of iron intoxication from accidental overdosage. Individuals with normal iron balance should not chronically take iron.

Precautions: When anemia is diagnosed, the type of anemia should be established. When iron-deficiency anemia is diagnosed, the cause of the iron deficiency should be established.
Ferrous iron compounds taken by mouth can impair the absorption of tetracycline and tetracycline derivatives. Antacids given concomitantly with iron compounds will decrease the absorption of iron.

Adverse Reactions: The incidence of adverse gastrointestinal reactions is reduced with Simron. Gastric irritation, nausea, constipation, and diarrhea are rarely observed.

Dosage and Administration: For the prevention and treatment of iron deficiency and iron-deficiency anemia the recommended dose is 1 Simron capsule three times a day *between meals*. This supplies 30 mg elemental iron. It should be noted that in patients with continued blood loss it may be necessary to exceed the recommended dose of Simron to obtain optimum therapeutic effect.

Overdosage: As little as 1 gram of elemental iron ingested orally may be toxic. Onset of symptoms usually occurs approximately 30 minutes after ingestion. Initially, gastrointestinal symptoms predominate (vomiting, diarrhea, melena). Shock, dyspnea, lethargy, and coma may follow. Metabolic acidosis may then occur.
Standard measures used to treat acute iron intoxication may include the following: 1) induced vomiting, 2) gastric lavage with 1% sodium bicarbonate, 3) general supportive measures for the treatment of shock and acidosis. Deferoxamine mesylate (Desferal®) should be given intramuscularly for patients not in shock, and intravenously for patients in shock. The manufacturer's recommendations should be consulted for details of administration. Some authors recommend 8000 mg deferoxamine in 50 ml of water via nasogastric tube.

How Supplied: Bottles of 100 soft-gelatin capsules

SIMRON PLUS®

Description: Each maroon, soft-gelatin capsule contains:
Elemental iron ....10 mg
(supplied by 86 mg ferrous gluconate USP)
Ascorbic acid.....................................50 mg
(supplied as sodium ascorbate)
Pyridoxine hydrochloride..............1.0 mg
Folic acid ....0.1 mg
Vitamin B$_{12}$.................................3.33 mcg
(supplied as cyanocobalamin)

Actions: Ferrous gluconate provides a source of elemental iron that will prevent and correct iron deficiency and iron-deficiency anemia.

In addition, factors necessary for normal hematopoiesis are supplied: ascorbic acid (as sodium ascorbate), pyridoxine hydrochloride, folic acid, and vitamin B$_{12}$ (as cyanocobalamin).

Indications: For the prevention and treatment of iron deficiency and iron deficiency anemia or anemia due to decreased erythrocyte formation except pernicious anemia or anemias due to bone marrow deficiencies. Simron Plus is indicated in the prevention and treatment of iron deficiency and iron-deficiency anemia of pregnancy.

Contraindications: Simron Plus is contraindicated in the treatment of patients with disease associated with increased iron storage (hemochromatosis).

Warnings: Simron Plus should be stored out of the reach of children because of the possibility of iron intoxication from accidental overdosage. Individuals with normal iron balance should not chronically take iron. Folic acid alone is improper therapy in the treatment of pernicious anemia and other megaloblastic anemias where vitamin B$_{12}$ is deficient.

Precautions: When anemia is diagnosed, the type of anemia should be established. When iron-deficiency anemia is diagnosed, the cause of the iron deficiency should be established.
Ferrous iron compounds taken by mouth can impair the absorption of tetracycline and tetracycline derivatives. Antacids given concomitantly with iron compounds will decrease the absorption of iron. This preparation is not a reliable substitute for parenterally administered cyanocobalamin (vitamin B$_{12}$) in the management of pernicious anemia.
Parenteral cyanocobalamin should be used in patients receiving folic acid unless pernicious anemia has been ruled out, since folic acid may correct blood disorders of pernicious anemia while nervous system changes progress. Periodic examinations and laboratory studies of pernicious anemia patients are essential.

Adverse Reactions: The incidence of adverse gastrointestinal reactions is reduced with Simron Plus. Gastric irritations, nausea, constipation, and diarrhea are rarely observed. Allergic sensitization has been reported following both oral and parenteral administration of folic acid.

Dosage and Administration: The recommended dose of Simron Plus is 1 capsule three times a day between meals.

Overdosage: As little as 1 gram of elemental iron ingested orally may be toxic. Onset of symptoms usually occurs approximately 30 minutes after ingestion. Initially, gastrointestinal symptoms predominate (vomiting, diarrhea, melena). Shock, dyspnea, lethargy, and coma may follow. Metabolic acidosis may then occur.
Standard measures used to treat acute iron intoxication may include the following: 1) induced vomiting, 2) gastric lavage with 1% sodium bicarbonate, 3)

general supportive measures for the treatment of shock and acidosis. Deferoxamine mesylate (Desferal®) should be given intramuscularly for patients not in shock, and intravenously for patients in shock. The manufacturer's recommendations should be consulted for details of administration. Some authors recommend 8000 mg deferoxamine in 50 ml of water via nasogastric tube.

How Supplied: Bottles of 100 soft-gelatin capsules

Merrick Medicine Company
P. O. BOX 1489 (76703)
501-503 S. 8TH STREET (76706)
WACO, TX

PERCY® MEDICINE
For relief of simple diarrhea and excess acid conditions of the stomach.

Active Ingredients: The active ingredients in an aqueous solution of 10 ml adult dose are as follows:
Bismuth Subnitrate NF .... 959.0 mg.
Calcium Hydroxide USP .... 21.9 mg.
The solution contains 5% alcohol, used as a preservative.

Indications: An antacid-astringent for simple diarrhea and for temporary relief of gastric discomfort due to overeating or other dietary indiscretions.

Drug Interaction Precautions: No known drug interaction.

Dosage and Directions For Use: Shake well before using. Administer orally 3 or 4 times daily as required. Vary dosage according to age. For use in infants and children under 6 years of age, consult your physician:

AGE BY YEARS	DOSAGE
6 to 12	1 to 1½ teaspoonfuls
12 to 18	1 to 2 teaspoonfuls
Over 18 and adults	2 teaspoonfuls

Normally, the clear liquid portion of this product (before shaking) is a light lemon color with a sweet palatable flavor. After a long period of time, the color may darken and flavor change. If the product is found to have lost its sweet agreeable flavor and light color, use is not recommended. PERCY MEDICINE may cause stool to darken temporarily.

Warning: Do not use for more than 2 days or in the presence of high fever or in infants or children under 6 years of age unless directed by a physician.
As with any drug, if you are pregnant or nursing a baby, seek professional advice before using this product.

Professional Labeling: Same as those outlined under indications.

How Supplied: Available only in 3 fl. oz. glass bottle encased in an outer carton (NDC 0322-2222-03), (UPC 0322-2222-03).

Shown in Product Identification Section, page 417

Miles Laboratories, Inc.
P. O. BOX 340
ELKHART, IN 46515

ALKA-MINTS® Chewable Antacid

Active Ingredient: Each ALKA-MINTS Chewable Antacid tablet contains calcium carbonate 850 mg. Each tablet contains less than .5 mg per tablet, and is dietarily sodium free.

Indications: ALKA-MINTS is an antacid for occasional use for relief of acid indigestion, heartburn and sour stomach.

Actions: ALKA-MINTS has a natural, clean, spearmint taste that leaves the mouth feeling refreshed. Measured by the in-vitro standard established by the Food and Drug Administration, one ALKA-MINTS tablet neutralizes 15.9 mEq of acid.

Warnings: Do not take more than 9 tablets in a 24 hour period, or use the maximum dosage of this product for more than 2 weeks, except under the advice and supervision of a physician. May cause constipation. As with any drug, if you are pregnant or nursing a baby, seek the advice of a health professional before using this product. Keep this and all drugs out of the reach of children.

Dosage and Administration: Chew 1 tablet every 2 hours or as directed by a physician.

How Supplied: Cartons of 30's and 60's. Each carton contains convenient pocket-sized packs with individually sealed tablets so ALKA-MINTS stay fresh wherever you go.

Product Identification Mark:
ALKA-MINTS embossed on each tablet.
Shown in Product Identification Section, page 417

ALKA-SELTZER® Effervescent Pain Reliever & Antacid With Specially Buffered Aspirin

Active Ingredient: Each tablet contains: aspirin 324 mg., heat treated sodium bicarbonate 1916 mg., citric acid 1000 mg. ALKA-SELTZER® in water contains principally the antacid sodium citrate and the analgesic sodium acetylsalicylate. Buffered pH is between 6 and 7.

Indications: ALKA-SELTZER® Effervescent Pain Reliever & Antacid is an analgesic and an antacid and is indicated for relief of sour stomach, acid indigestion or heartburn with headache or body aches and pains. Also for fast relief of upset stomach with headache from overindulgence in food and drink—especially recommended for taking before bed and again on arising. Effective for pain relief alone: headache or body and muscular aches and pains.

Actions: When the ALKA-SELTZER® Effervescent Pain Reliever & Antacid tablet is dissolved in water, the acetylsalicylate ion differs from acetylsalicylic acid chemically, physically and pharmacologically. Being fat insoluble, it is not absorbed by the gastric mucosal cells. Studies and observations in animals and man including radiochrome determinations of fecal blood loss, measurement of ion fluxes and direct visualization with gastrocamera, have shown that, as contrasted with acetylsalicylic acid, the acetylsalicylate ion delivered in the solution does not alter gastric mucosal permeability to permit back-diffusion of hydrogen ion, and gastric damage and acute gastric mucosal lesions are therefore not seen after administration of the product. ALKA-SELTZER® Effervescent Pain Reliever & Antacid has the capacity to neutralize gastric hydrochloric acid quickly and effectively. In-vitro, 154 ml. of 0.1 N hydrochloric acid are required to decrease the pH of one tablet of ALKA-SELTZER® Effervescent Pain Reliever & Antacid in solution to 4.0. Measured against the in vitro standard established by the Food and Drug Administration one tablet neutralizes 17.2 mEq of acid. In vivo, the antacid activity of two ALKA-SELTZER® Effervescent Pain Reliever & Antacid tablets is comparable to that of 10 ml. of milk of magnesia. ALKA-SELTZER® Effervescent Pain Reliever & Antacid is able to resist pH changes caused by the continuing secretion of acid in the normal individual and to maintain an elevated pH until emptying occurs.
ALKA-SELTZER® Effervescent Pain Reliever & Antacid provides highly water soluble acetylsalicylate ions which are fat insoluble. Acetylsalicylate ions are not absorbed from the stomach. They empty from the stomach and thereby become available for absorption from the duodenum. Thus, fast drug absorption and high plasma acetylsalicylate levels are achieved. Plasma levels of salicylate following the administration of ALKA-SELTZER® Effervescent Pain Reliever & Antacid solution (acetylsalicylate ion equivalent to 648 mg. acetylsalicylic acid) can reach 29 mg./liter in 10 minutes and rise to peak levels as high as 55 mg./liter within 30 minutes.

Warnings: Except under the advice and supervision of a physician, do not take more than, Adults: 8 tablets in a 24 hour period. (60 years of age or older: 4 tablets in a 24 hour period), Children (6–12), 4 tablets in a 24 hour period, (3–5), 2 tablets in a 24 hour period, or use the maximum dosage for more than 10 days (5 days for children). Do not use if you are allergic to aspirin or have asthma, if you have a coagulation (bleeding) disease, or if you are on a sodium restricted diet. Each tablet contains 554 mg. of sodium. As with any drug, if you are pregnant or nursing a baby, seek the advice of a health professional before using this product.
Keep this and all drugs out of the reach of children.

Continued on next page

Miles—Cont.

Dosage and Administration:
ALKA-SELTZER® Effervescent Pain Reliever and Antacid is taken in solution, approximately three ounces of water per tablet is sufficient.
Adults: 2 tablets every 4 hours. Children: (6–12) 1 tablet, (3–5) ½ tablet, every 4–6 hours; children under 3, as directed by a physician. CAUTION: If symptoms persist or recur frequently, or if you are under treatment for ulcer, consult your physician.

How Supplied: Tablets: in bottles of 8 and 26; foil sealed; box of 12; dispenser boxes of 36 tablets in 18 foil twin packs; 100 tablets in 50 foil twin packs; carton of 72 tablets in 36 foil twin packs. Product Identification Mark: "Alka-Seltzer" embossed on each tablet.
Shown in Product Identification Section, page 417

ALKA–SELTZER® Effervescent Antacid

Active Ingredient: Each tablet contains heat treated sodium bicarbonate 958 mg., citric acid 832 mg., potassium bicarbonate 312 mg. ALKA-SELTZER® Effervescent Antacid in water contains principally the antacids sodium citrate and potassium citrate.

Indications: ALKA-SELTZER® Effervescent Antacid is indicated for relief of acid indigestion, sour stomach or heartburn.

Actions: The ALKA-SELTZER® Effervescent Antacid solution provides quick and effective neutralization of gastric acid. Measured by the in vitro standard established by the Food and Drug Administration one tablet will neutralize 10.6 mEq of acid.

Warnings: Except under the advice and supervision of a physician, do not take more than: Adults: 8 tablets in a 24 hour period (60 years of age or older: 7 tablets in a 24 hour period), Children 4 tablets in a 24 hour period; or use the maximum dosage of this product for more than 2 weeks.
Do not use this product if you are on a sodium restricted diet. Each tablet contains 296 mg. of sodium.
Keep this and all drugs out of the reach of children. As with any drug, if you are pregnant or nursing a baby, seek the advice of a health professional before using this product.

Dosage and Administration:
ALKA-SELTZER® Effervescent Antacid is taken in solution; approximately 3 oz. of water per tablet is sufficient. Adults: one or two tablets every 4 hours as needed. Children: ½ the adult dosage.

How Supplied: Tablets: foil sealed, box of 12; dispenser boxes of 20 tablets in 10 foil twin packs; 36 tablets in 18 foil twin packs.
Shown in Product Identification Section, page 417

ALKA-SELTZER PLUS® Cold Medicine

Active Ingredients:
Each dry ALKA-SELTZER PLUS® Cold Tablet contains the following active ingredients: Phenylpropanolamine bitartrate 24 mg., chlorpheniramine maleate 2 mg., aspirin 324 mg. The product is dissolved in water prior to ingestion and the aspirin is converted into its soluble ionic form, sodium acetylsalicylate.

Indications: For relief of the symptoms of head colds, common flu, sinus congestion and hay fever.

Actions: Each tablet contains: A decongestant which helps restore free breathing, shrink swollen nasal tissue and relieve sinus congestion due to head colds or hay fever. An antihistamine which helps relieve the runny nose, sneezing, sniffles, itchy watering eyes that accompany colds or hay fever. Specially buffered aspirin which relieves headache, scratchy sore throat, general body aches and the feverish feeling of a cold and common flu.

Warnings: Do not use if you are allergic to aspirin or have asthma, or if you have a coagulation (bleeding) disease. If symptoms do not improve in 7 days or are accompanied by high fever or if fever persists for more than 3 days consult a physician before continuing use. Do not take this product if you have glaucoma or difficulty in urination due to enlargement of the prostate gland except under the advice and supervision of a physician. Avoid alcoholic beverages while taking this product.

Caution: Individuals with high blood pressure, diabetes, heart or thyroid disease or on a sodium restricted diet should use only as directed by a physician. Each tablet contains 515 mg. of sodium. Product may cause drowsiness: use caution if operating heavy machinery or driving a vehicle. Keep this and all drugs out of the reach of children. As with any drug, if you are pregnant or nursing a baby, seek the advice of a health professional before using this product.

Dosage and Administration:
ALKA-SELTZER PLUS® is taken in solution; approximately 3 ounces of water per tablet is sufficient. Adults: two tablets every 4 hours up to 8 tablets in 24 hours. Children (6–12): Half of adult dosage. Children under 6 years: Consult your physician.

How Supplied: Tablets: carton of 20 tablets in 10 foil twin packs; carton of 36 tablets in 18 foil twin packs.
Product Identification Mark:
"Alka-Seltzer Plus" embossed on each tablet.
Shown in Product Identification Section, page 417

BACTINE® Antiseptic·Anesthetic First Aid Spray

Active Ingredients: Benzalkonium Chloride 0.13% w/w, Lidocaine, HCl. 2.5% w/w, Alcohol 3.17% w/w*

* Alcohol is contained in aerosol spray but not in liquid spray. Aerosol ingredients are % w/w of concentrate.

Indications: Antiseptic/anesthetic for helping prevent infection, cleanse wounds, and for the temporary relief of pain and itching due to insect bites, minor burns, sunburn, minor cuts and minor skin irritations.

Warnings: (Aerosol Spray and Liquid Spray)
For external use only. Do not use in large quantities, particularly over raw surfaces or blistered areas. Avoid spraying in eyes, mouth, ears or on sensitive areas of the body. This product is not for use on wild or domestic animal bites. If you have an animal bite or puncture wound, consult your physician immediately. If condition worsens or if symptoms persist for more than 7 days, discontinue use of this product and consult a physician. Do not bandage tightly. Keep this and all drugs out of reach of children. In case of accidental ingestion, seek professional assistance or contact a Poison Control Center immediately.
(Aerosol Only): Contents under pressure. Do not puncture or incinerate. Do not store at temperature above 120° F. Use only as directed. Intentional misuse by deliberately concentrating and inhaling the contents can be harmful or fatal.

Dosage and Administration: For adults and children 2 years of age or older. For superficial skin wounds, cuts, scratches, scrapes, cleanse affected area thoroughly.

Directions: (Liquid) First Aid Spray
To spray, hold bottle upright 2 to 3 inches from injured area and squeeze repeatedly. To pour, hold bottle down. To aid in removing foreign particles, dab injured area with clean gauze saturated with product. For sunburn, minor burns, insect bites, and minor skin irritations, apply to affected area of skin for temporary relief. To spray, hold bottle upright 2 to 3 inches from affected area and squeeze repeatedly. To pour, hold bottle down. Product can be applied to affected area with clean gauze saturated with product.
(Aerosol First Aid Spray)
Shake well. For adults and children 2 years of age and older. For superficial skin wounds, cuts, scratches, scrapes, cleanse affected area thoroughly. Hold can upright 2 to 3 inches from injured area and spray until wet. To aid in removing foreign particles, dab injured area with clean gauze saturated with product. For sunburn, minor burns, insect bites, and minor skin irritations, hold can upright 2 to 3 inches from injured area and spray until wet. Product can be applied to affected area with clean gauze saturated with product.

How Supplied: 2 oz., 4 oz. liquid spray, 16 oz. liquid, 3 oz. aerosol.
Shown in Product Identification Section, page 417

BACTINE® Brand Hydrocortisone Skin Care Cream Antipruritic (Anti-Itch)

Active Ingredient: Hydrocortisone 0.5%

Indications: For the temporary relief of minor skin irritations, itching, and rashes due to eczema, dermatitis, insect bites, poison ivy, poison oak, poison sumac, soaps, detergents, cosmetics, and jewelry.

Warnings: For external use only. Avoid contact with the eyes. If condition worsens or if symptoms persist for more than seven days, discontinue use and consult a physician.
Do not use on children under 2 years of age except under the advice and supervision of a physician.
Keep this and all drugs out of the reach of children. In case of accidental ingestion, seek professional assistance or contact a Poison Control Center immediately.

Directions: For adults and children 2 years and older. Gently massage into affected skin area not more than 3 or 4 times daily.

How Supplied: ½ oz. plastic tube.
Shown in Product Identification Section, page 417

BIOCAL™ 250 mg Chewable Tablets Calcium Supplement

Each Tablet Contains: 625 mg of calcium carbonate, U.S.P. which provides: elemental calcium 250 mg.

Indication: Calcium supplementation

Description: BIOCAL™ 250 mg Tablets are round, white, pleasant-tasting mint flavored chewable tablets containing pure calcium carbonate. No sugar, salt, preservatives, or artificial colors added.

Directions: Four chewable tablets daily provide:

Elemental Calcium	For Adults and Children Over 4 % U.S. RDA
1000 mg	100%
	For Pregnant or Lactating Women
	77%

Chew 2 to 4 tablets daily or as recommended by a physician. Keep out of reach of children.

How Supplied: Bottles of 60 tablets in tamper-resistant package.
Shown in Product Identification Section, page 417

BIOCAL™ 500 mg Tablets Calcium Supplement

Each Tablet Contains: 1250 mg of calcium carbonate, U.S.P. which provides elemental calcium 500 mg.

Indications: Calcium supplementation.

BUGS BUNNY® Children's Chewable Vitamins Plus Iron (Sugar Free)
FLINTSTONES® Children's Chewable Vitamins Plus Iron
One Tablet Provides

Vitamins	Quantity	For Children 2 to 4 Years of Age	For Adults and Children over 4 Years of Age
		% of U.S. RDA	
Vitamin A	2500 I.U.	100	50
Vitamin D	400 I.U.	100	100
Vitamin E	15 I.U.	150	50
Vitamin C	60 mg.	150	100
Folic Acid	0.3 mg.	150	75
Thiamine	1.05 mg.	150	70
Riboflavin	1.20 mg.	150	70
Niacin	13.50 mg.	150	67
Vitamin B_6	1.05 mg.	150	52
Vitamin B_{12}	4.5 mcg.	150	75
Mineral:			
Iron (Elemental)	15 mg.	150	83

Description: BIOCAL™ 500 mg Tablets are white, capsule-shaped tablets containing pure calcium carbonate. No sugar, salt, preservatives, artificial colors or flavors added.

Directions: Two tablets daily provide:

Elemental Calcium	For Adults % U.S. RDA	For Pregnant or Lactating Women % U.S. RDA
1000 mg	100%	77%

Take one or two tablets daily or as recommended by a physician.
Keep out of reach of children.

How Supplied: Bottles of 60 tablets in tamper-resistant package.
Shown in Product Identification Section, page 417

BUGS BUNNY® Children's Chewable Vitamins (Sugar Free)
BUGS BUNNY® Children's Chewable Vitamins Plus Iron (Sugar Free)
FLINTSTONES® Children's Chewable Vitamins Plus Iron
FLINTSTONES® Children's Chewable Vitamins

Vitamin Ingredients: Each multivitamin supplement with iron contains the ingredients listed in the chart below. [See table above].
BUGS BUNNY® Children's Chewable Vitamins and FLINTSTONES® Children's Chewable Vitamins provide the same quantities of vitamins, but do not provide iron.

Indication: Dietary supplementation

Dosage and Administration: One chewable tablet daily. For adults and children two years and older; tablet must be chewed.

Precaution:
IRON SUPPLEMENTS ONLY.
Contains iron, which can be harmful in large doses. Close tightly and keep out of reach of children. In case of overdose contact a Poison Control Center immediately.

How Supplied: All four products are supplied in bottles of 60 and 100 with child resistant caps.
Shown in Product Identification Section, page 417

FLINTSTONES® With Extra C Children's Chewable Vitamins
BUGS BUNNY® With Extra C Children's Chewable Vitamins (Sugar Free)

Vitamin Ingredients: Each multivitamin supplement contains the ingredients listed in the chart below:
[See table bottom next page].

Indication: Dietary supplementation

Dosage and Administration: One chewable tablet daily for adults and children two years and older; tablet must be chewed.

How Supplied: Bottles of 60's & 100's with child resistant caps.

Shown in Product Identification Section, page 417

FLINTSTONES® COMPLETE With Iron, Calcium & Minerals Children's Chewable Vitamins
BUGS BUNNY® Children's Chewable Vitamins + Minerals With Iron and Calcium (Sugar Free)

Ingredients: Each supplement provides the ingredients listed in the chart below:
[See table top next page].

Indication: Dietary Supplementation

Dosage and Administration: One chewable tablet daily. For adults and children over 4 years of age; tablet must be chewed.

Precaution: Contains iron, which can be harmful in large doses. Close tightly and keep out of reach of children. In case of overdose, contact a physician or poison control center immediately.

How Supplied: Bottles of 60's with child resistant caps.
Shown in Product Identification Section, page 417

Continued on next page

Product Information

614

Miles—Cont.

MILES® Nervine
Nighttime Sleep–Aid

Active Ingredient: Each capsule-shaped tablet contains diphenhydramine HCl 25 mg.

Indications: Miles® Nervine helps you fall asleep and relieves occasional sleeplessness.

Actions: Antihistamines act on the central nervous system and produce drowsiness.

Warnings: Use only as directed. Do not give to children under 12 years of age. Take this product with caution if alcohol is being consumed. As with any drug, if you are pregnant or nursing a baby, seek the advice of a health professional before using this product. NOT FOR PROLONGED USE. If sleeplessness persists continuously for more than 2 weeks, consult your physician. Insomnia may be a symptom of serious underlying medical illness. Keep this and all drugs out of the reach of children. In case of accidental overdose, seek professional assistance or contact a Poison Control Center immediately. DO NOT TAKE THIS PRODUCT IF YOU HAVE ASTHMA, GLAUCOMA OR ENLARGEMENT OF THE PROSTATE GLAND EXCEPT UNDER THE ADVICE AND SUPERVISION OF A PHYSICIAN.

Dosage and Administration: Two tablets once daily at bedtime or as directed by a physician.

How Supplied: Blister pack 12's, bottles of 30's and 50's with child resistant caps.
Shown in Product Identification Section, page 418

ONE–A–DAY® Essential Vitamins
13 Essential Vitamins

Ingredients: One tablet daily of ONE-A-DAY® Essential provides:

Vitamins	Quantity	U.S. RDA
Vitamin A	5,000 I. U.	100
Vitamin C	60 mg.	100
Thiamine (B₁)	1.5 mg.	100
Riboflavin (B₂)	1.7 mg.	100
Niacin	20 mg.	100

BUGS BUNNY® With Extra C
Children's Chewable Vitamins
(Sugar Free)
FLINTSTONES® With Extra C
Children's Chewable Vitamins

One Tablet Provides

Vitamins	Quantity	% of U.S. RDA For Children 2 To 4 Years of Age	For Adults and Children Over 4 Years of Age
Vitamin A	2500 I.U.	100	50
Vitamin D	400 I.U.	100	100
Vitamin E	15 I.U.	150	50
Vitamin C	250 mg.	625	417
Folic Acid	0.3 mg.	150	75
Thiamine	1.05 mg.	150	70
Riboflavin	1.20 mg.	150	70
Niacin	13.50 mg.	150	67
Vitamin B₆	1.05 mg.	150	52
Vitamin B₁₂	4.5 mcg.	150	75

FLINTSTONES® COMPLETE Children's Chewable Vitamins
BUGS BUNNY® Children's Chewable Vitamins + Minerals
(Sugar Free)

One Tablet Provides:

Vitamins	Quantity	Percent U.S. RDA For Adults and Children Over 4 Years of Age
Vitamin A	5000 I.U.	100
Vitamin D	400 I.U.	100
Vitamin E	30 I.U.	100
Vitamin C	60 mg	100
Folic Acid	0.4 mg	100
Vitamin B-1 (Thiamine)	1.5 mg	100
Vitamin B-2 (Riboflavin)	1.7 mg	100
Niacin	20 mg	100
Vitamin B-6 (Pyridoxine)	2 mg	100
Vitamin B-12 (Cyanocobalamin)	6 mcg	100
Biotin	40 mcg	13
Pantothenic Acid	10 mg	100
Minerals		
Iron (Elemental)	18 mg	100
Calcium	100 mg	10
Phosphorus	100 mg	10
Iodine	150 mcg	100
Magnesium	20 mg	5
Manganese	2.5 mg	**
Zinc	15 mg	100

**No U.S. RDA established

Vitamin D	400 I.U.	100
Vitamin E	30 I.U.	100
Vitamin B₆	2 mg.	100
Folic Acid	0.4 mg.	100
Vitamin B₁₂	6 mcg.	100
Biotin	30 mcg.	10
Pantothenic Acid	10 mg.	100
Vitamin K	50 mcg.	*

Indication: Dietary supplementation.

Dosage and Administration: One tablet daily for adults and teens.

How Supplied: ONE-A-DAY® Essential, bottles of 60, 100, 250, and 365.
Shown in Product Identification Section, page 418

ONE–A–DAY® Maximum Formula
Vitamins and Minerals
Supplement for adults
The most complete leading brand.

Ingredients:
One tablet daily of ONE-A-DAY® Maximum Formula provides:

Vitamins	Quantity	% of U.S. RDA
Vitamin A	5,000 I.U.	100
Vitamin C	60 mg.	100
Thiamine (B₁)	1.5 mg.	100
Riboflavin (B₂)	1.7 mg.	100
Niacin	20 mg.	100
Vitamin D	400 I.U.	100
Vitamin E	30 I.U.	100
Vitamin B₆	2 mg.	100
Folic Acid	0.4 mg.	100
Vitamin B₁₂	6 mcg.	100
Biotin	30 mcg.	10
Pantothenic Acid	10 mg.	100
Vitamin K	50 mcg.	*

Minerals	Quantity	% of U.S. RDA
Iron (Elemental)	18 mg.	100
Calcium	129.6 mg.	13
Phosphorus	100 mg.	10
Iodine	150 mcg.	100
Magnesium	100 mg.	25
Copper	2 mg.	100
Zinc	15 mg.	100
Chromium	10 mcg.	*
Selenium	10 mcg.	*
Molybdenum	10 mcg.	*
Manganese	2.5 mg.	*
Potassium	37.5 mg.	*
Chloride	34 mg.	*

*No U.S. RDA established

Indication: Dietary supplementation.

Dosage and Administration: One tablet daily for adults.

Precaution: Contains iron, which can be harmful in large doses. Close tightly and keep out of reach of children. In case of overdose, contact a physician or Poison Control Center immediately.

How Supplied: Bottles of 30, 60, and 100 with child-resistant caps.
Shown in Product Identification Section, page 418

ONE-A-DAY® Plus Extra C
Vitamins. For adults and teens.

Vitamin ingredients: One tablet daily of ONE-A-DAY® Plus Extra C provides:

Vitamins	Quantity	% of U.S. RDA
Vitamin A	5,000 I.U.	100
Vitamin C	500 mg.	833
Thiamine (B$_1$)	1.5 mg.	100
Riboflavin (B$_2$)	1.7 mg.	100
Niacin	20 mg.	100
Vitamin D	400 I.U.	100
Vitamin E	30 I.U.	100
Vitamin B$_6$	2 mg.	100
Folic Acid	0.4 mg.	100
Vitamin B$_{12}$	6 mcg.	100
Biotin	30 mcg.	10
Pantothenic Acid	10 mg.	100
Vitamin K	50 mcg.	*

*No U.S. RDA established.

Indication: Dietary supplementation.

Dosage and Administration: One tablet daily.

How Supplied: Bottles of 60's with child resistant caps.

Shown in Product Identification Section, page 418

STRESSGARD®
High Potency B Complex and C plus A, D, E, Iron and Zinc
The most complete stress product.
Multivitamin/Multimineral Supplement For Adults

Ingredients:

Vitamins	Quantity	% of U.S. RDA
Vitamin A	5000 I.U.	100
Vitamin C	600 mg.	1000
Thiamine (B$_1$)	15 mg.	1000
Riboflavin (B$_2$)	10 mg.	588
Niacin	100 mg.	500
Vitamin D	400 I.U.	100
Vitamin E	30 I.U.	100
Vitamin B$_6$	5 mg.	250
Folic Acid	400 mcg.	100
Vitamin B$_{12}$	12 mcg.	200
Pantothenic Acid	20 mg.	200
Biotin	30 mcg.	10
Vitamin K	50 mcg.	*

Minerals	Quantity	% of U.S. RDA
Iron (Elemental)	18 mg.	100
Zinc	15 mg.	100
Copper	2 mg.	100

*No U.S. RDA established.

Indication: Dietary supplementation.

Dosage and Administration: Adults —one tablet daily with food.

Precaution: Contains iron, which can be harmful in large doses. Close tightly and keep out of reach of children. In case of overdose, contact a physician or Poison Control Center immediately.

How Supplied: Bottles of 60 with child-resistant caps.

Shown in Product Identification Section, page 418

WITHIN™ Advanced Multivitamin for women with calcium and extra iron.
Provides calcium and extra iron Plus the daily nutritional support of 13 essential vitamins.

Ingredients: One tablet daily of WITHIN™ provides:

Vitamins	Quantity	% of U.S. RDA
Vitamin A	5,000 I. U.	100
Vitamin C	60 mg.	100
Thiamine (B$_1$)	1.5 mg.	100
Riboflavin (B$_2$)	1.7 mg.	100
Niacin	20 mg.	100
Vitamin D	400 I.U.	100
Vitamin E	30 I.U.	100
Vitamin B$_6$	2 mg.	100
Folic Acid	0.4 mg.	100
Vitamin B$_{12}$	6 mcg.	100
Biotin	30 mcg.	10
Pantothenic Acid	10 mg.	100
Vitamin K	50 mcg.	*

Mineral	Quantity	% of U.S. RDA
Iron (Elemental)	27 mg.	150
Calcium (Elemental)	300 mg.	30

*No U.S. RDA established

Indication: Dietary supplementation.

Dosage and Administration: One tablet daily.

Precaution: Contains iron, which can be harmful in large doses. Close tightly and keep out of reach of children. In case of overdose, contact a physician or Poison Control Center immediately.

How Supplied: Bottles of 60 and 100 with child resistant caps.

Shown in Product Identification Section, page 418

Miller Pharmacal Group Inc.
245 W. ROOSEVELT ROAD
W. CHICAGO, IL 60185

AMINA-21

Description: Each capsule contains 600 mg of 21 free form amino acids without sugar, starch, yeast, wheat, soy, fillers, binders, colors or preservatives. AMINA-21 is composed of the following amino acids: L-Lysine, L-Leucine, L-Glutamine, L-Iso Leucine, L-Tryptophan, L-Alanine, L-Arginine, L-Threonine, L-Histidine, L-Aspartic Acid, L-Cystine, L-Tyrosine, L-Valine, L-Glycine, L-Glutamic Acid, L-Methionine, L-Phenylalanine, L-Citrulline, L-Proline, L-Serine, L-Hydroxyproline.

Indications: Effective as an adjunctive therapy in celiac disease, negative nitrogen balance, malabsorption syndrome, or other digestive disturbances. May also be useful for postoperative tissue and burn healing, catastrophic illness, and in alcoholic or psychiatric rehabilitation as an efficient source of nitrogen and protein.

Contraindications: AMINA-21 may be contraindicated in severe hepatic or renal impairment where blood ammonia levels should be closely monitored.

Dosage and Oral Administration: A protein supplement requires additional mineral, vitamin, fatty acid and carbohydrate intake sufficient to maintain homeostasis. Other dietary sources of calories are, therefore, essential. Recommended as a dietary supplement for adults and children 4 or more years of age, at 6 to 10 capsules per day, in divided doses, 20 minutes before meals, or as directed by a physician.

How Supplied: 600 mg Capsule: Bottles of 100 or 300. Powder: Bottles of 100 g and 250 g.

Muro Pharmaceutical, Inc.
890 EAST STREET
TEWKSBURY, MA 01876-9987

DUOLUBE®
Sterile Eye Lubricating Ointment

Contains: White petrolatum and mineral oil.

Supplied: 3.5 g tubes.

MURO TEARS®
Artificial Tears

Ingredients: Hydroxypropyl methylcellulose, dextran 40, sodium and potassium chlorides (total chlorides 0.85%). Also contains benzalkonium chloride 0.01% as a preservative, disodium EDTA and purified water. Buffered with sodium borate and boric acid.

How Supplied: 15 ml plastic dropper bottles.

MUROCEL™
(methylcellulose) 1%
Ocular Lubricant For Dry Eyes

How Supplied: 15 ml plastic dropper bottles.

SALINEX NASAL MIST AND DROPS
Buffered Isotonic Saline Solutions

Ingredients: Sodium Chloride 0.4%, polyethylene glycol, propylene glycol, hydroxypropyl methylcellulose, benzalkonium chloride 0.01% as preservative.

Indications: Rhinitis Medicamentosa and Rhinitis Sicca. For relief of nasal congestion associated with overuse of nasal sprays, drops and inhalers. To alleviate crusting due to nose bleeds; to compensate for nasal stuffiness and dryness due to lack of humidity.

Directions: Squeeze twice in each nostril as needed.

Continued on next page

Muro—Cont.

How Supplied: SPRAY: 50 ml plastic spray bottle. DROPS: 15 ml plastic dropper bottle.

National Magnesia Co., Inc.
70-32 83RD STREET
GLENDALE, NY 11385

CITROMA®
LOW SODIUM SUGAR FREE
FORMULA LEMON FLAVOR &
CHERRY FLAVOR MAGNESIUM
CITRATE ORAL SOLUTION
CITROMA®
REGULAR FORMULA LEMON
FLAVOR
MAGNESIUM CITRATE ORAL
SOLUTION

Description: Effervescent pasteurized liquid laxative. Also referred to as Citrate of Magnesia.

Active Ingredient: Each fluid ounce contains 1.745 grams of Magnesium Citrate.
LOW SODIUM SUGAR FREE FORMULAS CONTAIN ONLY 2 mg (0.085 mEq) OF SODIUM PER FL. OZ. AND ARE SUGAR FREE.

Indications: For the relief of constipation. Also for use as part of a bowel cleansing regimen in preparing the patients for surgery, or the colon for x-ray or endoscopic examination.

Actions: A mild saline laxative.

Warnings: Frequent and continued use may cause dependence upon laxatives. Do not use when abdominal pain, nausea or vomiting are present. As with any drug, if you are pregnant or nursing a baby, seek the advice of a health professional before using this product.

Dosage and Administration: Adult: one glassful (7 oz.) to one bottle (10 oz.). Children: (6 to 12 years): half a glassful. Infants: on the advice of a physician. Repeat dose if necessary.

How Supplied: Bottles of 10 fluid ounces.

IDENTIFICATION PROBLEM?
Consult the
Product Identifcation Section
where you'll find
products pictured
in full color.

Natra-Bio Company
2615 STANWELL DR.
CONCORD, CA 94520

NATRA-BIO
Homeopathic Medicines

Description: Natra-Bio homeopathic medicines are 100% natural. Each 1 Oz. dropper bottle contains approximately 50 doses of sublingual administration, 3–5 times daily. 20% alcohol solution.

Actions: Promotes relief by stimulating the body's defense mechanisms to accelerate the relief of symptoms naturally.

Contraindications: None.

Warnings: Can occasionally cause temporary worsening of symptoms. Homeopathically this is a positive sign that the body's defenses are working, however if excessive discomfort occurs reduce frequency.

The Natren Company, Inc.
10935 CAMARILLO STREET
NORTH HOLLYWOOD, CA 91602

BIFIDO FACTOR

Description: A highly viable, freeze-dried Bifidobacteria culture composed of milk solids, sweet dairy whey, and Bifidobacteria which naturally occurs in mother's milk. Completely free of preservatives, fillers, artificial colors and/or flavors.

Indications: Research indicates that Bifidobacteria inhibit the growth of many common pathogenic & toxin-producing bacteria including E. coli and Salmonella. Extremely effective for use in adults who are undergoing liver detoxification programs. Bifidobacteria is also indicated for use by pregnant women, lactating mothers, and children up to age 7. Establishes a vital, healthy intestinal microflora and stimulates the immune system.

Contraindications: In those adult patients with *milk fat intolerance,* administer in doses of ⅛ tsp. daily for first week. If no adverse reaction is observed, increase daily dose to ¼ tsp. for second week, until indicated dose has been reached. Where *lactose intolerance* is prevalent, product should be administered in same manner as above, until enzymatic build-up is in evidence. In cases of *casein intolerance,* use caution; patient might require support or other amino-acids in order to avoid possible adverse reactions.

Adverse Reactions: In extremely sensitive patients, initial reaction might be gas, bloating, diarrhea or constipation.

Dosage and Administration:
For infancy to age 7: ⅛ tsp. dissolved in 3 tsp. to 4 oz. of unchilled filtered or spring water, depending on age of child. Feed with dropper or water feeding in

case of infant, or in a glass with older children. Also to be administered before or after taking of meals or other solid foods.
For patients age 7 or above: GRAS—no known toxic levels.
Therapeutic dose: 6 grams (3 level tsp.) daily in up to 8 oz. of unchilled filtered or spring water. Drink immediately. *Always* consume Bifido Factor either 1 hour prior to or 3 hours following meal. *Preventive dose:* 1 gram (½ level tsp.) daily as described above.

How Supplied: Freeze-dried powder in 2½ oz. (150 cc.) or 4½ oz. (250 cc) bottle.
PERISHABLE—Must be kept refrigerated. DO NOT FREEZE.
Brochures, Technical data, Laboratory assays, and Research articles available at all times free of charge.

SUPERDOPHILUS™

Description: A selected, highly viable strain(s) of L. acidophilus especially formulated for adults. Highly potent freeze-dried culture of Lactobacillus acidophilus bacteria grown in a medium composed of milk solids, sweet dairy whey, and selected food extracts. Completely free of fillers, artificial colors, or artificial flavors.

Indications: Exhibits natural antibiotic activity against 11 common pathogens, stimulates the immune system, and maximizes nutrient absorption. Inhibits the growth of toxin-producing microorganisms in the colon. Extremely effective for use in detoxification programs, and against vaginitis and candidiasis.

Contraindications: In those patients with *milk fat intolerance,* administer in doses of ⅛ tsp. daily for first week. If no adverse reaction is observed, increase daily dosage to ¼ tsp. for second week, until indicated dosage has been reached. Where *lactose intolerance* is prevalent, product should also be administered in same manner as above, until enzymatic build-up is in evidence. In cases of *casein intolerance,* handle with caution; patient might need support of other amino acids to avoid possible adverse reaction.

Adverse reactions: In extremely sensitive patients, initial reactions might be gas, bloating, constipation, or diarrhea.

Dosage & Oral Administration: GRAS—no known toxic levels.
Therapeutic dose—6 grams (3 level tsp.) daily in up to 8 oz. of unchilled filtered or spring water. Drink immediately. *Always* consume Superdophilus either 1 hour prior to or 3 hours following meals. *Preventive dose*—1 gram (½ level tsp.) daily in same manner described above.

How Supplied: Freeze-dried powder in 2½ oz. (150 cc) bottle or 4½ oz. (250 cc) bottle.
PERISHABLE—Must be kept refrigerated. DO NOT FREEZE.
Brochures, Technical data, Laboratory assays, and Research articles available at all times free of charge.

Nature's Bounty, Inc.
105 ORVILLE DRIVE
BOHEMIA, NY 11716

ACEROLA "C" (100 mg.)
Each chewable tablet contains:
Vitamin C with
Rose Hips and Acerola ....100 mg.
Citrus Bioflavonoids
Complex .... 5 mg.

Supplied: Tablets, bottles of 100, 500.

ACIDOPHILUS
Aid in maintaining healthy balance of intestinal flora.
Each capsule contains live lactobacillus acidophilus

Supplied: Capsules, bottles of 100.

ALFALFA (500 mg.)

Supplied: Tablets, bottles of 100, 500.

B–1 (100 mg.)
Tablets, bottles of 100
B–1 (250 mg.)
Tablets, bottles of 100
B–1 (500 mg.)
Tablets, bottles of 100

B–2 (100 mg.)
Tablets, bottles of 100

B–6 (50 mg.)
Tablets, bottles of 100, 250
B–6 (100 mg.)
Tablets, bottles of 100, 250
B–6 (500 mg.)
Tablets, bottles of 100

B–12 (25 mcg.)
Tablets, bottles of 100, 500
B–12 (50 mcg.)
Tablets, bottles of 100, 500
B–12 (100 mcg.)
Tablets, bottles of 100, 250
B–12 (250 mcg.)
Tablets, bottles of 100, 250
B–12 (500 mcg.)
Tablets, bottles of 100, 250
B–12 (1000 mcg.)
Tablets, bottles of 100, 250
B–12 (1500 mcg.) Long Acting
Tablets, bottles of 100, 500
B–12 (2500 mcg.) Sublingual
Tablets, bottles of 50

B–50®
(Vitamin B Complex)
Tablets, bottles of 50, 100, 250

B-100®
Each tablet contains:

		% RDA*
Vitamin B-1	100 mg.	6,666
Vitamin B-2	100 mg.	5,882
Vitamin B-6	100 mg.	5,000
Vitamin B-12	100 mcg.	1,667
Niacinamide	100 mg.	500
Folic Acid	100 mcg.	25
Pantothenic Acid	100 mg.	1,000
d-Biotin	100 mcg.	33
Para Aminobenzoic Acid (PABA)	100 mg.	**
Choline Bitartrate	100 mg.	**
Inositol	100 mg.	**

*RDA—Recommended Daily Allowance
**RDA not established.

B-100®
Ultra B—Complex Vitamin
Sugar and Starch Free
[See table above].

Recommended Intake: Adults, 1 tablet daily or as directed by physician.

Supplied: Capsule-shaped tablets (protein-coated)—bottles of 50, 100 and 250.

B–100® (TIME RELEASE)
(Vitamin B Complex)
Tablets, bottles of 50, 100

B–125®
(Vitamin B Complex)
Tablets, bottles of 50, 100

B–150™
(Vitamin B Complex)

Supplied: Tablets bottles of 30, 100.

B & C LIQUID
Each teaspoon (5cc.) contains:
Vitamin C ....300 mg.
Vitamin B-1
(thiamine hydrochloride) ...... 15 mg.
Vitamin B-2
(riboflavin) .... 10 mg.
Vitamin B-6
(pyridoxine hydrochloride) ... 5 mg.
Vitamin B-12
(cobalamin concentrate) .... 5 mcg.
Niacinamide ....100 mg.
d-Panthenol .... 20 mg.

Supplied: 4 oz. bottle.

B–COMPLEX AND B–12
Each tablet contains:
Protease (from natural
Carica Papaya) .... 10 mg.
Vitamins:
B–12 (from Cobalamin) .... 25 mcg.
B–1 (Thiamine) .... 7 mg.
B–2 (Riboflavin) .... 14 mg.
Niacin .... 4.5 mg.

Supplied: Tablets, bottles of 90.

B–COMPLEX & C
(TIME RELEASE)
Each time release tablet contains vitamins:
C (with rose hips) ....200 mg.
B-1 (Thiamine) .... 10 mg.
B-2 (Riboflavin) .... 10 mg.
B-6 (Pyridoxine HCl) .... 5 mg.
B-12 (Cobalamin) .... 10 mcg.
Niacinamide .... 50 mg.
Calcium Pantothenate .... 10 mg.

Supplied: Tablets, bottles of 100.

BEE POLLEN (500 mg.)
Tablets, bottles of 100, 250
BEE POLLEN "1000" ™
Tablets, bottles of 100

BETA–CAROTENE
(25,000 I.U. Vitamin A)

Supplied: Capsules, bottles of 90.

BIOTIN (300 mcg.)
Tablets, bottles of 100

BONE MEAL W/VIT. D
Tablets, bottles of 100, 250, 500

BREWER'S YEAST POWDER (DEBITTERED)
A specially cultivated brewer's yeast containing B complex vitamins in natural high potency.

Supplied: 16 oz. can.

BREWER'S YEAST
Tablets, bottles of 250, 500, 1000

C–250 W/ROSE HIPS
Tablets, bottles of 100, 500
C–300 W/ROSE HIPS (CHEWABLE)
Tablets, bottles of 100, 250
C–500 W/ROSE HIPS
Tablets, bottles of 100, 250, 500
C–1000 W/ROSE HIPS
Tablets, bottles of 100, 250

C–COMPLEX
Each tablet contains:
Vitamin C with rose hips ......500 mg.
Bioflavonoids ....100 mg.
Rutin (Buckwheat) .... 50 mg.
Hesperidin Complex .... 25 mg.
Acerola .... 1.0 mg.

Supplied: Tablets, bottles of 100, 250.

VITAMIN C CRYSTALS
One teaspoonful provides:
Vitamin C ....5000 mg.

Supplied: 6 oz. bottle.

Continued on next page

Natures Bounty—Cont.

C–LIQUID

One teaspoon supplies:
Vitamin C with Rose Hips ...... 300 mg.

Supplied: 4 oz. bottles.

C–TIME 500™
with Rose Hips
Sustained Release Tablets
Sugar and Starch Free

Each tablet contains: (U.S.R.D.A.)
Vitamin C
   with Rose Hips .... 500 mg. (833%)

Recommended Intake: Adults, 1 tablet daily or as directed by physician.

Supplied: Capsule-shaped tablets (protein-coated to provide gradual release of Vitamin C over a prolonged period of time). Bottles of 100, 500.

C–TIME 750™ (TIME RELEASE)
Tablets, bottles of 100, 250

C–TIME 1500™
with Rose Hips
Sustained Release Tablets
Sugar and Starch Free

Each tablet contains: (U.S.R.D.A.)
Vitamin C
   with Rose Hips ..... 1500 mg. (2500%)

Recommended Intake: Adults, 1 tablet daily or as directed by physician.

Supplied: Capsule-shaped tablets (protein-coated to provide gradual release of Vitamin C over a prolonged period of time). Bottles of 30, 100 and 250.

CALCIDAY–667™

Each tablet contains:
Calcium Carbonate......................667 mg.

Supplied: Tablets, bottles of 60.

CALCIUM ASCORBATE (500 mg.)
Tablets, bottles of 100

CALCIUM LACTATE (10 gr.)
Tablets, bottles of 100, 250

CALMTABS™

Each tablet contains:
Ext. Valerian ....1 grain
Passiflora ....1 grain
Celery Seed ....1 grain
Catnip ....1 grain
Hops ....½ grain
Dried Orange Peel ....½ grain

Supplied: Tablets, bottles of 100.

CENTRAFREE™
Tablets, bottles of 100

CHELATED CALCIUM

Each tablet contains:
Calcium Amino Acid
   Chelate .... 750 mg.
(equivalent to 150 mg. elemental Calcium)

Supplied: Tablets, bottles of 100.

CHELATED CHROMIUM

Each tablet contains:
Chromium Amino Acid
   Chelate .... 50 mg.
(equivalent to 1000 mcg. of elemental Chromium)

Supplied: Tablets, bottles of 100.

CHELATED COPPER

Each tablet contains:
Copper Amino Acid Chelate ...... 20 mg.
(equivalent to 2 mg. of elemental Copper)

Supplied: Tablets, bottles of 100.

CHELATED MAGNESIUM

Each tablet contains:
Magnesium Amino Acid
   Chelate .... 500 mg.
(equivalent to 100 mg. of elemental Magnesium)

Supplied: Tablets, bottles of 100.

CHELATED MANGANESE

Each tablet contains:
Manganese Amino Acid
   Chelate .... 50 mg.
(equivalent to 5 mg. of elemental Manganese)

Supplied: Tablets, bottles of 100.

CHELATED MULTI–MINERALS

A multiple mineral amino acid chelate of 10 minerals.

Supplied: Tablets, bottles of 100, 250.

CHELATED POTASSIUM

Each tablet contains:
Potassium Amino Acid
   Complex .... 495 mg.
(equivalent to 99 mg. of elemental Potassium)

Supplied: Tablets, bottles of 100.

CHELATED ZINC

Each tablet contains:
Zinc Amino Acid Chelate .... 150 mg.
(equivalent to 15 mg. of elemental Zinc)

Supplied: Tablets, bottles of 100.

CHEW–IRON

Each chewable tablet contains:
Ferrous Fumarate .... 150 mg.
(elemental iron 50 mg)
B–12 (Cobalamin) .... 33 mcg.
B–1 (Thiamine) .... 10 mg.
Protease (from natural
   Papaya) .... 10 mg.

Supplied: Tablets, bottles of 100.

CHILDREN'S CHEWABLE VITAMINS

A popular chewable vitamin formula containing 10 essential vitamins.

Supplied: Tablets, bottles of 100, 250.

CHILDREN'S CHEWABLE VITAMINS WITH IRON

A popular chewable vitamin formula containing 10 essential vitamins with iron (15 mg.).

Supplied: Tablets, bottles of 100, 250.

CHOLINE (650 mg.)
Tablets, Bottles of 100, 500

CHROMIUM, GTF (50 mcg.)
Tablets, bottles of 100, 500
CHROMIUM, GTF (200 mcg.)
Tablets, bottles of 50, 100

CITRUS BIOFLAVONOIDS (1000 mg.)

Supplied: Tablets, bottles of 100.

DOLOMITE
Tablets, bottles of 100, 250, 500, 1000

E–200 (d–ALPHA TOCOPHEROL ACETATE)
Capsules, Bottles of 100, 250
E–400 (d–ALPHA TOCOPHEROL ACETATE)
Capsules, bottles of 100, 250, 1000

E–200 (NATURAL COMPLEX)
Capsules, bottles of 100
E–400 (NATURAL COMPLEX)
Capsules, bottles of 100, 250
E–600 (NATURAL COMPLEX)
Capsules, bottles of 50, 100
E–1000 (NATURAL COMPLEX)
Capsules, bottles of 50, 100, 250

EMULSIFIED E–200
Capsules, bottles of 100

EVENING PRIMROSE OIL (500 mg.)
Capsules, bottles of 30

FERROUS SULFATE (5 gr.)
Tablets, bottles of 100

FOLIC ACID (400 mcg.)
Tablets, bottles of 250
FOLIC ACID (800 mcg.)
Tablets, bottles of 250

GARLIC OIL (15 gr.)
Capsules, bottles of 100, 500
GARLIC OIL (77 gr.)
Capsules, bottles of 100

GARLIC & PARSLEY
(7½ minim)

Each capsule contains:
Concentrated garlic oil ....10 mg.
Concentrated parsley .... 1 mg.

Supplied: Capsules, bottles of 100.

GINSENG, MANCHURIAN™
(250 mg.)
Capsules, bottles of 50, 100
GINSENG, MANCHURIAN™
(500 mg.)
Tablets, bottles of 50, 100, 250

GLUCOMANNAN 500 mg.

Supplied: Capsules, bottles of 90.

GLUTAMIC ACID (500 mg.)
Tablets, bottles of 100, 500

HALIBUT LIVER OIL

Each capsule contains:
Vitamin A (from halibut
  liver oil) .... 5000 USP Units
Vitamin D (from halibut
  liver oil) .... 85 USP Units

Supplied: Capsules, bottles of 100.

HERBAL LAXATIVE

A gentle vegetable and herb laxative.

Supplied: Tablets, bottles of 100.

INOSITOL (650 mg.)
Tablets, bottles of 100

IRON
(Ferrous Gluconate, 5 gr.)
Tablets, bottles of 100, 250

KELP
Tablets, bottles of 250, 500

KLB6®
Natural Diet Aid

Six capsules contain:
Vitamin B-6
  (Pyridoxine HCl) .... 21 mg.
Cider Vinegar ....240 mg.
Soya Lecithin ....600 mg.
Kelp ....150 mg.

Supplied: Capsules, bottles of 100, 250.

KLB6 COMPLETE®

The famous KLB6® formula with wheat bran (500 mg) and 100% of RDA of 10 essential vitamins.

Supplied: Capsules, bottles of 100, 250.

KLB6 DIET MIX®
Regular and Carob Flavor

Balanced low-calorie meal replacement fortified with fiber, fructose, kelp, lecithin & Vitamin B-6.

Supplied: 14 oz. can.

L-ARGININE (500 mg.)
Tablets, bottles of 50

L-CYSTEINE (500 mg.)
Tablets, bottles of 50

L-GLUTAMINE (500 mg.)
Tablets, bottles of 50, 100

L-HISTIDINE (500 mg.)
Tablets, bottles of 50

L-LYSINE (500 mg.)
Tablets, bottles of 100, 500

L-ORNITHINE (500 mg.)
Tablets, bottles of 50

L-PHENYLALANINE (500 mg.)
Tablets, bottles of 50

L-TRYPTOPHAN (200 mg.)

Supplied: Tablets, bottles of 30, 100.

L-TRYPTOPHAN (500 mg.)

Supplied: Tablets, bottles of 30, 100.

L-TRYPTOPHAN (667 mg.)

Supplied: Tablets, bottles of 30, 100.

LECITHIN (1200 mg.)
Capsules, bottles of 100, 250

LECITHIN, CHEWABLE (1200 mg)

Supplied: Tablets, bottles of 100, 250.

LECITHIN W/VIT. D

Each capsule contains:
Soya Lecithin ....259.2 mg.
Soy Bean Oil ....170.2 mg.
Vitamin D ....150 USP units

Supplied: Capsules, bottles of 100.

LECITHIN GRANULES

Each tablespoon contains 7.5 gms of lecithin.

Supplied: 14 oz. can.

LIVER W/B-12
Tablets, bottles of 100, 250

MAGNESIUM
(Magnesium Gluconate, 30 mg.)

Supplied: Tablets, bottles of 100.

MANGANESE
(Manganese Gluconate, 50 mg.)

Supplied: Tablets, bottles of 100.

MEGA B® W/C

High B-Complex formula with Vitamin C (500 mg).

Supplied: Tablets, bottles of 60, 180.

MEGA V & M™

Mega potency multiple vitamin and mineral formula.

Supplied: Tablets, bottles of 30, 60, 100.

MEMORY BOOSTER™
Tablets, bottles of 50
Each two tablets contain:
L-Glutamine..................................250 mg.
RNA (Ribonucleic Acid)...............250 mg.
L-Phenylalanine...........................250 mg.
Choline Bitartrate ....250 mg.
Gota Kola ....250 mg.
Lecithin ....1000 mg.

MULTI-MINERALS

A multiple mineral formula containing nine essential minerals.

Supplied: Tablets, bottles of 100, 250.

NATURE'S BOUNTY HAIR BOOSTER™

Vitamin-Mineral Complex for the hair.

Supplied: Tablets, bottles of 60, 250.

NATURE'S BOUNTY 1™

[See table on next page].

Supplied: Tablets, bottles of 30, 60.

NATURE'S BOUNTY SLIM®

100% Natural High Protein Powder plus Vitamins.

Supplied: 16 oz. can.

NIACIN (100 mg.)
Tablets, bottles of 100
NIACIN (250 mg.)
Tablets, bottles of 100

NIACINAMIDE (500 mg.)
Tablets, bottles of 100, 250

OCTACOSANOL (1000 mcg.)
Capsules, bottles of 50

OYSTERCAL-D™ 250

Three tablets provide:		(U.S.R.D.A.)
Calcium	750 mg.	(94%)
Vitamin D.....	375 I.U.	(75%)

Supplied: Tablets, bottles of 100, 250.

OYSTERCAL™ 500

Two tablets provide:		(U.S.R.D.A.)
Calcium	1000 mg.	(100%)

Supplied: Tablets, bottles of 60.

OYSTER CALCIUM (375 mg.)

Each tablet contains:
Calcium ....375 mg.
Vitamin A ....800 I.U.
Vitamin D-2 ....200 I.U.

Supplied: Tablets, bottles of 100, 500.

PABA
(Para-Aminobenzoic Acid, 100 mg.)
Tablets, bottles of 250, 500

Continued on next page

Natures Bounty—Cont.

PABA
(Para-Aminobenzoic Acid, 500 mg.)
Tablets, bottles of 100

PANTOTHENIC ACID (100 mg.)
Tablets, bottles of 100, 250
PANTOTHENIC ACID (200 mg.)
Tablets, bottles of 100, 250

PAPAYA ENZYME (1 gr.)
Aid to starch and protein digestion.

Supplied: Tablets, bottles of 100, 250.

POTASSIUM
(Potassium Gluconate, 99 mg.)
Tablets, bottles of 100, 250

POTASSIUM & B–6
Each tablet contains:
Potassium ....30 mg.
Vitamin B-6
(pyridoxine HCl) ....50 mg.

Supplied: Tablets, bottles of 90, 250.

PROTEIN (250 mg.)
A food supplement from soya, dried malt extract and dry milk powder.

Supplied: Tablets, bottles of 100, 250, 500.

PROTEIN FOR BODY BUILDING™
100% Natural High Protein Powder

Supplied: 16 oz. cans

RNA
(100 mg from brewer's yeast)

Supplied: Tablets, bottles of 100.

RNA/DNA
(100 mg of each from brewer's yeast)

Supplied: Tablets, bottles of 100.

RUTIN (50 mg.)
Tablets, bottles of 250

SELENIUM (50 mcg.)
Tablets, bottles of 100, 250
SELENIUM (200 mcg.)
Tablets, bottles of 50, 100

SPIRULINA (500 mg.)
Tablets, bottles of 90

STRESS FORMULA "605" ™
Hi-potency stress formula vitamins.

Supplied: Tablets, bottles of 60, 250.

STRESS FORMULA "605" ™ W/IRON
Hi-potency stress formula vitamins with iron (27 mg).

Supplied: Tablets, bottles of 60, 250.

STRESS FORMULA "605" ™ W/ZINC
Hi-potency stress formula with zinc (23.9 mg.).

Supplied: Tablets, bottles of 60, 250.

STRESS "1000"™
Sugar, Starch and Preservative Free

		%USRDA*
Vitamin C (with Rose Hips)	1000 mg.	1667
Vitamin E (d-alpha Tocopheryl Acetate)	30 I.U.	100
Thiamine (Vitamin B-1) (as Thiamine Mononitrate)	15 mg.	1000
Riboflavin (Vitamin B-2)	15 mg.	882
Niacinamide	100 mg.	500
Vitamin B-6 (as Pyridoxine Hydrochloride)	5 mg.	205
Vitamin B-12 (Cyanocobalamin)	12 mcg.	200
Pantothenic Acid (Calcium Pantothenate USP)	20 mg.	183

Each tablet provides:

*Percentage of the U.S. government recommended daily allowance for adults and children four or more years of age.

Supplied: Tablets, bottles of 30, 60, 90, 250.

SUPEROXIDE DISMUTASE (SOD)
2000 Units

Supplied: Tablets, bottles of 50, 100, 500.

ULTRA "A"
(Vitamin A, 25,000 USP Units)
Capsules, bottles of 100, 250
ULTRA "A"
(Vitamin A, 25,000 USP Units)
Tablets, bottles of 100

ULTRA "A & D"
(25,000 UNITS OF VIT. A & 1,000 UNITS OF VIT. D)
Tablets, bottles of 100

ULTRA "D"
(1000 USP units Vit. D)

Supplied: Tablets, bottles of 100.

ULTRA KLB6®
Three tablets contain:
Lecithin ....1200 mg.
Vitamin B-6 .... 350 mg.
Kelp .... 100 mg.
Cider Vinegar .... 240 mg.

Supplied: Tablets, bottles of 100, 250.

ULTRA VITA–TIME™
Ultra potency vitamins, minerals, amino acids and lipotropic formula.

Supplied: Tablets, bottles of 50, 100, 250.

VITAMIN A (10,000 USP UNITS)
Capsules, bottles of 100, 250
VITAMIN A (10,000 USP UNITS)
Tablets, bottles of 100, 250

VITAMIN A & D
(10,000 UNITS VIT. A & 400 UNITS VIT. D)
Tablets, bottles of 100

VITAMIN D (400 USP UNITS)
Tablets, bottles of 100

NATURE'S BOUNTY 1™
Each tablet contains:

		%US RDA
VITAMIN A Fish Liver Oil and Beta-Carotene	25,000 I.U.	500
VITAMIN D Fish Liver Oil	800 I.U.	200
VITAMIN E	30 I.U.	100
† VITAMIN C Ascorbic Acid and Rose Hips	250 mg.	417
† VITAMIN B-1 Thiamine HCl Yeast	25 mg.	1667
† VITAMIN B-2 Riboflavin Yeast	25 mg.	1471
† VITAMIN B-6 Pyridoxine HCl Yeast	50 mg.	2500
† Vitamin B-12 Cobalamin Conc. Yeast	50 mcg.	833
† NIACINAMIDE	50 mg.	250
† CALCIUM PANTOTHENATE	50 mg.	500
† FOLIC ACID	400 mcg.	100
† BIOTIN	50 mcg.	17
† CHOLINE	15 mg.	*
† INOSITOL	15 mg.	*
† PABA	50 mg.	*
VITAMIN K	10 mcg.	*
IODINE Potassium Iodide, Kelp	150 mcg.	100
IRON Ferrous Fumarate	10 mg.	56
CALCIUM, Bone Meal	50 mg.	5
PHOSPHOROUS, Bone Meal	23 mg.	2
CHROMIUM, Chromium Chelate	100 mcg.	*
MAGNESIUM, Magnesium Oxide Dolomite	100 mg.	25
ZINC	15 mg.	100
MANGANESE, Manganese Sulfate	5 mg.	*
SELENIUM, Yeast	25 mcg.	*
COPPER Copper Sulfate	2 mg.	100
POTASSIUM Potassium Chloride	1 mg.	*
CHLORIDE, Potassium Chloride	1 mg.	*
MOLYBDENUM, Sodium Molybdate	15 mcg.	*

All in a base of Bioflavonoids, Rutin, Rose Hips, Yeast, Kelp and Dolomite
† Timed-release B-Complex and C vitamins to supply the availability and benefits of prolonged absorption of the mega-vitamins.

VITAMIN K (100 mcg.)
Tablets, bottles of 100, 500

VITA–TIME™
High potency vitamins, minerals and amino acids.

Supplied: Tablets, bottles of 100, 250.

WATER PILL W/IRON (NATURAL DIURETIC)
Capsules, bottles of 50, 100, 250

WATER PILL W/POTASSIUM (NATURAL DIURETIC)
Each tablet contains:
Buchu Leaves Powder ....50 mg.
Uva Ursi Leaves Powder ....50 mg.
Parsley Leaves Powder ....50 mg.
Juniper Berries Powder ....10 mg.
Potassium ....20 mg.

Supplied: Tablets, bottles of 50, 100, 250.

WHEAT GERM OIL (6 minim)
Capsules, bottles of 100
WHEAT GERM OIL (14 minim)
Capsules, bottles of 100
WHEAT GERM OIL (20 minim)
Capsules, bottles of 100, 250

YEAST PLUS VITAMIN
B12, B-Complex with minerals and amino acids.

Supplied: Tablets, bottles of 100, 250.

ZACNE®
Each tablet contains:
Zinc Gluconate .... 25 mg.
Vitamin C
with Rose Hips .... 75 mg.
B–6 (Pyridoxine HCl) .... 10 mg.
Vitamin A
(fish liver oils) .... 500 I.U.
Vitamin E .... 25 I.U.

Directions: As a dietary supplement, two tablets three times daily before meals.

Supplied: Tablets, bottles of 100, 500.

ZINC (10 mg.)
(Zinc Gluconate)
Tablets, bottles of 100, 250
ZINC (25 mg.)
Tablets, bottles of 100
ZINC (50 mg.)
Tablets, bottles of 100, 500
ZINC (100 mg.)
Tablets, bottles of 100, 500

Products are cross-indexed
by product classifications
in the
BLUE SECTION

Norcliff Thayer Inc.
**303 SOUTH BROADWAY
TARRYTOWN, NY 10591**

A–200 Pyrinate® Pediculicide Shampoo
Liquid, Gel

A-200 Pyrinate® Liquid

Description: Active ingredients: pyrethrins 0.17%, piperonyl butoxide technical 2% (equivalent to 1.6% (butylcarbityl) (6-propylpiperonyl) ether and 0.4% related compounds). Inert ingredients: petroleum distillate 5%, other inert ingredients 92.83%.

A-200 Pyrinate® Gel

Description: Active ingredients: pyrethrins 0.33%, piperonyl butoxide technical 4% (equivalent to 3.2% (butylcarbityl) (6-propylpiperonyl) ether and 0.8% related compounds). Inert ingredients: petroleum distillate 5.33%, other inert ingredients 90.34%.

Actions: A-200 Pyrinate is an effective pediculicide for control of head lice (Pediculus humanus capitis), pubic lice (Phthirus pubis) and body lice (Pediculus humanus corporis), and their nits.

Indications: A-200 Pyrinate Liquid and Gel are indicated for the treatment of human pediculosis—head lice, body lice and pubic lice, and their eggs. A-200 Pyrinate Gel is specially formulated for pubic lice and head lice in children, where control of application is desirable.

Contraindications: A-200 Pyrinate is contraindicated in individuals hypersensitive to any of its ingredients or allergic to ragweed.

Precautions: A-200 Pyrinate is for external use only. It is harmful if swallowed or inhaled. It may be irritating to the eyes and mucous membranes. In case of accidental contact with eyes, they should be immediately flushed with water. In order to prevent reinfestation with lice, all clothing and bedding must be sterilized or treated concurrent with the application of this preparation. If skin irritation or signs of infection are present, a physician should be consulted.

Dosage and Administration: Apply sufficient A-200 Pyrinate to completely "wet" the hair and scalp or skin of any infested area. Allow application to remain no longer than 10 minutes. Wash and rinse with plenty of warm water. Remove dead lice and eggs from hair with fine comb. To restore body and luster to hair following scalp applications, follow with a good shampoo. If necessary, this treatment may be repeated, but should not exceed two applications within 24 hours.

How Supplied: A-200 Pyrinate Liquid in 2 and 4 fl. oz. bottles with special comb. A-200 Pyrinate Gel in 1 oz. tubes.

Literature Available: Patient literature available upon request.

*Shown in Product Identification
Section, page 418*

ASTHMAHALER®
(brand of epinephrine bitartrate)
FOR TEMPORARY RELIEF FROM ACUTE PAROXYSMS OF BRONCHIAL ASTHMA

FOR ORAL INHALATION ONLY.
Each inhalation delivers 0.3 mg of epinephrine bitartrate equivalent to 0.16 mg of epinephrine base.

How Supplied: ½ fl. oz. (15 ml.) Available as combination package metal vial plus plastic mouthpiece, or as refill metal vial only.

ASTHMANEFRIN® SOLUTION INHALANT ANTI-ASTHMATIC
(brand of racemic epinephrine hydrochloride)
FOR TEMPORARY RELIEF OF THE PAROXYSMS OF BRONCHIAL ASTHMA
A solution of Racepin® (brand of bioassayed specially purified racemic epinephrine) as the hydrochloride, equivalent to 2.25% epinephrine base. Contains 0.5% chlorobutanol as a preservative.

How Supplied: ½ fl. oz. (15 ml.) and 1 fl. oz. (30 ml.) Solutions. FOR USE WITH ASTHMANEFRIN® NEBULIZER.

ESOTÉRICA® MEDICATED FADE CREAM
Regular
Facial with Sunscreen
Fortified Scented with Sunscreen
Fortified Unscented with Sunscreen

Description:
Regular:
Active Ingredient: Hydroquinone 2%. Other Ingredients: Water, glyceryl stearate, isopropyl palmitate, propylene glycol, ceresin, mineral oil, stearyl alcohol, propylene glycol stearate, PEG-6-32 stearate, poloxamer 188, steareth-20, laureth-23, dimethicone, sodium lauryl sulfate, citric acid, sodium bisulfite, methylparaben, propylparaben, trisodium EDTA, BHA.
Facial with Sunscreen:
Active Ingredients: Hydroquinone 2.0%, padimate O 3.3%, oxybenzone 2.5%. **Other Ingredients:** Water, isopropyl myristate, stearyl alcohol, glyceryl stearate, propylene glycol, ceresin, poloxamer 188, steareth-20, ceteareth-3, dimethicone, sodium lauryl sulfate, citric acid, fragrance, trisodium EDTA, BHA, sodium bisulfite, methylparaben, propylparaben.
Fortified Scented and Unscented with Sunscreen:
Active Ingredients: Hydroquinone 2%, padimate O 3.3%, oxybenzone 2.5%. Other Ingredients: Water, glyceryl stearate, isopropyl palmitate, ceresin, propylene glycol, stearyl alcohol, PEG-6-32 stearate, poloxamer 188, mineral oil, steareth-20, laureth-23, steareth-10, allantoin ascorbate, dimethicone, sodium lauryl sulfate, methylparaben, propylparaben, sodium bisulfite, BHA, trisodium EDTA.

Continued on next page

Norcliff Thayer—Cont.

Fragrance in all except Fortified Unscented with Sunscreen.

Indications: Regular and Fortified Scented and Unscented with Sunscreen: Indicated for helping fade darkened skin areas including age spots, liver spots, freckles and melasma on the face, hands, legs and body and when used as directed helps prevent their recurrence. Facial with Sunscreen: Specially designed to help fade darkened skin areas including age spots, liver spots, freckles and melasma on the face and when used as directed helps prevent their recurrence. It has emollients to help moisturize while it lightens, so it makes an excellent night cream as well.

Actions: Esotérica Medicated helps bleach and lighten hyperpigmented skin.

Contraindications: Should not be used by persons with known sensitivity to hydroquinone.

Warnings: Do not use if skin is irritated. Some individuals may be sensitive to the active ingredient(s) in this cream. Discontinue use if irritation appears. Avoid contact with eyes. Excessive exposure to the sun should be avoided. For external use only.
Facial and Fortified Scented and Unscented with Sunscreen: Not for use in the prevention of sunburn.

Directions: Apply Esotérica to areas you wish to lighten and rub in well. Use cream in the morning and at bedtime for at least six weeks for maximum results. Esotérica is greaseless and may be used under makeup.

How Supplied: 3 oz. glass jars.

LIQUIPRIN®
(acetaminophen)

Description: Liquiprin is a nonsalicylate analgesic and antipyretic particularly suitable for children. Each 1.66 ml (top mark on dropper) contains 80 mg (1.23 gr.) of acetaminophen. Liquiprin is raspberry flavored, reddish pink solution, and does not contain alcohol.

Actions: Liquiprin safely and effectively reduces fever and pain at any age without the hazards of salicylate therapy (e.g., gastric mucosal irritation).

Indications: Liquiprin is indicated for use in the treatment of infants and children with conditions requiring reduction of fever and/or relief of pain such as mild upper respiratory infections (tonsillitis, common cold, flu), teething, headache, myalgia, postimmunization reactions, post-tonsillectomy discomfort and gastroenteritis. As adjunctive therapy with antibiotics or sulfonamides, Liquiprin may be useful as an analgesic and antipyretic in bacterial or viral infections, such as bronchitis, pharyngitis, tracheobronchitis, sinusitis, pneumonia, otitis media and cervical adenitis.

Precautions and Adverse Reactions: If a sensitivity reaction occurs, the drug should be discontinued. Liquiprin Drops has rarely been found to produce side effects. It is usually well tolerated by patients who are sensitive to products containing aspirin.

Usual Dosage: Liquiprin should be administered at 4-hour intervals 3 to 4 times daily in the following dosages:
Under 3 years: Up to 160 mg (two dropperfuls filled to 80 mg top mark)
3 years: 160 mg (two dropperfuls filled to 80 mg top mark)
4 to 5 years: 240 mg (three dropperfuls filled to 80 mg top mark)

How Supplied: Liquiprin is available in a 1.16 fl. oz. (35 ml) plastic bottle with a calibrated dropper and child-resistant cap, and safety sealed package.
Shown in Product Identification Section, page 418

NATURE'S REMEDY®
Laxative

Active Ingredients: Cascara sagrada 150 mg, aloe 100 mg.

Indications: For gentle, overnight relief of constipation.

Actions: Nature's Remedy has two natural active ingredients that give gentle, overnight relief of constipation. These ingredients, cascara sagrada and aloe, gently stimulate the body's natural function.

Warnings: Do not take any laxative when nausea, vomiting, abdominal pain, or other symptoms of appendicitis are present. Frequent or prolonged use of laxatives may result in dependence on them. If pregnant or nursing, consult your physician before using this or any medicine.

Dosage and Administration: Adults, swallow two tablets daily along with a full glass of water; children (8–15 yrs.), one tablet daily; or as directed by a physician.

How Supplied: Beige, film-coated tablets with foil-backed blister packaging in boxes of 12s, 30s and 60s.
Shown in Product Identification Section, page 418

NOSALT™
Salt Alternative Regular and Seasoned

Description: Food seasoning to be used as an alternative or substitute for salt (NaCl) at the table and in cooking to help regulate dietary sodium intake.

Regular Ingredients: Contains potassium chloride, potassium bitartrate, adipic acid, mineral oil, fumaric acid. Looks, sprinkles and tastes like salt, contains less than 10 mg of sodium per 100 g (0.01%) which is considered sodium free. Contains approximately 32 mEq (1,251 mg) of potassium per ½ level teaspoon.

Seasoned Ingredients: Potassium chloride, dextrose, onion and garlic, spices and other natural flavors, lactose, cream of tartar, paprika, silica, disodium inosinate and disodium guanylate, turmeric and extratives of paprika. Contains less than 5 mg sodium per teaspoon which is considered salt free. Contains approximately 664 mg potassium (17 mEq) per ½ level teaspoon.

Uses: Sprinkled on food or in cooking, in the same proportion or less than regular salt, gives food salt flavor while helping to reduce sodium intake. Appropriate for persons on low sodium diets, as for example, those whose sodium intake has been restricted for medical reasons.

Caution to Physicians: The potassium intake of persons receiving potassium-sparing diuretics or potassium supplementation should be evaluated. Potassium chloride should not be used in patients with hyperkalemia, oliguria, and severe kidney disease.

Consumer Warning: For normal, healthy people. Persons having diabetes, heart or kidney disease, or persons receiving medical treatment should consult a physician before using a salt alternative or substitute.

How Supplied: Regular: 11 oz. container with shaker top. **Seasoned:** 8 oz. container with shaker top.
Shown in Product Identification Section, page 418

OXY CLEAN™
Medicated Cleanser, Pads, Soap

Active Ingredient:
Oxy Clean™ Medicated Cleanser: Salicylic Acid* 0.5%, SD Alcohol 40B 40%
Oxy Clean™ Medicated Pads: Salicylic Acid* 0.5%, SD Alcohol 40B 40%
Oxy Clean™ Medicated Soap: Salicylic Acid* 3.5%
*Salicylic Acid (2-Hydroxybenzoic Acid)

Indications: These medicated skin products are useful for opening plugged pores and for removing excess dirt and oil. Also helps remove and prevent blackheads.

Additional Benefits: When used regularly cleanses acne prone skin and removes dirt, grime and excess skin oil. For a complete anti-acne program, after using Oxy Clean™ follow use with Oxy-5®, Oxy-10®, or Oxy-10® Cover acne pimple medication.

Caution: For external use only. If skin irritation develops, discontinue use and consult a physician. May be irritating to eyes or mucous membranes. If contact occurs, flush thoroughly with water. Keep this and all drugs out of reach of children. Store at room temperature. Keep away from flame, fire and heat.

Dosage and Administration: See labeling instructions for use.

How Supplied:
Medicated Liquid Cleanser—4 fl. oz.
Medicated Pads—Plastic Jar/50 pads

Medicated Soap—3.25 oz. soap bar.
Shown in Product Identification Section, page 418

OXY CLEAN™
Lathering Facial Scrub

Description: Oxy Clean Scrub is a skin cleanser containing dissolving abradant granules and is useful for opening plugged pores and for removing excess oil. Oxy Clean Scrub can't over-abrade as can cleansers with non-dissolving abradant particles.

Composition: Contains dissolving abradant granules (sodium tetraborate decahydrate) in a base containing a unique combination of surface active soapless cleaning agents.

Directions: Use in place of your usual soap or cleanser. Wet face with warm water. Squeeze Oxy Clean Scrub onto fingertips and gently massage into face. Continue massaging and adding water until abradant granules are completely dissolved. (About one minute.) Rinse thoroughly with warm water and dry. Use once or twice daily, or as required.

Caution: Avoid contact with eyes. If particles get into eyes, flush thoroughly with water and avoid rubbing eyes. Discontinue use if skin irritation or excessive dryness develops. Not to be used on infants or children under 3 years of age. Do not use on inflamed skin. Keep out of reach of children.

How Supplied: 2.65 oz. plastic tubes.
Shown in Product Identification Section, page 418

OXY-5® and OXY-10® with SORBOXYL™
Benzoyl peroxide lotion 5% and 10% with silica oil absorber

Description: Active Ingredient: Oxy-5: Benzoyl peroxide 5%. Oxy-10: Benzoyl peroxide 10%.
Other Ingredients: Water, cetyl alcohol, silica (Sorboxyl™), propylene glycol, citric acid, sodium citrate, sodium lauryl sulfate, methylparaben, propylparaben.

Indications: Topical medication for the treatment of acne vulgaris.

Action: Provides antibacterial activity against Propionibacterium acnes.

Additional benefits: Absorbs excess skin oil up to 12 hours. It is colorless, odorless, greaseless lotion that vanishes upon application.

Directions for Use: Shake well before using. Wash skin thoroughly and dry well. Since some people are sensitive to the active ingredients of acne medications, first determine whether you are sensitive to this product by testing on a small affected area once a day for two days. If no excessive dryness or undue irritation develops, dab on lotion, smoothing into oily acne-pimple areas of face, neck and body. Apply once a day initially, then two or three times a day, or as directed by a physician.

Contraindications: Should not be used by persons with known sensitivity to benzoyl peroxide.

Caution: Persons with sensitive skin or known allergy to benzoyl peroxide should not use this medication. First test on a small affected area by applying this product once a day for two days. If discomforting irritation or undue dryness occurs during treatment, reduce frequency of use or dosage. If excessive itching, redness, burning, swelling, irritation or dryness occurs, discontinue use and consult a physician. Avoid contact with eyes, lips and mouth. May bleach hair or dyed fabrics. Keep tightly closed. Keep this and all drugs out of reach of children. Store at room temperature; avoid excessive heat. For external use only.

How Supplied: 1 fl. oz. plastic bottles.
Shown in Product Identification Section, page 418

OXY 10® COVER with SORBOXYL
Benzoyl peroxide lotion 10% with silica oil absorber

Description: Active Ingredient: Benzoyl peroxide 10%.

Other Ingredients: Water, titanium dioxide, cetyl alcohol, silica (Sorboxyl™), glyceryl stearate, propylene glycol, stearic acid, iron oxides, sodium lauryl sulfate, citric acid, sodium citrate, methylparaben, propylparaben.

Indications: Topical medication for the treatment of acne vulgaris.

Action: Provides antibacterial activity against Propionibacterium acnes.

Additional Benefits: Absorbs excess skin oil up to 12 hours. It is a flesh tone, odorless, greaseless lotion that covers up acne pimples while it treats them.

Directions: Wash thoroughly and dry well. Since some people are sensitive to the active ingredients of acne medications, first determine whether you are sensitive to this product by applying lotion on a small affected area once a day for two days. If no excessive dryness or undue irritation develops, smooth on evenly on oily acne-pimple areas. Put an extra dab of Oxy 10 Cover on particularly troublesome areas. Apply once a day initially, then two or three times a day, or as directed by a physician.

Contraindications: Should not be used by persons with known sensitivity to benzoyl peroxide.

Caution: Persons with sensitive skin or known allergy to benzoyl peroxide should not use this medication. First test on a small affected area by applying this product once a day for two days. If discomforting irritation or undue dryness occurs during treatment, reduce frequency of use or dosage. If excessive itching, redness, burning, swelling, irritation or dryness occurs, discontinue use and consult a physician. Avoid contact with eyes, lips and mouth. May bleach hair or dyed fabrics. Keep tightly closed. Keep this and all drugs out of reach of children. Store at room temperature; avoid excessive heat. For external use only.

How Supplied: 1 fl. oz. plastic bottles.
Shown in Product Identification Section, page 418

OXY 10® WASH Antibacterial Skin Wash

Active Ingredient: Benzoyl peroxide 10%.

Indications: Antibacterial skin wash used as an aid in the treatment of acne vulgaris.

Actions: Promotes antibacterial activity against Propionibacterium acnes.

Additional Benefits: When used instead of regular soap, cleanses acne-prone skin and removes dirt, grime and excess skin oil.
For a complete anti-acne program, follow Oxy 10® Wash with Oxy-5® acne-pimple medication. Or for stubborn and adult acne, use Oxy-10® or Oxy 10® Cover maximum strength acne-pimple medication.

Contraindications: Should not be used by persons with known sensitivity to benzoyl peroxide.

Caution: Persons with sensitive skin or known allergy to benzoyl peroxide should not use this medication. First test on a small affected area by applying this product as directed once a day for two days. If discomforting irritation or undue dryness occurs during treatment, reduce frequency of use or dosage. If excessive itching, redness, burning, swelling, irritation or dryness occurs, discontinue use and consult a physician. Avoid contact with eyes, lips and mouth. May bleach hair or dyed fabrics. **For external use only.**

Directions: Shake well. Wet area to be washed. Apply Oxy 10® Wash massaging gently for 1 to 2 minutes. Rinse thoroughly. Use 2 to 3 times daily or as directed by physician.

How supplied: 4 fl. oz. plastic bottles.
Shown in Product Identification Section, page 418

TUMS® Antacid Tablets
Regular and Extra Strength

Description: Regular Tums: Active Ingredient: Calcium carbonate, precipitated U.S.P. 500 mg.
An antacid composition providing liquid effectiveness in a low cost, pleasant-tasting tablet. Tums tablets are free of the chalky aftertaste usually associated with calcium carbonate therapy and remain pleasant tasting even during long-term therapy. Tums is a dietetically sodium free antacid. Each tablet contains less than 3 mg of sodium.
Extra Strength Tums: Active Ingredient: Calcium Carbonate, 750 mg.

Continued on next page

Norcliff Thayer—Cont.

Contains less that 4.5 mg sodium per tablet, considered dietetically sodium free. Non-laxative/non-constipating.

Indications: For fast relief of acid indigestion, heartburn, sour stomach and upset stomach associated with these symptoms.

Actions: Regular Tums lowers the upper limit of the pH range without affecting the innate antacid efficiency of calcium carbonate. One tablet, when tested *in vitro* according to the *Federal Register* procedure (*Fed. Reg.* 39-19862, June 4, 1974), neutralizes 10 mEq of 0.1N HCl. This high neutralization capacity combined with a rapid rate of reaction makes Tums an ideal antacid for management of conditions associated with hyperacidity. It effectively neutralizes free acid yet does not cause systemic alkalosis in the presence of normal renal function. A double-blind placebo controlled clinical study demonstrated that calcium carbonate taken at a dosage of 16 Tums tablets daily for a two-week period was non-constipating/non-laxative.

Warnings: Regular Tums: Do not take more than 16 tablets in a 24-hour period or use the maximum dosage of this product for more than 2 weeks, except under the advice and supervision of a physician.
Extra Strength Tums: Do not take more than 10 tablets in a 24 hour period or use the maximum dosage of this product for more than two weeks, except under the advice and supervision of a physician. Keep this and all drugs out of the reach of children.

Dosage and Administration: Chew 1 or 2 TUMS tablets as symptoms occur. Repeat hourly if symptoms return, or as directed by a physician. No water is required. Simulated Drip Method: The pleasant-tasting TUMS tablet may be kept between the gum and cheek and allowed to dissolve gradually by continuous sucking to prolong the effective relief time.

Professional Labeling: Indicated for the symptomatic relief of hyperacidity associated with the diagnosis of peptic ulcer, gastritis, peptic esophagitis, gastric hyperacidity, and hiatal hernia.

How Supplied: Regular Tums: Peppermint and Assorted Flavors of Cherry, Lemon, Orange and Wintergreen are available in 12-tablet rolls, 3-roll wraps, and bottles of 75 and 150 tablets. **Extra Strength Tums:** Cartons of 48s, blister packs of 12s.
Shown in Product Identification Section, page 418

Products are cross-indexed by generic and chemical names in the **YELLOW SECTION**

Noxell Corporation
**11050 YORK ROAD
HUNT VALLEY, MARYLAND
21030-2098**

NOXZEMA
Medicated Skin Cream

Active Ingredients: Camphor, phenol (less than 0.5%), clove oil, eucalyptus oil, menthol.

Other Ingredients: Water, stearic acid, linseed oil, soybean oil, fragrance, propylene glycol, gelatin, ammonium hydroxide, calcium hydroxide.

Actions: Antipruritic, counterirritant and antiseptic.

Indications: This medicated skin product is an effective facial cleanser and has been demonstrated to be more effective than soap in an acne washing regimen. When used on sunburned skin, this medicated cream actually reduces the surface temperature of the skin to relieve pain almost instantly.

Additional Benefits: Noxzema is also an effective moisturizer for an effective anti-acne program. Instead of soap, wash with Noxzema and treat acne prone areas with Noxzema Acne-12.

Directions: (Wash) Morning and night wash your face with Noxzema Skin Cream. Scoop out some Noxzema and spread over your face with a wet washcloth, gently work in using a circular motion. Rinse. (Sunburn) Apply Noxzema Skin Cream liberally to areas of burn or discomfort.

Contraindications: None.

Cautions: For persistent skin problems or serious burn, consult physician. Keep out of the reach of children.
Shown in Product Identification Section, page 418

NuAge Laboratories, Ltd.
**4200 LACLEDE AVENUE
ST. LOUIS, MO 63108**

BIOCHEMIC TISSUE SALTS

Ingredients: Each tissue salt tablet provides Schuessler homoeopathic ingredients as the recommended triturated tablet in the required Lactose base per U.S.H.P.

Action: Biochemic Tissue Salts (or Cell Salts) work homoeopathically to help the body achieve relief and maintain health and fitness by stimulating the body's healing process.

History: The NuAge Biochemic Tissue Tablets were developed over one hundred years ago by Dr. Wm. Schuessler. Their use is explained in THE BIOCHEMIC HANDBOOK and many other publications. The Tissue Salts are "official" when made in accordance with the United States Homoeopathic Pharmacopoeia.

Contraindications: None

Warning: As with any drug, if nursing or pregnant seek the advice of a professional before using. Keep this and all medicine out of the reach of children. If symptoms persist or recur, consult a licensed medical practitioner.

Instructions: Use according to standard Homoeopathic indications.

Nutritional Factors
**2615 STANWELL DR.
CONCORD, CA 94520**

ACIDAID
Natural Antacid

Description: All natural antacid includes aloe vera, and contains no aluminum, sodium, or sugar. Safe for pregnant women.

Active Ingredients: Each teaspoonful (5 ml.) contains calcium carbonate 500 mg., and magnesium hydroxide 166 mg.

Indications: ACIDAID provides fast, effective relief of acid indigestion, heartburn, and sour stomach.

Warnings: Do not take more than 12 teaspoonfuls in 24 hour period, or use the maximum dosage for more than 2 weeks except under the supervision of a physician. Keep out of the reach of children. Also available in tablets.

Nutritional Specialty Products
**2210 WILSHIRE BLVD.
SUITE 159
SANTA MONICA, CA 90403**

GERIAVIT PHARMATON®
**Exclusive Swiss
Multivitamin/Multimineral Plus
G115® Formula**

Description: Each of the easy-to-take soft-gelatine capsules contains an exactly-balanced combination of active ingredients: vitamins, minerals, and G115® standardized Ginseng extract.

Composition:

Each capsule provides:			Percent US RDA
Vitamin A	5000	IU	100
Vitamin D	400	IU	100
Vitamin E	45	IU	150
Vitamin C	60	mg	100
Vitamin B$_1$	2	mg	133
Vitamin B$_2$	2	mg	118
Vitamin B$_6$	2	mg	100
Vitamin B$_{12}$	6	mcg	100
Niacinamide	20	mg	100
Pantothenic Acid	14	mg	140
Calcium	90	mg	9
Phosphorus	70	mg	7
Iron	18	mg	100
Copper	2	mg	100
Magnesium	40	mg	10
Zinc	4	mg	27
Manganese	1	mg	**

Potassium	8 mg	**
Rutin	20 mg	***
Lecithin	50 mg	***
Ginseng	40 mg	***
(standardized extract G115®)		

*US Recommended Daily Allowance to Adults
**US RDA not established
***US RDA not applicable

Indications: Created to provide a vitamin and mineral supplement which may be taken by adults at those certain times in life to help maximize health and to maintain the physical and mental well-being, and to counteract the nutritional deficiencies caused by modern day stress, poor eating habits, slimming cures, excessive smoking, alcohol and menopausal symptoms.

Dosage and Administration: One capsule in the morning with breakfast and one capsule at noon during 2 to 4 weeks. Then one capsule with the breakfast is usually sufficient.

How Supplied: Available in tamper resistant blister packs of 30, 60, and 100 capsules.

Literature: Sample and literature available on request. For more information contact: Nutritional Specialty Products, a division of Nutrition Associates Inc., 2210 Wilshire Blvd Suite 159, Santa Monica, Ca. 90403 Telephone: (213) 393 0827, Telex: 4995300 burx lsa (att: nsp*)

Reference: Comprehensive series of analytical, toxicological, pharmacological and clinical tests, Geriavit Pharmaton is now the most thoroughly proven preparation of its kind. Millions of capsules are sold through pharmacies throughout the world. Recommended by pharmacists and physicians in over 60 countries and for over 15 years.
Shown in Product Identification Section, page 419

Optimox, Inc.
**2720 MONTEREY STEEET
SUITE 406
TORRANCE, CA 90503**

OPTIVITE® for Women
(Multiple Megavitamin Formula with Amino Acid Chelated Minerals and Digestive Aids)

Composition:
Six (6) Tablets Provide:

Vitamins

Liposoluble

Vitamin A (Palmitate) (Water Dispersed)	12,500 I.U.
Vitamin E (d'Alpha Tocopherol)	100 I.U.
Vitamin D3 (Cholecalciferol)	100 I.U.

Hydrosoluble (Sustained Release)

Folic Acid	200 mcg
Vitamin B1 (Thiamin HCl)	25 mg
Vitamin B2 (Riboflavin)	25 mg
Niacinamide	25 mg
Vitamin B6 (Pyridoxine HCl)	300 mg
Vitamin B12	62.5 mcg
Biotin	62.5 mcg
Pantothenic Acid (d'Cal. Pan)	25 mg
Choline Bitartrate	312.5 mg
Inositol	25 mg
Para Amino Benzoic Acid	25 mg
Vitamin C (Ascorbic Acid)	1,500 mg
Bioflavonoid	250 mg
Rutin	25 mg

Minerals

Calcium (Amino Acid Chelate)	125 mg
Magnesium (Amino Acid Chelate)	250 mg
Iodine (Hydrolyzed Protein Complex)	75 mcg
Iron (Amino Acid Chelate)	15 mg
Copper (Amino Acid Chelate)	0.5 mg
Zinc (Amino Acid Chelate)	25 mg
Manganese (Amino Acid Chelate)	10 mg
Potassium (Hydrolyzed Protein Complex)	47.5 mg
Selenium (Hydrolyzed Protein Complex)	100 mcg
Chromium (Hydrolyzed Protein Complex)	100 mcg

Digestive Aids

Amylase Activity	15,000 NF Units
Protease Activity	15,000 NF Units
Lipase Activity	1,200 NF Units
Betaine Acid HCl	100 mg

Indications: OPTIVITE for Women has been formulated for the adult premenopausal woman to help her cope with the tensions and stresses of every-day living. This is a multi-vitamin-mineral combination with emphasis on vitamin C, vitamin B-6 and the minerals magnesium and zinc. These nutrients are most susceptible to loss and poor utilization in women on hormonal contraceptive pills and with premenstrual distress.
OPTIVITE for Women does not replace but works together with a good nutritional program, adequate exercise, preferably outdoor, and proper rest.

Dosage and Administration: Since vitamins and minerals come naturally with food and our digestive system is accustomed to handle them together with food, OPTIVITE for Women works best when taken with a full meal. The effect lasts 8–12 hours and it is best taken with breakfast for day workers. It is recommended to build up the dose slowly by starting with 2 pills a day and increasing by 2 pills every week. Adjust the dose according to need. Most women need 2–6 tablets a day except one week before periods when the need increases. Do not exceed 12 tablets a day.

How Supplied: Yellow and modified capsule shaped tablets (riboflavin coated) in bottles of 126 and 252 tablets.

References:
1. Abraham, G.E.: Premenstrual tension, In Current Problems in OB Gyn. August 1980, page 1. Yearbook Medical Publishers, Chicago Levanthal, M. (Ed.).
2. Abraham, G.E.: Primary dysmenorrhea, Clin. Obstet. Gynecol. 21:139, 1978.
3. Abraham, G.E. and Hargrove, J.T.: Effect of vitamin B-6 on premenstrual symtomatology in women with premenstrual tension syndromes: A double blind crossover study. Infertility 3:155, 1980.
4. Abraham, G.E. and Lubran, M.M.: Serum and red cell magnesium levels in patients with premenstrual tension. Am. J. Clin. Nutr. 34:2364–2366, 1981.
Shown in Product Identification Section, page 419

Ortho Pharmaceutical Corporation
**Advanced Care Products Division
RARITAN, NJ 08869**

CONCEPTROL®
Birth Control Cream

Description: A contraceptive cream containing the active spermicide Nonoxynol-9 (5%), in an oil-in-water emulsion at pH 4.5.

Indication: Contraception.

Action and Uses: A spermicidal cream for intravaginal contraception.

Warning: Occasional burning and/or irritation of the vagina or penis have been reported. In such cases, the medication should be discontinued and a physician consulted. Not effective if taken orally. Keep out of reach of children. When pregnancy is contraindicated, the contraceptive program should be discussed with a health care professional.

Dosage and Administration: One applicatorful of CONCEPTROL should be inserted deeply into the vagina just before intercourse. An additional applicatorful is required each time intercourse is repeated. If intercourse has not occurred within one hour after application of CONCEPTROL, repeat the application before intercourse. If a douche is desired for cleansing purposes, wait at least six hours following intercourse. Refer to directions and diagrams for detailed instructions.
CONCEPTROL is an easy to use, pleasant and reliable method of birth control. While no method of contraception can provide an absolute guarantee against becoming pregnant, for maximum protection, CONCEPTROL Cream must be used according to directions.

How Supplied: CONCEPTROL Cream is available in a 2.46 oz. tube with re-usable applicator.

Continued on next page

Ortho Pharm.—Cont.

Storage: Conceptrol Cream should be stored at room temperature.

Shown in Product Identification Section, page 419

CONCEPTROL®
Contraceptive Gel

Description: An unscented, unflavored, colorless, greaseless and non-staining gel containing the active spermicide Nonoxynol-9 (4%) at pH 4.5.

Indications: Contraception

Actions: A spermicidal gel for use whenever control of conception is desirable.

Warnings: Occasional burning and/or irritation of the vagina or penis have been reported. If this occurs, discontinue use and consult a physician. Not effective if taken orally. Keep out of reach of children. When pregnancy is contraindicated, the contraceptive program should be discussed with a health care professional.

Dosage and Administration: One applicatorful of CONCEPTROL should be inserted deeply into the vagina just before intercourse. An additional applicatorful is required each time intercourse is repeated. If intercourse has not occurred within one hour after the application of CONCEPTROL, repeat the application of CONCEPTROL before intercourse.

Douching is not recommended after using CONCEPTROL Gel. However, if desired for cleansing purposes, wait at least six hours following last intercourse to allow for full spermicidal activity of CONCEPTROL Gel.

While no method of contraception can provide an absolute guarantee against becoming pregnant, for maximum protection, CONCEPTROL Gel must be used according to directions.

How Supplied: CONCEPTROL Gel is available in a 2.46 oz. tube with re-usable applicator.

Storage: CONCEPTROL Gel should be stored at room temperature.

Shown in Product Identification Section, page 419

CONCEPTROL® Disposable
Contraceptive Gel

Description: An unscented, unflavored, colorless, greaseless and non-staining gel in convenient, easy-to-use disposable plastic applicators. Each applicator is filled with a single, pre-measured dose containing the active spermicide Nonoxynol-9 (4%) at pH 4.5.

Indication: Contraception

Actions and Uses: A spermicidal gel for use whenever control of conception is desirable.

Warning: Occasional burning and/or irritation of the vagina or penis have

been reported. If this occurs, discontinue use and consult a physician. Not effective if taken orally. Keep out of reach of children. When pregnancy is contraindicated, the contraceptive program should be discussed with a health care professional.

Dosage and Administration: One applicatorful of CONCEPTROL should be inserted deeply into the vagina just before intercourse. An additional applicatorful is required each time intercourse is repeated. If intercourse has not occurred within one hour after the application of CONCEPTROL, repeat the application of CONCEPTROL before intercourse.

Douching is not recommended after using CONCEPTROL Gel. However, if desired for cleansing purposes, wait at least six hours following last intercourse to allow for full spermicidal activity of CONCEPTROL Gel.

While no method of contraception can provide an absolute guarantee against becoming pregnant, for maximum protection, CONCEPTROL Gel must be used according to directions.

How Supplied: CONCEPTROL Gel is available in packages of 6 and 10 disposable applicators, premeasured, prefilled, prewrapped.

Storage: Conceptrol Gel should be stored at room temperature.

Shown in Product Identification Section, page 419

DELFEN®
Contraceptive Foam

Description: A contraceptive foam in an aerosol dosage formulation containing 12.5% Nonoxynol-9 and buffered to normal vaginal pH 4.5.

Indication: Contraception.

Action and Uses: A spermicidal foam for intravaginal contraception.

Warning: Occasional burning and/or irritation of the vagina or penis have been reported. In such cases, the medication should be discontinued and a physician consulted. Not effective if taken orally. Keep out of reach of children. When pregnancy is contraindicated, the contraceptive program should be discussed with a health care professional.

Dosage and Administration: Insert DELFEN Contraceptive Foam just prior to each intercourse. You may have intercourse any time up to one hour after you have inserted the foam. If you repeat intercourse, insert another applicatorful of DELFEN Foam. After shaking the vial, place the measured-dose (5cc) applicator over the top of the vial, then press applicator down very gently. Fill to the top of the barrel threads. Remove applicator to stop flow of foam. Insert the filled applicator well into the vagina and depress the plunger. Remove the applicator with the plunger in depressed position. If a douche is desired for cleansing purposes, wait at least six hours after intercourse. Refer to directions and dia-

grams for detailed instructions. DELFEN Foam is a reliable method of birth control. While no method of birth control can provide an absolute guarantee against becoming pregnant, for maximum protection, DELFEN Foam must be used according to directions.

How Supplied: DELFEN Contraceptive Foam 0.70 oz. Starter vial with applicator. Also available in 0.70 oz. and 1.75 oz. Refill vials without applicator.

Storage: Contents under pressure. Do not puncture or incinerate container. Do not expose to heat or store at temperatures above 120°F.

Shown in Product Identification Section, page 419

DIMENSYN™
Maximum Strength
Menstrual Discomfort Relief

Description: Each DIMENSYN capsule contains the maximum strength levels of each of three ingredients for symptomatic relief of menstrual discomfort: acetaminophen 500mg, pamabrom 25mg, and pyrilamine maleate 15mg.

Indications: For the temporary relief of: emotional changes related to the premenstrual period such as irritability, nervous tension, and anxiety; pain of the premenstrual and menstrual periods; and temporary water weight gain, bloating, swelling and/or full feeling associated with the premenstrual and menstrual periods.

Actions and Uses: Each DIMENSYN capsule contains a non-aspirin analgesic (acetaminophen), a non-caffeine diuretic (pamabrom), and an antihistamine (pyrilamine maleate) to help relieve common menstrual discomfort symptoms.

Warning: Do not use for more than 10 days consecutively without seeking the advice of your physician. As with any medication, if you are or may be pregnant or are nursing a baby, seek advice of a health care professional before using this product. May cause drowsiness. If this occurs, do not operate a motor vehicle or heavy machinery. Keep this and all medication out of the reach of children. Do not exceed recommended dosages. In case of accidental overdose, seek professional assistance or contact a poison control center immediately.

Dosage and Administration: 2 capsules orally every 3 to 4 hours, as needed, up to 8 capsules in any 24-hour period.

How Supplied: Packages of 24 or 48 capsules each.

Shown in Product Identification Section, page 419

GYNOL II®
Contraceptive Jelly

Description: A colorless, unscented, unflavored, greaseless and non-staining contraceptive jelly containing the active spermicide Nonoxynol-9 (2%) and having a pH of 4.5

Indication: Contraception

Actions and Uses: An aesthetically pleasing spermicidal jelly to be used in conjunction with a diaphragm whenever control of conception is desired.

Warning: Occasional burning and/or irritation of the vagina or penis have been reported. In such cases, the medication should be discontinued and a physician consulted. Not effective if taken orally. Keep out of reach of children. When pregnancy is contraindicated, the contraceptive program should be discussed with a health care professional.

Dosage and Administration: Used in conjunction with a vaginal diaphragm. Prior to insertion, put about a teaspoonful of GYNOL II Contraceptive Jelly into the cup of the dome of the diaphragm and spread a small amount around the edge with your fingertip. This will aid in insertion and provide protection.
Some doctors recommend that the diaphragm be inserted every night to avoid unprotected intercourse.
It is also important to remember that if intercourse occurs more than six hours after insertion, or if repeated intercourse takes place, an additional application of GYNOL II is necessary. DO NOT REMOVE THE DIAPHRAGM—simply add more GYNOL II with the applicator provided in the applicator package, being careful not to dislodge the diaphragm.
Remember, another application of GYNOL II is required each time intercourse is repeated, regardless of how little time has transpired since the diaphragm has been in place. In addition, it is essential that the diaphragm remain in place for at least 6 hours after intercourse. Removal of the diaphragm before this time may increase the risk of becoming pregnant. The diaphragm should not be worn continuously for more than 24 hours. If a douche is desired for cleansing purposes, wait at least six hours after intercourse. While no method of contraception can provide an absolute guarantee against becoming pregnant, for maximum protection, GYNOL II must be used according to directions.

How Supplied: 81 gm starter tube with measured dose applicator and large size 126 gm refill package.

Storage: Gynol II should be stored at room temperature.
Shown in Product Identification Section, page 419

INTERCEPT®
Contraceptive Inserts

Description: An effervescent, single dose vaginal contraceptive insert containing the active spermicide Nonoxynol-9, (100 mg) at pH 4.5.

Indication: Contraception

Action: A spermicidal insert for intravaginal contraception.

Warning: Occasional burning and/or irritation of the vagina or penis have been reported. Should sensitivity to the ingredients or irritation of the vagina or penis develop, discontinue use and consult a physician. Not effective if taken orally. Keep out of reach of children. When pregnancy is contraindicated, the contraceptive program should be discussed with a health care professional.

Dosage and Administration: INTERCEPT should be inserted into the vagina at least ten minutes prior to male penetration to insure proper dispersion. INTERCEPT provides protection from ten minutes to one hour after product insertion. Insert a new INTERCEPT Contraceptive Insert each time intercourse is repeated. If a douche is desired for cleansing purposes, wait at least six hours following intercourse.
INTERCEPT is an effective method of contraception. While no method of birth control can provide an absolute guarantee against becoming pregnant, for maximum protection, Intercept must be used according to directions.

How Supplied: INTERCEPT Contraceptive Inserts are available in a starter package containing 12 inserts with applicator and in a 12 insert refill package.

Storage: Avoid exposing Intercept to excessive heat (over 86°F or 30°C).
Shown in Product Identification Section, page 419

MASSÉ®
Breast Cream

Composition: MASSE Breast Cream.

Action and Uses: MASSE Breast Cream is especially designed for care of the nipples of pregnant and nursing women.

Administration and Dosage:
BEFORE BIRTH
During the last two or three months of pregnancy, it is often desirable to prepare the nipple and the nipple area of the breast for eventual nursing. In these cases, MASSE is used once or twice daily in the following manner: Carefully cleanse the breast with a soft, clean cloth and plain water and dry. Squeeze a ribbon of MASSE, approximately an inch long, and lightly massage into the nipple and immediate surrounding area. Do so until the cream has completely disappeared. The massage motion should be gentle and outward.
AFTER BABY IS BORN
During the nursing period MASSE is used as follows: BEFORE AND AFTER EACH NURSING cleanse the breasts with a clean cloth and water. After drying squeeze a ribbon of MASSE, approximately an inch long, and gently massage into the nipple and the immediate surrounding area.

Contraindications: MASSE should not be used in cases of acute mastitis or breast abscess.

Caution: In cases of excessive tenderness or irritation of any kind, consult your physician.

How Supplied: MASSE Breast Cream is available in a 2 oz. tube.

Storage: Massé should be stored at room temperature.
Shown in Product Identification Section, page 419

MICATIN®
Antifungal For Athlete's Foot

Description: An antifungal containing the active ingredient miconazole nitrate 2%, clinically proven to cure athlete's foot, jock itch and ringworm.

Indications: Athlete's foot (tinea pedis), jock itch (tinea cruris), and ringworm (tinea corporis).

Actions and Uses: Proven clinically effective in the treatment of athlete's foot (tinea pedis), jock itch (tinea cruris), and ringworm (tinea corporis). For effective relief of the itching, scaling, burning and discomfort that can accompany these conditions.

Directions: Cleanse skin with soap and water and dry thoroughly. Apply a thin layer of MICATIN over affected area morning and night or as directed by a doctor. For athlete's foot, pay special attention to the spaces between the toes. It is also helpful to wear well-fitting, ventilated shoes and to change shoes and socks at least once daily. Best results in athlete's foot and ringworm are usually obtained with 4 weeks' use of this product and in jock itch with 2 weeks' use. If satisfactory results have not occurred within these times, consult a doctor or pharmacist. Children under 12 years of age should be supervised in the use of this product. This product is not effective on the scalp or nails.
Do not use on children under 2 years of age except under the advise and supervision of a doctor. For external use only. If irritation occurs, or if there is no improvement within 4 weeks (for athlete's foot or ringworm) or within 2 weeks (for jock itch), discontinue use and consult a doctor or pharmacist. Keep this and all drugs out of the reach of children. In case of accidental ingestion, seek professional assistance or contact a Poison Control Center immediately.

How Supplied:
MICATIN® Antifungal Cream is available in a 0.5 oz. tube and a 1.0 oz. tube.
MICATIN Antifungal Spray Powder is available in a 3.0 oz. aerosol can.
MICATIN Antifungal Powder is available in a 1.5 oz. plastic bottle.
MICATIN Antifungal Spray Liquid is available in a 3.5 oz. aerosol can.

Storage: Store at room temerature.
Shown in Product Identification Section, page 419

MICATIN®
Antifungal For Jock Itch

Description: An antifungal containing the active ingredient miconazole nitrate 2%, clinically proven to cure jock itch.

Continued on next page

Ortho Pharm.—Cont.

Indications: Jock itch (tinea cruris).

Actions and Uses: Proven clinically effective in the treatment of jock itch (tinea cruris). For effective relief of the itching, scaling, burning and discomfort that can accompany this condition.

Directions: Cleanse skin with soap and water and dry thoroughly. Apply a thin layer of product over affected area morning and night or as directed by a doctor. Best results are usually obtained within 2 weeks' use of this product. If satisfactory results have not occurred within this time, consult a doctor or pharmacist. Children under 12 years of age should be supervised in the use of this product. This product is not effective on the scalp or nails.

Warnings: Do not use on children under 2 years of age except under the advice and supervision of a doctor. For external use only. If irritation occurs, or if there is no improvement of jock itch within 2 weeks, discontinue use and consult a doctor or pharmacist. Keep this and all drugs out of the reach of children. In case of accidental ingestion, seek professional assistance or contact a Poison Control Center immediately.

How Supplied:
MICATIN® Jock Itch Cream is available in a 0.5 oz. tube.
MICATIN Jock Itch Spray Powder is available in a 3.0 oz. aerosol can.

Storage: Store at room temperature.
Shown in Product Identification Section, page 419

ORTHO–CREME®
Contraceptive Cream

Description: ORTHO-CREME Contraceptive Cream is a white, pleasantly scented cream of cosmetic consistency. ORTHO-CREME is a greaseless, non-staining and non-irritating spermicidal cream containing the active spermicide Nonoxynol-9 (2%), at pH 4.5.

Indication: Contraception.

Action and Uses: An aesthetically pleasing spermicidal vaginal cream for use with a vaginal diaphragm when control of conception is desirable.

Warning: Occasional burning and/or irritation of the vagina or penis have been reported. In such cases, the medication should be discontinued and a physician consulted. Not effective if taken orally. Keep out of reach of children. When pregnancy is contraindicated the contraceptive program should be discussed with a health care professional.

Dosage and Administration: Used in conjunction with a vaginal diaphragm. Prior to insertion, put about a teaspoonful of ORTHO-CREME Contraceptive Cream into the cup of the dome of the diaphragm and spread a small amount around the edge with the fingertip. This

will aid in insertion and provide protection.
Some doctors recommend that the diaphragm be inserted every night to avoid unprotected intercourse.
It is also important to remember that if intercourse occurs more than six hours after insertion, or if repeated intercourse takes place, an additional application of ORTHO-CREME is necessary. DO NOT REMOVE THE DIAPHRAGM—simply add more ORTHO-CREME with the applicator provided in the applicator package, being careful not to dislodge the diaphragm.
Remember, another application of OR-THO-CREME is required each time intercourse is repeated, regardless of how little time has transpired since the diaphragm has been in place.
In addition, it is essential that the diaphragm remain in place for at least six hours after intercourse. Removal of the diaphragm before this time may increase the risk of becoming pregnant. The diaphragm should not be worn continuously for more than 24 hours. If a douche is desired for cleansing purposes, wait at least 6 hours after intercourse. Refer to directions and diagrams for detailed instructions. While no method of contraception can provide an absolute guarantee against becoming pregnant, for maximum protection, ORTHO-CREME must be used according to directions.

How Supplied: 2.46 oz. Starter tube with measured-dose applicator. Regular size 2.46 oz. Refill tube only. Large size 4.05 oz. Refill tube only.

Storage: Ortho-Creme should be stored at room temperature.
Shown in Product Identification Section, page 419

ORTHO® Disposable
Vaginal Applicators

Action and Uses: ORTHO Disposable applicators are made of paperboard and are designed to provide a simple, clean, accurate method for inserting tubed vaginal jellies and creams into the vagina. The applicator may be readily filled directly from the tube used and then discarded.

How Supplied: Packages of 18 applicators each.
Shown in Product Identification Section, page 420

ORTHO–GYNOL®
Contraceptive Jelly

Description: ORTHO-GYNOL Contraceptive Jelly is a water dispersible spermicidal jelly having a pH of 4.5 and contains the active spermicide p-diisobutyl-phenoxypolyethoxyethanol (1%).

Indication: Contraception.

Action and Uses: An aesthetically pleasing spermicidal vaginal jelly for use with a vaginal diaphragm whenever the control of conception is desirable.

Warning: Occasional burning and/or irritation of the vagina or penis have been reported. In such cases, the medication should be discontinued and a physician consulted. Not effective if taken orally. Keep out of reach of children. When pregnancy is contraindicated, the contraceptive program should be discussed with a health care professsional.

Dosage and Administration: Used in conjunction with a vaginal diaphragm. Prior to insertion, put about a teaspoonful of ORTHO-GYNOL Contraceptive Jelly into the cup of the dome of the diaphragm and spread a small amount around the edge with the fingertip. This will aid in insertion and provide protection.
Some doctors recommend that the diaphragm be inserted every night to avoid unprotected intercourse.
It is also important to remember that if intercourse occurs more than six hours after insertion, or if repeated intercourse takes place, an additional application of ORTHO-GYNOL is necessary. DO NOT REMOVE THE DIAPHRAGM—simply add more ORTHO-GYNOL with the applicator provided in the applicator package, being careful not to dislodge the diaphragm.
Remember, another application of OR-THO-GYNOL is required each time intercourse is repeated, regardless of how little time has transpired since the diaphragm has been in place.
In addition, it is essential that the diaphragm remain in place for at least six hours after intercourse. Removal of the diaphragm before this time may increase the risk of becoming pregnant. The diaphragm should not be worn continuously for more than 24 hours. If a douche is desired for cleansing purposes, wait at least 6 hours after intercourse. Refer to directions and diagrams for complete instructions. While no method of contraception can provide an absolute guarantee against becoming pregnant, for maximum protection ORTHO-GYNOL must be used according to directions.

How Supplied: 2.85 oz. Starter tube with measured-dose applicator. Regular size 2.85 oz. Refill tube only. Large size 4.44 oz. Refill tube only.

Storage: Ortho-Gynol should be stored at room temperature.
Shown in Product Identification Section, page 420

ORTHO® PERSONAL LUBRICANT

Description: ORTHO PERSONAL LUBRICANT is a non-staining, water soluble lubricating jelly that is safe for delicate tissues.

Indications: ORTHO PERSONAL LUBRICANT is especially formulated as a sexual lubricant that is designed to be gentle and non-irritating for both women and men. It may also be used for easy insertion of rectal thermometers, tampons, douche nozzles and enema nozzles.

Dosage and Administration: Apply a one (1″) to two (2″) inch ribbon of product, or desired amount, to external vaginal area and/or penis. Repeat applications may be used by one or both partners. If desired, this product may be used inside the vagina.

Precaution: ORTHO PERSONAL LUBRICANT does not contain spermicide. It is not a contraceptive.

How Supplied: ORTHO PERSONAL LUBRICANT is available in 2 oz. and 4 oz. tubes.

Storage: Store at room temperature (59–86°F). Do not freeze.
Shown in Product Identification Section, page 420

Ortho Pharmaceutical Corporation
DERMATOLOGICAL DIVISION
RARITAN, NJ 08869

PURPOSE® Dry Skin Cream

Composition: Contains purified water, petrolatum, propylene glycol, glyceryl stearate, sodium lactate, almond oil, steareth-20, cetyl alcohol, cetyl esters wax, mineral oil, steareth-2, xanthan gum, sorbic acid, lactic acid and fragrance.

Action and Uses: PURPOSE Dry Skin Cream is formulated especially to meet the need for an effective dry skin cream that dermatologists can recommend. PURPOSE Dry Skin Cream moisturizes dry, chapped and irritated skin and provides effective, lasting relief from drying and scaling. PURPOSE Dry Skin Cream smoothes easily into skin for all-over body care.

Administration and Dosage: Instruct patients to use PURPOSE Dry Skin Cream as any other dry skin cream.

How Supplied: 3 oz. tube.
Shown in Product Identification Section, page 420

PURPOSE® Shampoo

Composition: Contains water, amphoteric 19, PEG-44 sorbitan laurate, PEG-150 distearate, sorbitan laurate, boric acid, fragrance, and benzyl alcohol.

Action and Uses: PURPOSE Shampoo is formulated especially to meet the need for a mild shampoo that dermatologists can recommend. PURPOSE Shampoo helps control oily scalp and hair and helps remove the scales of dandruff leaving hair clean and manageable. Safe for color-treated hair. PURPOSE Shampoo works into a rich, pleasant lather. It may be used daily.

Administration and Dosage: Instruct patients to use PURPOSE Shampoo as any other shampoo.

How Supplied: 8 fluid oz. plastic bottle.
Shown in Product Identification Section, page 420

PURPOSE® Soap

Composition: Contains sodium and potassium salts of fatty acids, glycerin, water and mild fragrance.

Action and Uses: Extraordinary mild PURPOSE Soap was created to wash tender, sensitive skin. Formulated especially to meet the need for a mild soap that dermatologists can recommend. This translucent washing bar is non-medicated and completely free of harsh detergents or other ingredients that might dry or irritate skin.

Administration and Dosage: Wash face with PURPOSE Soap two or three times a day or as directed by your physician. Rinse with warm water. For complete skin care, use it also for bath and shower.

How Supplied: 3.6 oz. and 6 oz. bars.
Shown in Product Identification Section, page 420

Paddock Laboratories, Inc.
3101 LOUISIANA AVE. NORTH
MINNEAPOLIS, MN 55427

EMULSOIL®
Castor Oil

Emulsoil is a self-emulsifying, flavored castor oil formulated to instantly mix with any beverage.

Active Ingredient: Each 2-ounce bottle contains 95% w/w Castor Oil, USP with self-emulsifying and natural sugarless flavoring agents.

Indications: Emulsoil is used in the preparation of the small and large bowel for radiography, colonoscopy, surgery, proctologic procedures and exploratory IVP use. Can also be used for isolated bouts of constipation.

Warnings: Not to be used when abdominal pain, nausea, vomiting or other symptoms of appendicitis are present. Frequent or prolonged use may result in dependence on laxatives. Do not use during pregnancy except under competent advice.

Dosage and Administration: Adults: 1–4 tablespoonfuls. Children: 1–2 teaspoonfuls.

How Supplied: Available in 2-ounce bottles. Packaged 12 and 48 bottles per case.

GLUTOSE®
Dextrose Gel

Active Ingredient: Dextrose 40%, Each 80-gram bottle contains 32 grams dextrose in a dye free jel base.

Indications: Glutose is a concentrated glucose (40% Dextrose) used for insulin reactions and hypoglycemic states.

Dosage and Administration: Usual dose is $\frac{1}{3}$ bottle Glutose (10 grams dextrose) orally, which can be repeated in 10 minutes if necessary. Response should be noticed in 10 minutes. The physician should then be notified when a hypoglycemic reaction occurs so that the insulin dose can be accurately adjusted. Glutose should not be given to children under 2 years of age unless otherwise directed by physician.

How Supplied: Packaged in an 80-gram squeeze bottle with a quick open dispenser top. Packaged in 6 and 12 bottles per case.

IPECAC SYRUP

Active Ingredients: Ipecac Syrup, USP contains in each 30 ml, not less than 36.9 mg and not more than 47.1 mg of the total ether soluble alkaloids of ipecac. The content of emetine and cephaeline together is not less than 90.0% of the amount of the total ether-soluble alkaloids.

Indications: Ipecac Syrup is indicated for emergency use to cause vomiting in poisoning.

Warnings: Do not use in unconscious persons. Ordinarily, this drug should not be used if strychnine, corrosives such as alkalies, lye and strong acids, or petroleum distillates such as kerosene, gasoline, coal oil, fuel oil, paint thinners, or cleaning fluids have been ingested.

Dosage and Administration: Usual Dosage: One tablespoonful (15 ml) followed by one to two glasses of water, in persons over 1 year of age. Repeat dosage in 20 minutes if vomiting does not occur.

How Supplied: Available in 1-ounce bottles. Packaged 12 bottles per case.

Products are indexed alphabetically in the
PINK SECTION

Products are cross-indexed by product classifications in the
BLUE SECTION

Products are cross-indexed by generic and chemical names in the
YELLOW SECTION

Parke-Davis
Division of Warner-Lambert
Company
201 TABOR ROAD
MORRIS PLAINS, NJ 07950

AGORAL® Plain
AGORAL® Raspberry
AGORAL® Marshmallow

Description: Each tablespoonful (15 ml) of Agoral Plain (white) contains 4.2 grams mineral oil in a thoroughly homogenized emulsion with agar, tragacanth, acacia, egg albumin, glycerin and water.
Each tablespoonful (15 ml) of Agoral Raspberry (pink) or of Agoral Marshmallow (white) contains 4.2 grams mineral oil and 0.2 grams phenolphthalein in a thoroughly homogenized emulsion with agar, tragacanth, acacia, egg albumin, glycerin and water.

Actions: Agoral, containing mineral oil, facilitates defecation by lubricating the fecal mass and softening the stool. More effective than nonemulsified oil in penetrating the feces, Agoral thereby greatly reduces the possibility of oil leakage at the anal sphincter. Phenolphthalein gently stimulates motor activity of the lower intestinal tract. Agoral's combined lubricating-softening and peristaltic actions can help to restore a normal pattern of evacuation.

Indications: Relief of constipation. Agoral may be especially required when straining at stool is a hazard, as in hernia, cardiac, or hypertensive patients; during convalescence from surgery; before and after surgery for hemorrhoids or other painful anorectal disorders; for patients confined to bed.
The management of chronic constipation should also include attention to fluid intake, diet and bowel habits.

Contraindication: Sensitivity to phenolphthalein.

Dosage and Management:
(Taken at bedtime, laxation may be expected the next morning.)

	Adults	Children over 6 years
Agoral Plain (without phenolphthalein)	1 to 2 tblsp.	2 to 4 tsp.
Agoral Raspberry	½ to 1 tblsp.	1 to 2 tsp.
Agoral Marshmallow	½ to 1 tblsp.	1 to 2 tsp.

Take at bedtime only, unless other time is advised by physician.
Agoral may be taken alone or in milk, water, fruit juice, or any miscible food. Expectant or nursing mothers, bedridden or aged patients, young children or infants should use only on advice of physician.

Supplied: Agoral Plain (without phenolphthalein), plastic bottles of 16 fl oz (N 0071-2071-23). Agoral (raspberry flavor), plastic bottles of 16 fl oz (N 0071-2072-23). Agoral (marshmallow flavor), plastic bottles of 8 fl oz (N 0071-2070-20) and 16 fl oz (N 0071-2070-23).

ANUSOL®
Suppositories/Ointment

Description:

	Anusol Suppositories each contains	Anusol Ointment each gram
Bismuth subgallate	2.25%	—
Bismuth Resorcin Compound	1.75%	—
Benzyl Benzoate	1.2 %	12 mg
Peruvian Balsam	1.8 %	18 mg
Zinc Oxide	11.0 %	110 mg
Analgine™ (pramoxine hydrochloride)	—	10 mg

Also contain the following inactive ingredients: calcium phosphate dibasic; coconut oil base, FD&C blue No. 2 Lake and red No. 40 Lake, hydrogenated fatty acid.

Also contains the following inactive ingredients: calcium phosphate dibasic, NF; cocoa butter, NF; glyceryl monooleate; glyceryl monostearate; kaolin, NF; mineral oil, USP; polyethylene wax.

Actions: Anusol Suppositories and Anusol Ointment help to relieve pain, itching and discomfort arising from irritated anorectal tissues. They have a soothing, lubricant action on mucous membranes. Analgine (pramoxine hydrochloride) in Anusol Ointment is a rapidly acting local anesthetic for the skin and mucous membranes of the anus and rectum. Analgine is also chemically distinct from procaine, cocaine, and dibucaine and can often be used in the patient previously sensitized to other surface anesthetics. Surface analgesia lasts for several hours.

Indications: Anusol Suppositories and Anusol Ointment are adjunctive therapy for the symptomatic relief of pain and discomfort in: external and internal hemorrhoids, proctitis, papillitis, cryptitis, anal fissures, incomplete fistulas, and relief of local pain and discomfort following anorectal surgery.
Anusol Ointment is also indicated for pruritus ani.

Contraindications: Anusol Suppositories and Anusol Ointment are contraindicated in those patients with a history of hypersensitivity to any of the components of the preparations.

Precautions: Symptomatic relief should not delay definitive diagnoses or treatment.
If irritation develops, these preparations should be discontinued. Keep this and all drugs out of the reach of children. In case of accidental ingestion seek professional assistance or contact a Poison Control Center immediately.

Adverse Reactions: Upon application of Anusol Ointment, which contains Analgine (pramoxine HCl), a patient may occasionally experience burning, especially if the anoderm is not intact. Sensitivity reactions have been rare; discontinue medication if suspected.

Dosage and Administration: Anusol Suppositories—Adults: Remove foil wrapper and insert suppository into the anus. Insert one suppository in the morning and one at bedtime, and one immediately following each evacuation.
Anusol Ointment—Adults: After gentle bathing and drying of the anal area, remove tube cap and apply freely to the exterior surface and gently rub in. Ointment should be applied every 3 or 4 hours, or, when necessary, every 2 hours. NOTE: If staining from either of the above products occurs, the stain may be removed from fabric by hand or machine washing with household detergent.

How Supplied: Anusol Suppositories—boxes of 12 (N 0071-1088-07), 24 (N 0071-1088-13) and 48 (N 0071-1088-18); in silver foil strips.
Anusol Ointment—1-oz tubes (N 0071-3075-13) and 2-oz tubes (N 0071-3075-15) with plastic applicator.
Store between 15° and 30°C (59° and 86°F).
Shown in Product Identification Section, page 420

BENADRYL® Antihistamine Cream

Description: Greaseless disappearing cream contains 2% Benadryl (diphenhydramine hydrochloride) in a water-miscible ointment base.

Indications: For relief of itching due to insect bites and other minor skin irritations (rashes, inflammation). FOR EXTERNAL USE ONLY.

Warning: Should not be applied to blistered, raw or oozing areas of the skin. If burning sensation results, discontinue use. In case of accidental ingestion, seek professional assistance or contact a Poison Control Center immediately.

Caution: Do not use in eyes. If condition persists or a rash or irritation develops, discontinue use and consult a physician.

Directions: Apply locally for itching three or four times daily or as directed by the physician.

How Supplied:
1-oz tubes (N 0071-3058-13)
2-oz tubes (N 0071-3058-15)
Shown in Product Identification Section, page 420

BENYLIN®
Cough Syrup

Description: Each teaspoonful (5 ml) contains Benadryl® (diphenhydramine hydrochloride), 12.5 mg. Alcohol, 5%. Also contains: ammonium chloride, USP; caramel, NF; citric acid anhydrous, USP; D&C Red No. 33; FD&C Red No. 40; Glycerin, USP; glucose liquid, NF; menthol,

USP; Raspberry Imitation flavor; sodium citrate, USP; sodium saccharin, USP; sugar, NF; water, purified, USP.

Indications: For the temporary relief of cough due to minor throat and bronchial irritation as may occur with the common cold or with inhaled irritants.

Warnings: May cause marked drowsiness. Keep this and all drugs out of the reach of children. In case of accidental overdosage, seek professional assistance or contact a poison control center immediately. Do not give to children under 6 years of age except under the advice and supervision of a physician. May cause excitability, especially in children. Do not take this product for persistent or chronic cough such as occurs with smoking, asthma, emphysema, or when cough is accompanied by excessive secretions, or if you have epilepsy, glaucoma, or difficulty in urination due to enlargement of the prostate gland except under the advice and supervision of a physician. As with any drug, if you are pregnant or nursing a baby, seek the advice of a health professional before using this product.

Caution: Avoid driving a motor vehicle or operating heavy machinery, or drinking alcoholic beverages. A persistent cough may be a sign of a serious condition. If cough persists for more than one week, tends to recur, or is accompanied by high fever, rash, or persistent headache, consult a physician.

Directions: Adults—two teaspoonfuls every four hours, not to exceed twelve teaspoonfuls in twenty-four hours; Children (6 to under 12 years), one teaspoonful every four hours not to exceed six teaspoonfuls in twenty-four hours; or as directed by a physician. Children (2 to under 6 years), one half teaspoonful every four hours not to exceed three teaspoonfuls in twenty-four hours. Use in children under 2 years of age is only at the discretion of the physician.

How Supplied: N 0071-2195-Benylin Cough Syrup is supplied in 4-oz, 8-oz, 1-pt, and 1-gal bottles.
Store below 30°C (86°F). Protect from freezing.
Shown in Product Identification Section, page 420

BENYLIN DM®
dextromethorphan cough syrup

Description: Each teaspoonful (5 ml) contains 10 mg dextromethorphan hydrobromide and 5% alcohol; also contains, ammonium chloride, USP; caramel, NF; citric acid, anhydrous, USP; D&C Red No. 33, glucose liquid, NF; glycerin, USP; menthol, USP; raspberry flavor; sodium citrate, USP; sugar; water, purified USP.
Nonnarcotic; Contains No Antihistamine

Indications: Antitussive—For the temporary relief of coughs due to minor throat and bronchial irritation as may

occur with the common cold or with inhaled irritants

Warnings: Keep this and all drugs out of the reach of children. In case of accidental overdosage, seek professional assistance or contact a poison control center immediately. Do not give this product to children under 2 years of age, except under the advice and supervision of a physician. Do not take this product for persistent or chronic cough such as occurs with smoking, asthma, or emphysema, or where cough is accompanied by excessive secretions, except under the advice and supervision of a physician. As with any drug, if you are pregnant or nursing a baby, seek the advice of a health professional before using this product.

Caution: A persistent cough may be a sign of a serious condition. If cough persists for more than 1 week, tends to recur, or is accompanied by high fever, rash, or persistent headache, consult a physician.

Dosage: For the temporary relief of cough—
Adults—1 to 2 teaspoonfuls every 4 hours, or 3 teaspoonfuls every 6 to 8 hours, not to exceed 12 teaspoonfuls in 24 hours
Children 6 to under 12 years—½ to 1 teaspoonful every 4 hours, or 1½ teaspoonfuls every 6 to 8 hours, not to exceed 6 teaspoonfuls in 24 hours
Children 2 to under 6 years—¼ to ½ teaspoonful every 4 hours, or ¾ teaspoonful every 6 to 8 hours, not to exceed 3 teaspoonfuls in 24 hours
Children under 2 years—there is no recommended dosage, except under the advice and supervision of a physician

How Supplied: N 0071-2401: 4-oz and 8-oz bottles.
Store below 30°C (86°F). Protect from freezing.
Shown in Product Identification Section, page 420

CALADRYL® Lotion
CALADRYL Cream

Description: Caladryl Lotion—A drying, calamine-antihistamine lotion containing calamine, 1% Benadryl® (diphenhydramine hydrochloride), camphor, and 2% alcohol. Also contains: fragrance; glycerin USP; sodium carboxymethyl-cellulose, USP; and water, purified, USP.
Caladryl Cream—a drying, calamine-antihistaminic cream containing calamine, 1% Benadryl (diphenhydramine hydrochloride) and camphor. Also contains: cetyl alcohol, NF; cresin white; fragrance; propylene glycol, USP; proplyparaben, USP; polysorbate 60; sorbitan monostearate; water, purified USP.

Indications: For relief of itching due to mild poison ivy or oak, insect bites, or other minor skin irritations, and soothing relief of mild sunburn

Warnings: Should not be applied to blistered, raw, or oozing areas of the skin.

Discontinue use if burning sensation or rash develops or condition persists. Remove by washing with soap and water. Use on extensive areas of the skin or for longer than seven days only as directed by a physician.

Caution: Keep away from eyes or other mucous membranes.
FOR EXTERNAL USE ONLY
Keep this and all drugs out of the reach of children. In case of accidental ingestion, seek professional assistance or contact a Poison Control Center immediately.

Directions: Caladryl Cream—Apply topically three or four times daily. Cleanse skin with soap and water and dry area before each application.
Caladryl Lotion—SHAKE WELL. Apply topically three or four times daily. Cleanse skin with soap and water and dry area before each application.

How Supplied: N 0071-3226-14: Caladryl Cream; 1½-oz tubes
N0071-3181: Caladryl Lotion—2½ fl.-oz. (75 ml) squeeze bottles and 6 fl.-oz. bottles.
Shown in Product Identification Section, page 420

GELUSIL®
Antacid–Anti-gas
Liquid/Tablets

Each teaspoonful (5 ml) or tablet contains:
200 mg aluminum hydroxide
200 mg magnesium hydroxide
25 mg simethicone

Advantages:
- High acid-neutralizing capacity
- Low sodium content
- Simethicone for antiflatulent activity
- Good taste for better patient compliance
- Fast dissolution of chewed tablets for prompt relief

Indications: Gelusil, a carefully balanced combination of two widely used antacids and the antiflatulent simethicone, is effective for the relief of symptoms associated with heartburn, sour stomach, and acid indigestion with gas. Gelusil provides symptomatic relief of hyperacidity associated with the diagnosis of peptic ulcer, gastritis, peptic esophagitis, gastric hyperacidity and hiatal hernia, and it alleviates or relieves the symptoms of gas and postoperative gas pain.

Actions and Uses: The proven neutralizing powers of aluminum hydroxide and of magnesium hydroxide combine to give Gelusil dependable antacid action with-

Continued on next page

This product information was prepared in December 1984. On these and other Parke-Davis Products, detailed information may be obtained by addressing PARKE-DAVIS, Division of Warner-Lambert Company, Morris Plains, NJ 07950.

Parke-Davis—Cont.

out the acid rebound sometimes associated with calcium carbonate.

The pleasant peppermint-flavored taste of Gelusil Liquid and Tablets encourages patient acceptance of, and compliance with, recommended antacid-anti-gas regimens.

Gelusil Tablets are easy to chew and are specifically formulated to dissolve readily, providing prompt onset of action and reliable relief of symptoms.

Gelusil is appropriate whenever there is a need for well-accepted, effective antacid-anti-gas therapy.

Dosage and Administration: Two or more teaspoonfuls or tablets one hour after meals and at bedtime, or as directed by a physician.

Tablets should be chewed.

The following information is provided to facilitate treatment:

Gelusil	LIQUID	TABLETS
Acid-neutral-izing capacity	24 mEq/ 10 ml	22 mEq/ 2 tabs
Sodium	0.7 mg/ 5 ml	0.8 mg/ tab
Lactose	0	0

Warnings: Do not take more than 12 tablets or teaspoonfuls in a 24-hour period, or use this maximum dosage for more than two weeks, or use this product if you have kidney disease, except under the advice and supervision of a physician.

Keep this and all drugs out of the reach of children.

Drug Interaction Precaution: Do not take this product if you are presently taking a prescription antibiotic drug containing any form of tetracycline.

All aluminum-containing antacids, including Gelusil, may prevent proper absorption of tetracycline.

How Supplied:

N 0071-2036—Liquid—In plastic bottles of 6 fl oz and 12 fl oz.

N 0071-0034—Tablets—White, embossed Gelusil P-D 034—individual strips of 10 in boxes of 50, 100 and 1000; 165 tablets loose-packed in plastic bottles.

Shown in Product Identification Section, page 420

GELUSIL–M®
Antacid–Anti-gas
Liquid/Tablets

Each teaspoonful (5 ml) or tablet contains:
300 mg aluminum hydroxide
200 mg magnesium hydroxide
25 mg simethicone

Advantages:
- High acid-neutralizing capacity
- Low sodium content
- Simethicone for antiflatulent activity
- Good taste for better patient compliance

- Fast dissolution of chewed tablets for prompt relief

Indications: Gelusil-M, a carefully balanced combination of two widely used antacids and the antiflatulent simethicone, is effective for the relief of symptoms associated with heartburn, sour stomach, and acid indigestion with gas. Gelusil-M provides symptomatic relief of hyperacidity associated with the diagnosis of peptic ulcer, gastritis, peptic esophagitis, gastric hyperacidity and hiatal hernia, and it alleviates or relieves the symptoms of gas and postoperative gas pain.

Actions and Uses: The proven neutralizing power of aluminum hydroxide and magnesium hydroxide combine to give Gelusil-M dependable antacid action without the acid rebound sometimes associated with calcium carbonate. The pleasant spearmint-flavored taste of Gelusil-M Liquid and Tablets encourages patient acceptance of, and compliance with, recommended antacid-anti-gas regimens.

Gelusil-M Tablets are easy to chew and are specifically formulated to dissolve readily, providing prompt onset of action and reliable relief of symptoms.

Gelusil-M is appropriate whenever there is a need for well-accepted, effective antacid-anti-gas therapy.

Dosage and Administration: Two or more teaspoonfuls or tablets one hour after meals and at bedtime, or as directed by a physician.

Tablets should be chewed.

The following information is provided to facilitate treatment:

Gelusil-M	LIQUID	TABLETS
Acid-neutral-izing capacity	30 mEq/ 10 ml	25 mEq/ 2 tabs
Sodium	1.2 mg/ 5 ml	1.3 mg/ tab
Lactose	0	0

Warnings: Do not take more than 10 teaspoonfuls or tablets in a 24-hour period, or use this maximum dosage for more than two weeks, or use this product if you have kidney disease, except under the advice and supervision of a physician.

Keep this and all drugs out of the reach of children.

Drug Interaction Precaution: Do not take this product if you are presently taking a prescription antibiotic drug containing any form of tetracycline.

All aluminum-containing antacids, including Gelusil-M, may prevent proper absorption of tetracycline.

How Supplied:

N 0071-2043—Liquid—In plastic bottles of 12 fl oz.

N 0071-0045—Tablets—White, embossed P-D 045— individual strips of 10 in boxes of 100.

GELUSIL–II®
Antacid–Anti-gas
Liquid/Tablets
High Potency

Each teaspoonful (5 ml) or tablet contains:
400 mg aluminum hydroxide
400 mg magnesium hydroxide
30 mg simethicone

Advantages:
- High acid-neutralizing capacity
- Low sodium content
- Simethicone for antiflatulent activity
- Good taste for better patient compliance
- Fast dissolution of chewed tablets for prompt relief
- Double strength antacid

Indications: Gelusil-II, a carefully balanced, high-potency combination of two widely used antacids and the antiflatulent simethicone, is effective for the relief of symptoms associated with heartburn, sour stomach, and acid indigestion with gas. Gelusil-II provides symptomatic relief of hyperacidity associated with the diagnosis of peptic ulcer, gastritis, peptic esophagitis, gastric hyperacidity and hiatal hernia, and it alleviates or relieves the symptoms of gas and postoperative gas pain.

Actions and Uses: The proven neutralizing powers of aluminum hydroxide and magnesium hydroxide combine to give Gelusil-II dependable antacid action without the acid rebound sometimes associated with calcium carbonate. The higher potency of Gelusil-II is achieved by greater concentration of antacid ingredients per dosage unit.

The pleasant taste of Gelusil-II Liquid (citrus-flavored) and Tablets (orange-flavored) encourages patient acceptance of, and compliance with, recommended antacid-anti-gas regimens.

Gelusil-II Tablets are easy to chew and are specifically formulated to dissolve readily, providing prompt onset of action and reliable relief of symptoms.

Gelusil-II is appropriate whenever there is a need for well-accepted, effective antacid-anti-gas therapy.

Dosage and Administration: Two or more teaspoonfuls or tablets one hour after meals and at bedtime, or as directed by a physician. Tablets should be chewed.

The following information is provided to facilitate treatment:

Gelusil-II	LIQUID	TABLETS
Acid-neutral-izing capacity	48 mEq/ 10 ml	42 mEq/ 2 tabs
Sodium	1.3 mg/ 5 ml	2.1 mg/ tab
Lactose	0	0

Warnings: Do not take more than 8 tablets or teaspoonfuls in a 24-hour period, or use this maximum dosage for more than two weeks, or use this product if you have kidney disease, except under the advice and supervision of a physician.

Keep this and all drugs out of the reach of children.

Drug Interaction Precaution: Do not take this product if you are presently taking a prescription antibiotic containing any form of tetracycline.
All aluminum-containing antacids, including Gelusil-II, may prevent proper absorption of tetracycline.

How Supplied:
N 0071-0042—Liquid—In plastic bottles of 12 fl oz.
N 0071-0043—Tablets—Double-layered white/orange, embossed P-D 043—individual strips of 10 in boxes of 80.

GERIPLEX-FS® KAPSEALS®

Composition: Each Kapseal represents:
Vitamin A ....(1.5 mg) 5,000 IU*
   (acetate)
Vitamin C........................ 50 mg
   (ascorbic acid)†
Vitamin B$_1$ .... 5 mg
   (thiamine mononitrate)
Vitamin B$_2$........................ 5 mg
   (riboflavin)
Vitamin B$_{12}$, crystalline
   (cyanocobalamin)........................ 2 mcg
Choline dihydrogen
   citrate........................ 20 mg
Nicotinamide .... 15 mg
   (niacinamide)
Vitamin E (dl-alpha tocoph-
   eryl acetate) .... (5 mg) 5 IU*
Iron‡ .... 6 mg
Copper sulfate................................ 4 mg
Manganese sulfate
   (monohydrate)........................ 4 mg
Zinc sulfate .... 2 mg
Calcium phosphate, dibasic
   (anhydrous)........................ 200 mg
Taka-Diastase® (aspergillus
   oryzae enzymes)........................2½ gr.
Docusate sodium .... 100 mg

* International Units
†Supplied as sodium ascorbate
‡Supplied as dried ferrous sulfate equivalent to the labeled amount of elemental iron

Action and Uses: A preparation containing vitamins, minerals, and a fecal softener for middle-aged and older individuals. The fecal softening agent, docusate sodium, acts to soften stools and make bowel movements easier.

Administration and Dosage: USUAL DOSAGE —One capsule daily, with or immediately after a meal.

How Supplied: N 0071-0544-24—Bottles of 100. Parcode® No. 544.

GERIPLEX-FS®
LIQUID
Geriatric Vitamin Formula with Iron and a Fecal Softener

Composition: Each 30 ml represents vitamin B$_1$ (thiamine hydrochloride), 1.2 mg; vitamin B$_2$ (as riboflavin-5'-phosphate sodium), 1.7 mg; vitamin B$_6$ (pyridoxine hydrochloride), 1 mg; vitamin B$_{12}$ (cyanocobalamin) crystalline, 5 mcg; niacinamide, 15 mg; iron (as ferric ammonium citrate, green), 15 mg; Pluronic® F-68,* 200 mg; alcohol, 18%.

Administration and Dosage: USUAL ADULT DOSAGE—Two tablespoonfuls (30 ml) daily or as recommended by the physician.

How Supplied: N 0071-2454-23—16-oz bottles.

*Pluronic is a registered trademark of BASF Wyandotte Corporation for polymers of ethylene oxide and propylene oxide.

MYADEC®

Each tablet represents:		% of US Recommended Daily Allowances (US RDA)
Vitamins		
Vitamin A	10,000 IU*	200%
Vitamin D	400 IU	100%
Vitamin E	30 IU	100%
Vitamin C	250 mg	417%
Folic Acid	0.4 mg	100%
Thiamine	10 mg	667%
Riboflavin	10 mg	588%
Niacin†	100 mg	500%
Vitamin B$_6$	5 mg	250%
Vitamin B$_{12}$	6 mcg	100%
Pantothenic Acid	20 mg	200%
Minerals		
Iodine	150 mcg	100%
Iron	20 mg	111%
Magnesium	100 mg	25%
Copper	2 mg	100%
Zinc	20 mg	133%
Manganese	1.25 mg	‡

Ingredients: Sodium ascorbate, magnesium oxide, microcrystalline cellulose, niacinamide, ferrous fumarate, ascorbic acid, zinc sulfate monohydrate, gelatin, vitamin E acetate, polyvinylpyrrolidone, calcium pantothenate, hydroxypropyl methylcellulose, silicon dioxide, riboflavin, thiamine mononitrate, magnesium stearate, pyridoxine hydrochloride, propylene glycol, cupric sulfate anhydrous, sugar, manganese sulfate monohydrate, vitamin A acetate, ethylcellulose, citric acid anhydrous, polysorbate 80, folic acid, wax, potassium iodide, vitamin D$_2$, titanium dioxide, vanillin, FD&C Yellow No. 6, FD&C Blue No. 2, FD&C Red No. 40, and vitamin B$_{12}$.

* International Units
† Supplied as niacinamide
‡ No US Recommended Daily Allowance (US RDA) has been established for this nutrient.

Actions and Uses: High potency vitamin supplement with minerals for adults.

Dosage: One tablet daily

How Supplied: N 0071-0335. In bottles of 130 and 250.

Shown in Product Identification Section, page 420

NATABEC® KAPSEALS®

Each capsule represents:

Vitamins	
Vitamin A	4,000 IU*
Vitamin D	400 IU
Vitamin C	50 mg
Vitamin B$_1$	3 mg
Vitamin B$_2$	2.0 mg
Nicotinamide†	10 mg
Vitamin B$_6$	3 mg
Vitamin B$_{12}$	5 mcg
Minerals	
Precipitated Calcium carbonate	600 mg
Iron	30 mg

*IU = International Units
†Supplied as niacinamide

Action and Uses: A multivitamin and mineral supplement for use during pregnancy and lactation.

Dosage: One capsule daily, or as directed by physician.

How Supplied: N 0071-0390-24. In bottles of 100. Parcode® 390.
The color combination of the banded capsule is a Warner-Lambert trademark.

THERA-COMBEX H-P®
High-Potency Vitamin B Complex with 500 mg Vitamin C

Composition: Each Kapseal contains:
Ascorbic acid
   (vitamin C)................................ 500 mg
Thiamine (vitamin B$_1$)
   mononitrate................................ 25 mg
Riboflavin
   (vitamin B$_2$)................................ 15 mg
Pyridoxine hydrochloride
   (vitamin B$_6$)................................ 10 mg
Vitamin B$_{12}$
   (cyanocobalamin)........................ 5 mcg
Niacinamide................................ 100 mg
dl-Panthenol .... 20 mg

Uses: For the prevention or treatment of vitamin B complex and vitamin C deficiencies.

Dosage: One or two capsules daily

How Supplied: N 0071-0550-24—Bottles of 100. Parcode® No. 550

TUCKS®
Pre-moistened Hemorrhoidal/Vaginal Pads

Indications: Temporarily relieve external discomfort of simple hemorrhoids. —Soothe, cool, and comfort itching, burning, and irritation of sensitive rectal and outer vaginal areas.

Continued on next page

This product information was prepared in December 1984. On these and other Parke-Davis Products, detailed information may be obtained by addressing PARKE-DAVIS, Division of Warner-Lambert Company, Morris Plains, NJ 07950.

Parke-Davis—Cont.

—As a compress, to help relieve discomfort from rectal/vaginal surgical stitches.

—Effective hygienic wipe to cleanse rectal area of irritation-causing residue.

—Solution buffered to help prevent further irritation.

Directions: For external use only. Use as a wipe following bowel movement, during menstruation, or after napkin or tampon change. Or, as a compress, apply to affected area 10 to 15 minutes as needed. Change compresses every 5 minutes.

Warnings: In case of rectal bleeding, consult physician promptly. In case of continued irritation, discontinue use and consult a physician. Keep this and all medication out of the reach of children. In case of accidental ingestion seek professional assistance or contact a Poison Control Center immediately.

Contains: Soft pads pre-moistened with a solution containing 50% Witch Hazel; 10% Glycerin USP; also contains: Benzalkonium Chloride NF 0.003%, Citric acid, USP ; Methylparaben NF 0.1%; sodium citrate, USP; water, purified USP. Buffered to acid pH.

How Supplied: Jars of 40 and 100. Also available as Tucks Take-Alongs®, individual, foil-wrapped, nonwoven wipes, 12 per box
Tucks—N 0071-1703
Tucks Take-Alongs—N 0071-1704-01
Shown in Product Identification Section, page 420

TUCKS® OINTMENT, CREAM

Composition: Tucks Ointment and Cream contain a specially formulated aqueous phase of 50% Witch Hazel (hamamelis water). Tucks Ointment also contains: arlacel; benzethonium chloride, NF; lanolin anhydrous, USP; sorbitol, USP; and white petrolatum, USP. Tucks Cream also contains: arlacel; benzethonium chloride, NF; cetyl alcohol; lanolin anhydrous, USP; polyethylene stearate; polysorbate; sorbitol solution, USP; and white petrolatum, USP.

Action and Uses: Both nonstaining Tucks Ointment and Tucks Cream exert a temporary soothing, cooling, mildly astringent effect on such superficial irritations as simple hemorrhoids, vaginal and rectal area itch, postepisiotomy discomfort and anorectal surgical wounds. Neither the Ointment nor the Cream contains steroids or skin sensitizing "caine" type topical anesthetics.

Warning: If itching or irritation continue, discontinue use and consult your physician. In case of rectal bleeding, consult physician promptly. Keep this and all drugs out of the reach of children. In case of accidental ingestion seek professional assistance or contact a Poison Control Center immediately.

Dosage and Administration:
Anal or vaginal itching—Apply to affected area and rub in gently. Pay particular attention to rectal and vaginal hygiene to help prevent recurrent itching and irritation.
Hemorrhoids and anorectal wounds—Apply Tucks Ointment or Cream following bowel movements and as often as needed for temporary relief of itching and discomfort. A special applicator is provided for rectal instillation. Tucks Ointment or Cream may also be used with anorectal dressings or pads.
Postpartum discomfort—Apply to tender perineal area or hemorrhoids as needed for temporary relief of discomfort and itching.

How Supplied: Tucks Ointment and Tucks Cream (water-washable) in 40-g tubes with rectal applicators. Tucks Ointment—N 0071-3021-14; Tucks Cream—N 0071-3022-14.

ZIRADRYL® Lotion

Description: A zinc oxide-antihistaminic lotion of 2% Benadryl® (diphenhydramine hydrochloride) and 2% zinc oxide; contains 2% alcohol. Also contains: camphor, USP; chlorophylline sodium; fragrances; glycerin, USP; methocel; polysorbate 40; and water, purified, USP.

Indications: For relief of itching in ivy or oak poisoning.

Warning: Should not be applied to extensive, or raw, oozing areas, or for a prolonged time, except as directed by a physician. Hypersensitivity to any of the components may occur.

Caution: Do not use in the eyes. If the condition for which this preparation is used persists or if a rash or irritation develops, discontinue use and consult physician.
FOR EXTERNAL USE ONLY
Keep this and all drugs out of the reach of children. In case of accidental ingestion seek professional assistance or contact a Poison Control Center immediately.

Directions: *SHAKE WELL*
For relief of itching, cleanse affected area and apply generously three or four times daily. Temporary stinging sensation may follow application. Discontinue use if stinging persists. Easily removed with water.

How Supplied: N 0071-3224-19: 6-oz bottles Protect from freezing.
Shown in Product Identification Section, page 420

Products are cross-indexed by generic and chemical names in the
YELLOW SECTION

The Parthenon Co., Inc.
3311 W. 2400 SOUTH
SALT LAKE CITY, UTAH 84119

DEVROM® CHEWABLE TABLETS

Active Ingredients: Bismuth Subgallate 200 mg/tablet

Indications: Devrom Chewable Tablets are used as an aid to reduce odor from colostomies or ileostomies.

Warnings: This product cannot be expected to be effective in the reduction of odor due to faulty personal hygiene. Keep this and all medication out of reach of children.
Note: The beneficial ingredient in these tablets may coat the tongue which may also darken in color. This condition is harmless and temporary. Darkening of the stool is also possible and is equally harmless.

Dosage and Administration: Take one or two tablets three times a day with meals or as directed by physician. Chew or swallow whole if desired. Keep bottle tightly closed in cool, dry place. Protect from light.

How Supplied: 100 tablets per bottle.

Pfipharmecs Division
PFIZER INC.
235 EAST 42ND STREET
NEW YORK, NY 10017

BONINE®
(meclizine hydrochloride)
Chewable Tablets

Actions: BONINE is an antihistamine which shows marked protective activity against nebulized histamine and lethal doses of intravenously injected histamine in guinea pigs. It has a marked effect in blocking the vasodepressor response to histamine, but only a slight blocking action against acetylcholine. Its activity is relatively weak in inhibiting the spasmogenic action of histamine on isolated guinea pig ileum.

Indications: BONINE is effective in the management of nausea, vomiting and dizziness associated with motion sickness.

Contraindications: Meclizine HCl is contraindicated in individuals who have shown a previous hypersensitivity to it.

Warnings: Since drowsiness may, on occasion, occur with the use of this drug, patients should be warned of this possibility and cautioned against driving a car or operating dangerous machinery.
Patients should avoid alcoholic beverages while taking this drug. Due to its potential anticholinergic action, this drug should be used with caution in patients with asthma, glaucoma, or enlargement of the prostate gland.
Usage in Children:
Clinical studies establishing safety and effectiveness in children have not been done; therefore, usage is not recom-

mended in children under 12 years of age.

Usage in Pregnancy:
As with any drug, if you are pregnant or nursing a baby, seek advice of a health care professional before taking this product.

Adverse Reactions: Drowsiness, dry mouth, and on rare occasions, blurred vision have been reported.

Dosage and Administration: For motion sickness 1 or 2 tablets of BONINE should be taken one hour prior to embarkation. Thereafter, the dose may be repeated every 24 hours for the duration of the journey.

How Supplied: BONINE (meclizine HCl) is available in convenient packets of 8 chewable tablets of 25 mg. meclizine HCl.

Shown in Product Identification Section, page 420

CORYBAN®-D CAPSULES
Decongestant Cold Capsules

Composition: Each capsule contains:
Caffeine U.S.P. ....30 mg.
Chlorpheniramine maleate
U.S.P...2 mg.
Phenylpropanolamine HCl ....25 mg.

How Supplied: In bottles of 24 light and dark blue capsules.

Shown in Product Identification Section, page 421

CORYBAN®-D COUGH SYRUP
With Decongestant

Composition: Each 5 ml (1 teaspoonful) contains:
Dextromethorphan HBr U.S.P....7.5 mg.
Guaifenesin ....50 mg.
Phenylephrine HCl..........................5 mg.
Acetaminophen ....120 mg.
Alcohol* 7.5%
* Small loss unavoidable

How Supplied: Coryban-D Cough Syrup is available in 4-ounce dripless spout bottles. Sorbitol, which is contained in this product, is a nutritive, carbohydrate sweetening agent which is metabolized more slowly than sugar.
Do not refrigerate.

Shown in Product Identification Section, page 421

LI-BAN® Spray
Lice Control Spray

THIS PRODUCT IS NOT FOR USE ON HUMANS OR ANIMALS

Active Ingredient:
(5-Benzyl-3-Furyl) methyl 2, 2-dimethyl-3-(2-methylpropenyl) cyclopropanecarboxylate

	0.500%
Related Compounds	0.068%
Aromatic petroleum	
hydrocarbons	0.664%
Inert Ingredients	98.768%
	100.000%

Actions: A highly active synthetic pyrethroid for the control of lice and louse

eggs on garments, bedding, furniture and other inanimate objects.

Warnings: Avoid contamination of feed and foodstuffs. Cover or remove fishbowls. **HARMFUL IF SWALLOWED.** This product is not for use on humans or animals. If lice infestations should occur on humans, consult either your physician or pharmacist for a product for use on humans.

Physical and Chemical Hazards:
Contents under pressure. Do not use or store near heat or open flame. Do not puncture or incinerate container. Exposure to temperatures above 130° F may cause bursting.

Direction For Use: It is a violation of Federal law to use this product in a manner inconsistent with its labeling.
Shake well before each use. Remove protective cap. Aim spray opening away from person. Push button to spray. **Caution: Avoid spraying in eyes. Avoid breathing spray mist. Use only in well ventilated areas. Avoid contact with skin. In case of contact wash immediately with soap and water. Vacate room and ventilate before reoccupying.**
To kill lice and louse eggs: Spray in an inconspicuous area to test for possible staining or discoloration. Inspect again after drying, then proceed to spray entire area to be treated.
Hold container upright with nozzle away from you. Depress valve and spray from a distance of 8 to 10 inches.
Spray each square foot for 3 seconds. Spray only those garments, parts of bedding, including mattresses and furniture that cannot be either laundered or dry cleaned.
Allow all sprayed articles to dry thoroughly before use. Repeat treatment as necessary.
Buyer assumes all risks of use, storage or handling of this material not in strict accordance with direction given herewith.
DISPOSAL OF CONTAINER
Wrap container and dispose of in trash. Do not incinerate.

How Supplied: 5 oz. aerosol can.
Shown in Product Identification Section, page 421

RID®
Liquid Pediculicide

Description: Rid is a liquid pediculicide whose active ingredients are: pyrethrins 0.3%, piperonyl butoxide, technical 3.00%, equivalent to 2.4% (butylcarbityl) (6-propylpiperonyl) ether and to 0.6% related compounds, petroleum distillate 1.20% and benzyl alcohol 2.4%. Inert ingredients 93.1%.

Actions: RID kills head lice (Pediculus humanus capitis), body lice (Pediculus humanus humanus), and pubic or crab lice (Phthirus pubis), and their eggs. The pyrethrins act as a contact poison and affect the parasite's nervous system, resulting in paralysis and death. The effi-

cacy of the pyrethrins is enhanced by the synergist, piperonyl butoxide.

Indications: RID is indicated for the treatment of infestations of head lice, body lice and pubic (crab) lice, and their eggs.

Warning: RID should be used with caution by ragweed sensitized persons.

Precautions: This product is for external use only. It is harmful if swallowed. It should not be inhaled. It should be kept out of the eyes and contact with mucous membranes should be avoided. If accidental contact with eyes occurs, flush immediately with water. In case of infection or skin irritation, discontinue use and consult a physician. Consult a physician if infestation of eyebrows or eyelashes occurs. Avoid contamination of feed or foodstuffs. Do not reuse container. Destroy when empty.
Do not transport or store below 32°F (0°C).

Dosage and Administration: (1) Apply RID undiluted to hair and scalp or to any other infested area until entirely wet. Do not use on eyelashes or eyebrows. (2) Allow RID to remain on area for 10 minutes but no longer. (3) Wash thoroughly with warm water and soap or shampoo. (4) Dead lice and eggs may require removal with fine-toothed comb provided. A second application should be made in 7–10 days to kill any newly hatched lice. Do not exceed two consecutive applications within 24 hours.
Since lice infestations are spread by contact, each family member should be examined carefully. If infested, he or she should be treated promptly to avoid spread or reinfestation of previously treated individuals. Contaminated clothing and other articles, such as hats, etc. should be dry cleaned, boiled or otherwise treated until decontaminated to prevent reinfestation or spread.

How Supplied: In 2 and 4 fl. oz. bottles and one gallon plastic containers. Special fine-tooth comb that removes all the nits and patient instruction booklet are included in each package of RID.
Shown in Product Identification Section, page 421

WART-OFF™

Active Ingredient: Salicylic Acid, U.S.P., 17%, in Flexible Collodion, U.S.P. Wart-Off™ Solution contains approx. 20.5% Alcohol and 54.2% Ether—small losses are unavoidable.

Indications: Removal of Warts

Warnings: Keep this and all medications out of reach of children to avoid accidental poisoning.
Flammable—Do not use near fire or flame. For external use only. In case of accidental ingestion, contact a physician or a Poison Control Center immediately. Do not use near eyes or on mucous membranes. Diabetics or other people with impaired circulation should not use

Continued on next page

Pfipharmecs—Cont.

Wart-Off™. Do not use on moles, birthmarks or unusual warts with hair growing from them. If wart persists, see your physician. If pain should develop, consult your physician.

Instructions For Use: Read warning and enclosed instructional brochure. Apply Wart-Off™ to warts only. Do not apply to surrounding skin. Make sure that surrounding skin is protected from accidental application. Before applying, soak affected area in hot water for several minutes. If any tissue has been loosened, remove by rubbing surface of wart gently with special brush enclosed in Wart-Off™ package. Dry thoroughly. Warts are contagious, so don't share your towel. Apply once or twice daily. Using plastic applicator attached to cap, apply one drop at a time until entire wart is covered. Lightly cover with small adhesive bandage. Replace cap tightly to avoid evaporation. This treatment may be used daily for three to four weeks if necessary.

How Supplied: 0.5 fluid ounce bottle with pinpoint plastic applicator, special cleaning brush and instructional brochure.

Shown in Product Identification Section, page 421

Pharmacraft Division
PENNWALT CORPORATION
755 JEFFERSON ROAD
ROCHESTER, NY 14623

ALLEREST® TABLETS, CHILDREN'S CHEWABLE TABLETS, HEADACHE STRENGTH TABLETS, SINUS PAIN FORMULA TABLETS, TIMED RELEASE CAPSULES

Active Ingredients:
acetaminophen
  Headache Strength, 325 mg.
  Sinus Pain Formula, 500 mg.
chlorpheniramine maleate
  Tablets, 2 mg.
  Children's Chewables, 1 mg.
  Sinus Pain Formula, 2 mg.
  Headache Strength, 2 mg.
  Timed Release, 4 mg.
phenylpropanolamine HCl
  Tablets, 18.7 mg.
  Children's Chewables, 9.4 mg.
  Sinus Pain Formula, 18.7 mg.
  Headache Strength, 18.7 mg.
  Timed Release, 50 mg.

Other Ingredients:
Allerest Tablets — Dibasic Calcium Phosphate; Dye, FD&C Blue #1 Aluminum Lake; Magnesium Stearate; Microcrystalline Cellulose; Povidone; Pregelatinized Starch; Sodium Starch Glycolate.
Children's Chewable Tablets—Calcium Stearate; Citric Acid; Dye, FD&C Blue #1 Aluminum Lake; Dye, FD&C Red #3 Aluminum Lake; Flavor; Magnesium Trisilicate Mannitol; Saccharin Sodium; Sorbitol.

Headache Strength Tablets—Magnesium Stearate; Microcrystalline Cellulose; Povidone; Pregelatinized Starch.
Sinus Pain Formula Tablets—Magnesium Stearate; Microcrystalline Cellulose; Povidone; Pregelatinized Starch; Sodium Starch Glycolate.

Indications: Allerest is indicated for symptomatic relief of hay fever, pollen allergies, upper respiratory allergies (perennial allergic rhinitis), allergic colds, sinusitis and nasal passage congestion. Those symptoms include headache pain, sneezing, runny nose, itching or watery eyes and itching nose and throat.

Actions: Allerest contains the antihistamine chlorpheniramine maleate which acts to suppress the symptoms of allergic rhinitis. In addition, it contains the decongestant phenylpropanolamine which acts to reduce swelling of the upper respiratory tract mucosa. Headache Strength and Sinus Pain Formula also contain acetaminophen to relieve headache pain.

Contraindications: Known hypersensitivity to the ingredients in this drug.

Warnings: Allerest should be used with caution in patients with cardiac disorders, hypertension, hyperthyroidism or diabetes. Since drowsiness may occur, patients should be instructed not to operate a car or machinery.

Adverse Reactions: Drowsiness; excitability, especially in children; nervousness; and dizziness.

Dosage and Administration: TABLETS AND HEADACHE STRENGTH —Adults, 2 tablets every 4 hours. Not to exceed 8 tablets in 24 hours. Children (6–12)—half the adult dose. Dosage for children under 6 should be individualized under the supervision of a physician. SINUS PAIN FORMULA—Adults, 2 tablets every 6 hours. Not to exceed 8 tablets in 24 hours. Not recommended for children 12 and under. CHILDREN'S CHEWABLE TABLETS — Children (6–12) 2 tablets every 4 hours. Not to exceed 8 tablets in 24 hours. Children under 6 consult a physician. Adults double the children's dose. TIMED RELEASE CAPSULES—Adults, 1 capsule in the morning and one capsule in the evening. If symptoms are especially severe, one capsule every 8 hours may be taken. Not to exceed 3 capsules in 24 hours. Do not give to children under 12 years without physician's approval.

Overdosage: Acetaminophen in massive overdosage may cause hepatotoxicity.

Drug Interaction Precautions: Not to be taken by patients currently taking a prescription antihypertensive or antidepressant drug containing a monoamine oxidase inhibitor except under the advice and supervision of a physician.
Antihistamines and oral nasal decongestants have additive effects with alcohol and other CNS depressants.

How Supplied: TABLETS packaged on blister cards in 24, 48 and 72 count cartons. CHILDREN'S CHEWABLE

TABLETS packaged on blister cards in 24 count cartons. SINUS PAIN FORMULA TABLETS packaged on blister cards in 20 count cartons. HEADACHE STRENGTH TABLETS packaged on blister cards in 24 count cartons. CAPSULES supplied in bottles of 10 count.

Shown in Product Identification Section, page 421

CaldeCORT® ANTI-ITCH CREAM AND SPRAY

Active Ingredient: *Cream*—Hydrocortisone Acetate (equivalent to Hydrocortisone 0.5%). *Spray*—Hydrocortisone 0.5%.

Other Ingredients: *Cream*—Glyceryl Monostearate; Lanolin Alcohol; Methylparaben; Mineral Oil; Polyoxyl 40 Stearate; Propylparaben; Sodium Metabisulfite; Sorbitol Solution; Stearyl Alcohol; Water; White Petrolatum; White Wax. *Spray*—Isobutane (propellant); Isopropyl Myristate; SD Alcohol 40-B 89.5% by volume.

Indications: For the temporary relief of itching associated with minor skin irritations, inflammation and rashes due to eczema, insect bites, poison ivy, poison oak, poison sumac, soaps, detergents, cosmetics and jewelry; and for external genital and anal itching.

Actions: Antidermatitis cream and spray for the temporary relief from itching and minor skin irritations.

Warnings: For external use only. Avoid contact with the eyes. If condition worsens, or if symptoms persist for more than 7 days or clear up and occur again within a few days, discontinue use and consult a doctor. Do not use if you have a vaginal discharge. Consult a doctor. Keep this and all drugs out of the reach of children. In case of accidental ingestion, seek professional assistance or contact a Poison Control Center immediately. *For Spray only*—Avoid spraying in eyes or on other mucous membranes. Contents under pressure. Do not puncture or incinerate. Flammable mixture, do not use near fire or flame. Do not store at temperature above 120°F. Use only as directed. Intentional misuse by deliberately concentrating and inhaling the contents can be harmful or fatal.

Directions: Adults and children 2 years of age and older: Apply to affected area not more than 3 to 4 times daily. Children under 2 years of age: Consult a doctor.

How Supplied: *Anti-Itch Cream*—½ and 1 oz. tubes. *Anti-Itch Spray*—1½ oz. can.

Shown in Product Identification Section, page 421

CALDESENE® MEDICATED POWDER AND OINTMENT

Active Ingredients: *Powder*—Calcium Undecylenate 10%. *Ointment*—Petrolatum 53.9%; Zinc Oxide 15%.

Other Ingredients: *Powder* — Fragrance; Talc. *Ointment*—Cod Liver Oil; Fragrance; Lanolin Oil; Methylparaben; Propylparaben; Talc.

Indications: Caldesene Medicated Powder is indicated to help heal, relieve and prevent diaper rash, prickly heat and chafing. Medicated Ointment helps prevent diaper rash and soothe minor skin irritations.

Actions: Antifungal and antibacterial Medicated Powder inhibits the growth of bacteria and fungi which cause diaper rash. Also, forms a protective coating to repel moisture, soothe and comfort minor skin irritations, helps heal and prevent chafing and prickly heat. Medicated Ointment forms a protective skin coating to repel moisture and promote healing of diaper rash, while its natural ingredients protect irritated skin against wetness. Soothes minor skin irritations, superficial wounds and burns.

Warnings: For external use only. Avoid contact with eyes. If condition worsens or does not improve within 7 days, consult a doctor. Do not apply ointment over deep or puncture wounds, infections and lacerations. Keep this and all drugs out of the reach of children. In case of accidental ingestion, seek professional assistance or contact a Poison Control Center immediately.

Directions: Cleanse and thoroughly dry affected area. Smooth on Caldesene 3–4 times daily, after every bath or diaper change, or as directed by a physician.

How Supplied: *Medicated Powder*—2.0 oz. and 4.0 oz. shaker containers. *Medicated Ointment*—1.25 oz. collapsible tubes.

Shown in Product Identification Section, page 421

COLD FACTOR 12™
Liquid and Capsules

Active Ingredients:
Liquid
Each teaspoonful (5 ml) contains phenylpropanolamine polistirex equivalent to 37.5 mg phenylpropanolamine HCl and chlorpheniramine polistirex equivalent to 4 mg chlorpheniramine maleate.

Other Ingredients:
Dye, D&C Red #33; Flavors; High Fructose Corn Syrup; Methylparaben; Polysorbate 80; Pregelatinized Starch; Propylparaben; Saccharin Sodium; Simethicone; Vegetable Oil; Water; Xanthan Gum.
Capsules
phenylpropanolamine HCl, 75 mg chlorpheniramine maleate, 8 mg

Indications: For temporary relief of nasal congestion due to the common cold. For temporary relief of nasal congestion associated with sinusitis. For temporary relief of running nose, sneezing, itching of the nose or throat and itchy and watery eyes as may occur in allergic rhinitis (such as hay fever).

Actions: Cold Factor 12 provides 12 hour symptomatic relief. It contains an antihistamine (chlorpheniramine) which acts to suppress the symptoms of allergic rhinitis, and a nasal decongestant (phenylpropanolamine) which acts to reduce swelling of the upper respiratory tract mucosa.

Warnings: Do not exceed recommended dosage because at higher doses nervousness, dizziness, or sleeplessness may occur. May cause excitability, especially in children. Do not take this product if you have asthma, glaucoma, high blood pressure, heart disease, diabetes, thyroid disease, or difficulty in urination due to enlargement of the prostate gland, except under the advice and supervision of a physician. Do not give this product to children under 6, except under the advice and supervision of a physician. If symptoms do not improve within 7 days or are accompanied by high fever, consult a physician before continuing use. May cause drowsiness. As with any drug, if you are pregnant or nursing a baby, seek the advice of a health professional before using this product. Keep this and all drugs out of the reach of children. In case of accidental overdose, seek professional assistance or contact a Poison Control Center immediately. Avoid driving a motor vehicle or operating heavy machinery. Avoid alcoholic beverages while taking this product.
Drug interaction precaution:
Do not take this product if you are presently taking a prescription antihypertensive or antidepressant drug containing a monoamine oxidase inhibitor except under the advice and supervision of a physician.

Dosage and Administration: *Liquid*—*Shake well before using.* Adults: 2 teaspoonfuls every 12 hours; do not exceed 4 teaspoonfuls in 24 hours. Children 6–12: 1 teaspoonful every 12 hours; do not exceed 2 teaspoonfuls in 24 hours. Children under 6: Use only under the advice and supervision of a physician. *Capsules*—Adults and children over 12: 1 capsule every 12 hours; do not exceed 2 capsules in 24 hours.

Professional Labeling: Dosage of Cold Factor 12 Liquid for children 2 to under 6: ½ teaspoonful every 12 hours; do not exceed 1 teaspoonful in 24 hours.

How Supplied: Liquid in bottles of 1.7 fl. oz. and 3 fl. oz. Capsules on blister cards in 10 count cartons.
Shown in Product Identification Section, page 421

CRUEX® ANTIFUNGAL POWDER, SPRAY POWDER AND CREAM

Active Ingredients: *Powder*—Calcium Undecylenate 10%. *Spray Powder*—Total Undecylenate 19%, as Undecylenic Acid and Zinc Undecylenate. *Cream*—Total Undecylenate 20%, as Undecylenic Acid and Zinc Undecylenate.

Other Ingredients: *Powder*—Colloidal Silicon Dioxide; Fragrance; Isopropyl Myristate; Talc. *Spray Powder*—Fragrance; Isobutane (propellant); Isopropyl Myristate; Menthol; Talc; Trolamine. *Cream*—Anhydrous Lanolin; Fragrance; Glycol Stearate SE; Methylparaben; PEG-6 Stearate; PEG-8 Cocoate; Propylparaben; Sorbitol Solution; Stearic Acid; Trolamine; Water; White Petrolatum.

Indications: For the treatment of Jock Itch (tinea cruris) and relief of itching, chafing, burning rash and irritation in the groin area. Cruex powders also absorb perspiration.

Actions: Antifungal Powder, Spray Powder and Cream are proven clinically effective in the treatment of superficial fungus infections of the skin.

Warnings: Do not use on children under 2 years of age except under the advice and supervision of a doctor. For external use only. If irritation occurs, or if there is no improvement within 2 weeks, discontinue use and consult a doctor or pharmacist. Keep this and all drugs out of the reach of children. In case of accidental ingestion, seek professional assistance or contact a Poison Control Center immediately. *For Spray Powder only*—Avoid spraying in eyes or on other mucous membranes. Contents under pressure. Do not puncture or incinerate. Flammable mixture, do not use near a fire or flame. Do not store at temperature above 120° F. Use only as directed. Intentional misuse by deliberately concentrating and inhaling the contents can be harmful or fatal.

Directions: Cleanse skin with soap and water and dry thoroughly. Apply Cruex to affected area morning and night, before and after athletic activity, or as directed by a doctor. Best results are usually obtained with 2 weeks' use of this product. If satisfactory results have not occurred within this time, consult a doctor or pharmacist. Children under 12 years of age should be supervised in the use of this product. This product is not effective on the scalp or nails.

How Supplied: *Powder*—1.5 oz. plastic squeeze bottle. *Spray Powder*—1.8 oz., 3.5 oz. and 5.5 oz. aerosol containers. *Cream*—½ oz. tube.
Shown in Product Identification Section, page 421

DESENEX® ANTIFUNGAL POWDER, SPRAY POWDER, CREAM, OINTMENT, LIQUID AND PENETRATING FOAM; SOAP; FOOT & SNEAKER SPRAY

Active Ingredients: *Powder, Spray Powder*—Total Undecylenate 19%, as Undecylenic Acid and Zinc Undecylenate. *Cream*—Total Undecylenate 20%, as Undecylenic Acid and Zinc Undecylenate. *Ointment*—Total Undecylenate 22%, as Undecylenic Acid and Zinc Undecylenate. *Liquid, Penetrating Foam*—Undecylenic Acid 10%. *Foot & Sneaker Spray*—Aluminum Chlorohydrex.

Continued on next page

Pharmcraft—Cont.

Other Ingredients: *Powder* — Fragrance; Talc. *Spray Powder*—Fragrance; Isobutane (propellant); Isopropyl Myristate; Menthol; Talc; Trolamine. *Cream, Ointment*—Anhydrous Lanolin; Fragrance; Glycol Stearate SE; Methylparaben; PEG-6 Stearate; PEG-8 Cocoate; Propylparaben; Sorbitol Solution; Stearic Acid; Trolamine; Water; White Petrolatum. *Liquid*—Fragrance; Isopropyl Alcohol 47.1% by volume; Polysorbate 80; Propylene Glycol; Trolamine; Water. *Penetrating Foam*—Emulsifying Wax; Fragrance; Isobutane (propellant); Isopropyl Alcohol 35.2% by volume; Sodium Benzoate; Trolamine; Water. *Foot & Sneaker Spray*—Colloidal Silicon Dioxide; Diisopropyl Adipate; Fragrance; Isobutane (propellant); Menthol; SD Alcohol 40-B 89.3% by volume; Talc; Tartaric Acid.

Indications: Desenex Antifungal Products cure athlete's foot (tinea pedis) and body ringworm (tinea corporis) exclusive of the ails and scalp. Relieves itching and burning. With daily use, prevents athlete's foot from coming back. Desenex Foot & Sneaker Spray helps stop odor and reduces wetness.

Actions: Desenex Antifungal Powders, Cream, Ointment, Liquid and Penetrating Foam are proven effective in the treatment of superficial fungus infections of the skin caused by the three major types of dermatophytic fungi (T. rubrum, T. mentagrophytes, E. floccosum). Penetrating Foam quickly dissolves into a highly concentrated liquid. Foot & Sneaker Spray is a formulated liquid that dries to a fine powder to protect feet from odor causing perspiration. Powder also helps keep feet dry and comfortable.

Warnings: Do not use on children under 2 years of age except under the advice and supervision of a doctor. For external use only. If irritation occurs, or if there is no improvement within 4 weeks, discontinue use and consult a doctor or pharmacist. Keep this and all drugs out of the reach of children. In case of accidental ingestion, seek professional assistance or contact a Poison Control Center immediately. *For Spray Powder, Penetrating Foam and Foot & Sneaker Spray only*—Avoid spraying in eyes or on other mucous membranes. Contents under pressure. Do not puncture or incinerate. Flammable mixture, do not use near fire or flame. Do not store at temperature above 120° F. Use only as directed. Intentional misuse by deliberately concentrating and inhaling the contents can be harmful or fatal.

Directions: *Powder, Spray Powder, Cream, Ointment, Liquid and Penetrating Foam*—Cleanse skin with soap and water and dry thoroughly. Apply over affected area morning and night or as directed by a doctor, paying special attention to the spaces between the toes. It is also helpful to wear well-fitting, ventilated shoes and to change shoes and socks at least once daily. Best results are usually obtained with 4 weeks' use of this product. If satisfactory results have not occurred within this time, consult a doctor or pharmacist. Children under 12 years of age should be supervised in the use of this product. This product is not effective on the scalp or nails. To prevent athlete's foot from coming back, use Desenex Powder or Spray Powder daily. For persistent cases of athlete's foot, use Desenex Ointment or Cream at night and Desenex Powder or Spray Powder during the day. *Soap*—Use in conjunction with Desenex Antifungal Products. *Foot & Sneaker Spray*—Spray on soles of feet and between toes daily. To fight offensive odor, spray liberally over entire inside area of shoes and sneakers before and after wearing.

How Supplied: *Powder*—1.5 oz. and 3.0 oz. shaker containers. *Spray Powder*—2.7 oz. and 5.5 oz. aerosol containers. *Cream*—½ oz. tubes. *Ointment*—0.9 oz. and 1.8 oz. tubes. *Liquid*—1.5 oz. pump spray bottle. *Penetrating Foam*—1.5 oz. aerosol container. *Soap*—3.25 oz. bar. *Foot & Sneaker Spray*—2.7 oz. aerosol container.

Shown in Product Identification Section, page 421

SINAREST® TABLETS

Active Ingredients:
acetaminophen:
    Tablets, 325 mg.
    Extra Strength, 500 mg.
chlorpheniramine maleate
    Tablets 2 mg.
    Extra Strength, 2 mg.
phenylpropanolamine HCl
    Tablets, 18.7 mg.
    Extra Strength, 18.7 mg.

Other Ingredients: Dye, D&C Yellow No. 10 Aluminum Lake; Dye, FD&C Yellow No. 6 Aluminum Lake; Magnesium Stearate; Microcrystalline Cellulose; Povidone; Pregelatinized Starch.

Indications: Sinarest is indicated for symptomatic relief from the headache pain, pressure and congestion associated with sinusitis, allergic rhinitis or the common cold.

Actions: Sinarest contains an antihistamine (chlorpheniramine maleate) and a decongestant (phenylpropanolamine) for the relief of sinus and nasal passage congestion as well as an analgesic (acetaminophen) to relieve pain and discomfort.

Contraindications: Known hypersensitivity to any of the ingredients in this compound.

Warnings: Sinarest should be used with caution in patients with high blood pressure, heart disease, diabetes or thyroid disease. Since drowsiness may occur, patients should be instructed not to operate a car or machinery. This product should not be taken for more than 10 consecutive days.

Adverse Reactions: Drowsiness; excitability, especially in children; nervousness; and dizziness.

Dosage and Administration: SINAREST TABLETS—Adults—take 2 tablets every 4 hours. Not to exceed 8 tablets in 24 hours. Children (6–12 years)—One half of adult dosage. Dosage for children under 6 should be individualized under the supervision of a physician. EXTRA STRENGTH TABLETS—Adults and Children over 12—take 2 tablets every 6 hours. Not to exceed 8 tablets in 24 hours. Not recommended for children 12 and under.

Overdosage: Acetaminophen in massive overdosage may cause hepatotoxicity.

Drug Interaction Precaution: Not to be taken by patients currently taking a prescription antihypertensive or antidepressant drug containing a monoamine oxidase inhibitor except under the advice and supervision of a physician. Antihistamines and oral nasal decongestants have additive effects with alcohol and other CNS depressants.

How Supplied: Blister packages of 20, 40 and 80 tablets. Extra Strength tablets: package of 24 tablets.

Pharmaderm
a division of Altana Inc.
60 BAYLIS ROAD
MELVILLE, NY 11747

ANALGESIC BALM

Active Ingredient: Methyl-salicylate 10% (wintergreen) and menthol 0.5%.

How Supplied: Available in 1 oz tubes and 1 lb jars.

ATHLETE'S FOOT CREAM and SOLUTION
(Tolnaftate Cream 1% and Tolnaftate Solution 1%)

Tolnaftate, the active ingredient in this medication, was synthesized in 1960. It is the first topically applied chemical compound effective against tinea pedis (athlete's foot), tinea cruris (jock itch) and tinea corporis (body ringworm)[1]. Fungal infections are caused by microorganisms that grow best in dark, moist areas such as showers and locker rooms as well as swimming pools. Body heat and perspiration also provide an ideal environment for fungi. As a result, fungi may often breed in articles of clothing, particularly shoes, socks and underwear. Pharmaderm Athlete's Foot Cream and Solution are effective in the treatment of superficial fungus infections of the skin which cause athlete's foot, jock itch and ringworm. Wash and dry the infected area thoroughly in the morning and evening. Apply the medication evenly to the infected area and gently rub in. To help prevent recurrence, continue treatment for 2 weeks after disappearance of all symptoms.

ATHLETE'S FOOT (tinea pedis)

Athlete's foot is characterized by the cracking and peeling of the skin between the toes often accompanied by itching and sometimes, stinging and burning. It may spread to other areas of the foot and body. Special attention should be given to personal hygiene as follows:

1. Don't go barefooted in public areas especially in locker rooms, showers or around swimming pools.
2. Bathe daily and use a clean dry towel.
3. Wear clean cotton socks. They should be changed frequently.
4. Wear shoes that allow proper air circulation. Sneakers and plastic or rubber footwear which enclose the foot and cause excessive perspiration should be avoided.
5. Launder all towels and socks promptly to avoid further spreading of the infection.
6. Use Pharmaderm Athlete's Foot Cream or Solution as directed on the package to kill athlete's foot fungi and help prevent reinfection.

JOCK ITCH (tinea cruris)

Jock itch is characterized by red, scaling patches which may be present in the groin, scrotum and the anal area. Itching and burning are usually accompanying symptoms. The condition is aggravated by friction or rubbing and the wearing of tight or constrictive apparel or protective equipment. Special attention should be given to personal hygiene as follows:

1. Bathe daily. Rinse the body well and dry with a clean, dry towel.
2. Try to keep the affected area dry and free of perspiration.
3. Wear clean, cotton underwear that is not tight.
4. Wear clothing that is clean, dry and soft and not tight fitting. Change clothes daily.
5. Launder all clothing and towels promptly to avoid further spreading of the infection.
6. Use Pharmaderm Athlete's Foot Cream or Solution as directed in the package to kill jock itch fungi and help prevent reinfection.

BODY RINGWORM (tinea corporis)

Ringworm is a popular name for a group of fungal diseases of the skin of man and domestic animals. It is marked by the formation of ring-shaped pigmented patches covered with vesicles or scales. When treating this condition, special attention should be given to personal hygiene as follows:

1. Bathe daily. Tub baths rather than showers are recommended for thorough cleansing of the trunk and skin folds.
2. Try to keep the affected area dry and free of perspiration.
3. Wear clean, dry, loose fitting clothes; change clothes daily.
4. Launder all clothing and towels promptly to avoid spreading the infection.
5. Use Pharmaderm Athlete's Foot Cream or Solution as directed on the package to kill body ringworm fungi and help prevent reinfection.

Pharmaderm Athlete's Foot Cream and Solution are greaseless, odorless and will not stain the skin. They are not for use in the eyes nor are they recommended for nail or scalp infections. Symptoms are usually cleared in 2 or 3 weeks. If skin is thickened, treatment may take 4 to 6 weeks. If burning or itching do not improve within 10 days or if irritation occurs, discontinue use and consult your physician or podiatrist. Do not use in children under 2 years of age except under the advice and supervision of a physician.

Available as:

Pharmaderm Athlete's Foot Cream
NDC 0462-0008-15, 15 gram tube
Pharmaderm Athlete's Foot Solution
NDC 0462-0009-10, 10 ml bottle

(1) Goodman, L.S., Gilman, A.G. and Gilman, A., The Pharmacologic Basis of Therapeutics, Fifth Edition, page 1241

Shown in Product Identification Section, page 421

BACITRACIN OINTMENT, U.S.P.

Active Ingredient: Bacitracin 500 units per gram.

How Supplied: Available in ½ oz and 1 oz tubes.

BACITRACIN–NEOMYCIN–POLY-MYXIN OINTMENT
Triple Antibiotic Ointment

Active Ingredient: Bacitracin 400 units, neomycin sulfate 5 mg, polymyxin B sulfate 5,000 units per gram.

How Supplied: Available in ½ oz and 1 oz tubes.

BACITRACIN–POLYMYXIN OINTMENT
Double Antibiotic Ointment

Active Ingredient: Bacitracin zinc 500 units, polymyxin B sulfate 10,000 units per gram.

How Supplied: Available in ½ oz and 1 oz tubes.

BORIC ACID OINTMENT

Active Ingredient: Boric Acid 10%.

How Supplied: Available in 1 oz and 2 oz tubes.

BORIC ACID OPHTHALMIC OINTMENT 5%

Active Ingredient: Boric Acid 5% in a base of White Petrolatum and Mineral Oil.

How Supplied: Available in ⅛ oz tube.

COLD CREAM USP

Active Ingredient: White Wax U.S.P. (Bee's Wax) with other Emollients.

How Supplied: Available in one pound jars.

DIBUCAINE OINTMENT USP 1%

Active Ingredient: Dibucaine 1% in a special base with Acetone Sodium Bisulfate 0.5% as a preservative.

How Supplied: Available in 1 oz tubes with pile pipe.

HYDROCORTISONE CREAM and OINTMENT, U.S.P., 0.5%

Active Ingredient: Hydrocortisone, U.S.P. 0.5%.

How Supplied: Available in 1 oz tubes.

HYDROPHILIC OINTMENT

Active Ingredient: Stearyl Alcohol, White Petrolatum, Propylene Glycol, Mineral Oil, Sodium Lauryl Sulfate, Purified Water and Preserved with Methyl and Propyl Paraben.

How Supplied: Available in one pound jars.

ICHTHAMMOL OINTMENT 10% and 20%

Active Ingredient: Ichthammol 10% and 20%.

How Supplied: Available in 1 oz tubes.

LANOLIN USP

Active Ingredient: Lanolin Anhydrous and Purified Water.

How Supplied: Available in one pound jars.

LANOLIN ANHYDROUS USP

Active Ingredient: Lanolin Anhydrous.

How Supplied: Available in one pound jars.

PETROLATUM WHITE, U.S.P.

Active Ingredient: Petrolatum White, U.S.P. Pharmaceutical grade.

How Supplied: Available in 1 oz tubes and 1 lb jars.

VITAMIN A + VITAMIN D OINTMENT

Composition: Vitamin A 1750 u/gm and Vitamin D 350 u/gm in a lanolin-petrolatum ointment base.

How Supplied: Available in 2 oz and 4 oz tubes; 1 lb jars.

WHITFIELD'S OINTMENT, U.S.P.

Active Ingredient: Benzoic Acid 6%, Salicylic Ointment 3% in a Polyethylene Glycol Ointment base.

How Supplied: Available in 1 oz tubes.

Continued on next page

Pharmaderm—Cont.

YELLOW MERCURIC OXIDE OPHTHALMIC OINTMENT 1% and 2%

Active Ingredient: Yellow Mercuric Oxide 1% and 2%.

How Supplied: Available in ⅛ oz tubes with eye tip and tamper evident caps to assure sterility.

ZINC OXIDE OINTMENT, U.S.P.

Active Ingredient: Zinc Oxide 20%.

How Supplied: Available in 1 oz and 2 oz tubes.

Plough, Inc.
**3030 JACKSON AVENUE
MEMPHIS, TN 38151**

AFTATE® Antifungal
**Aerosol Liquid
Aerosol Powder
Gel
Powder**

Active Ingredients: Tolnaftate 1% (Also contains: Aerosol Spray Liquid-36% alcohol; Aerosol Spray Powder-14% alcohol.)

Indications: Aftate affords excellent topical treatment and prophylaxis (prevention) of tinea pedis (Athlete's foot), tinea cruris (Jock Itch), tinea corporis (body ringworm). All forms begin to relieve burning, itching and soreness within 24 hours. Symptoms are usually cleared in 2 to 3 weeks. Aftate powder and Aerosol powder aid in the drying of moist areas.

Actions: AFTATE is a highly active synthetic fungicidal agent that is effective in the treatment of superficial fungus infections of the skin. It is inactive systemically, virtually nonsensitizing, and does not ordinarily sting or irritate intact or broken skin, even in the presence of acute inflammatory reactions.

Warnings: For external use only. Keep out of eyes. Not recommended for nail and scalp infections. If symptoms do not improve in ten (10) days or if irritation occurs, discontinue use unless directed otherwise by a physician.

Dosage and Administration: Wash and dry infected area before use. Then apply liberally and evenly on infected areas. To prevent recurrence, continue treatment for 2 weeks after symptoms disappear. To help prevent recurrence of Athlete's Foot and Jock Itch, apply Aftate Powder daily.

How Supplied:
AFTATE for Athlete's Foot
Sprinkle Powder—2.25 oz. bottle
Aerosol Spray Powder—3.5 oz can
Gel—.5 oz. tube.
Aerosol Spray Liquid—4 oz. can.
AFTATE for Jock Itch
Aerosol Spray Powder—3.5 oz. can

Sprinkle Powder—1.5 oz. bottle.
Gel—.5 oz. tube.
Shown in Product Identification Section, page 421

ASPERGUM®
**Analgesic
Gum Tablet**

Active Ingredients: Each gum tablet contains aspirin 3½ gr.

Indications: For temporary relief of minor sore throat pain, simple headache, aches and pains of colds and muscular aches and pains.

Actions: ASPERGUM is a convenient way to administer aspirin to children and adults who cannot or will not gargle properly or who cannot readily swallow tablets.

Caution: Do not use more than 2 days or administer to children under 3 years of age unless directed by a physician. Do not exceed maximum dosage (in adults) of 16 tablets in 24 hours; (in children 6–12 years) of 8 tablets in 24 hours, unless directed by physician; (in children 3–6 years) of 3 tablets in 24 hours.

Warning: Reye Syndrome is a rare but serious disease which can follow flu or chicken pox in children and teenagers. While the cause of Reye Syndrome is unknown, some reports claim aspirin may increase the risk of developing this disease. Consult doctor before use in children or teenagers with flu or chicken pox.
As with any drug, if you are pregnant or nursing a baby, seek the advice of a health professional before using this product.

Precaution: ASPERGUM is not intended for treatment of severe or persistent sore throat pain, high fever, headache, nausea or vomiting.

Dosage and Administration: Adults—chew 2 tablets; repeat every 4 hours as required up to a maximum of 16 tablets in any 24 hour period, or as directed by physician. Children—6 to 12 years—chew 1 to 2 tablets every 4 hours as required up to 8 tablets daily, or as directed by physician. Children—3 to 6 years—chew 1 tablet every 4 hours as required up to 3 tablets daily. Children under 3 years of age, consult physician.

How Supplied:
ASPERGUM tablets in chewing gum form. Individual safety sealed blister packaging.
Orange flavored: boxes of 16 and 40 tablets.
Cherry flavored: boxes of 16 and 40 tablets.
Shown in Product Identification Section, page 421

COPPERTONE® Sunscreens
**COPPERTONE® Sunscreen Lotion
SPF 6
COPPERTONE® Sunscreen Lotion
SPF 8**

COPPERTONE® Sunblocking Lotion SPF 15

Active Ingredients: Padimate O and Oxybenzone

Indications: Sunscreens to help prevent sunburn. COPPERTONE sunscreens 6, 8 and 15 provide 6, 8, and 15 times your natural sunburn protection. For allover application or for spot use on unprotected areas. Liberal and regular use may help reduce chances of premature aging and wrinkling of skin and skin cancer, due to long term over exposure to the sun. Excellent for use on children.

Actions: Sunscreen

Warnings: Avoid contact with eyes or mouth. Discontinue use if signs of irritation or rash appear.

Dosage and Administration: Apply evenly and liberally to exposed skin. COPPERTONE SPF 8 is water resistant and should be reapplied after 40 minutes in the water. To insure maximum protection of COPPERTONE SPF 6 or 15, reapply after swimming or exercise.

How Supplied: 4 fl. oz. Plastic Bottles
Shown in Product Identification Section, page 422

CORRECTOL®
**Laxative
Tablets/Liquid**

Active Ingredients: Tablets—Yellow phenolphthalein, 65 mg. and docusate sodium, 100 mg. per tablet. Liquid—Yellow phenolphthalein, 65 mg per tablespoonful.

Indications: For temporary relief of constipation.

Actions: Yellow phenolphthalein—stimulant laxative; docusate sodium—fecal softener.

Warnings: Not to be taken in case of nausea, vomiting, abdominal pain, or signs of appendicitis. Take only as needed —as frequent or continued use of laxatives may result in dependence on them. If skin rash appears, do not use this or any other preparation containing phenolphthalein. As with any drug, if you are pregnant or nursing a baby, seek the advice of a health professional before using this product.

Dosage and Administration
Dosage: Adults—1 or 2 tablets or tablespoonfuls daily as needed, at bedtime or on arising.
Children over 6 years—1 tablet or tablespoonful daily as needed.

How Supplied: Tablets—Individual foil-backed safety sealed blister packaging in boxes of 15, 30, 60 and 90 tablets. Liquid—8 and 16 fl. oz. bottles, safety sealed.
Shown in Product Identification Section, page 421

CUSHION GRIP®
Thermoplastic Denture Adhesive

Indications: A soft pliable thermoplastic adhesive which creates a secure seal to help reduce looseness, shifting, clicking of dentures.

Actions: Securely holds dentures comfortably for up to 4 days. Won't wash off in water. Even after repeated cleaning. CUSHION GRIP remains in place, remains soft and pliable... recreates a secure seal each time dentures are reinserted. CUSHION GRIP is safe for plastic and porcelain plates.

Caution: Intended for use only on non-defective dentures. Ill-fitting, broken or irritating dentures may impair health of patient. Periodic dental examination is recommended at least every six months.

Directions for Use: Refer patient to detailed instructions supplied with each package.

How Supplied: In tubes of ¼, ½ and 1 oz. In safety sealed cartons.

DI–GEL®
Antacid · Anti-Gas
Tablets/Liquid

Active Ingredients: DI-GEL Tablets: Each tablet contains: Simethicone 25 mg., aluminum hydroxide-magnesium carbonate codried gel 282 mg., magnesium hydroxide 85 mg.
Sodium Content: Less than 5 mg. per tablet.
DI-GEL Liquid: Each teaspoonful contains: Simethicone 20 mg., aluminum hydroxide (equivalent to aluminum hydroxide dried gel, U.S.P.) 282 mg., magnesium hydroxide 87 mg.
Sodium Content: 8.5 mg. per teaspoonful.

Indications: For fast, temporary relief of acid indigestion, heartburn, sour stomach and accompanying painful gas symptoms.

Actions: The antacid system in DI-GEL relieves and soothes acid indigestion, heartburn and sour stomach. At the same time, the simethicone "defoamers" eliminate gas.
When air becomes entrapped in the stomach, heartburn and acid indigestion can result, along with sensations of fullness, pressure and bloating.

Warnings: Do not take more than 20 teaspoonfuls or tablets in a 24 hour period, or use the maximum dosage of this product for more than 2 weeks, except under the advice and supervision of a physician. If you have kidney disease or if you are on a sodium restricted diet, do not use this product except under the advice and supervision of a physician. May cause constipation or have a laxative effect.

Drug Interaction: This product should not be taken if patient is presently taking a prescription antibiotic drug containing any form of tetracycline.

Dosage and Administration: Two teaspoonfuls or tablets every 2 hours, or after or between meals and at bedtime, not to exceed 20 teaspoonfuls or tablets per day, or as directed by a physician.

How Supplied:
DI-GEL Liquid in Mint and Lemon/Orange Flavors - 6 and 12 fl. oz. bottles, safety sealed.
DI-GEL Tablets in Mint and Lemon/Orange Flavors - In boxes of 30, 60 and 90 in handy portable safety sealed blister packaging.
Shown in Product Identification Section, page 421

DURATION®
12 Hour Nasal Spray
12 Hour Mentholated Nasal Spray
Mild 4 Hour Nasal Spray
Topical Nasal Decongestant

Active Ingredients:
12 Hour Nasal Spray:
Oxymetazoline HCl 0.05%
Mild 4 Hour Nasal Spray:
Phenylephrine HCl 0.5%

Other Ingredients:
12 Hour Nasal Spray: Preservative Phenylmercuric Acetate 0.4222% (Mentholated Nasal Spray also contains the following aromatics: menthol, camphor, eucalyptol).
Mild 4 Hour Nasal Spray: Preservative: Cetyl pyridimium chloride .04%.

Indications: Temporary relief for up to 12 hours or 4 hours, of nasal congestion due to colds, hay fever and sinusitis.

Actions: The sympathomimetic action of DURATION constricts the smaller arterioles of the nasal passages, producing a gentle and predictable decongesting effect.

Warnings: Do not exceed recommended dosage because symptoms may occur such as burning, stinging, sneezing, or increase of nasal discharge. Do not use this product for more than 3 days. If symptoms persist, consult a physician. The use of dispenser by more than one person may spread infection.

Dosage and Administration:
DURATION 12 Hour Nasal Spray—With head upright, spray 2 or 3 times in each nostril twice daily—morning and evening. To spray, squeeze bottle quickly and firmly. Not recommended for children under 6.
DURATION Mild 4 Hour Nasal Spray—With head upright, spray 2 or 3 times into each nostril. Repeat every 4 hours as needed. Not recommended for children under 12.

How Supplied:
DURATION 12 Hour Nasal Spray—½ and 1 fl. oz. plastic squeeze bottle.
DURATION 12 Hour Mentholated Nasal Spray—½ fl. oz. plastic squeeze bottle.
DURATION Mild 4 Hour Nasal Spray—½ fl. oz. plastic squeeze bottle.
All bottles in safety sealed cartons.
Shown in Product Identification Section, page 422

FEEN-A-MINT®
Laxative Gum/Pills

Active Ingredient: Gum—yellow phenolphthalein 97.2 mg. per tablet. Pills—yellow phenolphthalein, 65 mg., and docusate sodium 100 mg. per pill.

Indications: For temporary relief of constipation.

Actions: Yellow phenolphthalein—stimulant laxative; docusate sodium—fecal softener

Warnings: Not to be taken in case of nausea, vomiting, abdominal pain, or signs of appendicitis. Take only as needed—as frequent or continued use of laxatives may result in dependence on them. If skin rash appears, do not use this or any other preparation containing phenolphthalein. As with any drug, if you are pregnant or nursing a baby, seek the advice of a health professional before using this product. In case of accidental overdose, contact a physician immediately.

Dosage and Administration: Gum and Pills—Adults: 1 or 2 tablets/pills per day, as needed, at bedtime or on arising. Children over 6 years: ½ gum tablet or 1 pill per day, as needed.

How Supplied: Gum—Individual foil-backed safety sealed blister packaging in boxes of 5, 16, and 40 tablets.
Pills—Safety sealed boxes of 15, 30, and 60 tablets.
Shown in Product Identification Section, page 422

MUSKOL® INSECT REPELLENT
Aerosol Liquid
Lotion

Active Ingredients: Aerosol—DEET 25% (N,N,-diethyl-m-toluamide 23.75%, related isomers 1.25%)
Lotion—DEET 100% (N,N,-diethyl-m-toluamide 95%, related isomers 5%)

Indications: MUSKOL affords long lasting protection against mosquitos, biting flies, chiggers, ticks, fleas and gnats. Aerosol provides hours of protection; lotion up to 10 hours.

Actions: Insect repellent.

Warnings: Harmful if swallowed. Avoid contact with eyes and lips. In case of contact with eyes, flush with plenty of water. Get medical attention if irritation persists. May cause skin reaction in rare cases.
Avoid contact with plastic and fabric such as acetate, rayon and dynel. Will not damage nylon, cotton or wool. May damage some plastics, furniture finishes, paints and linoleum. Do not reuse empty container. Wrap container and put in trash collection.
For Aerosol
Flammable. Contents under pressure. Keep away from heat, sparks, and open flame. Do not puncture or incinerate container. Exposure to temperatures above 130°F may cause bursting.

Continued on next page

Plough—Cont.

Dosage and Administration:
Aerosol—Spray over clothing and exposed skin except face. To apply to face, spray into palms of hands and spread evenly on the face and neck except near eyes and mouth.
Lotion—Squeeze a few drops into hands and apply to all exposed skin. Rub in well and wipe or wash palms after applying. For chiggers and ticks, apply around all clothing openings.

How Supplied: Aerosol—6 oz
Lotion—1¼ fl oz and 2 fl oz
Shown in Product Identification Section, page 422

REGUTOL®
Stool Softener Tablets

Active Ingredient: Each tablet contains 100 mg. docusate sodium.

Indications: Regutol relieves constipation without cramping sometimes associated with stimulant laxative products.

Actions: REGUTOL contains docusate sodium which aids natural regularity and promotes easier elimination by moistening and softening dry, hard, constipating waste. REGUTOL does not cause cramps.

Warning: As with any drug, if you are pregnant or nursing a baby, seek the advice of a health professional before using this product.

Dosage and Administration: Adults and children over 12 years old, 1–3 tablets daily as needed. Children 2–12, 1 tablet daily as needed. Usually requires 1–3 days for full effect.

How Supplied: REGUTOL tablets in boxes of 30, 60 and 90 individually safety sealed blister packaging.
Shown in Product Identification Section, page 422

ST. JOSEPH® Aspirin for Children
Pediatric Analgesic/Antipyretic
Chewable Tablets

Active Ingredient: Aspirin 81 mg. (1¼ grain) per tablet.

Indications: For temporary reduction of fever, relief of minor aches and pains of colds.

Actions: Analgesic/Antipyretic

Precaution: Do not administer this product for more than 5 days. If symptoms persist or new ones occur, consult physician. If fever persists for more than three days, or recurs, consult physician. Severe or persistent sore throat, high fever, headaches, nausea or vomiting may be serious. Discontinue use and consult physician if not relieved in 24 hours.

Warning: Reye Syndrome is a rare but serious disease which can follow flu or chicken pox in children and teenagers. While the cause of Reye Syndrome is unknown, some reports claim aspirin may increase the risk of developing this disease. Consult doctor before use in children or teenagers with flu or chicken pox. As with any drug, if you are pregnant or nursing a baby, seek the advice of a health professional before using this product.

Dosage and Administration:
Dosage by Age and Weight
To be administered only under adult supervision.
[See St. Joseph Children's Dosage Chart next page].
ST. JOSEPH Aspirin for Children may be given one of five ways. Always follow with ½ glass of water, milk, or fruit juice.
1. CHEWED, followed by liquid.
2. SWALLOWED whole, followed by liquid.
3. DISSOLVED on tongue, followed by liquid.
4. CRUSHED or dissolved in a teaspoon of liquid.
5. POWDERED for infant use, when so directed by physician.

How Supplied: Chewable orange flavored tablets in plastic bottles of 36 tablets. Child-resistant, safety sealed packaging.
Shown in Product Identification Section, page 422

ST. JOSEPH® Aspirin–Free
for Children
Chewable Tablets, Liquid, Drops

Active Ingredient: Each Children's St. Joseph Aspirin-Free Chewable Tablet contains 80 mg. acetaminophen in a fruit-flavored tablet. Children's St. Joseph Aspirin-Free Liquid is stable, cherry flavored, red in color and alcohol-free and sugar-free. Each 5 ml. contains 160 mg. acetaminophen. Infant's St. Joseph Aspirin-Free Drops are stable, fruit flavored, orange in color and alcohol-free and sugar-free. Each 0.8 ml. (one calibrated dropperful) contains 80 mg. acetaminophen.

Indications: For temporary reduction of fever, relief of minor aches and pains of colds and flu.

Actions: Analgesic/Antipyretic

Warnings: Do not administer this product for more than 5 days. If symptoms persist or new ones occur, consult physician. If fever persists for more than three days, or recurs, consult physician. When using St. Joseph Aspirin-Free products do not give other medications containing acetaminophen unless directed by your physician. NOTE: SEVERE OR PERSISTENT SORE THROAT, HIGH FEVER, HEADACHES, NAUSEA OR VOMITING MAY BE SERIOUS. DISCONTINUE USE AND CONSULT PHYSICIAN IF NOT RELIEVED IN 24 HOURS. Do not exceed recommended dosage because severe liver damage may occur. As with any drug, if you are pregnant or nursing a baby, seek the advice of a health professional before using this product.

Dosage and Administration:
[See table on next page].
ST. JOSEPH Aspirin-Free Tablets for Children may be given one of three ways. Always follow with ½ glass of water, milk or fruit juice.
1. Chewed, followed by liquid.
2. Crushed or dissolved in a teaspoon of liquid (for younger children).
3. Powdered for infant use, when so directed by physician.

How Supplied: Chewable fruit flavored tablets in plastic bottles of 30 tablets. Cherry tasting Elixir in 2 and 4 fl. oz. plastic bottles. Fruit flavored drops in ½ fl. oz. plastic bottles, with calibrated plastic dropper.
All packages have child resistant safety caps and safety sealed packaging.
Shown in Product Identification Section, page 422

ST. JOSEPH® Cold Tablets for Children
Pediatric Analgesic/Antipyretic/
Nasal Decongestant

Active Ingredients: Aspirin, 81 mg. (1¼ grain) and phenylpropanolamine hydrochloride 3.125 mg. per tablet.

Indications: Temporary reduction of fever, relief of minor aches and pains, nasal congestion, runny nose, difficult nasal breathing accompanying colds.

Actions: Aspirin provides analgesia and antipyresis. Phenylpropanolamine hydrochloride restricts the smaller arterioles of nasal passages resulting in a nasal decongestant effect. Helps decongest sinus openings and sinus passages, thus promoting sinus drainage.

Precaution: Do not administer this product for more than 5 days. If symptoms persist or new ones occur, consult physician. If fever persists for more than three days, or recurs, consult physician. Severe or persistent sore throat with high fever, headaches, nausea or vomiting may be serious. Discontinue use and consult physician if not relieved in 24 hours.

Warning: Reye Syndrome is a rare but serious disease which can follow flu or chicken pox in children and teenagers. While the cause of Reye Syndrome is unknown, some reports claim aspirin may increase the risk of developing this disease. Consult doctor before use in children or teenagers with flu or chicken pox. As with any drug, if you are pregnant or nursing a baby, seek the advice of a health professional before using this product.

Dosage and Administration:
Dosage by Age and Weight
To be administered only under adult supervision.
[See St. Joseph Children's Dosage chart next page].
ST. JOSEPH Cold Tablets for Children may be given one of three ways. Always follow with ½ glass of water, milk, or fruit juice.

ST. JOSEPH CHILDREN'S DOSAGE CHART

Age	0–3 (months)	4–11 (months)	12–23 (months)	2–3 (years)	4–5 (years)	6–8 (years)	9–10 (years)	11 (years)	12+ (years)
Weight (lbs.)	7–12	13–21	22–26	27–35	36–45	46–65	66–76	77–83	84+
Dose of St. Joseph Acetaminophen Drops Dropperfuls	½	1	1½	2	3	4	5	—	—
Acetaminophen Liquid Teaspoonfuls	—	½	¾	1	1½	2	2½	3	4
Chewable Tablets Acetaminophen (80 mg. each) Aspirin (81 mg. each)	—	—	1½	2	3	4	5	6	8
Cold Tablets (81 mg. aspirin, 3.125 mg. phenylpropanolamine HCl)	—	—	1½	2	3	4	5	6	8

All dosages may be repeated every 4 hours, but do not exceed 5 dosages daily except for Cold Tablet dosages which should not exceed 4 doses daily.

Note: Since St. Joseph pediatric products are available without prescription, parents are advised on the package label to consult a physician for use in children under two years.

---

1. CHEWED, followed by liquid.
2. SWALLOWED whole, followed by liquid.
3. CRUSHED or dissolved in a teaspoon of liquid.

How Supplied: Chewable orange flavored tablets in plastic bottles of 36 tablets. Child-resistant, safety sealed packaging.

Shown in Product Identification Section, page 422

ST. JOSEPH® Cough Syrup for Children
Pediatric
Antitussive Syrup

Active Ingredient: Dextromethorphan hydrobromide 7.5 mg. per 5 cc.

Indications: For relief of coughing of colds and flu for up to 8 hours.

Actions: Antitussive

Warning: Should not be administered to children for persistent or chronic cough such as occurs with asthma or emphysema or where cough is accompanied by excessive secretions except under physician's advice. As with any drug, if you are pregnant or nursing a baby, seek the advice of a health professional before using this product.

Dosage and Administration:
Dosage:
[See St Joseph Cough Syrup for Children Dosage Chart below.]

How Supplied: Cherry tasting syrup in plastic bottle of 2 and 4 fl. ozs. In safety sealed packaging.

Shown in Product Identification Section, page 422

SHADE® Sunscreens

SHADE® Sunscreen Lotion SPF 4
SHADE® Sunscreen Lotion SPF 6
SHADE® Sunscreen Lotion SPF 8
SUPERSHADE® Sunblock Lotion SPF 15

Active Ingredients: Padimate O and Oxybenzone.

Indications: Waterproof sunscreens to help prevent harmful effects from the sun. SHADE screens both UVB and UVA rays. SHADE Moderate, Extra, Maximal and Highest Degree of Protection provide 4, 6, 8, and 15 times your natural sunburn protection. Liberal and regular use may help reduce the chances of premature aging and wrinkling of skin, due to overexposure to the sun. All strengths are waterproof, maintaining their sun protection factor for up to 80 minutes in water. Excellent for use on children.

Actions: Sunscreen

Warnings: For external use only. Avoid contact with eyes. Discontinue use if signs of irritation or rash appear.

Dosage and Administration: Apply evenly and liberally to all exposed skin. Reapply after prolonged swimming or excessive perspiration.

How Supplied: 4 fl. oz. Plastic Bottles
Shown in Product Identification Section, page 422

SOLARCAINE®
Antiseptic·Topical Anesthetic Lotion/Cream/Aerosol Spray Liquid

Active Ingredients:
SOLARCAINE Aerosol Spray—to deliver benzocaine 9.4% (w/w), triclosan 0.18% (w/w). Also contains isopropyl alcohol 24% (w/w) in total contents.
SOLARCAINE Lotion—Benzocaine and triclosan.
SOLARCAINE Cream—Benzocaine and triclosan.

Indications: Medicated first aid to provide fast temporary relief of sunburn pain, minor burns, cuts, scrapes, chapping and skin injuries, poison ivy, detergent hands, insect bites (non-venomous).

Actions: Benzocaine provides local anesthetic action to relieve itching and pain. Triclosan provides antimicrobial activity.

Caution: Not for use in eyes. Not for deep or puncture wounds or serious burns, nor for prolonged use. If condition persists, or infection, rash or irritation develops, discontinue use.

Warnings: For Aerosol Spray—Flammable—Do not spray while smoking or near fire. Do not spray into eyes or mouth. Avoid inhalation. Contents under pressure. For external use only.

Dosage and Administration: Lotion and Cream—Apply freely as needed. Spray—Hold 3 to 5 inches from injured area. Spray until wet. To apply to face, spray on palm of hand. Use often for antiseptic protection.

How Supplied:
SOLARCAINE Aerosol Spray—3- and 5-oz. cans.
SOLARCAINE Lotion—3- and 6-fl oz. bottles.
SOLARCAINE Cream—1-oz. tube.
Shown in Product Identification Section, page 422

St. Joseph Cough Syrup for Children Dosage Chart

Age	Weight	Dosage
Under 2 years	below 27 lbs.	As directed by physician.
2 to under 6 yrs.	27 to 45 lbs.	1 teaspoonful every 6 to 8 hours. (Not to exceed 4 teaspoonfuls daily.)
6 to under 12 yrs.	46 to 83 lbs.	2 teaspoonfuls every 6 to 8 hours. (Not to exceed 8 teaspoonfuls daily.)
12 years and older	84 and greater	4 teaspoonfuls every 6 to 8 hours. (Not to exceed 16 teaspoonfuls daily.)

Procter & Gamble
P. O. BOX 171
CINCINNATI, OH 45201

CHILDREN'S CHLORASEPTIC® LOZENGES

Description: Each Children's Chloraseptic Lozenge contains 5 mg. benzocaine as anesthetic in a grape flavored base of sugar and corn syrup solids.

Indications: Children's Chloraseptic Lozenges provide prompt, temporary relief of minor sore throat pain which may accompany conditions such as tonsillitis, pharyngitis and in posttonsillectomy soreness, and discomfort of minor mouth and gum irritations.

Dosage and Administration: Allow one lozenge to dissolve slowly in the mouth. Repeat hourly if needed. Do not take more than 12 lozenges per day. Not for children under 3 unless directed by a physician.

In addition, consumer labeling carries the following statement:

Warning: Consult physician promptly if sore throat is severe or lasts more than 2 days or is accompanied by high fever, headache, nausea, or vomiting. Not for children under 3 years unless directed by physician.

Active Ingredient: benzocaine (5 mg per lozenge).
STORE BELOW 86°F (30°C). PROTECT FROM MOISTURE.
KEEP ALL MEDICINES OUT OF REACH OF CHILDREN.

Packaging: Carton of 18 lozenges.
Shown in Product Identification Section, page 422

CHLORASEPTIC® LIQUID
(oral anesthetic, antiseptic)

Description: An alkaline solution containing phenol and sodium phenolate (total phenol 1.4%). In addition, Menthol Chloraseptic and Cherry Chloraseptic 1.5-oz Spray contain compressed nitrogen as a propellant.

Indications: Pleasant-tasting Chloraseptic is an antiseptic, anesthetic, deodorizing mouthwash and gargle. It is an alkaline solution designed specifically to maintain oral hygiene and to relieve local soreness and irritation without "caines." Chloraseptic may be used as a topical anesthetic while antibacterials are used systemically in the treatment of infection.

Chloraseptic acts promptly, often providing effective surface anesthesia in minutes. It is a valuable adjunct for temporary relief of pain and discomfort and will reduce oral bacterial flora temporarily to improve oral hygiene.

Chloraseptic is indicated for prompt temporary relief of discomfort due to the following conditions: *Medical*—oropharyngitis and throat infections; acute tonsillitis; and posttonsillectomy soreness; *Dental*—minor irritation or injury of soft tissue of the mouth; minor oral surgery or extractions; irritation caused by dentures or orthodontic appliances; and aphthous ulcers.

Administration and Dosage: Chloraseptic Mouthwash and Gargle—*Irritated throat:* Spray 5 times (children 3–12 years of age, 3 times) and swallow. May be used as a gargle. Repeat every 2 hours if necessary. *After oral surgery:* Allow full-strength solution to run over affected areas for 15 seconds without swishing, then expel remainder. Repeat every 2 hours if necessary. Not for children under 3 years of age unless directed by a physician or dentist. *Adjunctive gingival therapy:* Rinse vigorously with full-strength solution for 15 seconds, working between teeth, then expel remainder. Repeat every 2 hours if necessary. *Daily deodorizing mouthwash and gargle:* Dilute with equal parts of water and rinse thoroughly, or spray full strength, then expel remainder.

Chloraseptic Spray: *Irritated throat:* Spray throat about 2 seconds (children 3–12 years about 1 second) and swallow. Repeat every 2 hours if necessary. *After oral surgery:* Spray affected area for 1 to 2 seconds, allow solution to remain for 15 seconds without swishing, then expel remainder. Repeat every 2 hours if necessary. *Adjunctive gingival therapy:* Spray affected area for about 2 seconds, swish for 15 seconds working between teeth, then expel remainder. Repeat every 2 hours if necessary. *Daily deodorizing spray:* Spray, rinse thoroughly, and expel remainder. Not for children under 3 years of age unless directed by a physician or dentist.

Consumer labeling contains the following caution statement:

Caution: Severe or persistent sore throat or sore throat accompanied by high fever, headache, nausea or vomiting may be serious. Consult your physician. If sore throat persists more than 2 days consult physician. Do not administer to children under 3 years unless directed by physician.

Warning: For 1.5 oz. Spray—Avoid spraying in eyes. Contents under pressure. Do not puncture or incinerate. (Do not burn or throw in fire, as can will burst). Do not store at temperature above 120°F. (Such high temperatures may cause bursting.) KEEP ALL MEDICINES OUT OF REACH OF CHILDREN.
To insure product quality, avoid excessive heat (over 104°F or 40°C). See bottom of can for expiration date and control number.

How Supplied: Available in menthol or cherry flavor—6 oz. size with sprayer, 12 oz. refill bottle, and 1.5 oz. nitrogen propelled spray.
Shown in Product Identification Section, page 422

CHLORASEPTIC® LOZENGES

Description: Each Chloraseptic Lozenge contains phenol, sodium phenolate (total phenol 32.5 mg).

Indications: Chloraseptic Lozenges provide prompt temporary relief of discomfort due to mouth and gum irritations and of minor sore throat due to colds. They also may be used for topical anesthesia as an adjunct to systemic antibacterial therapy. For prompt temporary relief of pain and discomfort associated with the following conditions: *Medical*—oropharyngitis and throat infections; acute tonsillitis; posttonsillectomy soreness; *Dental*—minor irritation or injury of soft tissue of the mouth; minor oral surgery; and aphthous ulcers.

Administration and Dosage: Adults: Dissolve 1 lozenge in the mouth every 2 hours; do not exceed 8 lozenges per day. Children 3–12 years: Dissolve 1 lozenge in the mouth every 3 hours; **do not exceed 4 lozenges per day.** Not for children under 3 unless directed by a physician or dentist.
Consumer labeling contains the following caution statement:

Caution: Consult physician if sore throat is severe or lasts more than 2 days or is accompanied by high fever, headache, nausea or vomiting. Not for children under 3 unless directed by physician.
KEEP ALL MEDICINES OUT OF REACH OF CHILDREN.
Avoid excessive heat (over 104°F or 40°C).

How Supplied: Available in choice of menthol or cherry flavor—packages of 18 and 45 lozenges.
No prescription necessary.
Shown in Product Identification Section, page 422

ENCAPRIN®
Arthritis Pain Reliever

Composition: Regular Strength Encaprin capsules contain 325 mg (5 grains) of aspirin. Maximum Strength Encaprin capsules contain 500 mg (7.7 grains) of aspirin.

Description: Each capsule contains hundreds of individually enteric-coated micrograins of aspirin. These enteric-coated micrograins are designed to pass through the stomach to the small intestine before dissolving. The small size of the micrograins enables them to pass readily through the pylorus. Encaprin enteric-coated micrograins are associated with significantly less gastric damage than plain or even buffered aspirin.

Indications: Encaprin is an excellent analgesic, antipyretic and anti-inflammatory agent, particularly where there is a need to protect the stomach from aspirin-induced damage during chronic aspirin regimens. Encaprin provides temporary relief from mild arthritis symptoms, headache, painful discomfort of colds and flu, fever, sore throat, muscular aches and pains, dental pain, and menstrual pain.

Usual Adult Dosage: The following dosages are the maximum daily doses recommended for self-medication.

Regular Strength: Two or three capsules with water every 4 hours. Do not exceed 12 capsules in 24 hours unless directed by a physician. Children under 12—as recommended by a physician.

Maximum Strength: Two capsules with water every 4 hours. Do not exceed 8 capsules in 24 hours unless directed by a physician. Children under 12—as recommended by a physician.

B.I.D. Dosage: Bioavailability and endoscopy studies conducted at 4 grams/day indicate Encaprin can be safely prescribed on a b.i.d. dosage regimen by the physician. Patients should be titrated gradually to a b.i.d. regimen to avoid exceeding the individual's maximum aspirin tolerance level.

Precautions: This aspirin product should not be used by persons allergic to aspirin or under medical care without consulting a physician. If pain persists more than 10 days or redness is present, or in arthritic or rheumatic conditions affecting children under 12, consult a physician immediately. Discontinue use if dizziness, ringing in ears, or impaired hearing occurs. KEEP THIS AND ALL MEDICINES OUT OF REACH OF CHILDREN. IN CASE OF ACCIDENTAL OVERDOSE, CONTACT A PHYSICIAN OR POISON CONTROL CENTER IMMEDIATELY. As with any drug, if you are pregnant or nursing a baby, seek the advice of a health professional before using this product.

How Supplied:
Regular Strength Encaprin 325 mg (5 grains):
NDC 37000-027-03   Bottle of 75 capsules
NDC 37000-027-04   Bottle of 150 capsules
Maximum Strength Encaprin 500 mg (7.7 grains):
NDC 37000-028-03   Bottle of 50 capsules
NDC 37000-028-04   Bottle of 100 capsules
NDC 37000-028-05   Bottle of 200 capsules
Easy opening cap available on Regular Strength 150's and Maximum Strength 200's for households without young children.
For further product information, contact Encaprin Professional Services Division, (513) 530-2153.

Shown in Product Identification Section, page 422

HEAD & CHEST™
DECONGESTANT/EXPECTORANT COLD MEDICINE

Active Ingredients:
Each TABLET and CAPSULE contains:
Phenylpropanolamine HCl ....25 mg
Guaifenesin ....200 mg
Each 5 ml (one teaspoonful) LIQUID contains:

Phenylpropanolamine HCl ....12.5 mg
Guaifenesin ....100 mg
Alcohol 5%

Indications: HEAD & CHEST is indicated in colds, sinusitis, bronchitis, and other respiratory conditions to reduce nasal congestion and promote drainage of bronchial passageways.

Actions: Phenylpropanolamine HCl is an effective vasoconstrictor that decongests swollen mucous membranes of the respiratory tract. The expectorant guaifenesin enhances the flow of respiratory tract fluid, promotes ciliary action and facilitates removal of viscous, inspissated mucus. As a result, sinus and bronchial drainage is improved, and dry, nonproductive coughs become more productive and less frequent.

Warnings: This product should not be taken by persons who are hypersensitive to any of its ingredients or those who have high blood pressure, heart disease, diabetes, thyroid disease or persistent or chronic cough such as occurs with smoking, asthma, or emphysema, or where cough is accompanied by excessive secretions, or by children under 2 years except under the advice and supervision of a physician. If symptoms do not improve within 7 days or are accompanied by fever, rash, or persistent headache, consult a physician before continuing use. Do not exceed recommended dosage because at higher doses nervousness, dizziness or sleeplessness are more likely to occur. Keep all medicines out of reach of children. In case of accidental overdose, seek professional assistance or contact a poison control center immediately. As with any drug, if you are pregnant or nursing a baby, seek the advice of a health professional before using the product.

Drug Interaction Precaution: Do not take this product if you are presently taking a prescription antihypertensive or antidepressant drug containing a monoamine oxidase inhibitor except under the advice and supervision of a physician.

Overdosage: Treatment of overdosage should be directed toward supporting the patient and reversing the effects of the drug.

Dosage:
Adults and children over 12 years—2 teaspoonfuls LIQUID or 1 TABLET or 1 CAPSULE
Children 6–12 years—1 teaspoonful LIQUID or ½ tablet
Children 2–6 years—½ teaspoonful LIQUID
Repeat above dosage every 4 hours as needed to maximum of 6 doses in 24 hours.

How Supplied: LIQUID, TABLETS, and CAPSULES

Shown in Product Identification Section, page 423

HEAD & SHOULDERS® SHAMPOO
Antidandruff Shampoo

In late 1983, New Improved Head & Shoulders Lotion Shampoo was introduced with a thicker, richer formula. It offers the consumer effective dandruff control and beautiful hair in a formula that is pleasant to use. Independently conducted clinical testing (double-blind and dermatologist-graded) has proved that the new lotion formula reduces dandruff flaking significantly more than the previous one. This new rich formula is also gentle enough to use every day for clean, manageable hair.

Active Ingredient: 1.0% pyrithione zinc suspended in an anionic detergent system. Cosmetic ingredients are also included.

Indications: For effective control of dandruff and seborrheic dermatitis of the scalp.

Actions: Pyrithione zinc is substantive to the scalp and remains after rinsing. Its mechanism of action has not been fully established, but it is believed to control the microorganisms associated with dandruff flaking and itching.

Precautions: Not to be taken internally. Keep out of children's reach. Avoid getting shampoo in eyes—if this happens, rinse eyes with water.

Dosage and Administration: For best results, Head & Shoulders should be used regularly. Head & Shoulders can be used not only to treat dandruff, but also regular use will help control the recurrence of symptoms. It is gentle enough to use for every shampoo. In treating seborrheic dermatitis, a minimum of four shampooings are needed to achieve full effectiveness.

How Supplied: Regular and Conditioning lotions available in 4.0 fl. oz., 7.0 fl. oz., 11.0 fl. oz., and 15.0 fl. oz. unbreakable plastic bottles. Cream form available in 2.5 oz., 4.0 oz., and 7.0 oz. tubes.

Composition: LOTION—Regular Formula: Pyrithione zinc in a shampoo base of water, TEA-lauryl sulfate, glycol distearate, cocamide MEA, sodium chloride, fragrance, citric acid, methylchloroisothiazolinone, methylisothiazolinone, and FD&C Blue No. 1. LOTION—Conditioning Formula: Pyrithione zinc in a shampoo base of water, TEA-lauryl sulfate, glycol distearate, cocamide MEA, sodium chloride, fragrance, citric acid, propylene glycol, methylchloroisothiazolinone, methylisothiazolinone, and FD&C Blue No. 1. CREAM: Pyrithione zinc in a shampoo base of water, sodium cocoglyceryl ether sulfonate, sodium chloride, sodium lauroyl sarcosinate, cocamide DEA, cocoyl sarcosine, fragrance, and FD&C Blue No. 1.

Continued on next page

Procter & Gamble—Cont.

NORWICH® Regular Strength Aspirin
Aspirin (acetylsalicylic acid) tablets

Active Ingredient: Each tablet contains 325 mg (5 grains) of pure aspirin.

Actions: Analgesic and antipyretic.

Indications: For fast effective relief of headaches, pains and fever from colds and flu, muscular and arthritic pains and aches, sprains, rheumatism, lower back pain, menstrual discomfort, toothaches, pains following dental procedures, and reduction of fever.

Warnings: Keep all medicines out of reach of children.

Contraindications: Do not take if asthmatic, pregnant or nursing except under advice and supervision of physician.

Caution: Do not take if you have ulcers, ulcer symptoms or bleeding problems. Consult physician if taking medicines for anticoagulation (thinning the blood), diabetes, gout or arthritis.
If pain persists for more than 10 days or if redness is present, or in conditions affecting children under 12, consult physician immediately. Discontinue use if ringing in the ears occurs.

Treatment of Oral Overdosage: In case of accidental overdose seek professional assistance or contact a poison control center immediately.

Dosage and Administration: Adults: 1 or 2 tablets every 3-4 hours up to 6 times a day. Children: under 3 years, consult physician; 3-6 years, ½-1 tablet; over 6 years, 1 tablet. May be taken every 3-4 hours up to 3 times a day.

Professional Labeling: Same as those outlined under Indications.

How Supplied: In bottles of 100, 250 and 500 tablets.
Shown in Product Identification Section, page 423

NORWICH® EXTRA-STRENGTH ASPIRIN
Aspirin (acetylsalicylic acid) tablets

Active Ingredient: Each tablet contains 500 mg (7.7 grains) of pure aspirin.

Actions: Analgesic and antipyretic.

Indications: For fast, effective relief of headaches, pains and fever from colds or flu, muscular and arthritic pains and aches, sprains, rheumatism, menstrual discomfort, lower back pain, toothaches, pains following dental procedure, and reduction of fever.

Warnings: Keep all medicines out of the reach of children.

Contraindications: Do not take if asthmatic, pregnant or nursing except under advice and supervision of physician.

Caution: Do not take if you have ulcers, ulcer symptoms or bleeding problems. Consult physician if taking medicines for anticoagulation (thinning the blood), diabetes, gout or arthritis.
If pain persists for more than 10 days or if redness is present, or in conditions affecting children under 12, consult physician immediately. Discontinue use if ringing in the ears occurs.

Treatment of Oral Overdosage: In case of accidental overdose seek professional assistance or contact a poison control center immediately.

Dosage and Administration: Adults: Initial dose 2 tablets followed by 1 tablet every 3½ hours or 2 tablets every 6 hours, not to exceed 8 tablets in any 24-hour period, or as directed by a physician. NOT RECOMMENDED FOR CHILDREN UNDER 12.

Professional Labeling: Same as outlined under Indications.

How Supplied: In bottles of 150 tablets.
Shown in Product Identification Section, page 423

PEPTO–BISMOL®
LIQUID AND TABLETS
For upset stomach, indigestion, nausea and heartburn.
Controls common diarrhea.

Active Ingredient: Bismuth subsalicylate, 300 mg per tablet or 262 mg per 15 ml (tablespoonful). Contains no sugar and is low in sodium.

Indications: Heartburn and indigestion—Pepto-Bismol soothes irritation with a protective coating action, without constipating. Nausea and upset stomach—Pepto-Bismol brings fast sure relief from distress of queasiness and that bloated feeling. Diarrhea—controls diarrhea within 24 hours, relieving associated abdominal cramps. Keep all medicines out of reach of children.

Caution: This product contains salicylates. If taken with aspirin and ringing of the ears occurs, discontinue use. If taking medicines for anticoagulation (thinning the blood), diabetes, or gout, consult physician before taking this product. If diarrhea is accompanied by high fever or continues more than 2 days, consult a physician.

Warning: As with any drug, if you are pregnant or nursing a baby, seek the advice of a health professional before using this product. Avoid excessive heat (over 140°F or 40°C).

Dosage Directions
Liquid—Shake well before using
Adults: 2 tablespoonfuls
Children (according to age):
  9–12 years—1 tablespoonful
  6–9 years—2 teaspoonsful
  3–6 years—1 teaspoonful
For children under 3 years, consult a physician.

Repeat above dosage every ½ to 1 hour, if needed to a maximum of 8 doses in 24 hour period.
Note: The beneficial medication may form a coating on the tongue which sometimes darkens in color. Darkening of the stool is also possible. Both conditions are harmless and temporary.
Tablets
Adults: 2 tablets
Children (according to age):
  9–12 years—1 tablet
  6–9 years—⅔ tablet
  3–6 years—⅓ tablet
For children under 3 years, consult a physician.
Chew or dissolve in mouth. Repeat every ½ to 1 hour as needed, to a maximum of 8 doses in 24-hour period. Each tablet dose is a full liquid dose in concentrated form.

How Supplied: Pepto-Bismol is available in Liquid and Tablets.
Shown in Product Identification Section, page 423

SCOPE®
Oral Rinse

Description: Scope is an oral rinse, green in color, with a pleasant tasting, fresh wintergreen flavor. It has a low surface tension, approximately ½ that of water. Scope refreshes the mouth and leaves it feeling clean.

Composition: Cetylpyridinium chloride (.045%), domiphen bromide (.005%) and SD alcohol 38F (18.5%) in a mouthwash base of water, glycerin, polysorbate 80, flavor, sodium saccharin, FD&C Blue No. 1 and FD&C Yellow No. 5.

Consumer Use: For mouth refreshment and as an aid to daily oral care. Scope also helps provide soothing, temporary relief of dryness and minor irritations of the mouth and throat.

Dental Office Use: Scope is used before, during and after instrumentation and dental prophylaxis in the interest of enhancing patient comfort, as well as to provide dentists with a more pleasant working environment. Scope's low surface tension also makes it ideal for preparing oral surfaces for impressions. A pre-impression rinse with Scope helps remove debris and ropy saliva from the oral cavity. It is also used for mouth freshening after taking impressions. Scope will not clog dental spray units (it contains no sugar).

Consumer Usage Instructions: Rinse or gargle for 20 seconds with one ounce of Scope first thing in the morning, after meals or when needed for mouth refreshment.

Consumer Precautions: Keep out of reach of children. Do not administer to any child under six years of age. Any sore throat may be serious; consult your doctor promptly.

Dental Office Precautions: Keep out of reach of children. Not to be used undiluted. Because of high alcohol content, avoid contact with eyes and ingestion of the undiluted concentrate.

How Supplied: Scope is supplied to consumers in 6, 12, 18, 24 and 40 fl. oz. bottles and is available to the dental profession in a ½ gallon concentrate (each ½ gallon makes 1.75 gallons of regular Scope). 18 oz. operatory decanters and a spray attachment for the decanter are available for office use.

The Purdue Frederick Company
100 CONNECTICUT AVENUE
NORWALK, CT 06856

BETADINE® Antiseptic Gel
(povidone-iodine, 10%)

Action and Uses: Applied at bedtime, BETADINE Antiseptic Gel works through the night to provide prompt, soothing symptomatic relief of minor vaginal irritation, itching and soreness. Its active ingredient — the broad-spectrum microbicide povidone-iodine — significantly and rapidly reduces the aerobic and anaerobic count, offering comfort on contact from annoying vaginal symptoms and odor. May also be used for preoperative degerming.

Advantages: Its gel formulation offers the advantage of prolonged contact with irritated vaginal tissue to help provide long-lasting relief. BETADINE Antiseptic Gel is gentle and virtually nonirritating to delicate vaginal tissue. It is nongreasy and nonsticky.

Directions for Use: Insert one applicatorful of BETADINE Antiseptic Gel. Leave medication in the vagina overnight. A sanitary napkin should be worn overnight. When external irritation is present, BETADINE Antiseptic Gel may be applied manually to the affected area. Treatment should be continued for seven days.

How Supplied: 18 g tubes and 3 oz. tubes, each packaged with a convenient, easy-to-use vaginal applicator.

BETADINE® SOLUTION
(povidone-iodine 10%)
Topical antiseptic, germicide

Action and Uses: For preoperative prepping of operative site, including the vagina, and as a general topical microbicide for: disinfection of wounds; emergency treatment of lacerations and abrasions; second– and third–degree burns; as a prophylactic anti-infective agent in hospital and office procedures, including postoperative application to incisions to help prevent infection; trichomonal, monilial, and nonspecific infectious vaginitis; oral moniliasis (thrush); bacterial and mycotic skin infections; decubitus and stasis ulcers; preoperatively, in the mouth and throat, as a swab. BETADINE Solution is microbicidal, and not merely bacteriostatic. It *kills* gram-positive and gram-negative bacteria (including antibiotic-resistant strains), fungi, viruses, protozoa and yeasts.

Administration: Apply full strength as often as needed as a paint, spray, or wet soak. May be bandaged.
Caution: In preoperative prepping, avoid "pooling" beneath the patient. Prolonged exposure to unabsorbed, wet solution may cause irritation.

How Supplied: ½ oz., 4 oz., 8 oz., 16 oz. (1 pt.), 32 oz. (1 qt.) and 1 gal. plastic bottles and 1 oz. packettes in foil or saran.

Also Available: BETADINE SOLUTION SWAB AIDS for degerming small areas of skin or mucous membranes prior to injections, aspirations, catheterization and surgery; boxes of 100 packettes. Also: disposable BETADINE SOLUTION SWABSTICKS, in packettes of 1's and 3's.

BETADINE® DOUCHE
(povidone-iodine)

A pleasantly scented solution, BETADINE Douche is clinically effective in the treatment of vaginitis. Also for the prompt symptomatic relief of minor vaginal irritation and itching, and as a cleansing douche.

Advantages: Low surface tension, with uniform wetting action to assist penetration into vaginal crypts and crevices. Active in the presence of blood, pus, or vaginal secretions. Virtually nonirritating to vaginal mucosa. Will not stain skin or natural fabrics.

Directions for Use: As a Therapeutic Douche: Two (2) tablespoonfuls to a quart of lukewarm water once daily. **As a Routine Cleansing Douche:** One (1) tablespoonful to a quart of lukewarm water once or twice per week. **As a Douche for Prompt Symptomatic Relief of Minor Vaginal Irritation and Itching.** One (1) tablespoonful to a quart of lukewarm water once daily for five days. Treatment should continue for the full five days, even if symptoms are relieved earlier.

How Supplied: 1 oz., 8 oz. plastic bottles. Disposable ½ oz. (1 tablespoonful) packettes.

Also Available: BETADINE Douche Kit is supplied as individual units, each containing:
(1) 8 oz. plastic bottle of BETADINE Douche concentrate;
(2) 14 oz., squeezable, plastic syringe bottle;
(3) anatomically-correct cannula;
(4) instruction booklet.
The 8 oz. bottle of BETADINE Douche concentrate is sufficient for up to 40 douches.

Directions for Use:
As a Therapeutic Douche: Add one (1) tablespoonful of BETADINE Douche concentrate to the 14 oz. syringe bottle which is then filled to the top with lukewarm water. Douche, then repeat the procedure. For daily use.
As a douche for prompt symptomatic relief of minor vaginal irritation and itching: Add BETADINE Douche concentrate to FIRST FILL-LINE on syringe bottle. Add lukewarm water up to WATER FILL-LINE. Use once daily for 5 days. Treatment should continue for the full 5 days, even if symptoms are relieved earlier.

As a Routine Cleansing Douche: Add BETADINE Douche concentrate to FIRST FILL-LINE on syringe bottle. Add lukewarm water up to WATER FILL-LINE. For use once or twice a week.

Also Available: BETADINE® Medicated Douche is a hygienic, **disposable,** convenient method to provide symptomatic relief of minor vaginal irritation, itching, and soreness. Also cleanses and deodorizes.
BETADINE Medicated Douche is supplied as individual units, each containing:
(1) 0.18 fl. oz. (5.2 ml) BETADINE Douche Concentrate;
(2) 6 fl. oz. (177 ml) of sanitized water in a squeezable, plastic syringe bottle with nozzle (when mixed, a 0.25% solution of povidone-iodine is formed);
(3) instruction booklet.
The syringe bottle and nozzle are completely disposable to avoid contamination from previously used douche accessories. Also supplied in a "Twin Pack."

BETADINE® SKIN CLEANSER
(povidone-iodine)

BETADINE Skin Cleanser is a sudsing antiseptic liquid cleanser. It essentially retains the nonselective microbicidal action of iodine, yet virtually without the undesirable features associated with iodine. BETADINE Skin Cleanser kills gram-positive and gram-negative bacteria (including antibiotic-resistant strains), fungi, viruses, protozoa and yeasts. It forms a rich golden lather; virtually nonirritating; nonstaining to skin and natural fabrics.

Indications: BETADINE Skin Cleanser aids in degerming the skin of patients with common pathogens, including Staphylococcus aureus. To help prevent the recurrence of acute inflammatory skin infections caused by iodine-susceptible pyogenic bacteria. In pyodermas, as a topical adjunct to systemic antimicrobial therapy. To help prevent spread of infection in acne pimples.

Directions for Use: Wet the skin and apply a sufficient amount of Skin Cleanser to work up a rich golden lather. Allow lather to remain about 3 minutes. Then rinse. Repeat 2-3 times a day or as needed.

Caution: In rare instances of local sensitivity, discontinue use by the individual.

How Supplied: 1 fl. oz. and 4 fl. oz. plastic bottles.

Note: Blue stains on starched linen will wash off with soap and water.

Continued on next page

Purdue Frederick—Cont.

BETADINE® OINTMENT
(povidone-iodine)

Action: BETADINE Ointment, in a water-soluble base, is a topical agent active against organisms commonly encountered in skin and wound infections. BETADINE Ointment kills gram-positive and gram-negative bacteria (including antibiotic-resistant strains), fungi, viruses, protozoa and yeasts.

The broad-spectrum activity of BETADINE Ointment provides microbicidal action against most commonly occurring skin bacteria. Its range of antibacterial activity encompasses many bacteria—including antibiotic-resistant forms.

The active ingredient in BETADINE Ointment substantially retains the broad-spectrum germicidal activity of iodine without the undesirable features or disadvantages of iodine. BETADINE Ointment is virtually nonirritating, does not block air from reaching the site of application, and washes easily off skin and natural fabrics. The site to which BETADINE Ointment is applied can be bandaged.

Indications: Therapeutically, BETADINE Ointment may be used as an adjunct to systemic therapy where indicated; for primary or secondary topical infections caused by iodine-susceptible organisms such as infected burns, infected surgical incisions, infected decubitus or stasis ulcers, pyodermas, secondarily infected dermatoses, and infected traumatic lesions.

Prophylactically: BETADINE Ointment may be used to prevent microbial contamination in burns, incisions and other topical lesions; for degerming skin in hyperalimentation, catheter care, the umbilical area or circumcision. The use of BETADINE Ointment for abrasions, minor cuts, and wounds, may prevent the development of infections and permit wound healing.

Administration: Apply directly to affected area as needed. May be bandaged.

How Supplied: $1/32$ oz. and $1/8$ oz. packettes; 1 oz. tubes; 16 oz. (1 lb.) and 5 lb. jars.

BETADINE® Vaginal Suppositories
(povidone-iodine, 10%)

Action and Uses: Applied at bedtime, BETADINE Vaginal Suppositories work through the night to provide prompt symptomatic relief of minor vaginal irritation, itching and soreness. Its active ingredient — the broad-spectrum microbicide povidone-iodine — significantly and rapidly reduces the aerobic and anaerobic count, offering soothing, nightlong relief from annoying vaginal symptoms and odor.

Advantages: BETADINE Vaginal Suppositories are easily and quickly inserted to provide prolonged contact with irritated vaginal tissue to help provide long-lasting relief. BETADINE Vaginal Suppositories are gentle and virtually non-irritating to delicate vaginal tissue. Non-staining to skin and natural fabrics, color can be washed off with soap and water.

Directions for Use: Unwrap a suppository and gently insert its smaller end into the applicator. Insert the suppository into the vagina. Leave medication in the vagina overnight. A sanitary napkin should be worn overnight. Treatment should be continued for seven days.

How Supplied: 7 Suppositories packaged with a convenient, easy-to-use applicator and patient instruction booklet.

FIBERMED®
High–Fiber Supplements
Fruit Flavor/Original Flavor
Also Fruit Flavor Snacks

Description: FIBERMED High-Fiber Supplements provide a measured quantity of natural dietary fiber in a palatable, ready-to-eat form. FIBERMED Supplements are standardized to provide concentrated dietary fiber in precise amounts—10 grams in two delicious biscuits. Original-Flavor FIBERMED contains natural dietary fiber from corn, wheat and oats. Fruit-Flavor FIBERMED contain natural dietary fiber from six sources: corn, oats, wheat, soy, apple and currants. Lack of fiber in the diet is a recognized cause of constipation, irritable bowel syndrome, diverticulosis and hemorrhoids.

Two FIBERMED High-Fiber Biscuits a day help provide the supplementary bulk that patients may need in their diet to avoid constipation.

FIBERMED also helps curb appetite. FIBERMED may help in weight control programs two ways. Fiber produces feelings of satiety and fullness, and can reduce one's desire for food. FIBERMED Supplements are superior to other fiber sources because of their uniform high-fiber content, convenience and good taste, qualities which encourage good compliance.

Ready-to-eat FIBERMED Supplements can be eaten any time, any place. Unlike most high-fiber foods or powdered bulks, FIBERMED requires no preparation and no mixing. They can be eaten with milk, coffee, tea, juice, soup or fruit; or dunked in a beverage.

NUTRITION INFORMATION PER SERVING OF ORIGINAL-FLAVOR FIBERMED:

Serving Size	1 Supplement
Servings per package	14
Calories	60
Protein	1 g
Carbohydrate	14 g*
Fat	2 g
Sodium	100 mg
Dietary Fiber	5 g

PERCENTAGE OF U.S. RECOMMENDED DAILY ALLOWANCE (% U.S. RDA):

Riboflavin (Vitamin B$_2$)	2
Niacin	2
Iron	4

Contains less than 2% of the U.S. RDA of Protein, Vitamin A, Vitamin C, Thiamine and Calcium.

*Includes 4.5 g of simple carbohydrates (brown sugar) and 8.5 g of complex carbohydrates.

Ingredients: Corn Bran, Brown Sugar, Wheat Flour, Corn Starch, Wheat Bran, Oat Flakes, Corn Germ Meal, Vegetable Shortening (Partially Hydrogenated Soybean Oil), Sodium Bicarbonate, Natural Vanilla Flavor, Ammonium Bicarbonate, Baking Acid, Salt, Cinnamon and Citric Acid.

NUTRITION INFORMATION PER SERVING OF FRUIT-FLAVOR FIBERMED:

Serving Size	1 Supplement
Servings per package	14
Calories	60
Protein	2 g
Carbohydrate	13 g*
Fat	2 g
Sodium	110 mg
Dietary Fiber	5 g

PERCENTAGE OF U.S. RECOMMENDED DAILY ALLOWANCES (% U.S. RDA):

Protein	2
Riboflavin (Vitamin B$_2$)	2
Niacin	4
Calcium	2
Iron	4

Contains less than 2% of the U.S. RDA of Vitamin A, Vitamin C and Thiamine.

*Includes 4.5 g of simple carbohydrates (brown sugar) and 8.5 g of complex carbohydrates.

Ingredients: Corn Bran, Brown Sugar, Whole Rolled Oats, Soy Flour, Vegetable Shortening (Partially Hydrogenated Soybean Oil), Currants, Wheat Bran, Dried Apple, Ammonium Bicarbonate, Citric Acid, Wheat Flour, Salt, Vanilla, Baking Acid, Cinnamon.

Usage: FIBERMED Supplements are indicated for those conditions, including constipation, in which it is desirable to regulate gastrointestinal transit time, increase stool weight and make elimination easier. Because of their taste and convenience, FIBERMED Supplements are the product of choice to significantly increase intake of dietary fiber in uniform amounts.

Two FIBERMED Supplements a day provide a high level of dietary fiber—10 grams—more dietary fiber than a serving of high-fiber cereal.

Directions: Two FIBERMED Biscuits per day provide the extra fiber required by most people. As with any healthful diet, adequate fluid intake is important.

Supplied: FIBERMED Supplements are available in Fruit Flavor as well as Original Flavor. FIBERMED Supplements are supplied in boxes of 14. For most individuals, 14 is a week's supply.

Also available: FIBERMED® High-Fiber SNACKS contain no preservatives.

FIBERMED SNACKS contain dietary fiber from six natural sources—corn, oats, wheat, soy, apples and currants. Thirteen bite-size FIBERMED SNACKS provide 5 grams of concentrated natural dietary fiber. Supplied in 8.5 oz. boxes.

SENOKOT® TABLETS/GRANULES
(standardized senna concentrate)

Action and Uses: Indicated for relief of functional constipation (chronic or occasional). SENOKOT Tablets/Granules contain a natural vegetable derivative, purified and standardized for uniform action. The current theory of the mechanism of action is that glycosides are transported to the colon, where they are changed to aglycones that stimulate Auerbach's plexus to induce peristalsis. This virtually colon-specific action is gentle, effective and predictable, usually inducing comfortable evacuation of well-formed stool within 8-10 hours. Found effective even in many previously intractable cases of functional constipation, SENOKOT preparations may aid in rehabilitation of the constipated patient by facilitating regular elimination. At proper dosage levels, SENOKOT preparations are virtually free of adverse reactions (such as loose stools or abdominal discomfort) and enjoy high patient acceptance. Numerous and extensive clinical studies show their high degree of effectiveness in varieties of functional constipation: chronic, geriatric, antepartum and postpartum, drug-induced, and pediatric, as well as in functional constipation concurrent with heart disease or anorectal surgery.

Contraindications: Acute surgical abdomen.

Administration and Dosage: Preferably at bedtime. GRANULES (deliciously cocoa-flavored): Adults: 1 level tsp. (maximum—2 level tsp. b.i.d.). For older, debilitated, and OB/GYN patients, the physician may consider prescribing ½ the initial adult dose. Children above 60 lb.: ½ level tsp. (maximum—1 level tsp. b.i.d.). TABLETS: Adults: 2 tablets (maximum—4 tablets b.i.d.). For older, debilitated, and OB/-GYN patients, the physician may consider prescribing ½ the initial dose. Children above 60 lb.: 1 tablet (maximum—2 tablets b.i.d.). To meet individual requirements, if comfortable bowel movement is not achieved by the second day, decrease or increase dosage daily by ½ level tsp. or 1 tablet (up to maximum) until optimal dose for evacuation is established.

How Supplied: Granules: 2, 6, and 12 oz. plastic canisters. Tablets: Box of 20, bottles of 50, 100 and 1000. SENOKOT Tablets Unit Strip Packs in boxes of 100 tablets; each tablet individually sealed in see-through pockets.

SENOKOT-S® TABLETS
(docusate sodium and standardized senna concentrate)
Stool Softener/Natural Laxative Combination

Action and Uses: SENOKOT-S Tablets are designed to relieve both aspects of functional constipation—dry, hard stools and bowel inertia. They provide a classic stool softener combined with a natural neuroperistaltic stimulant: docusate sodium softens the stool for smoother and easier evacuation, while standardized senna concentrate gently stimulates Auerbach's plexus in the colonic wall. This coordinated dual action of the two ingredients results in colon-specific, predictable laxative effect, usually in 8-10 hours. Administering the tablets at bedtime allows the patient an uninterrupted night's sleep, with a comfortable evacuation in the morning. Flexibility of dosage permits fine adjustment to individual requirements. At proper dosage levels, SENOKOT-S Tablets are virtually free from side effects. SENOKOT-S Tablets are highly suitable for relief of postsurgical and postpartum constipation, and effectively counteract drug-induced constipation. They facilitate regular elimination in impaction-prone and elderly patients, and are indicated in the presence of cardiovascular disease where straining must be avoided, as well as in the presence of hemorrhoids and anorectal disease.

Contraindications: Acute surgical abdomen.

Administration and Dosage: (preferably at bedtime) Recommended Initial Dosage: ADULTS—2 tablets (maximum dosage—4 tablets b.i.d.); CHILDREN (above 60 lbs.)—1 tablet (maximum dosage—2 tablets b.i.d.). For older or debilitated patients, the physician may consider prescribing half the initial adult dose. To meet individual requirements, if comfortable bowel movement is not achieved by the second day, dosage may be decreased or increased by 1 tablet, up to maximum, until the most effective dose is established.

Supplied: Bottles of 30 and 60 Tablets.

Reed & Carnrick
**1 NEW ENGLAND AVENUE
PISCATAWAY, NJ 08854**

PHAZYME® Tablets

Description: A pink coated two-phase tablet. Contains specially activated simethicone both in the outer layer for release in the stomach and in the inner enteric coated core for release in the small intestine, a total of 60 mg. Inactive ingredients include: Acacia, calcium sulfate, carnauba wax, crospovidone, FD&C Yellow #6 Lake, FD&C Red #40 Lake, gelatin, lactose, microcrystalline cellulose, polyoxyl-40 stearate, polyvinyl acetate phthalate, povidone, pregelatinized starch, rice starch, sodium benzoate, sucrose, titanium dioxide.

Actions: PHAZYME is the only dual approach to the problem of gastrointestinal gas. Simethicone minimizes gas formation and relieves gas entrapment in both the stomach and the lower G.I. tract. This action combats pain, due to gastrointestinal gas. Also, for relief of gas distress associated with other functional or organic conditions such as: diverticulitis, spastic colitis, hyperacidity, post-cholecystectomy syndrome and chronic cholecystitis.

Indications: PHAZYME is indicated for the relief of occasional or chronic pain caused by gas entrapped in the stomach or in the lower gastrointestinal tract—resulting from aerophagia, postoperative distention, dyspepsia and food intolerance.

Contraindications: A known sensitivity to any ingredient.

Dosage: One or two tablets with each meal and at bedtime or as required.

How Supplied: Pink coated two-phase tablet in bottles of 50, 100, and 1,000.
Shown in Product Identification Section, page 423

PHAZYME®–95 Tablets

Description: A red coated two-phase tablet with the highest dose of simethicone available in a single tablet. Contains specially activated simethicone both in the outer layer for release in the stomach and in the inner enteric coated core for release in the small intestine, a total of 95 mg. Inactive ingredients include: Acacia, calcium sulfate, carnauba wax, crospovidone, FD&C Yellow #6 Lake, FD&C Red #40 Lake, gelatin, lactose, microcrystalline cellulose, polyoxyl-40 stearate, polyvinyl acetate phthalate, povidone, pregelatinized starch, rice starch, sodium benzoate, sucrose, titanium dioxide.

Actions: PHAZYME is the only dual approach to the problem of gastrointestinal gas. Simethicone minimizes gas formation and relieves gas entrapment in both the stomach and the lower G.I. tract. This action combats pain, due to gastrointestinal gas. Also, for relief of gas distress associated with other functional or organic conditions such as: diverticulitis, spastic colitis, hyperacidity, post-cholecystectomy syndrome and chronic cholecystitis.

Indications: PHAZYME-95 is indicated for the relief of acute severe lower intestinal pain due to gas—resulting from aerophagia, postoperative distention, dyspepsia and food intolerance.

Contraindications: A known sensitivity to any ingredient.

Dosage: One tablet with each meal and at bedtime, or as required.

Continued on next page

Reed & Carnrick—Cont.

How Supplied: Red coated two-phase tablet in 10 pack, bottles of 50, 100 and 500.

Shown in Product Identification Section, page 423

proctoFoam®/non-steroid (pramoxine HCl 1%)

Description: proctoFoam is a foam for anal and perianal use containing Pramoxine hydrochloride 1%.

Actions: proctoFoam is an anesthetic mucoadhesive foam which medicates the anorectal mucosa, and provides prompt temporary relief from itching and pain. Its lubricating action helps make bowel evacuations more comfortable.

Indications: Prompt, temporary relief of anorectal inflammation, pruritus and pain associated with hemorrhoids, proctitis, cryptitis, fissures, postoperative pain and pruritus ani.

Contraindications: Contraindicated in persons hypersensitive to any of the ingredients.

Warning: Not for prolonged use. Do not use more than four consecutive weeks. If redness, pain, irritation or swelling persists or rectal bleeding occurs, discontinue use and consult a physician. Keep this and all medicines out of the reach of children.

Caution: Do not insert any part of the aerosol container into the anus. Contents of the container are under pressure, but not flammable. Do not burn or puncture the aerosol container. Store at room temperature. not over 120° F.

Dosage:
One applicatorful two or three times daily and after bowel evacuation.
1. To fill—Shake foam container vigorously before use. Hold container upright and insert into opening of applicator tip. With applicator drawn out all the way, press down on container cap. When the foam reaches fill line in the applicator, it is ready to use. CAUTION: The aerosol container should never be inserted directly into the anus.
2. To administer—Separate applicator from container. Hold applicator by barrel and gently insert tip into the anus. With applicator in place, push plunger in order to expel foam, then withdraw applicator. (Applicator parts should be pulled apart for thorough cleaning with warm water.)
Note: To relieve itching place some foam on a tissue and apply externally.

How Supplied: Available in 15 g aerosol container, with special plastic applicator. The aerosol supplies approximately 18 applications.

Literature Available: Instruction pads with directions for use available upon request.

Shown in Product Identification Section, page 423

R&C SHAMPOO® Shampoo Pediculicide

Description: R&C SHAMPOO is the only one-step pediculicide shampoo available without a prescription. Its active ingredients are: pyrethrins 0.30%, piperonyl butoxide technical 3.00%, equivalent to 2.40% (butycarbityl) (6-propylpiperonyl) ether and 0.60% related compounds, petroleum distillate 1.20%. Inert ingredients 95.50%.

Action: R&C SHAMPOO kills head lice (pediculus capitis), crab lice (phthirus pubis) and body lice (pediculus corporis) and their eggs on contact.

Indications: R&C SHAMPOO is indicated for the treatment of infestations with head lice, crab lice and body lice.

Warning: R&C SHAMPOO should not be used by ragweed sensitized persons.

Caution: R&C SHAMPOO is for external use only. It can be harmful if swallowed or inhaled. It should be kept out of eyes and avoid contact with mucous membranes. If accidental contact with eyes occurs, flush immediately with water. In case of infection or skin irritation, discontinue use and consult a physician. Consult a physician if louse infestation of eyebrows and eyelashes occurs. Avoid contamination of feed or foodstuffs.

Storage and Disposal:
Storage: Store below 120°F.
Disposal: Do not reuse container. Rinse thoroughly before discarding in trash.

Dosage and Administration: (1) Apply a sufficient quantity of R&C SHAMPOO to throughly wet dry hair and skin, paying particular attention to the infested and adjacent hairy areas. (2) Allow R&C SHAMPOO to remain on the area for 10 minutes. (3) Add small quantities of water, working the shampoo into the hair and skin until a lather forms. (4) Rinse thoroughly. Dead lice and eggs will require removal with fine-tooth comb. If necessary, treatment may be repeated but do not exceed two consecutive applications within 24 hrs.
Since lice infestations are spread by contact, each family member should be examined carefully. If infested, he or she should be treated promptly to avoid spreading or reinfestation of previously treated individuals.
To eliminate infestation, it is important to wash all clothing, bedding, towels and combs and brushes, used by the infested person in hot water (130°). Dry clean non-washable items.

How Supplied: In 2 and 4 fl oz. plastic bottles with pourable cap. Fine-tooth comb to aid in removal of dead lice and nits and patient booklet are included in each package of R&C SHAMPOO.

Literature Available: Patient information available on request.

Shown in Product Identification Section, page 423

R&C SPRAY® III Lice Control Insecticide

Description: Active ingredients: 3-Phenoxybenzyl d-cis and trans 2,2-dimethyl-3-(2-methylpropenyl) cyclopropanecarboxylate 0.382%
Other Isomers 0.018%
Petroleum Distillates 4.255%
Inert Ingredients: 95.345%
_____
100.000%

Actions: R&C SPRAY is specially formulated to kill lice and their nits on inanimate objects.

Indications: R&C SPRAY is recommended for use only on bedding, mattresses, furniture and other objects infested or possibly infested with lice which cannot be laundered or dry cleaned.

Warnings: Contents under pressure. Do not use or store near heat or open flame. Do not puncture or incinerate container. Exposure to temperatures above 130°F may cause bursting. It is a violation of Federal law to use this product in a manner inconsistent with its labeling. NOT FOR USE ON HUMANS OR ANIMALS.

Caution: Avoid spraying in eyes. Avoid breathing spray mist. Avoid contact with the skin. May be absorbed through the skin. In case of contact, wash immediately with soap and water. Harmful if swallowed. Vacate room after treatment and ventilate before reoccupying. Avoid contamination of feed and foodstuffs. Remove pets, birds and cover fish aquariums before spraying.

Directions: SHAKE WELL BEFORE AND OCCASIONALLY DURING USE. Spray on an inconspicuous area to test for possible staining or discoloration. Inspect after drying, then proceed to spray entire area to be treated.
Hold container upright with nozzle away from you. Depress valve and spray from a distance of 8 to 10 inches.
Spray each square foot for about three seconds. For mattresses, furniture, or similar objects (that cannot be laundered or dry cleaned): Spray thoroughly. Do not use article until spray is dry. Repeat treatment as necessary. Do not use in commercial food processing, preparation, storage or serving areas.

Storage and Disposal:
Storage: Store in a cool area away from heat or open flame.
Disposal: Wrap container and put in trash.

How Supplied: In 5 oz. and 10 oz. aerosol container.

Shown in Product Identification Section, page 423

Requa Manufacturing Company, Inc.
1 SENECA PLACE
GREENWICH, CT 06830

CHARCOAID*
Poison Antidote, liquid- has sweet, pleasant taste and feel; especially good for young patients.

Active Ingredient: Activated vegetable charcoal U.S.P., 30g per bottle, suspended in sorbitol solution U.S.P.

Indication: For the treatment of acute poisoning.

Action: Adsorbent

Warnings: Before using call a poison control center, emergency room, or a physician for advice. If the patient has been given Ipecac Syrup, do not give activated charcoal until after the patient has vomited. Do not use in a semi-conscious or unconscious person.

Precaution: May cause laxation.

Dosage and Administration: Shake well and drink entire contents (add water if too sweet). To insure a full dose, rinse bottle with water and drink. For adults, 2 to 3 bottles may be given.

Professional Labeling: Some dilution may be necessary for administration via lavage tube. Add a small amount of water to bottle and shake.

How Supplied: 5 fl. oz. unit dose bottle, 30g activated charcoal U.S.P., suspended in sorbitol solution U.S.P.
* U.S. Patent #4,122,169

CHARCOCAPS®
Activated Charcoal Capsules

Active Ingredient: Activated vegetable charcoal U.S.P., 260 mg per capsule

Indications: Relief of intestinal gas, diarrhea, gastrointestinal distress associated with indigestion. Also for the prevention of non-specific pruritus associated with kidney dialysis treatment.

Actions: Adsorbent, detoxicant, soothing agent. Reduces the volume of intestinal gas and allays related discomfort.

Warnings: As with all anti-diarrheals—not for children under 3 unless directed by physician. If diarrhea persists more than two days or is accompanied by high fever, consult physician.

Drug Interaction: Activated Charcoal USP can adsorb medication while they are in digestive tract.

Precaution: Take two hours before or one hour after medication including oral contraceptives.

Symptoms and Treatment of Oral Overdosage: Overdosage has not been encountered. Medical evidence indicates that high dosage or prolonged use does not cause side effect or harm the nutritional state of the patient.

Dosage and Administration: Two capsules after meals or at first sign of dis-

comfort. Repeat as needed up to eight doses (16 capsules) per day.

Professional Labeling: None.

How Supplied: Bottles of 36 capsules

Rexall Nutritional Products, Inc.
3901 N. KINGSHIGHWAY BLVD.
ST. LOUIS, MO 63115

PMS BALANCE™
Premenstrual Nutritional Supplement

Active Ingredients: Vitamin B-6 (100 mg), Vitamin E (300 IU) and Magnesium (200 mg).

Indications: Dietary Supplementation for better premenstrual nutritional balance.

Dosage and Administration: One swallowable tablet taken daily during premenstrual phase of monthly cycle.

How Supplied: Bottles of 45.

Sugar Free PAC-MAN™ Calcium for Kids™
Chewable Calcium Supplement

Active Ingredients: Provides the calcium equivalent of one 8 oz. glass of milk as 300 mg calcium carbonate. Each tablet is chocolate flavored with no artificial flavors or colors and no preservatives are added.

Indications: Dietary Supplementation

Dosage and Administration: One Tablet provides 30% U.S. RDA for children and adults 4 years and older.

How Supplied: Bottles of 30.

Sugar-Free PAC-MAN™
Chewable Multivitamins plus Iron
Pre-School and School Age Formulas

Active Ingredients: 100% U.S. RDA for 10 essential vitamins plus iron for under age 4 and over age 4 (no artificial flavors or colors, no preservatives added).

Indications: Dietary supplementation.

Precaution: Contains iron which can be harmful in large dosage. Close tightly and keep out of reach of children.

Dosage and Administration: One chewable tablet daily.

How Supplied: Bottles of 60.

Products are
indexed alphabetically
in the
PINK SECTION

Richardson-Vicks Inc.
PERSONAL CARE PRODUCTS
DIVISION
TEN WESTPORT ROAD
WILTON, CT 06897

CLEARASIL® Super Strength
Acne Treatment Cream
Vanishing and Covering

Active Ingredient: Benzoyl Peroxide 10% in an odorless, greaseless cream base, containing water, propylene glycol, aluminum hydroxide, bentonite, glyceryl stearate SE, isopropyl myristate, cellulose gum, dimethicone, PEG-12, potassium carbomer-940, methylparaben, and propylparaben. The covering formula also contains titanium dioxide and iron oxides.

Indications: For the topical treatment of acne vulgaris.

Actions: CLEARASIL Super Strength Acne Treatment Cream contains benzoyl peroxide, an antibacterial and keratolytic as well as bentonite and aluminum hydroxide as oil absorbants. The product 1) helps heal and prevent acne pimples, 2) helps absorb excess skin oil often associated with acne blemishes, 3) helps your skin look fresh. The Vanishing formula works invisibly. The Covering formula hides pimples while it works.

Warnings: Persons with a known sensitivity to benzoyl peroxide should not use this medication. Excessive dryness or peeling may occur especially when used by persons with unusually dry, sensitive, or maturing skin. If itching, redness, burning, swelling or undue dryness occurs, reduce dosage or discontinue use. If symptoms persist, consult a physician promptly. For external use only. Keep from eyes, lips, mouth and sensitive areas of the neck. Colored or dyed fabrics may be bleached by the oxidizing action of this product. Keep this and all medicine out of the reach of children.

Symptoms and Treatment of Ingestion: These symptoms are based upon medical judgement, not on actual experience. Theoretically, ingestion of very large amounts may cause nausea, vomiting, abdominal discomfort and diarrhea. Treatment is symptomatic, with bedrest and observation.

Directions For Use: 1. Wash thoroughly. (Clearasil® Antibacterial Soap and Clearasil® Pore Deep Cleanser are excellent products to use in your cleansing regimen.) **2.** Try this sensitivity test. Apply cream sparingly with fingertips to one or two small affected areas during the first three days. If no discomfort or reaction occurs, apply up to two times daily, wherever pimples and oil are a problem. **3.** If bothersome dryness or peeling occurs, reduce dosage to one application per day or every other day.

How Supplied: Available in both Vanishing and Covering formulas in 1 oz. and .65 oz. squeeze tubes.

Continued on next page

Richardson-Vicks—Cont.

*Shown in Product Identification
Section, page 423*

CLEARASIL® Adult Care—
Medicated Blemish Cream

Active Ingredient: Sulfur, resorcinol (alcohol 10%) in a cream base which contains water, bentonite, glyceryl stearate SE, propylene glycol, isopropyl myristate, sodium bisulfite, dimethicone, methylparaben, propylparaben, fragrance, iron oxides.

Indications: For the topical treatment of acne vulgaris in adults.

Actions: CLEARASIL Adult Care—Medicated Blemish Cream especially suited for adult usage since it dries acne lesions without overdrying or irritating the skin the way many benzoyl peroxide-containing products do. The product contains sulfur and resorcinol to help heal acne pimples, and bentonite to absorb excess sebum.

Warnings: For external use only. Other topical acne medications should not be used at the same time as this medication. Apply to affected areas only. Do not use on broken skin or apply to large areas of the body. Do not get into eyes. Some people with sensitive skin may experience slight irritation after use of this product. If condition persist, consult a doctor or pharmacist. Keep this and all medicine out of reach of children.

Symptoms and Treatment of Oral Overdosage: These symptoms are based upon medical judgement, not on actual experience. Theoretically, ingestion of very large amounts may cause nausea, vomiting, abdominal discomfort and diarrhea. Treatment is symptomatic, with bedrest and observation.

Dosage and Administration: Cleanse skin thoroughly before applying medication. To clear up the blemishes you have now, apply Clearasil Adult Care directly on and around the affected area two or three times daily. If excessive drying occurs, decrease usage to one or two applications per day.

How Supplied: Available in a .6 oz. tube.

*Shown in Product Identification
Section, page 423*

CLEARASIL®
10% Benzoyl Peroxide Lotion
Acne Medication

Active Ingredient: Benzoyl Peroxide 10% in a colorless, greaseless lotion which contains water, aluminum hydroxide, isopropyl stearate, PEG-100 stearate, glyceryl stearate, cetyl alcohol, glycereth-26, isocetyl stearate, glycerin, dimethicone copolyol, sodium citrate, citric acid, methylparaben, propylparaben, fragrance.

Indications: For the topical treatment of acne vulgaris.

Actions: CLEARASIL 10% Benzoyl Peroxide Lotion contains benzoyl peroxide, an antibacterial and keratolytic. The product **1. Helps heal and prevent acne pimples.** Benzoyl peroxide dries up existing pimples and kills acne causing bacteria to help prevent new ones.
2. Helps absorb excess skin oil often associated with acne blemishes. Contains aluminum hydroxide which is a special oil absorbing ingredient that allows Clearasil Lotion to absorb **more** excess skin oil than 10% benzoyl peroxide alone.
3. Helps your skin look fresh. Extra oil absorption helps your skin look less oily, more natural.

Warnings: Persons with a known sensitivity to benzoyl peroxide should not use this medication. Excessive dryness or peeling may occur especially when used by persons with unusually dry, sensitive, or maturing skin. If itching, redness, burning, swelling or undue dryness occurs, reduce dosage or discontinue use. If symptoms persist, consult a physician promptly. For external use only. Keep from eyes, lips, mouth and sensitive areas of the neck. Colored or dyed fabrics may be bleached by the oxidizing action of this product. Keep this and all medicine out of the reach of children.

Symptoms and Treatment of Ingestion: These symptoms are based upon medical judgement, not on actual experience. Theoretically, ingestion of very large amounts may cause nausea, vomiting, abdominal discomfort and diarrhea. Treatment is symptomatic, with bedrest and observation.

Directions For Use:
SHAKE WELL BEFORE USING.
1. Wash thoroughly. (Clearasil® Antibacterial Soap and Clearasil® Pore Deep Cleanser are excellent products to use in your cleansing regimen) **2.** Try this sensitivity test. Apply lotion sparingly with fingertips to one or two small affected areas during the first three days. If no discomfort or reaction occurs, apply up to two times daily, wherever pimples and oil are a problem **3.** If bothersome dryness or peeling occurs, reduce dosage to one application per day or every other day.

How Supplied: Available in a 1 fl. oz. squeeze bottle.

*Shown in Product Identification
Section, page 423*

CLEARASIL®
Pore Deep Cleanser

Active Ingredient: Salicylic Acid (0.5%), also contains ethyl alcohol (43%).

Indications: Topical Skin Cleanser for treatment of acne vulgaris.

Actions: Clearasil® Pore Deep Cleanser contains a comedolytic agent that penetrates deep into pores to clean out oil and dead skin cells that can clog pores and cause pimples.

Warnings: For external use only. May be irritating to the eyes. Keep away from extreme heat or flame.

Drug Interaction: None known.

Symptoms and Treatment of Ingestion: Product contains ethyl alcohol. If large amounts are ingested, nausea, vomiting, gastrointestinal irritation may develop. Bed rest and observation are indicated if ingested.

Directions for Use: Saturate cotton pad and apply 2-3 times per day. Do not rinse after use.

How Supplied: 4 and 8 oz. plastic bottles.

*Shown in Product Identification
Section, page 423*

DENQUEL® Sensitive Teeth
Toothpaste
Desensitizing Dentifrice

Each tube contains potassium nitrate (5%) in a low abrasion, pleasant mint flavored dentifrice.

Dental hypersensitivity is a condition in which pain or discomfort arises when various stimuli, such as hot, cold, sweet or sour contact exposed dentin. Exposure of dentin often occurs as a result of either gingival recession or periodontal surgery.

Daily use of Denquel can provide, within the first 2 weeks of regular brushing, a significant decrease in hypersensitivity. As regular use continues, greater improvement will be noticed. The Council on Dental Therapeutics of the American Dental Association has given Denquel the ADA Seal of Acceptance as an effective desensitizing dentifrice for teeth sensitive to hot and cold.

Contraindications: See a dentist if tooth sensitivity is not reduced after 4 weeks of regular use, as this may indicate a dental condition other than hypersensitivity.

Dosage: Use twice a day or as directed by a dentist.

How Supplied: Denquel Sensitive Teeth Toothpaste is supplied in tubes containing 1.6, 3.0, or 4.5 ounces.

Riker Laboratories, Inc.
**225-1S-07/3M CENTER
ST. PAUL, MN 55144**

CAL·SUP™
Calcium Supplement 300 mg

Composition: Each tablet contains 750 mg calcium carbonate (equivalent to 300 mg elemental calcium) with glycine.

Indications: For use in the prevention of calcium deficiency when needed or recommended by a physician.

Directions: Take three or four tablets daily, or as directed by your physician. Chew, swallow or melt in the mouth.

Three tablets daily provide:

Quantity	U.S. RDA†	
Calcium 900 mg	90%*	69%**

Four tablets daily provide:

Quantity	U.S. RDA†	
Calcium 1200 mg	120%*	92%**

† U.S. recommended daily allowance
* For adults and children 12 or more years of age
**For pregnant and lactating women

How Supplied: Bottles of 100 white tablets (NDC **0089-0110-10**).

MEDIHALER–EPI®
(epinephrine bitartrate)
FOR TEMPORARY RELIEF FROM ACUTE PAROXYSMS OF BRONCHIAL ASTHMA.

FOR ORAL INHALATION THERAPY ONLY

Each inhalation delivers 0.3 mg epinephrine bitartrate equivalent to 0.16 mg of epinephrine base.

How Supplied: 15 ml. size: Available as a combination package (vial with oral adapter) or as a refill (vial only).

A. H. Robins Company, Inc.
**CONSUMER PRODUCTS DIVISION
3800 CUTSHAW AVENUE
RICHMOND, VIRGINIA 23230**

ALLBEE® C–800 TABLETS
ALLBEE® C–800 plus IRON TABLETS
Allbee C-800

One tablet daily provides:	Percentage of U.S. Recommended Daily Allowances (U.S. RDA)		
Vitamin E	150	45	I.U.
Vitamin C	1333	800	mg
Thiamine (Vitamin B₁)	1000	15	mg
Riboflavin (Vitamin B₂)	1000	17	mg
Niacin	500	100	mg
Vitamin B₆	1250	25	mg
Vitamin B₁₂	200	12	mcg
Pantothenic Acid	250	25	mg

Ingredients: Ascorbic Acid, Niacinamide Ascorbate, Starch, Vitamin E Acetate, Hydrolyzed Protein, Calcium Pantothenate, Hydroxypropyl Methylcellulose, Pyridoxine Hydrochloride, Riboflavin, Stearic Acid, Thiamine Mononitrate, Artificial Color, Silicon Dioxide, Lactose, Magnesium Stearate, Povidone, Polyethylene Glycol 400, Vanillin, Gelatin, Polysorbate 80, Sorbic Acid, Sodium Benzoate, Cyanocobalamin.

Allbee C-800 plus Iron

One tablet daily provides: Vitamin Composition	Percentage of U.S. Recommended Daily Allowances (U.S. RDA)		
Vitamin E	150	45.0	I.U.
Vitamin C	1333	800.0	mg
Folic Acid	100	0.4	mg
Thiamine (Vitamin B₁)	1000	15.0	mg
Riboflavin (Vitamin B₂)	1000	17.0	mg
Niacin	500	100.0	mg
Vitamin B₆	1250	25.0	mg
Vitamin B₁₂	200	12.0	mcg
Pantothenic Acid	250	25.0	mg
Mineral Composition			
Iron	150	27.0	mg

Ingredients: Ascorbic Acid, Niacinamide Ascorbate, Ferrous Fumarate, Starch, Vitamin E Acetate, Hydrolyzed Protein, Calcium Pantothenate, Hydroxypropyl Methylcellulose, Pyridoxine Hydrochloride, Riboflavin, Stearic Acid, Thiamine Mononitrate, Povidone, Silicon Dioxide, Artificial Color, Lactose, Magnesium Stearate, Polyethylene Glycol 400, Vanillin, Gelatin, Folic Acid, Polysorbate 80, Sorbic Acid, Sodium Benzoate, Cyanocobalamin.

Actions and Uses: The components of Allbee C-800 have important roles in general nutrition, healing of wounds, and prevention of hemorrhage. Allbee C-800 is recommended for nutritional supplementation of these components in conditions such as febrile diseases, chronic or acute infections, burns, fractures, surgery, physiologic stress, alcoholism, prolonged exposure to high temperature, geriatrics, gastritis, peptic ulcer, and colitis; and in weight-reduction and other special diets.
In dentistry, Allbee C-800 is recommended for nutritional supplementation of its components in conditions such as herpetic stomatitis, aphthous stomatitis, cheilosis, herpangina and gingivitis.
In addition, Allbee C-800 Plus Iron is recommended as a nutritional source of iron. The iron is present as ferrous fumarate, a well-tolerated salt. The ascorbic acid in the formulation enhances the absorption of iron.

Precautions: Do not take Allbee C-800 Plus Iron within two hours of oral tetracycline antibiotics, since oral iron products interfere with absorption of tetracycline. Not intended for treatment of iron-deficiency anemia.

Adverse Reactions: Iron-containing medications may occasionally cause gastrointestinal discomfort, nausea, constipation or diarrhea.

Dosage: The recommended OTC dosage for adults and children twelve or more years of age is one tablet daily. Under the direction and supervision of a physician, the dose and frequency of administration may be increased in accordance with the patient's requirements.

How Supplied: Allbee C-800—orange, film-coated, elliptically-shaped tablets in bottles of 60 (NDC 0031-0677-62). Allbee

C-800 Plus Iron—red, film-coated, elliptically-shaped tablets in bottles of 60 (NDC 0031-0678-62).

Shown in Product Identification Section, page 423 and 424

ALLBEE® WITH C CAPSULES

One capsule daily provides:	Percentage of U.S. Recommended Daily Allowance (U.S. RDA)		
Vitamin C	500	300.0	mg
Thiamine (Vitamin B₁)	1000	15.0	mg
Riboflavin (Vitamin B₂)	600	10.2	mg
Niacin	250	50.0	mg
Vitamin B₆	250	5.0	mg
Pantothenic Acid	100	10.0	mg

Ingredients: Ascorbic Acid; Gelatin; Niacinamide; Lactose; Corn Starch; Thiamine Mononitrate; Calcium Pantothenate; Riboflavin; Magnesium Stearate; Pyridoxine Hydrochloride; Light Mineral Oil; FD&C Yellow No. 5; Vanillin; Artificial Color.

Action and Uses: Allbee with C is a high potency formulation of B and C vitamins. Its components have important roles in general nutrition, healing of wounds, and prevention of hemorrhage. It is recommended for deficiencies of B-vitamins and ascorbic acid in conditions such as febrile diseases, chronic or acute infections, burns, fractures, surgery, toxic conditions, physiologic stress, alcoholism, prolonged exposure to high temperature, geriatrics, gastritis, peptic ulcer, and colitis; and in conditions involving special diets and weight-reduction diets.
In dentistry, Allbee with C is recommended for deficiencies of B-vitamins and ascorbic acid in conditions such as herpetic stomatitis, aphthous stomatitis, cheilosis, herpangina, gingivitis.

Precaution: This product contains FD&C Yellow No. 5 (tartrazine) which may cause allergic-type reactions (including bronchial asthma) in certain susceptible individuals. Although the overall incidence of FD&C Yellow No. 5 (tartrazine) sensitivity in the general population is low, it is frequently seen in patients who have aspirin hypersensitivity.

Dosage: The recommended OTC dosage for adults and children twelve or more years of age, other than pregnant or lactating women, is one capsule daily. Under the direction and supervision of a physician, the dose and frequency of administration may be increased in accordance with the patient's requirements.

Continued on next page

Robins—Cont.

How Supplied: Yellow and green capsules, monogrammed AHR and 0674, in bottles of 100 (NDC 0031-0674-63), 1,000 capsules (NDC 0031-0674-74) and in Dis-Co® Unit Dose Packs of 100 (NDC 0031-0674-64).

Shown in Product Identification Section, page 424

CHAP STICK® Lip Balm

Active Ingredients: 44% Petrolatums, 1.5% Padimate O (2-ethyl-hexyl p-dimethylaminobenzoate, 1% Lanolin, 1% Isopropyl Myristate, .5% Cetyl Alcohol.

Indications: Aids prevention and healing of dry, chapped, sun and windburned lips.

Actions: A specially designed lipid complex hydrophobic base containing Padimate O which forms a barrier to prevent moisture loss and protect lips from the drying effects of cold weather, wind and sun which cause chapping. The special emollients soften the skin by forming an occlusive film thus inducing hydration, restoring suppleness to the lips, and preventing drying from evaporation of water that diffuses to the surface from the underlying layers of tissue. Chap Stick also protects the skin from the external environment and its sunscreen offers protection from exposure to the sun.

Warning: Discontinue use if signs of irritation appear.

Symptoms and Treatment of Oral Ingestion: The oral LD_{50} in rats is greater than 5 gm/kg. There have been no reported overdoses in humans. There are no known symptoms of overdosage.

Dosage and Treatment: For dry, chapped lips apply as needed. To help prevent dry, chapped sun or windburned lips, apply to lips as needed before, during and following exposure to sun, wind, water and cold weather.

Professional Labeling: None.

How Supplied: Available in 4.25 gm tubes in Regular, Mint, Cherry, Orange, and Strawberry flavors.

Shown in Product Identification Section, page 424

CHAP STICK® SUNBLOCK 15 Lip Balm

Active Ingredients: 44% Petrolatums, 7% Padimate O, 3% Oxybenzone, 0.5% Lanolin, 0.5% Isopropyl Myristate, 0.5% Cetyl Alcohol.

Indications: Ultra Sunscreen Protection (SPF-15). Aids prevention and healing of dry, chapped, sun and windburned lips. Overexposure to sun may lead to premature aging of skin and lip cancer. Liberal and regular use may help reduce the sun's harmful effects.

Actions: Ultra sunscreen protection for the lips, plus the attributes of Chap Stick® Lip Balm. The emollients in the specially-designed lipid complex hydrophobic base soften the lips by forming an occlusive film while the two sunscreens have specific ultraviolet absorption ranges which overlap to offer ultra sunscreen protection (SPF-15).

Warning: Discontinue use if signs of irritation appear.

Symptoms and Treatment of Oral Ingestion: Toxicity studies indicate this product to be extremely safe. The oral LD_{50} in rats is greater than 5 gm./kg. There are no known symptoms of overdosage.

Dosage and Treatment: For ultra sunscreen protection, apply evenly and liberally to lips before exposure to sun. Reapply as needed. For dry, chapped lips, apply as needed. To help prevent dry, chapped, sun, and windburned lips, apply to lips as needed before, during, and following exposure to sun, wind, water, and cold weather.

How Supplied: 4.25 gm. tube.
Shown in Product Identification Section, page 424

DIMACOL® CAPSULES

Composition: Each capsule contains:
Guaifenesin, USP ....100 mg
Pseudoephedrine
   Hydrochloride, USP ....30 mg
Dextromethorphan
   Hydrobromide, USP ....15 mg

Actions: Dimacol helps reduce nasal congestion and suppresses cough associated with the common cold and other upper respiratory disorders.
Guaifenesin enhances the output of lower respiratory tract fluid. The enhanced flow of less viscid secretions promotes ciliary action, and facilitates the removal of inspissated mucus. As a result, dry unproductive coughs become more productive and less frequent. *Pseudoephedrine hydrochloride* is an orally effective nasal decongestant. Through its vasoconstrictor action, pseudoephedrine gently but promptly reduces edema and congestion of nasal passages. *Dextromethorphan hydrobromide* is a synthetic, non-narcotic cough suppressant. The antitussive effectiveness of dextromethorphan has been demonstrated in both animal and clinical studies, and the incidence of toxic effects has been remarkably low.

Indications: Dimacol is indicated for the management of cough accompanied by nasal mucosal congestion and edema, and nasal hypersecretion, associated with the common cold, upper respiratory infection and sinusitis.

Contraindications: Hypersensitivity to any of the ingredients. Dimacol should not be administered to patients receiving MAO inhibitors.

Warnings: As with any drug, if you are pregnant or nursing a baby, seek the advice of a health professional before using this product.

Cautions: Administer with caution in the presence of hypertension, heart disease, peripheral vascular disease, diabetes or hyperthyroidism.
Note: Guaifenesin has been shown to produce a color interference with certain clinical laboratory determinations of 5-hydroxyindoleacetic acid (5-HIAA) and vanilmandelic acid (VMA).

Adverse Reactions: The following adverse reactions may possibly occur: nausea, vomiting, dry mouth, nervousness, insomnia.

Dosage and Administration: Adults and children over 12 years of age, one capsule three times a day.

How Supplied: Orange and green capsules in bottles of 100 (NDC 0031-1650-63), and 500 (NDC 0031-1650-70) and consumer packages of 12 (NDC 0031-1650-46) and 24 (NDC 0031-1650-54) (individually packaged).

Shown in Product Identification Section, page 424

DIMETANE®
brand of Brompheniramine Maleate, USP
Tablets—4 mg
Elixir—2 mg/5 ml (Alcohol, 3%)
Extentabs®—8 mg and 12 mg

Family Description: Dimetane® is Robins brand name for Brompheniramine Maleate, USP, an antihistamine. It comes in several oral dosage forms (tablets, elixir and Extentabs®) and can be used when an antihistamine is indicated.

Indications: For temporary relief of hay fever symptoms: itching of the nose or throat; itchy, watery eyes; sneezing; running nose.

Warnings: May cause drowsiness. May cause excitability, especially in children. This product should not be taken by patients who have asthma, glaucoma or difficulty in urination due to enlargement of the prostate gland. The tablets and liquid should not be given to children under six years, except under the advice and supervision of a physician. The Extentabs should not be given to children under 12 years, except under the advice and supervision of a physician. As with any drug, women who are pregnant or nursing a baby should seek the advice of a health professional before using these products.

Cautions: Driving a motor vehicle, operating heavy machinery and drinking alcoholic beverages should be avoided while this drug is being taken.
THIS AND ALL DRUGS SHOULD BE KEPT OUT OF THE REACH OF CHILDREN. IN CASE OF ACCIDENTAL OVERDOSE, PROFESSIONAL ASSISTANCE SHOULD BE OBTAINED OR A POISON CONTROL CENTER SHOULD BE CONTACTED IMMEDIATELY.

Directions For Use: Tablets and Liquid—The recommended OTC dosage is:

Adults and children 12 years of age and over: 1 tablet or 2 teaspoonfuls every four to six hours, not to exceed 6 tablets or 12 teaspoonfuls in 24 hours. **Children 6 to under 12 years:** ½ tablet or 1 teaspoonful every four to six hours, not to exceed 3 whole tablets or 6 teaspoonfuls in 24 hours. Children under 6 years: Use only as directed by a physician.

Extentabs®—The recommended OTC dosage is: **Adults and children 12 years of age and over:**

8 mg Extentab: One tablet every eight to twelve hours, NOT TO EXCEED 1 TABLET EVERY 8 HOURS OR 3 TABLETS IN A 24-HOUR PERIOD.

12 mg Extentab: One tablet every twelve hours, NOT TO EXCEED 1 TABLET EVERY 12 HOURS OR 2 TABLETS IN A 24-HOUR PERIOD.

Children under 12 years of age should use only as directed by a physician.

How Supplied:
[See table above].

Shown in Product Identification Section, page 424

DIMETANE® DECONGESTANT ELIXIR
DIMETANE® DECONGESTANT TABLETS

Elixir:
Each 5 ml (1 teaspoonful) contains:
Phenylephrine
   Hydrochloride, USP ....5 mg
Brompheniramine
   Maleate, USP ....2 mg
Alcohol 2.3 percent
Tablet:
Each tablet contains:
Phenylephrine
   Hydrochloride, USP ....10 mg
Brompheniramine
   Maleate, USP ....4 mg

Indications: For temporary relief of nasal congestion due to the common cold, sinusitis, hay fever or other upper respiratory allergies; runny nose, sneezing, itching of the nose or throat and itchy and watery eyes as may occur in allergic rhinitis (such as hay fever). Temporarily restores freer breathing through the nose.

Contraindications: Hypersensitivity to any of the ingredients; marked hypertension.

Warnings: May cause excitability, especially in children. Use with caution in children under 2 years. Prescribe cautiously for patients with asthma, glaucoma, difficulty in urination due to enlargement of the prostate gland, high blood pressure, heart disease, diabetes or thyroid disease and for patients who are receiving MAO inhibitors or antihypertensive medication. May cause drowsiness. Doses in excess of the recommended dosage may cause nervousness, dizziness or sleeplessness. As with any drug, if you are pregnant or nursing a baby, seek the advice of a health professional before using this product.

Product Name	NDC 0031-	Form	Strength	Package Size	Package Type
Dimetane Tablets	1857-54	Peach-colored, compressed	4 mg tablet	24	Blister Unit
	1857-63			100	Bottles
	1857-70	scored tablets		500	Bottles
Dimetane Elixir	1807-12	Peach-colored, liquid	2 mg/5 ml	4 fl. oz.	Bottles
	1807-25			1 Pint	Bottles
Dimetane Extentabs 8 mg	1868-46	Persian rose-colored, tablets	8 mg tablet	12	Blister Unit
	1868-63			100	Bottles
	1868-70			500	Bottles
Dimetane Extentabs 12 mg	1843-46	Peach-colored, coated tablets	12 mg tablets	12	Blister Unit
	1843-63			100	Bottles
	1843-70			500	Bottles

Cautions: Patients should be warned about driving a motor vehicle, operating heavy machinery, or consuming alcoholic beverages while taking this product.

Recommended Dosage: *Elixir:* Adults and children 12 years of age and over: 2 teaspoonfuls every 4 hours, not to exceed 12 teaspoonfuls in a 24-hour period; children 6 to under 12 years: 1 teaspoonful every 4 hours, not to exceed 6 teaspoonfuls in a 24-hour period; children 2 to under 6 years: ½ teaspoonful every 4 hours, not to exceed 3 teaspoonfuls in a 24-hour period.
Tablets: Adults and children 12 years of age and over: 1 tablet every 4 hours, not to exceed 6 tablets in a 24-hour period; children 6 to under 12 years: ½ tablet every 4 hours, not to exceed 3 tablets in a 24-hour period.

How Supplied: *Tablets*—light blue, capsule shaped tablets in cartons of 24 (NDC 0031-2117-54) and 48 (NDC 0031-2117-59) individually packaged blister units.
Elixir—red colored, grape flavored liquid in 4 fl. oz. bottle (NDC 0031-2127-12).
Shown in Product Identification Section, page 424

EXTEND 12® LIQUID
brand of Dextromethorphan Polistirex

Composition: Each 5 ml. (1 teaspoonful) contains dextromethorphan polistirex equivalent to 30 mg. dextromethorphan hydrobromide in a peach-colored, citrus-flavored suspension.

Actions and Uses: Extend 12 Liquid is a sustained-action, single-ingredient cough suppressant for the temporary relief of coughs due to minor throat and bronchial irritation as may occur with the common cold or with inhaled irritants. Extend 12 Liquid employs ion-exchange technology, whereby dextromethorphan is released steadily into the gastrointestinal tract when it is displaced from the resin complex by potassium or sodium ions.

Contraindications: Hypersensitivity to dextromethorphan, or in patients who are taking MAO inhibitors.

Warnings: This product should not be given to children under 2 years except under the advice and supervision of a physician. This product should not be taken for persistent or chronic cough such as occurs with smoking, asthma, or emphysema, or where cough is accompanied by excessive secretions except under the advice and supervision of a physician. As with any drug, if you are pregnant or nursing a baby, seek the advice of a health professional before using this product.

Cautions: A persistent cough may be a sign of a serious condition. If cough persists for more than 1 week, tends to recur or is accompanied by high fever, rash or persistant headache, a physician should be consulted.

Dosage: Adults and children over 12 years of age: 2 teaspoonfuls every 12 hours; do not exceed 4 teaspoonfuls in 24 hours. Children 6–12: 1 teaspoonful every 12 hours; do not exceed 2 teaspoonfuls in 24 hours. Children 2–5 ½ teaspoonful every 12 hours; do not exceed 1 teaspoonful in 24 hours. Children under 2: Use only under the advice and supervision of a physician.

How Supplied: Bottles of 2 fl. oz. (NDC 0031-5240-05) and 4 fl. oz. (NDC 0031-5240-12).
Shown in Product Identification Section, page 424

LIP SOOTHER™
Medicated Lip Cream

Active Ingredients: 1% Camphor, .25% Menthol, .5% Phenol

Indications: For temporary relief of pain caused by dry, chapped, sunburned lips, cold sores and fever blisters. The emollient base softens and lubricates the

Continued on next page

Prescribing information on A.H. Robins products listed here is based on official labeling in effect December 1, 1984 with Indications, Contraindications, Warnings, Precautions, Adverse Reactions, and Dosage stated in full.

Robins—Cont.

lips and helps prevent moisture loss from lip tissue.

Actions: Camphor is used to furnish slight local anesthetic action to sore and chapped lips.

Warning: For external use only. —Avoid contact with the eyes. If condition persists or if a rash, swelling or irritation develops, discontinue use and consult a physician. Keep out of reach of children.

Dosage and Administration: For dry, chapped lips apply as needed. At first sign of cold sore or fever blister, gently apply and massage Lip Soother into the immediate (sensitive) area.

How Supplied: .13 oz. tube
Shown in Product Identification Section, page 424

ROBITUSSIN®
ROBITUSSIN–CF®
ROBITUSSIN–DM®
ROBITUSSIN–PE®

Composition: *Robitussin* contains Guaifenesin, USP 100 mg in 5 ml (1 teaspoonful) of palatable aromatic syrup; alcohol 3.5%. *Robitussin-CF* contains in each 5 ml (1 teaspoonful): Guaifenesin, USP 100 mg, Phenylpropanolamine Hydrochloride, USP 12.5 mg, Dextromethorphan Hydrobromide, USP 10 mg; alcohol 4.75%. *Robitussin-DM* contains in each 5 ml (1 teaspoonful): Guaifenesin, USP 100 mg and Dextromethorphan Hydrobromide, USP 15 mg; alcohol 1.4%. *Robitussin-PE* contains in each 5 ml (1 teaspoonful): Guaifenesin, USP 100 mg and Pseudoephedrine Hydrochloride, USP 30 mg; alcohol 1.4%.

Action and Uses: All four preparations employ the expectorant action of guaifenesin which enhances the output of respiratory tract fluid (RTF). The enhanced flow of less viscid secretions promotes ciliary action, and facilitates the removal of inspissated mucus. As a result, unproductive coughs become more productive and less frequent. *Robitussin* is therefore, useful in combating coughs associated with the common cold, bronchitis, laryngitis, tracheitis, pharyngitis, pertussis, influenza and measles, and for coughs provoked by chronic paranasal sinusitis. In *Robitussin-CF* the guaifenesin is supplemented with phenylpropanolamine which provides mild vasoconstrictor action resulting in a nasal decongestant effect and dextromethorphan, a synthetic, non-narcotic, centrally-acting cough suppressant. In *Robitussin-DM*, the guaifenesin is supplemented by dextromethorphan. In *Robitussin-PE*, the expectorant action of guaifenesin is supplemented by a sympathomimetic amine, pseudoephedrine, which helps reduce mucosal congestion and edema in the nasal passages.

Contraindications: Hypersensitivity to any of the components. *Robitussin-DM* is also contraindicated in patients who

are receiving MAO inhibitors. *Robitussin-CF* and *Robitussin-PE* are also contraindicated in marked hypertension, hyperthyroidism or in patients who are receiving MAO inhibitors or antihypertensive medication.

Warnings: As with any drug, if you are pregnant or nursing a baby, seek the advice of a health professional before using this product.

Cautions: *Robitussin-CF* and *Robitussin-PE* should be administered with caution to patients with hypertension, cardiac disorders, diabetes or peripheral vascular disease. As with all products containing sympathomimetic amines, these products should be used with caution in patients with prostatic hypertrophy or glaucoma.
Note: Guaifenesin has been shown to produce a color interference with certain clinical laboratory determinations of 5-hydroxyindoleacetic acid (5-HIAA) and vanillylmandelic acid (VMA).

Adverse Reactions: No serious side effects have been reported from guaifenesin or dextromethorphan. Possible adverse reactions of *Robitussin-CF* and *Robitussin-PE* include nausea, vomiting, dry mouth, nervousness, insomnia, restlessness or headache.

Dosage: The following dosages are recommended for *Robitussin* and *Robitussin-CF:* Adults and children 12 years of age and over: 2 teaspoonfuls every four hours, not to exceed 12 teaspoonfuls in a 24-hour period; children 6 to under 12 years: 1 teaspoonful every four hours, not to exceed 6 teaspoonfuls in a 24-hour period; children 2 to under 6 years: ½ teaspoonful every four hours, not to exceed 3 teaspoonfuls in a 24-hour period; children under 2 years: use only as directed by physician. *Robitussin-DM:* Adults and children 12 years of age and over: 2 teaspoonfuls every six to eight hours, not to exceed 8 teaspoonfuls in a 24-hour period; children 6 to under 12 years: 1 teaspoonful every six to eight hours, not to exceed 4 teaspoonfuls in a 24-hour period; children 2 to under 6 years: ½ teaspoonful every six to eight hours, not to exceed 2 teaspoonfuls in a 24-hour period; children under 2 years: use only as directed by physician. *Robitussin-PE:* Adults and children 12 years of age and over: 2 teaspoonfuls every four hours, not to exceed 8 teaspoonfuls in a 24-hour period; children 6 to under 12 years: 1 teaspoonful every four hours, not to exceed 4 teaspoonfuls in a 24-hour period; children 2 to under 6 years: ½ teaspoonful every four hours, not to exceed 2 teaspoonfuls in a 24-hour period; children under 2 years: use as directed by physician.

How Supplied: *Robitussin* (wine-colored) in bottles of 4 fl. oz. (NDC 0031-8624-12), 8 fl. oz. (NDC 0031-8624-18), pint (NDC 0031-8624-25) and gallon (NDC 0031-8624-29). *Robitussin-DM* (cherry-colored) in bottles of 4 fl. oz. (NDC 0031-8684-12), 8 fl. oz. (NDC 0031-8684-18), pint (NDC 0031-8684-25), and gallon (NDC 0031-8684-29). *Robitussin-*

CF (red-colored) in bottles of 4 fl. oz. (NDC 0031-8677-12), 8 fl. oz. (NDC 0031-8677-18), and pint (NDC 0031-8677-25). *Robitussin-PE* (orange-red) in bottles of 4 fl. oz. (NDC 0031-8695-12), 8 fl. oz. (NDC 0031-8695-18) and pint (NDC 0031-8695-25). *Robitussin* also available in 1 fl. oz. bottles (4 x 25's-NDC 0031-8624-02) and Dis-Co® Unit Dose Packs of 10 x 10's in 5 ml (NDC 0031-8624-23), 10 ml (NDC 0031-8624-26) and 15 ml (NDC 0031-8624-28). *Robitussin-DM* also available in Dis-Co® Unit Dose Packs of 10 x 10's in 5 ml (NDC 0031-8684-23) and 10 ml (NDC 0031-8684-26).
Shown in Product Identification Section, page 424 and 425

ROBITUSSIN NIGHT RELIEF®
COLDS FORMULA

Composition:
Each fluid ounce contains:
    Acetaminophen, USP ....1,000 mg
    Phenylephrine HCl, USP ....10 mg
    Pyrilamine Maleate, USP ....50 mg
    Dextromethorphan
      Hydrobromide, USP ....30 mg
    Alcohol 25%

Ingredients:
Phenylephrine: An effective, safe, nasal decongestant. Provides temporary relief of nasal and sinus congestion by shrinking mucous membranes.
Acetaminophen: A commonly recommended non-aspirin analgesic which relieves the generalized aches and pains, malaise and fever often associated with a viral infection. Adverse reactions to acetaminophen are rare in recommended doses.
Pyrilamine: An antihistamine which is recognized to be safe and effective in relieving running nose; sneezing; itching, watery eyes, and post-nasal drip.
Dextromethorphan: A non-narcotic cough suppressant which temporarily reduces the frequency of cough especially the irritating, dry unproductive cough which so often disturbs sleep. Dextromethorphan is safe and effective at the recommended dosage.

Actions and Uses: Robitussin Night Relief Colds Formula is an adult strength multi-symptom colds product designed specifically for nighttime use. The combined action of the ingredients in Robitussin Night Relief provides temporary relief of major cold and flu symptoms: nasal and sinus congestion, aches and pains, minor sore throat pain, fever, coughs, running nose, sneezing, itchy and watery eyes.

Contraindications: Hypersensitivity to dextromethorphan, sympathomimetic amines, acetaminophen, or antihistamines.

Warnings: Keep this and all medicine out of the reach of children. In case of accidental overdose, consult a physician immediately. Persistent cough may indicate a serious condition. Persons with high fever, persistent cough, asthma, glaucoma, high blood pressure, diabetes, heart or thyroid disease or difficulty in urination due to enlargement of the prostate gland should not use this medication unless directed by a physician. Avoid alcoholic beverages while taking this product. Do not use for more than 10 days unless directed by a physician. As with any drug, if you are pregnant or nursng a baby, seek the advice of a health professional before using this product.

Cautions: If under medical care, do not take this medication without consulting a physician. Do not exceed recommended dosage. Do not give to children under 12 years of age unless directed by a physician. Do not operate machinery while taking this medication as it may cause drowsiness.

Administration and Dosage: Adults (12 years and over): one fluid ounce (2 tablespoonfuls) at bedtime. If your cold keeps you confined to bed or at home, take one dose every 6 hours not to exceed 4 doses per 24-hour period.

Overdosage: These symptoms are based on medical judgment and not on actual clinical experience, since there are no reports of overdose. Presenting symptom of overdosage is drowsiness. Large overdoses may cause emesis, ataxia, nausea, vomiting, restlessness, vertigo, dysuria, palpitations, sweating, and insomnia. Treatment is symptomatic. Acetaminophen may cause hepatotoxicity in certain patients. Since clinical and laboratory evidence may be delayed for up to one week, close clinical monitoring and serial hepatic enzyme determinations are recommended.

How Supplied: Bottles of 4 fl. oz. (NDC 0031-8640-12) and 8 fl. oz. (NDC 0031-8640-18).

Shown in Product Identification Section, page 425

Z-BEC® Tablets

One tablet daily provides:

Vitamin Composition	Percentage of U.S. Recommended Daily Allowance (U.S. RDA)	
Vitamin E	150	45.0 I.U.
Vitamin C	1000	600.0 mg
Thiamine (Vitamin B_1)	1000	15.0 mg
Riboflavin (Vitamin B_2)	600	10.2 mg
Niacin	500	100.0 mg
Vitamin B_6	500	10.0 mg
Vitamin B_{12}	100	6.0 mcg
Pantothenic Acid	250	25.0 mg
Mineral Composition		
Zinc	150	22.5 mg*

*22.5 mg zinc (equivalent to zinc content in 100 mg Zinc Sulfate, USP)

Ingredients: Niacinamide Ascorbate; Ascorbic Acid; Microcrystalline Cellulose; Zinc Sulfate; Vitamin E Acetate; Hydrolyzed Protein; Calcium Pantothenate; Modified Starch; Hydroxypropyl Methylcellulose; Thiamine Mononitrate; Stearic Acid; Pyridoxine Hydrochloride; Riboflavin; Silicon Dioxide; Polysorbate 20; Magnesium Stearate; Lactose; Povi-done; Propylene Glycol; Artificial Color; Vanillin; Hydroxypropyl Cellulose; Gelatin; Sorbic Acid; Sodium Benzoate; Cyanocobalamin.

Actions and Uses: Z-BEC is a high potency formulation. Its components have important roles in general nutrition, healing of wounds, and prevention of hemorrhage. It is recommended for deficiencies of these components in conditions such as febrile diseases, chronic or acute infections, burns, fractures, surgery, leg ulcers, toxic conditions, physiologic stress, alcoholism, prolonged exposure to high temperature, geriatrics, gastritis, peptic ulcer, and colitis; and in conditions involving special diets and weight-reduction diets.

In dentistry, Z-BEC is recommended for deficiencies of its components in conditions such as herpetic stomatitis, aphthous stomatitis, cheilosis herpangina and gingivitis.

Precaution: Not intended for the treatment of pernicious anemia.

Dosage: The recommended OTC dosage for adults and children twelve or more years of age, other than pregnant or lactating women, is one tablet daily with food or after meals. Under the direction and supervision of a physician, the dose and frequency of administration may be increased in accordance with the patient's requirements.

How Supplied: Green film-coated, capsule shaped tablets in bottles of 60 (NDC 0031-0689-62), 500 (NDC 0031-0689-70), and Dis-Co® Unit Dose Packs of 100 (NDC 0031-0689-64).

Shown in Product Identification Section, page 425

Vi-Penta Composition Table

Each 0.6 cc of Vi-Penta Infant Drops provides:	% minimum daily requirements (MDR)	
	Infants (under 1 year)	Young Children (1–6 years)
Vitamin A (as the palmitate) 5000 U.S.P. Units	333%	166%
Vitamin D_2 .... 400 U.S.P. Units	100%	100%
Vitamin C .... 50 mg	500%	250%
Vitamin E (as dl-α-tocopheryl acetate) 2 Int. Units	*	*

Each 0.6 cc of Vi-Penta Multivitamin Drops provides:	% minimum daily requirements (MDR)		
	Infants (under 1 year)	Children (1-6 years)	(6-12 years)
Vitamin A (as the palmitate) 5000 U.S.P. Units	333%	166%	166%
Vitamin D_2 .... 400 U.S.P. Units	100%	100%	100%
Vitamin C .... 50 mg	500%	250%	250%
Vitamin B_1 (as hydrochloride) .... 1 mg	400%	200%	133%
Vitamin B_2 (as riboflavin-5'-phosphate sodium) .... 1 mg	166%	111%	111%
Vitamin B_6 .... 1 mg	*	*	*
Vitamin E (as dl-α-tocopheryl acetate) 2 Int. Units	*	*	*
d-Biotin .... 30 mcg	†	†	†
Niacinamide .... 10 mg	*	200%	133%
Dexpanthenol (equiv. to 11.6 mg Calcium pantothenate) .... 10 mg	†	†	†

*MDR for these vitamins has not been determined.
†The need for these vitamins in human nutrition has not been established.

Roche Laboratories
Division of Hoffmann-La Roche Inc.
340 KINGSLAND STREET
NUTLEY, NJ 07110

VI-PENTA® INFANT DROPS
VI-PENTA® MULTIVITAMIN DROPS

The following text is complete prescribing information based on official labeling in effect December 1, 1984.

Composition: Vi-Penta Infant Drops and Vi-Penta Multivitamin Drops are designed to fill the vitamin needs of specific age groups. (See Composition Table below.)
[See table above].

Action and Uses: Vi-Penta Drops are water miscible and can be mixed with food or infant formula, or placed directly on the tongue.
Vi-Penta Infant Drops—a selective formula for prevention of vitamin deficiencies in infants and young children. *Vi-Penta Multivitamin Drops*—a comprehensive formula for daily nutritional support in adults as well as children of all ages. It is an especially convenient dosage form when a small volume liquid vitamin supplement is desired, such as to supplement the diets of those patients with conditions which permanently or temporarily impair their ability to swallow, chew or consume normal amounts and/or kinds of food.

Dosage: The average daily dose is 0.6 cc; therapeutic doses should be given according to the needs of the patient.

Continued on next page

Roche—Cont.

How Supplied: Vi-Penta Infant Drops and Vi-Penta Multivitamin Drops—fruit flavored, 50-cc bottles packaged with calibrated dropper.

Shown in Product Identification Section, page 425

William H. Rorer, Inc.
500 VIRGINIA DRIVE
FORT WASHINGTON, PA 19034

ASCRIPTIN®
Aspirin, Alumina and Magnesia Tablets, Rorer
Aspirin with Maalox®

Formula: Each tablet contains:
Aspirin...........................(5 grains) 325 mg
Maalox®:
  Magnesium Hydroxide................75 mg
  Dried Aluminum Hydroxide
  Gel...............................75 mg

Description: Ascriptin® is an excellent analgesic, antipyretic, and anti-inflammatory agent for general use, particularly where there is concern over aspirin-induced gastric distress. When large doses are used, as in arthritis and rheumatic disorders, gastric discomfort is rare.

Indications: As an analgesic for the relief of pain in such conditions as headache, neuralgia, minor injuries, and dysmenorrhea. As an analgesic and antipyretic in colds and influenza. As an analgesic and anti-inflammatory agent in arthritis and other rheumatic diseases. As an inhibitor of platelet aggregation, see TIA's indications.

Usual adult dose: Two or three tablets four times daily. For children under 12, at the discretion of the physician. As an inhibitor of platelet aggregation, see TIA's dosage information.

For Recurrent TIA's in Men

Indications: For reducing the risk of recurrent transient ischemic attacks (TIA's) or stroke in men who have had transient ischemia of the brain due to fibrin platelet emboli. There is inadequate evidence that aspirin or buffered aspirin is effective in reducing TIA's in women at the recommended dosage. There is no evidence that aspirin or buffered aspirin is of benefit in the treatment of completed strokes in men or women.

Precautions: (1) Patients presenting with signs and symptoms of TIA's should have a complete medical and neurologic evaluation. Consideration should be given to other disorders which resemble TIA's.
(2) Attention should be given to risk factors: It is important to evaluate and treat, if appropriate, other diseases associated with TIA's and stroke such as hypertension and diabetes.
(3) Concurrent administration of absorbable antacids at therapeutic doses may increase the clearance of salicylates in some individuals. The concurrent administration of nonabsorbable antacids may alter the rate of absorption of aspirin, thereby resulting in a decreased acetylsalicylic acid/salicylate ratio in plasma. The clinical significance on TIA's of these decreases in available aspirin is unknown.

Dosage: 1300 mg a day, in divided doses of 650 mg twice a day or 325 mg four times a day.

Warning: As with any drug, if you are pregnant or nursing a baby, seek the advice of a health professional before using this product.
Reye Syndrome Warning: Do not use in children, including teenagers, with chicken pox or flu.
In arthritis and rheumatism, if pain persists for more than 10 days, or redness is present, consult a physician immediately. Keep this and all drugs out of the reach of children. In case of accidental overdose, seek professional assistance or contact a poison control center immediately.

Supplied: Bottles of 50 tablets (NDC 0067-0135-50), 100 tablets (NDC 0067-0135-68), and 225 tablets (NDC 0067-0135-77) with child-resistant caps. Bottles of 500 tablets (NDC 0067-0135-74) without child-resistant closures (for arthritic patients). Military Stock #NSN 6505-00-135-2783. V.A. Stock #6505-00-890-1979A (bottles of 500).

Shown in Product Identification Section, page 425

ASCRIPTIN® A/D Arthritic Doses
Aspirin, Alumina and Magnesia Tablets, Rorer
Aspirin with Maalox® for increased buffering in Arthritic Doses
Aspirin, Alumina and Magnesia Tablets, Rorer

Formula: Each capsule shaped tablet contains:
Aspirin...........................(5 grains) 325 mg
Maalox®:
  Magnesium Hydroxide..............150 mg
  Dried Aluminum Hydroxide
  Gel..............................150 mg

Description: Ascriptin® A/D is a highly buffered analgesic, anti-inflammatory and antipyretic agent for use in the treatment of rheumatoid arthritis, osteoarthritis, and other arthritic conditions. It is formulated with added Maalox® to provide increased neutralization of gastric acid thus improving the likelihood of GI tolerance when large antiarthritic doses of aspirin are used.

Indications: As an analgesic, anti-inflammatory, and antipyretic agent in rheumatoid arthritis, osteoarthritis, and other arthritic conditions.

Usual Adult Dose: Two or three tablets, four times daily, or as directed by the physician for arthritis therapy. For children under twelve, at the discretion of the physician.

Drug Interaction Precaution: Do not use if patient is taking a tetracycline antibiotic.

Warning: As with any drug, if you are pregnant or nursing a baby, seek the advice of a health professional before using this product.
Reye Syndrome Warning: Do not use in children, including teenagers, with chicken pox or flu.
In arthritis and rheumatism, if pain persists for more than 10 days, or redness is present, consult a physician immediately. Keep this and all drugs out of the reach of children. In case of accidental overdose, seek professional assistance or contact a poison control center immediately.

Supplied: Available in bottles of 100 tablets (NDC 0067-0137-68), and 225 tablets (NDC 0067-0137-77) with child-resistant caps and in special bottles of 500 tablets (without child-resistant closures) for arthritic patients (NDC 0067-0137-74).

Shown in Product Identification Section, page 425

CAMALOX®
Magnesium and Aluminum Hydroxides with Calcium Carbonate Oral Suspension and Tablets, Rorer
High-potency antacid

Description: Camalox® Suspension is a carefully balanced formulation of 200 mg magnesium hydroxide, 225 mg aluminum hydroxide and 250 mg calcium carbonate per teaspoonful (5 ml). This combination of ingredients produces an antacid capability that exceeds that of other leading ethical products in terms of quantity of acid neutralized as well as the speed and duration of antacid activity as measured by laboratory tests. The formulation also minimizes the possibilities of both constipation and diarrhea. Camalox is prepared by a process which enhances its texture and vanilla-mint flavor, making it especially palatable even for patients who must take antacids for extended periods.
Camalox® Tablets contain 200 mg magnesium hydroxide, 225 mg aluminum hydroxide and 250 mg calcium carbonate per tablet and have a delicate vanilla-mint flavor. They compare favorably with Camalox Suspension in terms of potency, as well as speed and duration of antacid activity, thus, Camalox Tablets overcome the usual deficiencies of antacid tablets. As measured by the *in vitro* test for acid neutralizing capacity, Camalox Tablets exceed the antacid capabilities of the leading ethical antacid suspensions as well as tablets. In addition, the manufacturing process contributes importantly to the flavor and to the texture of the tablets. Patients can take Camalox Tablets in full dosage day after day without tiring of the taste.

Acid Neutralizing Capacity
Camalox Suspension—36.9 mEq/10 ml
Camalox Tablets—36.7 mEq/2 tablets
Sodium Content
Camalox Suspension—1.2 mg (0.05 mEq)/5 ml

Camalox Tablets—1.0 mg (0.04 mEq) tablet

Indications: A high potency antacid for the symptomatic relief of hyperacidity associated with the diagnosis of peptic ulcer, gastritis, peptic esophagitis, gastric hyperacidity, heartburn, or hiatal hernia.

Directions for Use: Camalox Suspension—two to four teaspoonfuls, four times a day, taken one-half hour after meals and at bedtime, or as directed by a physician.

Camalox Tablets—each Camalox Tablet is equivalent to one teaspoonful of Camalox Suspension. Two to four tablets, well-chewed, one-half to one hour after meals and at bedtime, or as directed by a physician.

Patient Warnings: Do not take more than 16 teaspoonfuls or tablets in a 24-hour period or use the maximum dosage for more than two weeks or use if you have kidney disease except under the advice and supervision of a physician. Keep this and all drugs out of the reach of children. In case of accidental overdose, seek professional assistance or contact a poison control center immediately.

Drug Interaction Precaution: Do not use with patients taking a prescription antibiotic drug containing any form of tetracycline. As with all aluminum-containing antacids, Camalox may prevent the proper absorption of tetracycline.

How Supplied: Camalox Suspension—white liquid in convenient 12 fluid ounce (355 ml) plastic bottles (NDC 0067-0180-71).

Camalox Tablets—Bottles of 50 tablets (NDC 0067-0185-50).

Rationale: Studies reveal that clinical symptoms of gastroesophageal reflux correlate with lower esophageal sphincter (LES) incompetency. Although the mechanism of action is unknown, gastric alkalinization has been shown to increase LES pressure.

Camalox is an ideal antacid for the treatment of reflux esophagitis. The balanced formulation of Camalox exerts its neutralizing effect faster and longer than the leading ethical antacids providing prompt symptomatic relief.

Camalox has been shown to produce significant increases in LES pressure providing a physiological barrier against reflux.*

Because Camalox is a high potency antacid with excellent acid neutralizing capacity, fewer and smaller doses are possible.

The refreshing vanilla-mint flavor and smooth texture of Camalox have earned a high level of patient acceptance and wearability. Available in equally effective dosage forms . . . physician-preferred suspension and convenient tablets.

Higgs, R.H., Smyth, R.D., and Castell, D.O., Gastric Alkalinization—Effect on Lower-Esophageal-Sphincter Pressure and Serum Gastrin, N. Engl. J. Med. 291:486-490, 1974.

EMETROL®
Phosphorated Carbohydrate Solution, Rorer
For nausea and vomiting

Description: Emetrol is an oral solution containing balanced amounts of levulose (fructose) and dextrose (glucose) and orthophosphoric acid with controlled hydrogen ion concentration. Pleasantly mint flavored.

Action: Emetrol quickly relieves nausea and vomiting by local action on the wall of the hyperactive G.I. tract. It reduces smooth-muscle contraction in direct proportion to the amount used. Unlike systemic antiemetics, Emetrol works almost immediately to control both nausea and active vomiting—and it is free from toxicity or side effects.

Indications: For nausea and vomiting.

Advantages:

1. Fast action—works almost immediately by local action on contact with the hyperactive G. I. tract.

2. Effectiveness—reported completely effective in epidemic vomiting—reduces smooth-muscle contractions in direct proportion to the amount used—stops both nausea and active vomiting.

3. Safety—no toxicity or side effects—won't mask symptoms of organic pathology.

4. Convenience—can be recommended over the phone for any member of the family, even the children—no Rx required.

5. Patient acceptance—a low cost that patients appreciate—a pleasant mint flavor that both children and adults like.

Usual dose: *Epidemic and other functional vomiting (intestinal "flu", G.I. grippe, etc.); or nausea and vomiting due to psychogenic factors:* Infants and children, one or two teaspoonfuls at 15 minute intervals until vomiting ceases; adults, one or two tablespoonfuls in same manner. If first dose is rejected, resume dosage schedule in five minutes. *Regurgitation in infants:* One or two teaspoonfuls ten or fifteen minutes before each feeding; in refractory cases, two or three teaspoonfuls one-half hour before feedings. *"Morning sickness":* One or two tablespoonfuls on arising, repeated every three hours or whenever nausea threatens.

Emetrol may also be used in motion sickness and in nausea and vomiting due to drug therapy or inhalation anesthesia; in teaspoonful dosage for young children, tablespoonful dosage for older children and adults.

Important: *DO NOT DILUTE or permit oral fluids immediately before or for at least 15 minutes after dose.*

Warning: Keep this and all drugs out of the reach of children. In case of accidental overdose, seek professional assistance or contact a poison control center immediately.

Supplied: Bottles of 3 fluid ounces (89 ml) (NDC 0067-0240-58) and 1 pint (473 ml) (NDC 0067-0240-74).
Shown in Product Identification Section, page 425

FERMALOX®
Hematinic

Formula: Each *uncoated* tablet contains: Ferrous Sulfate 200 mg; Maalox® (magnesium-aluminum hydroxide) 200 mg.

Advantages: "A less irritating, more easily tolerated medicinal iron compound (Fermalox) fills an important need in the treatment of iron-deficiency states. The demonstration of effective absorption by means of the radioactive iron tracer, plus thousands of clinical cases showing satisfactory rise of hemoglobin level, fully establishes the efficacy of this medicament. In addition, the almost complete absence of the common adverse reactions to ordinary iron medicaments enables the physician to continue use of the drug until a satisfactory therapeutic result is obtained."[1]

Indications: For use as a hematinic in iron-deficiency conditions as may occur with: rapid growth, pregnancy, blood loss, menorrhagia, post-surgical convalescence, pathologic bleeding.

Usual Adult Dose: Two tablets daily; in mild cases dosage may be reduced to one tablet daily.

Warning: As with any drug, if you are pregnant or nursing a baby, seek the advice of a health professional before using this product. Keep this and all drugs out of the reach of children. In case of accidental overdose, seek professional assistance or contact a poison control center immediately.

Supplied: Bottles of 100 tablets (NDC 0067-0260-68) with child-resistant caps.
1. *Price, A.H., Erf, L., and Bierly, J.: J.A.M.A. 167:1612 (July 26), 1958.*

GEMNISYN®
(acetaminophen and aspirin, Rorer)
Double Strength Analgesic For Pain

Description: Each Gemnisyn® tablet contains aspirin 325 mg (5 gr) and acetaminophen 325 mg (5 gr) for increased assurance of analgesia in adults compared to a standard analgesic dosage unit.

Indications: For relief of pain requiring increased analgesic strength when the usual doses of mild analgesics are inadequate.

Contraindications: Sensitivity to aspirin or acetaminophen.

Adult Dosage: 1 or 2 Gemnisyn tablets every 4 to 6 hours while pain persists, not to exceed 6 tablets in any 24-hour period.

Warning: As with any drug, if you are pregnant or nursing a baby, seek the advice of a health professional before using this product. Use with caution in the presence of peptic ulcer, asthma, liver damage or with anticoagulant therapy.

Continued on next page

Rorer—Cont.

Not recommended for children under 12. Patient Precaution: If pain persists for more than 10 days, consult your physician.

Reye Syndrome Warning: Do not use in children, including teenagers, with chicken pox or flu.

Keep this and all drugs out of the reach of children. In case of accidental overdose, seek professional assistance or contact a poison control center immediately.

Overdosage: A massive overdosage of acetaminophen may cause hepatotoxicity. Since clinical and laboratory evidence may be delayed for up to one week, close clinical monitoring and serial hepatic enzyme determinations are recommended.

Supplied: Plastic bottle of 100 tablets. NDC 0067-0171-68

KUDROX® SUSPENSION (DOUBLE-STRENGTH) ANTACID

Composition: A pleasantly flavored SUSPENSION containing a concentrated combination of aluminium hydroxide gel and magnesium hydroxide in d-sorbitol.

One teaspoonful of KUDROX Liquid contains not more than 0.65 mEq (15 mg.) of sodium.

Actions and Uses: A palatable antacid to alleviate acid indigestion, heartburn and/or sour stomach, or whenever antacid therapy is the treatment indicated for symptomatic relief of hyperacidity associated with the diagnosis of peptic ulcer, gastritis, peptic esophagitis, gastric hyperacidity, and hiatal hernia. The ratio of aluminium hydroxide to magnesium hydroxide is such that undesirable bowel effects are minimal. Each 5 ml dose of SUSPENSION will neutralize approximately 25 mEq of HCl. High concentration of the active ingredients produces prompt, long lasting neutralization without the acid rebound associated with calcium carbonate containing antacids.

Dosage: KUDROX SUSPENSION, half that ordinarily employed with other liquid antacids. Usual dose only 1 teaspoonful 30 minutes after meals and at bedtime. May be taken undiluted or mixed with water or milk. In peptic ulcer, 2 to 4 teaspoonfuls after meals and at bedtime.

Warning: Antacids containing magnesium hydroxide or magnesium salts should be administered cautiously in patients with renal insufficiency.

Drug Interaction Precaution: This product should not be taken if the patient is currently taking a prescription drug containing any form of tetracycline.

Supplied: KUDROX SUSPENSION, 12 oz. plastic bottles (NDC 0091-4475-42).

LACTRASE™ (Lactase Enzyme) A Dietary Aid in the Digestion of Milk and Other Lactose-Containing Foods

Description: LACTRASE, also known as lactase, is a natural ezyme produced by a unique fermentation process. LACTRASE is biochemically beta-D-galactosidase. Each light brown and white capsule contains 125 mg of standardized enzyme dispersed in malto-dextrins.

Action: Lactose is a non-absorbable disaccharide found as a common constituent in most dairy products. Under normal conditions, dietary lactose is hydrolyzed in the jejunum and proximal ileum by beta-D-glactosidase or lactase. Lactase is produced in the brush border of the columnar epithelial cells of the intestinal villi. Lactase hydrolyzes lactose into two monosaccharides, glucose and galactose, that are readily absorbed by the intestine.

Lactose Intolerance: Though lactase is normally present in adequate quantities in infants, in several populations its concentration naturally declines starting at about 4–5 years of age and is low in a substantial number of individuals by their teens or early 20's. Within certain geographic and ethnic groups, especially in adult Blacks, Orientals, American Indians and eastern European Jews, the lactase activity may be low even earlier. Although many of them can easily digest smaller quantities of lactose in milk, after consumption of excessive volume of milk or dairy products, they may exhibit symptoms of lactose intolerance.
When available lactase is insufficient to split the lactose, the unabsorbable sugar remains in the small intestine for an extended period, presenting an osmotic load that increases and retains intraluminal fluid and intensifies intestinal motility; thus the individual reports a bloated feeling and cramps. The undigested lactose is decomposed by the intestinal flora in the lower intestine and excessive carbon dioxide and hydrogen is produced. These gases contribute to flatulence and increased abdominal discomfort. The lactic acid and other short chain acids raise the osmolality, hinder fluid reabsorption and decrease transit time of the contents of the colon, leading to diarrhea. Often hydrogen is noticed in the expired breath of a lactase deficient patient.

Indications: LACTRASE is indicated for individuals exhibiting symptoms of lactose intolerance or lactase insufficiency as identified by lactose tolerance test or by symptoms of gastrointestinal disturbances after consumption of milk or dairy products.

Precautions: It should be noted that in diabetic persons who use LACTRASE, the milk sugar will be metabolically available and must be taken into account (25 g of glucose and 25 g of galactose per quart of milk). Individuals with galactos-

emia may not have milk in any form, lactose enzyme modified or not.

Directions For Use: Milk may be pretreated with LACTRASE; simply add contents from one or two capsules to each quart of milk, shake gently, and store the milk in the refrigerator for 24 hours. The LACTRASE will break down milk sugar to digestible simple sugars. LACTRASE powder will not alter the appearance of milk, however the taste may be slightly sweeter than untreated milk.
Alternatively, one or two LACTRASE Capsules swallowed with milk or dairy products is all that is necessary to digest the milk sugar contained in a normal serving. If the individual is severely intolerant to lactose, additional capsules may be taken until a satisfactory response is achieved as recognized by resolution of the symptoms. LACTRASE Capsules are safe to take and higher quantities in severe cases will be well tolerated.
If the individual cannot swallow capsules, the contents of the capsules may be sprinkled onto diary products before consuming. LACTRASE will not alter the taste of the dairy product when used in this manner.

How Supplied: LACTRASE Capsules are brown and white and are imprinted "KREMERS-URBAN 500". They are supplied in bottles of 100 capsules (NDC 0091-3500-01).
Shown in Product Identification Section, page 425

MAALOX® Magnesia and Alumina Oral Suspension and Tablets, Rorer Antacid A Balanced Formulation of Magnesium and Aluminum Hydroxides

Description: Maalox Suspension is a balanced combination of magnesium and aluminum hydroxides. . . first in order of preference for all routine purposes of antacid medication. The high neutralizing power of magnesium hydroxide and the established acid binding capacity of aluminum hydroxide support the reputation of Maalox for reliable antacid action.
MAALOX® SUSPENSION: 225 mg Aluminum Hydroxide Equivalent to Dried Gel, USP, and 200 mg Magnesium Hydroxide per 5 ml.
MAALOX® No. 1 TABLETS: (200 mg Magnesium Hydroxide, 200 mg Dried Aluminum Hydroxide Gel) per tablet
MAALOX® No. 2 TABLETS: (400 mg Magnesium Hydroxide, 400 mg Dried Aluminum Hydroxide Gel) per tablet
Acid Neutralizing Capacity
Maalox® Suspension—26.6 mEq/10 ml
Maalox No. 1 Tablets—19.4 mEq/2 tablets
Maalox No. 2 Tablets—23.4 mEq/tablet
Sodium Content
Maalox Suspension and Tablets are dietetically sodium-free*. Each teaspoonful (5 ml) of Maalox Suspension contains approximately 0.06 mEq sodium (1.4 mg

and Maalox No. 1 and No. 2 Tablets contain approximately 0.03 mEq (0.7 mg) and 0.06 mEq (1.4 mg) sodium respectively per tablet.

Indications: As an antacid for symptomatic relief of hyperacidity associated with the diagnosis of peptic ulcer, gastritis, peptic esophagitis, gastric hyperacidity, heartburn or hiatal hernia.

Advantages: Many patients prefer Maalox whether they are taking it for occasional heartburn or routinely on an ulcer therapy regimen. Once started on Maalox, patients tend to stay on Maalox because of effectiveness, taste, and non-constipating characteristics... three important reasons for Maalox when prolonged therapy is necessary. In addition, Maalox Suspension and Tablets are sodium-free.

Directions for use:
MAALOX® SUSPENSION: Two to four teaspoonfuls, four times a day, taken twenty minutes to one hour after meals and at bedtime, or as directed by a physician.
MAALOX NO. 1 TABLETS: Two to four tablets, well chewed, twenty minutes to one hour after meals and at bedtime, or as directed by a physician.
MAALOX NO. 2 TABLETS: One or two tablets, well chewed, twenty minutes to one hour after meals and at bedtime, or as directed by a physician. May be followed with milk or water.

Patient Warnings: Do not take more than 16 teaspoonfuls of Maalox Suspension, 16 Maalox No. 1 Tablets or 8 Maalox No. 2 Tablets in a 24-hour period or use the maximum dosage for more than 2 weeks or use if you have kidney disease, except under the supervision of a physician.

Drug Interaction Precaution: Do not use with patients taking a prescription antibiotic drug containing any form of tetracycline. As with all aluminum-containing antacids, Maalox® may prevent the proper absorption of the tetracycline. Keep this and all drugs out of the reach of children.

Supplied:
MAALOX SUSPENSION is available in plastic bottles of 12 fluid ounces (355 ml) (NDC 0067-0330-71), 5 fluid ounces (148 ml) (NDC 0067-0330-62), and 26 fluid ounces (769 ml) (NDC 0067-0330-44). Military Stock #NSN 6505-00-680-0133; V.A. Stock #6505-00-074-0993A [bottles of 6 fluid ounces (177 ml)].
MAALOX NO. 1 TABLETS (400 mg) available in bottles of 100 tablets (NDC 0067-0335-68).
MAALOX NO. 2 TABLETS (800 mg) available in bottles of 50 (NDC 0067-0337-50) and 250 tablets (NDC 0067-0337-70). Also available in boxes of 24 (NDC 0067-0337-24) and 100 tablets (NDC 0067-0337-67) in easy-to-carry strips.
V.A. Stock #6505-00-993-3507A [boxes of 100 tablets (in cellophane strips)].
*dietetically insignificant
Shown in Product Identification Section, page 425

MAALOX® PLUS
Alumina, Magnesia and Simethicone Oral Suspension and Tablets, Rorer Antacid-Antiflatulent

☐ **Lemon swiss-creme flavor... the taste preferred by physician and patient.**
☐ **Physician-proven Maalox® formula for antacid effectiveness.**
☐ **Simethicone, at a recognized clinical dose, for antiflatulent action.**

Description: Maalox® Plus, a balanced combination of magnesium and aluminum hydroxides plus simethicone, is a non-constipating, lemon-flavored, antacid-antiflatulent.

Composition: To provide symptomatic relief of hyperacidity plus alleviation of gas symptoms, each teaspoonful/tablet contains:

Active Ingredients	Maalox Plus Per Tsp. (5 ml)	Per Tablet
Magnesium Hydroxide	200 mg	200 mg
Aluminum Hydroxide	225 mg	200 mg
Simethicone	25 mg	25 mg

To aid in establishing proper dosage schedules, the following information is provided:

Minimum Recommended Dosage:	Per 2 Tsp. (10 ml)	Per 2 Tablets
Acid neutralizing capacity	26.7 mEq	22.8 mEq
Sodium content*	2.4 mg	1.6 mg
Sugar content	None	1.1 g
Lactose content	None	None

Indications: As an antacid for symptomatic relief of hyperacidity associated with the diagnosis of peptic ulcer, gastritis, peptic esophagitis, gastric hyperacidity, heartburn or hiatal hernia. As an antiflatulent to alleviate the symptoms of gas, including postoperative gas pain.

Advantages: Among antacids, Maalox Plus is uniquely palatable—an important feature which encourages patients to follow your dosage directions. Maalox Plus has the time proven, nonconstipating, sodium-free* Maalox formula—useful for those patients suffering from the problems associated with hyperacidity. Additionally, Maalox Plus contains simethicone to alleviate discomfort associated with entrapped gas.
*Dietetically insignificant. Contains approximately 0.05 mEq sodium per teaspoonful of Suspension. Each Maalox Plus Tablet contains approximately 0.03 mEq sodium per Tablet.

Directions for Use:
MAALOX® PLUS SUSPENSION: Two to four teaspoonfuls, four times a day, taken twenty minutes to one hour after meals and at bedtime, or as directed by a physician.
MAALOX® PLUS TABLETS: Two to four tablets, well chewed, four times a day, taken twenty minutes to one hour after meals and at bedtime, or as directed by a physician.

Patient Warnings: Do not take more than 16 teaspoonfuls or 16 tablets in a 24-hour period or use the maximum dosage for more than two weeks or use if you have kidney disease except under the advice and supervision of a physician.

Drug Interaction Precaution: Do not use with patients taking a prescription antibiotic containing any form of tetracycline. As with all aluminum-containing antacids, Maalox Plus may prevent the proper absorption of the tetracycline. Keep this and all drugs out of the reach of children.

Supplied:
MAALOX PLUS SUSPENSION is available in a plastic 12 fluid ounce (355 ml) bottle (NDC 0067-0332-71).
MAALOX PLUS TABLETS are available in bottles of 50 tablets (NDC 0067-0339-50) and boxes of 100 tablets (NDC 0067-0339-67) in handy portable strips, convenience packs of 12 tablets (NDC 0067-0339-29), and Roll Packs of 12 tablets (NDC 0067-0339-23).
Shown in Product Identification Section, page 425

MAALOX® TC Suspension and Tablets
Therapeutic Concentrate (Magnesium & Aluminum Hydroxides Oral Suspension and Tablets, Rorer)

Description: Maalox® TC Suspension is a potent, concentrated, balanced formulation of 300 mg magnesium hydroxide and 600 mg aluminum hydroxide per teaspoonful (5 ml). This formulation produces a therapeutically concentrated antacid that exceeds standard antacids in acid neutralizing capacity. Maalox® TC Suspension is formulated to reduce the need to alter therapy due to treatment-induced changes in bowel habits. Palatability is enhanced by a pleasant-tasting peppermint flavor.
Maalox® TC Tablets contain 300 mg magnesium hydroxide and 600 mg aluminum hydroxide per tablet, with a pleasant-tasting peppermint-lemon-creme flavor. *In vivo* testing demonstrates a longer duration of action for the tablets when compared with equivalent doses of suspension. Maalox® TC tablets thus overcome the usual deficiencies of antacid tablets.

Continued on next page

Rorer—Cont.

Acid Neutralizing Capacity
Maalox® TC Suspension—27.2 mEq 5 ml
Maalox® TC Tablets—28.0 mEq/tablet
Sodium Content:
Maalox® TC Suspension—0.8 mg/5 ml (0.03 mEq)
Maalox® TC Tablets—0.5 mg/tablet (0.2 mEq)

Indications: Maalox® TC Suspension and Tablets are indicated for the symptomatic relief of hyperacidity associated with the diagnosis of peptic ulcer and other gastrointestinal conditions where a high degree of acid neutralization is desired.

Directions for Use: Maalox® TC Suspension—one or two teaspoonsful one hour after meals and at bedtime. Higher dosage regimens may be employed under the direct supervision of a physician in the treatment of active peptic ulcer disease.
Maalox® TC Tablets—each Maalox® tablet is equivalent to one teaspoon of Maalox® TC Suspension. One or two Maalox® TC tablets, well chewed one hour after meals and at bedtime. Higher dosage regimens may be employed under the direct supervision of a physician in the treatment of active peptic ulcer disease.

Patient Warning: Do not take more than 8 teaspoonsful of the suspension or 8 tablets in a 24-hour period, or use the maximum dosage of this product for more than two weeks except under the advice and supervision of a physician. Also, if you have kidney disease, do not use except under the advice and supervision of a physician.

Drug Interaction Precaution: Antacids may decrease the absorption of certain prescription drugs particularly tetracyclines, phenytoin, digoxin, hypoglycemic agents and H_2 antagonists. Administer antacids at least one hour before or after administration of these drugs.

How Supplied: Maalox® TC Suspension is available in a 12-fluid ounce (355 ml) plastic bottle.
Maalox® TC Tablets are available in plastic bottles of 48 tablets.
* Dietetically Insignificant
Shown in Product Identification Section, page 425

MILKINOL®

Composition: MILKINOL is a unique formulation containing liquid petrolatum for lubrication, a special emulsifier to aid in penetration and softening of the fecal mass, and to make oil and water mix for complete dispersion.

Action and Uses: Pleasant, dependable MILKINOL provides safe, gentle lubrication for the constipation problem. No oily taste, no purgative griping, not habit forming, sugar free. MILKINOL is an agent of choice for the correction of simple constipation in older children and adults. At the discretion of the physician it may also be employed in the management of constipation in younger children, in pregnant patients and in elderly or bedridden persons.

Dosage: Adults 1 to 2 tablespoonfuls. Children over 6: 1 to 2 teaspoonfuls. Infants, young children, expectant mothers, aged or bedridden patients, use only as directed by physician.

Directions: Pour desired dosage of MILKINOL into a dry drinking glass. Add just a small amount (about ¼ glass or less) of water, milk, fruit juice or soft drink. Stir and drink. Follow with additional liquid if desired.

Precautions: Prolonged usage, without intermission is not advised. Should be given at bedtime ONLY.

Supplied: 8-oz. glass bottles (NDC 0091-7580-08).

PERDIEM®

Actions: Perdiem®, with its gentle action provides comfortable relief from constipation. The vegetable mucilages of Perdiem® soften the stool and provide pain-free evacuation of the bowel. Perdiem® is effective as an aid to elimination for the hemorrhoid or fissure patient prior to and following surgery.

Composition: Perdiem® contains as its active ingredients, 82% psyllium (Plantago Hydrocolloid) and 18% senna (Cassia Pod Concentrate) which are natural vegetable derivatives. Each rounded teaspoonful (6.0 g) contains 3.25 g psyllium, 0.74 g senna, 1.8 mg of sodium, 35.5 mg of potassium, and 4 calories. Perdiem® is "Dye-Free". Inactive ingredients: acacia, iron oxides, natural flavors, paraffin, sucrose, talc.

Indication: For relief of constipation.

Patient Warning: Should not be used in the presence of undiagnosed abdominal pain. Frequent or prolonged use without the direction of a physician is not recommended, as it may lead to laxative dependence. Do not use in patients with a history of psyllium allergy. Psyllium allergy is rare but can be severe. If an allergic reaction occurs, discontinue use.
Bulk forming agents have the potential to obstruct the esophagus, particularly in the presence of esophageal narrowing or when consumed with insufficient fluid. Patients should be made aware of the symptoms of esophageal obstruction, including chest pain/pressure, regurgitation, and difficulty swallowing. Patients experiencing these symptoms should seek immediate medical attention. Patients with esophageal narrowing or dysphagia should not use Perdiem®.
As with any drug, if you are pregnant or nursing a baby, seek the advice of a health professional before using this product. Keep this and all drugs out of the reach of children. In case of accidental overdose, seek professional assistance or contact a poison control center immediately.

Directions For Use—Adults: In the evening and/or before breakfast, 1–2 rounded teaspoonfuls of Perdiem® granules (in single or partial teaspoon doses) should be placed in the mouth and swallowed with at least 8 fl oz of cool beverage after the dose. Additional liquid would be helpful. Perdiem® granules should not be chewed.
After Perdiem® takes effect (usually after 24 hours, but possibly not before 36–48 hours): reduce the morning and evening doses to one rounded teaspoonful. Subsequent doses should be adjusted after adequate laxation is obtained.

Note: It is extremely important that Perdiem® Plain be taken with at least 8 fl oz of cool liquid.

In Obstinate Cases: Perdiem® may be taken more frequently, up to two rounded teaspoonfuls every six hours.

For Patients Habituated to Strong Purgatives: Two rounded teaspoonfuls of Perdiem® in the morning and evening may be required along with half the usual dose of the purgative being used. The purgative should be discontinued as soon as possible and the dosage of Perdiem® granules reduced when and if bowel tone shows lessened laxative dependence.

For Colostomy Patients: To ensure formed stools, give one to two rounded teaspoonfuls of Perdiem® in the evening.

For Clinical Regulation: For patients confined to bed, for those of inactive habits, and in the presence of cardiovascular disease where straining must be avoided, one rounded teaspoonful of Perdiem® taken once or twice daily will provide regular bowel habits.

For Children: From age 7–11 years, give one rounded teaspoonful one to two times daily. From age 12 and older, give adult dosage.

How Supplied: Granules: 100-gram (3.5-oz) and 250-gram (8.8-oz) canisters, Hospital Unit Dose 50 6-gram packets in a gravity feed dispenser.
Shown in Product Identification Section, page 425

PERDIEM® PLAIN

100% Bulk Forming Action: Perdiem® Plain is a light brown, minty tasting, granular, non-irritating bulk laxative which gently softens the stool and promotes normal elimination of the bowels. Perdiem® Plain is effective in the treatment of constipation, contains no irritants, and when used under the direction of a physician, can safely be taken for prolonged periods.

Composition: Perdiem® Plain contains as its active ingredient 100% psyllium (Plantago Hydrocolloid), a natural vegetable derivative. Each rounded teaspoonful (6.0 g) contains 4.03 g of psyllium, 1.8 mg of sodium, 36.1 mg of potassium and 4 calories. Perdiem® Plain is "Dye-Free". Inactive ingredients: acacia, iron oxides, natural flavors, paraffin, sucrose, talc.

Indications: Perdiem® Plain provides gentle relief from simple, chronic, and spastic constipation. In addition, it relieves constipation associated with convalescence, pregnancy, and advanced age. Perdiem® Plain is also indicated for use in special diets lacking in residue fiber and in the management of constipation associated with irritable bowel syndrome, diverticular disease, hemorrhoids, and anal fissures.

Patient Warning: Should not be used in the presence of undiagnosed abdominal pain. Frequent or prolonged use without the direction of a physician is not recommended.
Do not use in patients with a history of psyllium allergy. Psyllium allergy is rare but can be severe. If an allergic reaction occurs, discontinue use.
Bulk forming agents have the potential to obstruct the esophagus, particularly in the presence of esophageal narrowing or when consumed with insufficient fluid. Patients should be made aware of the symptoms of esophageal obstruction, including chest pain/pressure, regurgitation, and difficulty swallowing. Patients experiencing these symptoms should seek immediate medical attention. Patients with esophageal narrowing or dysphagia should not use Perdiem® Plain. Keep this and all drugs out of the reach of children. In case of accidental overdose, seek professional assistance or contact a poison control center immediately.

Directions For Use—Adults: In the evening and/or before breakfast, 1 to 2 rounded teaspoonfuls (6.0 to 12.0 g) of Perdiem® Plain granules (in full or partial teaspoon doses) should be placed in the mouth and swallowed with at least 8 fl oz of cool beverage after the dose. Additional liquid would be helpful. Perdiem® Plain granules should not be chewed. Children: For children age 7–11, give 1 rounded teaspoonful 1–2 times daily. Age 12 and older, give adult dosage.

Note: It is extremely important that Perdiem® Plain be taken with at least 8 fl oz of cool liquid.

In Obstinate Cases: Perdiem® Plain may be taken more frequently, up to 2 rounded teaspoonfuls every 6 hours depending upon need and response. Perdiem® Plain generally takes effect after 24 hours, however, in resistant cases, 48 to 72 hours may be required to provide optimal benefit.

After Rectal Surgery: The vegetable mucilages of Perdiem® Plain soften the stool and ensure pain-free evacuation of the bowel. Perdiem® Plain is effective as an aid to elimination for the hemorrhoid or fissure patient prior to and following surgery.

For Clinical Regulation: For patients confined to bed—after an operation for example—and for those of inactive habits, 1 rounded teaspoonful of Perdiem®

Plain taken 1–2 times daily will ensure regular bowel habits.

During Pregnancy: Because of its natural ingredient and bulking action, Perdiem® Plain is effective for expectant mothers when used under a physician's care. In most cases 1–2 rounded teaspoonfuls taken each evening is sufficient.

How Supplied: Granules: 100-gram (3.5-oz) and 250-gram (8.8-oz) canisters, Hospital Unit Dose 50 6-gram packets in a gravity feed dispenser.
Shown in Product Identification Section, page 426

Ross Laboratories
COLUMBUS, OH 43216

ADVANCE®
Nutritional Beverage

Usage: As a fortified milk/soy-based feeding more appropriate than 2% low-fat milk for feeding older babies and toddlers.

Availability:
Concentrated Liquid: 13-fl-oz cans; 12 per case; No. 3313.
Ready To Feed: (Prediluted, 16 Cal/fl oz) 32-fl-oz cans; 6 per case; No. 3301.

Preparation: Standard dilution (16 Cal/fl oz) is one part Concentrated Liquid to one part water. Ready To Feed requires no dilution. For hospital use, ADVANCE in disposable nursing bottles is available in the Ross Hospital Formula System.

Composition: Concentrated Liquid

Ingredients: Ⓤ-D Water, corn syrup, nonfat milk, soy oil, soy protein isolate, corn oil, mono- and diglycerides, soy lecithin, minerals (calcium phosphate tribasic, potassium citrate, magnesium chloride, ferrous sulfate, zinc sulfate, cupric sulfate, manganese sulfate), vitamins (ascorbic acid, alpha-tocopheryl acetate, niacinamide, calcium pantothenate, vitamin A palmitate, thiamine chloride hydrochloride, pyridoxine hydrochloride, riboflavin, folic acid, phylloquinone, vitamin D_3, cyanocobalamin), carrageenan and taurine.

Nutrients (wt/liter):	Concen-trated		Standard Dilution*	
Protein	40.0	g	20.0	g
Fat	54.0	g	27.0	g
Carbohydrate	110.0	g	55.0	g
Minerals (Ash)	7.0	g	3.5	g
Calcium	1020	mg	510	mg
Phosphorus	780	mg	390	mg
Magnesium	128	mg	64	mg
Iron	24	mg	12	mg
Iodine	120	mcg	60	mcg
Zinc	10	mg	5.0	mg
Copper	1.2	mg	0.6	mg
Manganese	68	mcg	34	mcg
Sodium	460	mg	230	mg
Potassium	1800	mg	900	mg
Chloride	1040	mg	520	mg
Water	843	g	920	g
Crude Fiber	0	g		

Calories per fl oz	32	16
Calories per liter	1080	540

Vitamins Per Liter (Standard Dilution*):

Vitamin A	2000	I.U.
Vitamin D	400	I.U.
Vitamin E	20	I.U.
Vitamin K_1	55	mcg
Vitamin C	50	mg
Thiamine (Vit. B_1)	0.75	mg
Riboflavin (Vit. B_2)	0.90	mg
Vitamin B_6	0.60	mg
Vitamin B_{12}	2.5	mcg
Niacin	10	mg
Folic Acid	100	mcg
Pantothenic Acid	4.0	mg

*Standard dilution is equal parts Advance Concentrated Liquid and water. (FAN 341-01)

Composition: Ready To Feed

Ingredients: Ⓤ-D Water, corn syrup, nonfat milk, soy oil, soy protein isolate, corn oil, mono- and diglycerides, soy lecithin, minerals (calcium phosphate tribasic, potassium citrate, magnesium chloride, ferrous sulfate, zinc sulfate, cupric sulfate, manganese sulfate), vitamins (ascorbic acid, alpha-tocopheryl acetate, niacinamide, calcium pantothenate, vitamin A palmitate, thiamine chloride hydrochloride, pyridoxine hydrochloride, riboflavin, folic acid, phylloquinone, vitamin D_3, cyanocobalamin), carrageenan and taurine.

Nutrients (wt/liter):

Protein	20.0	g
Fat	27.0	g
Carbohydrate	55.0	g
Minerals (Ash)	3.5	g
Calcium	510	mg
Phosphorus	390	mg
Magnesium	64	mg
Iron	12	mg
Iodine	60	mcg
Zinc	5.0	mg
Copper	0.6	mg
Manganese	34	mcg
Sodium	230	mg
Potassium	900	mg
Chloride	520	mg
Water	920	g
Crude Fiber	0	g
Calories per fl oz	16	
Calories per liter	540	

Vitamins Per Liter:

Vitamin A	2000	I.U.
Vitamin D	400	I.U.
Vitamin E	20	I.U.
Vitamin K_1	55	mcg
Vitamin C	50	mg
Thiamine (Vit. B_1)	0.75	mg
Riboflavin (Vit. B_2)	0.90	mg

Continued on next page

If desired, additional information on any Ross Product will be provided upon request to Ross Laboratories.

Ross—Cont.

Vitamin B$_6$	0.60	mg
Vitamin B$_{12}$	2.5	mcg
Niacin	10	mg
Folic Acid	100	mcg
Pantothenic Acid	4.0	mg

The addition of iron to this beverage conforms to the recommendation of the Committee on Nutrition of the American Academy of Pediatrics.
(FAN 341-01)

CLEAR EYES®
Eye Drops

Description: Clear Eyes is a sterile isotonic buffered solution containing naphazoline hydrochloride 0.012%, boric acid, sodium borate, and water. Edetate disodium 0.1% and benzalkonium chloride 0.01% are added as preservatives. (Contains vasoconstrictor.)

Indications: Clear Eyes is a decongestant ophthalmic solution specially designed to soothe as it removes redness from eyes irritated due to swimming, plant allergies (pollen), colds, smog, sun glare, wind, dust, wearing contact lenses, and overuse of eyes in reading, driving, TV and close work. Clear Eyes contains laboratory tested, and scientifically blended ingredients including an effective vasoconstrictor which narrows swollen blood vessels and rapidly whitens reddened eyes in a formulation which produces a refreshing, soothing effect. Clear Eyes is a sterile, isotonic solution compatible with the natural fluids of the eye.

Warning: Clear Eyes should only be used for minor eye irritations.
Clear Eyes should not be used by individuals with glaucoma and serious eye diseases. In some instances redness or inflammation may be due to serious eye conditions such as acute iritis, acute glaucoma, or corneal trauma. When redness, pain, or blurring persist, discontinue use. A physician should be consulted at once.

Dosage and Administration: One or two drops in eye(s) up to 4 times daily or as directed by physician. Do not touch bottle tip to any surface, since this may contaminate the solution. Remove contact lenses before using. Keep this and all medicines out of the reach of children. Replace cap after using.

How Supplied: In 0.5 fl oz and 1.5 fl oz plastic dropper bottle.
Shown in Product Identification Section, page 426
(FAN 2021-02)

EAR DROPS BY MURINE
See Murine Ear Wax Removal System/Murine Ear Drops
Shown in Product Identification Section, page 426

ISOMIL®
Soy Protein Formula

Usage: As a beverage for infants, children and adults with an allergy or sensitivity to cow's milk. A feeding for patients with disorders where lactose should be avoided: lactase deficiency, lactose intolerance and galactosemia. A feeding following diarrhea.

Availability:
Powder: 14-oz cans, measuring scoop enclosed; 6 per case; No. 00107. 1.07-oz packets; 12 four-packet cartons per case; No. 00219.
Concentrated Liquid: 13-fl-oz cans; 24 per case; No. 02110.
Ready To Feed: (Prediluted, 20 Cal/fl oz)
32-fl-oz cans; 6 per case; No. 00230.
8-fl-oz cans; 4 six-packs per case; No. 00173.
For hospital use, Isomil in disposable nursing bottles is available in the Ross Hospital Formula System.

Preparation:
Powder: Standard dilution (20 Cal/fl oz) is one level, unpacked scoop of Isomil Powder for each 2 fl oz of warm water; or, one packet (1.07 oz) for each 7 fl oz of warm water.
Concentrated Liquid: Standard dilution (20 Cal/fl oz) is one part Concentrated Liquid to one part water.
Note: All forms of Isomil should be shaken well before feeding.

Composition: Powder

Ingredients: (Pareve, Ⓤ) 30.7% corn syrup solids, 20.5% sucrose, 16.1% soy protein isolate, 14.0% corn oil, 14.0% coconut oil, minerals (1.6% calcium phosphate tribasic, 0.9% potassium citrate, 0.3% potassium chloride, 0.3% magnesium chloride, 0.2% sodium chloride, calcium carbonate, ferrous sulfate, zinc sulfate, cupric sulfate, manganese sulfate, potassium iodide), vitamins (ascorbic acid, choline chloride, alpha-tocopheryl acetate, niacinamide, calcium pantothenate, vitamin A palmitate, thiamine chloride hydrochloride, riboflavin, pyridoxine hydrochloride, phylloquinone, folic acid, biotin, vitamin D$_3$, cyanocobalamin), L-methionine and taurine.

Nutrients:	Powder (wt/100 g)		Standard Dilution* (wt/liter)	
Protein	13.7	g	18.0	g
Fat	28.1	g	36.9	g
Carbohydrate	51.7	g	68.0	g
Minerals (Ash)	3.5	g	4.6	g
Calcium	530	mg	700	mg
Phosphorus	380	mg	500	mg
Magnesium	38	mg	50	mg
Iron	9.1	mg	12	mg
Iodine	80	mcg	100	mcg
Zinc	3.8	mg	5.0	mg
Copper	0.38	mg	0.50	mg
Manganese	150	mcg	200	mcg
Sodium	240	mg	320	mg
Potassium	580	mg	770	mg
Chloride	450	mg	590	mg
Moisture	2.5	g	902	g

Crude Fiber	0	g		
Calories	514		676	
Calories per fl oz			20	

Vitamins Per Liter (Standard Dilution*):

Vitamin A	2000	I.U.
Vitamin D	400	I.U.
Vitamin E	17	I.U.
Vitamin K$_1$	100	mcg
Vitamin C	55	mg
Thiamine (Vit. B$_1$)	0.40	mg
Riboflavin (Vit. B$_2$)	0.60	mg
Vitamin B$_6$	0.40	mg
Vitamin B$_{12}$	3.0	mcg
Niacin	9.0	mg
Folic Acid	100	mcg
Pantothenic Acid	5.0	mg
Biotin	30	mcg
Choline	53	mg
Inositol	32	mg

*Standard dilution is one level unpacked scoop of Isomil Powder for each 2 fl oz of warm water; or, one packet (1.07 oz) for each 7 fl oz of warm water, or 131.5 g of Powder diluted to 1 liter.
(FAN 341-03)

Composition: Concentrated Liquid

Ingredients: (Pareve, Ⓤ) 74% water, 7.2% corn syrup, 5.8% sucrose, 4.1% soy oil, 3.8% soy protein isolate, 2.7% coconut oil, 1.0% modified corn starch, minerals (calcium phosphate tribasic, potassium citrate, potassium chloride, magnesium chloride, sodium chloride, ferrous sulfate, zinc sulfate, cupric sulfate, manganese sulfate, potassium iodide), mono- and diglycerides, soy lecithin, vitamins (ascorbic acid, choline chloride, alpha-tocopheryl acetate, niacinamide, calcium pantothenate, vitamin A palmitate, thiamine chloride hydrochloride, riboflavin, pyridoxine hydrochloride, phylloquinone, folic acid, biotin, vitamin D$_3$, cyanocobalamin), L-methionine, carrageenan and taurine.

Nutrients (wt/liter):	Concentrated		Standard Dilution*	
Protein	36.0 g		18.0 g	
Fat	73.8 g		36.9 g	
Carbohydrate	136.0 g		68.0 g	
Minerals (Ash)	7.5 g		3.8 g	
Calcium	1400	mg	700	mg
Phosphorus	1000	mg	500	mg
Magnesium	100	mg	50	mg
Iron	24	mg	12	mg
Iodine	200	mcg	100	mcg
Zinc	10	mg	5.0	mg
Copper	1.0	mg	0.50	mg
Manganese	400	mcg	200	mcg
Sodium	640	mg	320	mg
Potassium	1540	mg	770	mg
Chloride	1180	mg	590	mg
Water	806	g	902	g
Crude Fiber	0	g		
Calories per fl oz	40		20	
Calories per liter	1352		676	

Vitamins Per Liter (Standard Dilution*):

Vitamin A	2000	I.U.

Vitamin D	400	I.U.
Vitamin E	20	I.U.
Vitamin K$_1$	100	mcg
Vitamin C	55	mg
Thiamine (Vit. B$_1$)	0.40	mg
Riboflavin (Vit. B$_2$)	0.60	mg
Vitamin B$_6$	0.40	mg
Vitamin B$_{12}$	3.0	mcg
Niacin	9.0	mg
Folic Acid	100	mcg
Pantothenic Acid	5.0	mg
Biotin	30	mcg
Choline	53	mg
Inositol	32	mg

*Standard dilution is equal amounts Isomil Concentrated Liquid and water. (FAN 341-03)

Composition: Ready To Feed

Ingredients: (Pareve, Ⓤ) 86.4% water, 4.1% corn syrup, 3.2% sucrose, 2.1% soy oil, 2.0% soy protein isolate, 1.4% coconut oil, minerals (calcium citrate, calcium phosphate tribasic, potassium phosphate monobasic, potassium chloride, potassium citrate, magnesium chloride, potassium phosphate dibasic, sodium chloride, ferrous sulfate, zinc sulfate, cupric sulfate, manganese sulfate, potassium iodide), mono- and diglycerides, soy lecithin, vitamins (ascorbic acid, choline chloride, alpha-tocopheryl acetate, niacinamide, calcium pantothenate, vitamin A palmitate, thiamine chloride hydrochloride, riboflavin, pyridoxine hydrochloride, phylloquinone, folic acid, biotin, vitamin D$_3$, cyanocobalamin), carrageenan, L-methionine and taurine.

Nutrients (wt/liter):

Protein	18.0	g
Fat	36.9	g
Carbohydrate	68.0	g
Minerals (Ash)	3.8	g
Calcium	700	mg
Phosphorus	500	mg
Magnesium	50	mg
Iron	12	mg
Iodine	100	mcg
Zinc	5.0	mg
Copper	0.50	mg
Manganese	200	mcg
Sodium	320	mg
Potassium	950	mg
Chloride	430	mg
Water	902	g
Crude Fiber	0	g
Calories per fl oz	20	
Calories per liter	676	

Vitamins Per Liter:

Vitamin A	2000	I.U.
Vitamin D	400	I.U.
Vitamin E	20	I.U.
Vitamin K$_1$	100	mcg
Vitamin C	55	mg
Thiamine (Vit. B$_1$)	0.40	mg
Riboflavin (Vit. B$_2$)	0.60	mg
Vitamin B$_6$	0.40	mg
Vitamin B$_{12}$	3.0	mcg
Niacin	9.0	mg
Folic Acid	100	mcg
Pantothenic Acid	5.0	mg
Biotin	30	mcg

Choline	53	mg
Inositol	32	mg

The addition of iron to this formula conforms to the recommendation of the Committee on Nutrition of the American Academy of Pediatrics. (FAN 341-02)

ISOMIL® SF
Sucrose–Free Soy Protein Formula

Usage: As a beverage for infants, children and adults with an allergy or sensitivity to cow's milk or an intolerance to sucrose or lactose. A feeding for patients following acute diarrhea. A feeding for patients with disorders where lactose and sucrose should be avoided.

Availability:
Concentrated Liquid: 13-fl-oz cans; 12 per case; No. 00119.
Ready To Feed: (Prediluted, 20 Cal/fl oz) 32-fl-oz cans; 6 per case; No. 00128. For hospital use, Isomil SF in disposable nursing bottles is available in the Ross Hospital Formula System.

Preparation:
Concentrated Liquid: Standard dilution (20 Cal/fl oz) is one part Isomil SF Concentrated Liquid to one part water. Note: All forms of Isomil SF should be shaken well before feeding.

Composition: Concentrated Liquid

Ingredients: (Pareve, Ⓤ) 75.7% water, 13.2% corn syrup solids, 4.2% soy protein isolate, 4.0% soy oil, 2.6% coconut oil, minerals (calcium phosphate tribasic, potassium citrate, potassium chloride, magnesium chloride, calcium carbonate, sodium chloride, ferrous sulfate, zinc sulfate, cupric sulfate, manganese sulfate, potassium iodide), mono- and diglycerides, soy lecithin, vitamins (ascorbic acid, choline chloride, alpha-tocopheryl acetate, niacinamide, calcium pantothenate, vitamin A palmitate, thiamine chloride hydrochloride, riboflavin, pyridoxine hydrochloride, phylloquinone, folic acid, biotin, vitamin D$_3$, cyanocobalamin), L-methionine and taurine.

Nutrients (wt/liter):	Concentrated		Standard Dilution*	
Protein	40.0	g	20.0	g
Fat	72.0	g	36.0	g
Carbohydrate	136.0	g	68.0	g
Minerals (Ash)	7.5	g	3.8	g
Calcium	1400	mg	700	mg
Phosphorus	1000	mg	500	mg
Magnesium	100	mg	50	mg
Iron	24	mg	12	mg
Iodine	200	mcg	100	mcg
Zinc	10	mg	5.0	mg
Copper	1.0	mg	0.50	mg
Manganese	400	mcg	200	mcg
Sodium	640	mg	320	mg
Potassium	1540	mg	770	mg
Chloride	1180	mg	590	mg
Water	806	g	902	g
Crude Fiber	0	g		
Calories per fl oz	40		20	

Calories per		
liter	1352	676

Vitamins Per Liter (Standard Dilution*):

Vitamin A	2000	I.U.
Vitamin D	400	I.U.
Vitamin E	20	I.U.
Vitamin K$_1$	100	mcg
Vitamin C	55	mg
Thiamine (Vit. B$_1$)	0.40	mg
Riboflavin (Vit. B$_2$)	0.60	mg
Vitamin B$_6$	0.40	mg
Vitamin B$_{12}$	3.0	mcg
Niacin	9.0	mg
Folic Acid	100	mcg
Pantothenic Acid	5.0	mg
Biotin	30	mcg
Choline	53	mg
Inositol	32	mg

*Standard dilution is equal amounts Isomil SF Concentrated Liquid and water. (FAN 341-01)

Composition: Ready To Feed
Ingredients: (Pareve, Ⓤ) 87.3% water, 6.7% corn syrup solids, 2.3% soy protein isolate, 2.0% soy oil, 1.4% coconut oil, minerals (calcium phosphate dibasic, potassium citrate, calcium carbonate, potassium chloride, calcium phosphate monobasic, magnesium chloride, ferrous sulfate, sodium chloride, zinc sulfate, cupric sulfate, manganese sulfate, potassium iodide), mono- and diglycerides, soy lecithin, vitamins (ascorbic acid, choline chloride, alpha-tocopheryl acetate, niacinamide, calcium pantothenate, vitamin A palmitate, thiamine chloride hydrochloride, riboflavin, pyridoxine hydrochloride, phylloquinone, folic acid, biotin, vitamin D$_3$, cyanocobalamin), carrageenan, L-methionine and taurine.

Nutrients (wt/liter):

Protein	20.0	g
Fat	36.0	g
Carbohydrate	68.0	g
Minerals (Ash)	3.8	g
Calcium	700	mg
Phosphorus	500	mg
Magnesium	50	mg
Iron	12	mg
Iodine	100	mcg
Zinc	5.0	mg
Copper	0.50	mg
Manganese	200	mcg
Sodium	320	mg
Potassium	770	mg
Chloride	590	mg
Water	902	g
Crude Fiber	0	g
Calories per fl oz	20	
Calories per liter	676	

Vitamins Per Liter:

Vitamin A	2000	I.U.
Vitamin D	400	I.U.
Vitamin E	20	I.U.

Continued on next page

If desired, additional information on any Ross Product will be provided upon request to Ross Laboratories.

Ross—Cont.

Vitamin K_1	100	mcg
Vitamin C	55	mg
Thiamine (Vit. B_1)	0.40	mg
Riboflavin (Vit. B_2)	0.60	mg
Vitamin B_6	0.40	mg
Vitamin B_{12}	3.0	mcg
Niacin	9.0	mg
Folic Acid	100	mcg
Pantothenic Acid	5.0	mg
Biotin	30	mcg
Choline	53	mg
Inositol	32	mg

The addition of iron to this formula conforms to the recommendation of the Committee on Nutrition of the American Academy of Pediatrics.
(FAN 341-01)

MURINE® EAR WAX REMOVAL SYSTEM/MURINE® EAR DROPS

Description: Carbamide peroxide 6.5% in anhydrous glycerin and a 1.0 fl oz soft rubber bulb ear washer. The MURINE EAR WAX REMOVAL SYSTEM is the only self-treatment method on the market for ear wax removal. Application of carbamide peroxide drops followed by warm water irrigation is an effective, medically recommended way to help loosen hardened ear wax.

Actions: The carbamide peroxide formula in MURINE EAR DROPS is an aid in the removal of hardened cerumen from the ear canal. Anhydrous glycerin penetrates and softens wax while the release of oxygen from carbamide peroxide provides a mechanical action resulting in the loosening of the softened wax accumulation. It is usually necessary to remove the loosened wax by gently flushing the ear with warm water using the soft rubber bulb ear washer provided.

Indications: The MURINE EAR WAX REMOVAL SYSTEM is indicated as an aid in the removal of hardened or tightly packed cerumen from the ear canal.

Caution: If redness, tenderness, pain, dizziness or ear drainage are present or develop, the medication should not be used or continued until a physician is seen. Do not use if ear drum is known to be perforated.

Dosage and Administration: For wax removal—Adults and children over 12 years: Tilt head sideways and place 5 to 10 drops into ear. Tip of bottle should not enter ear canal. Keep drops in ear for several minutes by keeping head tilted or placing cotton in ear. Wax remaining after treatment may be removed by gently flushing ear with warm water, using soft rubber bulb ear washer placed on edge of ear canal. Use twice daily, up to 4 days if needed, or as directed by a doctor. Children under 12 years: Consult a doctor.
Used regularly, the Murine Ear Wax Removal System helps keep the ear canal free from blockage due to accumulated ear wax.

How Supplied: The MURINE EAR WAX REMOVAL SYSTEM contains 0.5 fl oz drops and a 1.0 fl oz soft rubber bulb ear washer.
Also available in 0.5 fl oz drops only, MURINE EAR DROPS.
Shown in Product Identification Section, page 426
(FAN 2014-02)

MURINE® REGULAR FORMULA
Eye Drops

Description: Murine Regular Formula is a sterile isotonic buffered solution containing glycerin, potassium chloride, sodium chloride, sodium phosphate (monobasic and dibasic), and water. Edetate disodium 0.05% and benzalkonium chloride 0.01% are added as preservatives. (No vasoconstrictor.)

Indications: Murine is a non-staining, clear solution formulated to closely match the natural fluid of the eye for gentle, soothing relief from minor eye irritation. Use whenever desired to cleanse or refresh the eyes and to relieve minor irritation due to smog, sun glare, wind, dust, wearing contact lenses and eyestrain from reading, driving, TV and close work.

Warning: Murine Regular Formula should only be used for minor eye irritations. If irritation persists or increases, discontinue use and consult your physician.

Dosage and Administration: Tilt head back and squeeze 2 or 3 drops into each eye as needed. Do not touch bottle tip to any surface since this may contaminate solution. Remove contact lenses before using. Keep this and all medicines out of the reach of children. Replace cap after using.

How Supplied: In 0.5 fl oz and 1.5 fl oz plastic dropper bottle.
Shown in Product Identification Section, page 426
(FAN 2021-03)

MURINE® PLUS
Eye Drops

Description: Murine Plus is a sterile isotonic buffered solution containing tetrahydrozoline hydrochloride 0.05%, boric acid, sodium borate and water. Edetate disodium 0.1% and benzalkonium chloride 0.01% are added as preservatives. (Contains vasoconstrictor.)

Indications: Murine Plus is a sterile, isotonic decongestant ophthalmic solution, compatible with the natural fluids of the eye. Its primary ingredient is a sympathomimetic agent, tetrahydrozoline hydrochloride, which produces local vasoconstriction in the eye. Thus, the drug effectively narrows swollen blood vessels locally and provides symptomatic relief of edema and hyperemia of conjunctival tissues due to eye allergies, minor local irritations and catarrhal (or "nonspecific") conjunctivitis. The formula of the solution includes other ingredients designed to produce a refreshing, soothing effect in addition to decongestion. Desirable effects comprise attenuation of burning, irritant and itching sensations, redness, and excessive lacrimation (tearing). Eyes reddened by swimming, plant allergies (pollen), overindulgence, colds, smog, sun glare, wind, dust, wearing contact lenses, and eyestrain from reading, driving, TV and close work are quickly whitened by the vasoconstrictor action noted above. Its effect is prompt (apparent within minutes) and sustained. Although other vasoconstrictors may dilate the pupil (mydriasis) or result in rebound hyperemia, the use of tetrahydrozoline in MURINE PLUS is not known to cause either of these effects.

Warning: Murine Plus should only be used for minor eye irritations. Murine Plus should not be used by individuals with glaucoma and serious eye diseases. In some instances redness or inflammation may be due to serious eye conditions such as acute iritis, acute glaucoma, or corneal trauma.
MURINE PLUS Eye Drops have been shown by various studies to be both safe and efficacious for minor eye irritations. If irritation or redness persists or increases, discontinue use and consult physician.

Dosage and Administration: Tilt head back and squeeze 1 or 2 drops into each eye, up to 4 times daily, or as directed by physician. Do not touch bottle tip to any surface since this may contaminate the solution. Remove contact lenses before using. Keep this and all medicines out of the reach of children. Replace cap after using.

How Supplied: In 0.5 fl oz and 1.5 fl oz plastic dropper bottle.
Shown in Product Identification Section, page 426
(FAN 2021-03)

RCF®
Ross Carbohydrate Free
Soy Protein Formula Base

Usage: For use in the dietary management of persons unable to tolerate the type or amount of carbohydrate in milk or conventional infant formulas; many of these patients have intractable diarrhea and are not able to tolerate other formulas. This product has been formulated to contain no carbohydrate, which must be added before feeding.

Availability:
Concentrated Liquid only: 13-fl-oz cans; 12 per case; No. 108.

Preparation:
RCF is for use only under the direction of a physician. Physician's instructions must include the type and amount of carbohydrate and the amount of water to be added to RCF. Standard dilution is one part Formula Base to one part prescribed carbohydrate and water solution.

A full-strength formula, 20 Calories per fluid ounce, may be prepared with one of the following typical carbohydrates: [See table right].

Composition: Concentrated Liquid

Ingredients: (Pareve, Ⓤ) 87% water, 4.4% soy protein isolate, 4.2% soy oil, 2.8% coconut oil, minerals (calcium phosphates [mono- and tribasic], potassium citrate, potassium chloride, magnesium chloride, calcium carbonate, sodium chloride, zinc sulfate, cupric sulfate), carrageenan, mono- and diglycerides, soy lecithin, vitamins (ascorbic acid, choline chloride, alpha-tocopheryl acetate, niacinamide, calcium pantothenate, vitamin A palmitate, riboflavin, thiamine chloride hydrochloride, pyridoxine hydrochloride, phylloquinone, biotin, folic acid, vitamin D₃, cyanocobalamin), L-methionine and taurine.

Nutrients (wt/liter):	Concentrated	Standard Dilution†
Protein	40.0 g	20.0 g
Fat	72.0 g	36.0 g
Carbohydrate	0.1 g	*
Minerals (Ash)	7.5 g	3.8 g
Calcium	1400 mg	700 mg
Phosphorus	1000 mg	500 mg
Magnesium	100 mg	50 mg
Iron	3.0 mg	1.5 mg

(This product is deficient in iron; an additional 5.3 mg iron per liter should be supplied from other sources.)

Iodine	200 mcg	100 mcg
Zinc	10 mg	5.0 mg
Copper	1.0 mg	0.50 mg
Manganese	400 mcg	200 mcg
Sodium	640 mg	320 mg
Potassium	1540 mg	770 mg
Chloride	1180 mg	590 mg
Water	885 g	*
Crude Fiber	0 g	
Calories per fl oz	24	*
Calories per liter	810	*

Vitamins Per Liter (Standard Dilution†):

Vitamin A	2000	I.U.
Vitamin D	400	I.U.
Vitamin E	20	I.U.
Vitamin K₁	100	mcg
Vitamin C	55	mg
Thiamine (Vit. B₁)	0.40	mg
Riboflavin (Vit. B₂)	0.60	mg
Vitamin B₆	0.40	mg
Vitamin B₁₂	3.0	mcg
Niacin	9.0	mg
Folic Acid	100	mcg
Pantothenic Acid	5.0	mg
Biotin	30	mcg
Choline	53	mg
Inositol	32	mg

*Varies depending on quantity of carbohydrate and water used. If carbohydrate is not added to this product, a 1:1 dilution with water provides approximately 12 Cal/fl oz (40.5 Cal/100 ml).

†Standard dilution is one part Formula Base to one part prescribed carbohydrate and water solution.

(FAN 341-01)

Carbohydrate Source	Amount of Carbohydrate	Water	RCF Formula Base
Table Sugar (sucrose)	4 level tablespoonfuls*	12 fl oz	one 13-fl-oz can
Dextrose Powder (hydrous)	6 level tablespoonfuls*	12 fl oz	one 13-fl-oz can
Polycose® Glucose Polymers Powder	See Polycose label	12 fl oz	one 13-fl-oz can

* Approximately the 52 grams needed for 20 Cal/fl oz formula.

SELSUN BLUE®
Dandruff Shampoo
(selenium sulfide lotion, 1%)

Selsun Blue is a non-prescription antidandruff shampoo containing a 1% concentration of selenium sulfide in a freshly scented, pH balanced formula to leave hair clean and manageable. Available in formulations for dry, oily or normal hair types.

Clinical testing has shown it to be safe and more effective than other leading shampoos in helping control dandruff symptoms with regular use.

Directions: Shake well before using. Lather, rinse thoroughly and repeat. Use regularly, once or twice weekly, for effective dandruff control.

Caution: For external use only. Keep out of eyes—if this happens, rinse thoroughly with water. If used just before or after bleaching, tinting or permanent waving, rinse hair for at least five minutes in cool running water. If irritation occurs, discontinue use.

Warning: Keep out of the reach of children.

How Supplied: 4, 7 and 11 fl oz plastic bottles.
Shown in Product Identification Section, page 426

SIMILAC®
Infant Formula

Usage: When an infant formula is needed if the decision is made to discontinue breast-feeding before age 1 year, if a supplement to breast-feeding is needed, or as a routine feeding if breast-feeding is not adopted.

Availability:
Powder: 1-lb cans, measuring scoop enclosed; 6 per case; No. 03139.
1.06-oz packets; 12 four-packet cartons per case; No. 00231.
Concentrated Liquid: 13-fl-oz cans; 24 per case; No. 00264.
Ready To Feed: (Prediluted, 20 Cal/fl oz)
32-fl-oz cans; 6 per case; No. 00232.
8-fl-oz cans; 4 six-packs per case; No. 00177.
4-fl-oz nursing bottles; 6 per carry-home carton, 8 cartons per case; No. 00480.
8-fl-oz nursing bottles; 6 per carry-home carton, 4 cartons per case; No. 00880.
For hospital use, Similac in disposable nursing bottles is available in the Ross Hospital Formula System.

Preparation:
Powder: Standard dilution (20 Cal/fl oz) is one level, unpacked scoop Powder

(8.74 g) for each 2 fl oz water, or, one packet (30.1 g) for each 7 fl oz water.
Concentrated Liquid: Standard dilution (20 Cal/fl oz) is one part Concentrated Liquid to one part water.

Composition: Powder
Ingredients: Ⓤ-D Nonfat milk, lactose, corn oil, coconut oil, vitamins (ascorbic acid, alpha-tocopheryl acetate, niacinamide, calcium pantothenate, vitamin A palmitate, thiamine chloride hydrochloride, pyridoxine hydrochloride, riboflavin, folic acid, phylloquinone, vitamin D₃, cyanocobalamin), minerals (zinc sulfate, ferrous sulfate, cupric sulfate, manganese sulfate) and taurine.

Nutrients:	Powder (wt/100 g)	Standard Dilution* (wt/liter)
Protein	11.4 g	15.0 g
Fat	27.6 g	36.3 g
Carbohydrate	54.9 g	72.3 g
Minerals (Ash)	3.1 g	4.1 g
Calcium	390 mg	510 mg
Phosphorus	300 mg	390 mg
Magnesium	31 mg	41 mg
Iron	1.1 mg	1.5 mg

(This product, like milk, is deficient in iron; an additional 5.3 mg iron per liter should be supplied from other sources.)

Iodine	76 mcg	100 mcg
Zinc	3.8 mg	5.0 mg
Copper	0.46 mg	0.60 mg
Manganese	26 mcg	34 mcg
Sodium	170 mg	230 mg
Potassium	610 mg	800 mg
Chloride	380 mg	500 mg
Water	2.0 g	902 g
Crude Fiber	0 g	
Calories	513	676
Calories per fl oz		20

Vitamins Per Liter (Standard Dilution*):

Vitamin A	2000	I.U.
Vitamin D	400	I.U.
Vitamin E	17	I.U.
Vitamin K₁	55	mcg
Vitamin C	55	mg
Thiamine (Vit. B₁)	0.65	mg
Riboflavin (Vit. B₂)	1.0	mg
Vitamin B₆	0.40	mg
Vitamin B₁₂	1.5	mcg
Niacin	7.0	mg

Continued on next page

If desired, additional information on any Ross Product will be provided upon request to Ross Laboratories.

Ross—Cont.

Folic Acid	100	mcg
Pantothenic Acid	3.0	mg

*Standard dilution is one level, unpacked scoop of Powder for each 2 fluid ounces of warm water, or 131.7 g of Powder diluted to 1 liter.
(FAN 341-02)

Composition: Concentrated Liquid
Ingredients: Ⓓ-D Water, nonfat milk, lactose, soy oil, coconut oil, mono- and diglycerides, soy lecithin, vitamins (ascorbic acid, alpha-tocopheryl acetate, niacinamide, calcium pantothenate, vitamin A palmitate, thiamine chloride hydrochloride, pyridoxine hydrochloride, riboflavin, folic acid, phylloquinone, vitamin D_3, cyanocobalamin), carrageenan, minerals (zinc sulfate, ferrous sulfate, cupric sulfate, manganese sulfate) and taurine.

Nutrients (wt/liter):	Concentrated	Standard Dilution*
Protein	30.0 g	15.0 g
Fat	72.6 g	36.3 g
Carbohydrate	144.6 g	72.3 g
Minerals (Ash)	6.6 g	3.3 g
Calcium	1.0 g	510 mg
Phosphorus	0.78 g	390 mg
Magnesium	82 mg	41 mg
Iron	3.0 mg	1.5 mg

(This product, like milk, is deficient in iron; an additional 5.3 mg iron per liter should be supplied from other sources.)

Iodine	200	mcg	100	mcg
Zinc	10	mg	5.0	mg
Copper	1.2	mg	0.60	mg
Manganese	68	mcg	34	mcg
Sodium	460	mg	230	mg
Potassium	1600	mg	800	mg
Chloride	1000	mg	500	mg
Water	806	g	902	g
Crude Fiber	0	g		
Calories per fl oz	40		20	
Calories per liter	1352		676	

Vitamins Per Liter (Standard Dilution*):

Vitamin A	2000	I.U.
Vitamin D	400	I.U.
Vitamin E	20	I.U.
Vitamin K_1	55	mcg
Vitamin C	55	mg
Thiamine (Vit. B_1)	0.65	mg
Riboflavin (Vit. B_2)	1.0	mg
Vitamin B_6	0.40	mg
Vitamin B_{12}	1.5	mcg
Niacin	7.0	mg
Folic Acid	100	mcg
Pantothenic Acid	3.0	mg

*Standard dilution is equal parts Similac Concentrated Liquid and water.
(FAN 341-02)

Composition: Ready To Feed
Ingredients: Ⓓ-D Water, nonfat milk, lactose, soy oil, coconut oil, mono- and diglycerides, soy lecithin, vitamins (ascorbic acid, alpha-tocopheryl acetate, niacinamide, calcium pantothenate, vitamin A palmitate, thiamine chloride hydrochloride, pyridoxine hydrochloride, riboflavin, folic acid, phylloquinone, vitamin D_3, cyanocobalamin), carrageenan, minerals (zinc sulfate, ferrous sulfate, cupric sulfate, manganese sulfate) and taurine.

Nutrients (wt/liter):

Protein	15.0	g
Fat	36.3	g
Carbohydrate	72.3	g
Minerals (Ash)	3.3	g
Calcium	510	mg
Phosphorus	390	mg
Magnesium	41	mg
Iron	1.5	mg

(This product, like milk, is deficient in iron; an additional 5.3 mg iron per liter should be supplied from other sources.)

Iodine	100	mcg
Zinc	5.0	mg
Copper	0.60	mg
Manganese	34	mcg
Sodium	230	mg
Potassium	800	mg
Chloride	500	mg
Water	902	g
Crude Fiber	0	g
Calories per fl oz	20	
Calories per liter	676	

Vitamins Per Liter:

Vitamin A	2000	I.U.
Vitamin D	400	I.U.
Vitamin E	20	I.U.
Vitamin K_1	55	mcg
Vitamin C	55	mg
Thiamine (Vit. B_1)	0.65	mg
Riboflavin (Vit. B_2)	1.0	mg
Vitamin B_6	0.40	mg
Vitamin B_{12}	1.5	mcg
Niacin	7.0	mg
Folic Acid	100	mcg
Pantothenic Acid	3.0	mg

(FAN 341-01)

SIMILAC® PM 60/40
Infant Formula

Usage: For infants in the lower range of homeostatic capacity; for those who are problem feeders; those who are predisposed to hypocalcemia; and those whose renal, digestive or cardiovascular functions would benefit from lowered mineral levels. Similac PM 60/40 should be used only under the supervision of a physician.

Availability: Powder only: 1-lb cans, measuring scoop enclosed; 6 per case; No. 00850. For hospital use, Ready To Feed Similac PM 60/40 in disposable nursing bottles is available in the Ross Hospital Formula System. (Ready To Feed has composition and nutrient values similar to Powder. For specific information see bottle tray.)

Preparation: Standard dilution (20 Cal/fl oz) is one level, unpacked scoop (8.56 g) Powder for each 2 fl oz of water. Higher caloric feedings are prepared by adding 8.56 g (1 level, unpacked scoopful) of Similac PM 60/40 to the following amounts of water:

For:	Water:	Yields:
24 Cal/fl oz	48 ml	55 ml (1.8 fl oz)
27 Cal/fl oz	42 ml	49 ml (1.6 fl oz)
30 Cal/fl oz	37 ml	44 ml (1.5 fl oz)

Composition: Powder

Ingredients: Ⓓ-D Lactose, corn oil, coconut oil, whey protein concentrate, sodium caseinate, minerals (calcium phosphate tribasic, potassium citrate, potassium chloride, magnesium chloride, sodium chloride, calcium carbonate, zinc sulfate, ferrous sulfate, cupric sulfate, manganese sulfate), vitamins (m-inositol, ascorbic acid, choline chloride, alpha-tocopheryl acetate, niacinamide, calcium pantothenate, vitamin A palmitate, thiamine chloride hydrochloride, riboflavin, pyridoxine hydrochloride, folic acid, phylloquinone, vitamin D_3, biotin, cyanocobalamin) and taurine.

Nutrients:	Powder (wt/100 g)	Standard Dilution* (wt/liter)
Protein (Lactalbumin and Lactoglobulin 60%, Casein 40%)	11.4 g	15.0 g
Fat	28.7 g	37.8 g
Carbohydrate	52.4 g	69.0 g
Minerals (Ash)	1.7 g	2.2 g
Calcium	304 mg	400 mg
Phosphorus	152 mg	200 mg
Magnesium	32 mg	42 mg
Iron	1.1 mg	1.5 mg

(This product, like milk, is deficient in iron; an additional 5.3 mg iron per liter should be supplied from other sources.)

Iodine	32	mcg	42	mcg
Zinc	3.8	mg	5.0	mg
Copper	0.46	mg	0.60	mg
Manganese	26	mcg	34	mcg
Sodium	121	mg	160	mg
Potassium	440	mg	580	mg
Chloride	304	mg	400	mg
Water	2.5	g	905	g
Crude Fiber	0	g		
Calories	513		676	
Calories per fl oz			20	

Vitamins Per Liter (Standard Dilution*):

Vitamin A	2000	I.U.
Vitamin D	400	I.U.
Vitamin E	17	I.U.
Vitamin K_1	55	mcg
Vitamin C	55	mg
Thiamine (Vit. B_1)	0.65	mg
Riboflavin (Vit. B_2)	1.0	mg
Vitamin B_6	0.40	mg
Vitamin B_{12}	1.5	mcg
Niacin	7.3	mg
Folic Acid	100	mcg
Pantothenic Acid	3.0	mg
Biotin	30	mcg
Choline	82	mg
Inositol	165	mg

*Standard dilution is one level, unpacked scoop of Powder for each 2 fl oz water, or 131.7 g of Powder diluted to 1 liter.

Precautions: In conditions where the infant is losing abnormal quantities of one or more electrolytes, it may be necessary to supply electrolytes from sources other than the formula. With premature infants weighing less than 1500 g at birth, it may be necessary to supply an additional source of sodium, calcium and phosphorus during the period of very rapid growth.
(FAN 341-01)

SIMILAC® WITH IRON
Infant Formula

Usage: When an iron-containing infant formula is needed if the decision is made to discontinue breast-feeding before age 1 year, if a supplement to breast-feeding is needed, or as a routine feeding if breast-feeding is not adopted.

Availability:
Powder: 1-lb cans, measuring scoop enclosed; 6 per case; No. 03360. 1.06-oz packets; 12 four-packet cartons per case; No. 00235.
Concentrated Liquid: 13-fl-oz cans; 24 cans per case; No. 00414.
Ready To Feed: (Prediluted, 20 Cal/fl oz) 32-fl-oz cans; 6 per case; No. 00241. 8-fl-oz cans; 4 six-packs per case; No. 00179.
4-fl-oz nursing bottles; 6 per carry-home carton, 8 cartons per case; No. 06201.
8-fl-oz nursing bottles; 6 per carry-home carton, 4 cartons per case; No. 06202.
For hospital use, Similac With Iron in disposable nursing bottles is available in the Ross Hospital Formula System.

Preparation:
Powder: Standard dilution (20 Cal/fl oz) is one level, unpacked scoop Powder (8.74 g) for each 2 fl oz of water; or, one packet (30.1 g) for each 7 fl oz water.
Concentrated Liquid: Standard dilution (20 Cal/fl oz) is one part Concentrated Liquid to one part water.

Composition: Powder
Ingredients: Ⓤ-D Nonfat milk, lactose, corn oil, coconut oil, vitamins (ascorbic acid, alpha-tocopheryl acetate, niacinamide, calcium pantothenate, vitamin A palmitate, thiamine chloride hydrochloride, pyridoxine hydrochloride, riboflavin, folic acid, phylloquinone, vitamin D_3, cyanocobalamin), minerals (ferrous sulfate, zinc sulfate, cupric sulfate, manganese sulfate) and taurine.

Nutrients:	Powder (wt/100 g)		Standard Dilution* (wt/liter)	
Protein	11.4	g	15.0	g
Fat	27.6	g	36.3	g
Carbohydrate	54.9	g	72.3	g
Minerals (Ash)	3.1	g	4.1	g
Calcium	390	mg	510	mg
Phosphorus	300	mg	390	mg
Magnesium	31	mg	41	mg
Iron	9.1	mg	12	mg
Iodine	76	mcg	100	mcg
Zinc	3.8	mg	5.0	mg
Copper	0.46	mg	0.60	mg
Manganese	26	mcg	34	mcg
Sodium	170	mg	230	mg

Potassium	610	mg	800	mg
Chloride	380	mg	500	mg
Water	2.0	g	902	g
Crude Fiber	0	g		
Calories	513		676	
Calories per fl oz			20	

Vitamins Per Liter (Standard Dilution*):

Vitamin A	2000	I.U.
Vitamin D	400	I.U.
Vitamin E	17	I.U.
Vitamin K_1	55	mcg
Vitamin C	55	mg
Thiamine (Vit. B_1)	0.65	mg
Riboflavin (Vit. B_2)	1.0	mg
Vitamin B_6	0.40	mg
Vitamin B_{12}	1.5	mcg
Niacin	7.0	mg
Folic Acid	100	mcg
Pantothenic Acid	3.0	mg

*Standard dilution is one level, unpacked scoop of Powder for each 2 fluid ounces of warm water, or 131.7 g of Powder diluted to 1 liter.
(FAN 341-02)

Composition: Concentrated Liquid
Ingredients: Ⓤ-D Water, nonfat milk, lactose, soy oil, coconut oil, mono- and diglycerides, soy lecithin, vitamins (ascorbic acid, alpha-tocopheryl acetate, niacinamide, calcium pantothenate, vitamin A palmitate, thiamine chloride hydrochloride, pyridoxine hydrochloride, riboflavin, folic acid, phylloquinone, vitamin D_3, cyanocobalamin), carrageenan, minerals (ferrous sulfate, zinc sulfate, cupric sulfate, manganese sulfate) and taurine.

Nutrients (wt/liter):	Concentrated		Standard Dilution*	
Protein	30.0	g	15.0	g
Fat	72.6	g	36.3	g
Carbohydrate	144.6	g	72.3	g
Minerals (Ash)	6.6	g	3.3	g
Calcium	1.0	g	510	mg
Phosphorus	0.78	g	390	mg
Magnesium	82	mg	41	mg
Iron	24	mg	12	mg
Iodine	200	mcg	100	mcg
Zinc	10	mg	5.0	mg
Copper	1.2	mg	0.60	mg
Manganese	68	mcg	34	mcg
Sodium	460	mg	230	mg
Potassium	1600	mg	800	mg
Chloride	1000	mg	500	mg
Water	806	g	902	g
Crude Fiber	0	g		
Calories per fl oz	40		20	
Calories per liter	1352		676	

Vitamins Per Liter (Standard Dilution*):

Vitamin A	2000	I.U.
Vitamin D	400	I.U.
Vitamin E	20	I.U.
Vitamin K_1	55	mcg
Vitamin C	55	mg
Thiamine (Vit. B_1)	0.65	mg
Riboflavin (Vit. B_2)	1.0	mg
Vitamin B_6	0.40	mg
Vitamin B_{12}	1.5	mcg
Niacin	7.0	mg
Folic Acid	100	mcg
Pantothenic Acid	3.0	mg

*Standard dilution is equal amounts Similac With Iron Concentrated Liquid and water.
(FAN 341-02)

Composition: Ready To Feed
Ingredients: Ⓤ-D Water, nonfat milk, lactose, soy oil, coconut oil, mono- and diglycerides, soy lecithin, vitamins (ascorbic acid, alpha-tocopheryl acetate, niacinamide, calcium pantothenate, vitamin A palmitate, thiamine chloride hydrochloride, pyridoxine hydrochloride, riboflavin, folic acid, phylloquinone, vitamin D_3, cyanocobalamin), carrageenan, minerals (ferrous sulfate, zinc sulfate, cupric sulfate, manganese sulfate) and taurine.

Nutrients (wt/liter):

Protein	15.0	g
Fat	36.3	g
Carbohydrate	72.3	g
Minerals (Ash)	3.3	g
Calcium	510	mg
Phosphorus	390	mg
Magnesium	41	mg
Iron	12	mg
Iodine	100	mcg
Zinc	5.0	mg
Copper	0.60	mg
Manganese	34	mcg
Sodium	230	mg
Potassium	800	mg
Chloride	500	mg
Water	902	g
Crude Fiber	0	g
Calories per fl oz	20	
Calories per liter	676	

Vitamins Per Liter:

Vitamin A	2000	I.U.
Vitamin D	400	I.U.
Vitamin E	20	I.U.
Vitamin K_1	55	mcg
Vitamin C	55	mg
Thiamine (Vit. B_1)	0.65	mg
Riboflavin (Vit. B_2)	1.0	mg
Vitamin B_6	0.40	mg
Vitamin B_{12}	1.5	mcg
Niacin	7.0	mg
Folic Acid	100	mcg
Pantothenic Acid	3.0	mg

The addition of iron to this formula conforms to the recommendation of the Committee on Nutrition of the American Academy of Pediatrics.
(FAN 341-01)

Continued on next page

If desired, additional information on any Ross Product will be provided upon request to Ross Laboratories.

Ross—Cont.

SIMILAC® WITH WHEY + IRON
Infant Formula

Usage: When an iron-fortified, whey-predominant-protein formula is desired for feeding term infants if the decision is made to discontinue breast-feeding before age 1 year, if a supplement to breast-feeding is needed, or as a routine feeding if breast-feeding is not adopted.

Availability:
Powder: 1-lb cans, measuring scoop enclosed; 6 per case; No. 00372.
Concentrated Liquid: 13-fl-oz cans; 12 per case; No. 00352.
Ready To Feed: (Prediluted, 20 Cal/fl oz) 32-fl-oz cans; 6 per case; No. 00312.
For hospital use, Similac With Whey + Iron in disposable nursing bottles is available in the Ross Hospital Formula System.

Preparation:
Powder: Standard dilution (20 Cal/fl oz) is one level, unpacked scoop Powder (8.74 g) for each 2 fl oz of water.
Concentrated Liquid: Standard dilution (20 Cal/fl oz) is one part Concentrated Liquid to one part water.

Composition: Powder
Ingredients: Ⓤ-D Nonfat milk, lactose, corn oil, coconut oil, whey protein concentrate, minerals (calcium phosphate tribasic, sodium chloride, magnesium chloride, potassium citrate, ferrous sulfate, zinc sulfate, cupric sulfate, manganese sulfate), vitamins (ascorbic acid, alpha-tocopheryl acetate, niacinamide, calcium pantothenate, vitamin A palmitate, thiamine chloride hydrochloride, riboflavin, pyridoxine hydrochloride, folic acid, phylloquinone, vitamin D_3, biotin, cyanocobalamin) and taurine.

Nutrients:	Powder (wt/100 g)		Standard Dilution (wt/liter)	
Protein	11.4	g	15.0	g
(Lactoglobulin and Lactalbumin 60%, Casein 40%)				
Fat	27.6	g	36.3	g
Carbohydrate	54.9	g	72.3	g
Minerals (Ash)	2.6	g	3.4	g
Calcium	300	mg	400	mg
Phosphorus	230	mg	300	mg
Magnesium	38	mg	50	mg
Iron	9.1	mg	12	mg
Iodine	76	mcg	100	mcg
Zinc	3.8	mg	5.0	mg
Copper	0.46	mg	0.60	mg
Manganese	26	mcg	34	mcg
Sodium	175	mg	230	mg
Potassium	570	mg	750	mg
Chloride	325	mg	430	mg
Water	2.5	g	902	g
Crude fiber	0	g		
Calories	513		676	
Calories per fl oz			20	

Vitamins Per Liter (Standard Dilution*):

Vitamin A	2000	I.U.
Vitamin D	400	I.U.
Vitamin E	17	I.U.
Vitamin K_1	55	mcg
Vitamin C	55	mg
Thiamine (Vit. B_1)	0.65	mg
Riboflavin (Vit. B_2)	1.0	mg
Vitamin B_6	0.40	mg
Vitamin B_{12}	1.5	mcg
Niacin	7.0	mg
Folic Acid	100	mcg
Pantothenic Acid	3.0	mg
Biotin	11	mcg

*Standard dilution is one level, unpacked scoop of Powder for each 2 fluid ounces of warm water, or 131.7 g of Powder diluted to 1 liter. (FAN 341-02)

Composition: Concentrated Liquid
Ingredients: Ⓤ-D Water, nonfat milk, lactose, soy oil, coconut oil, whey protein concentrate, minerals (calcium phosphate tribasic, sodium chloride, potassium citrate, ferrous sulfate, magnesium chloride, zinc sulfate, cupric sulfate, manganese sulfate), soy lecithin, mono- and diglycerides, vitamins (ascorbic acid, alpha-tocopheryl acetate, niacinamide, calcium pantothenate, vitamin A palmitate, thiamine chloride hydrochloride, riboflavin, pyridoxine hydrochloride, folic acid, phylloquinone, vitamin D_3, biotin, cyanocobalamin), carrageenan and taurine.

Nutrients (wt/liter):	Concentrated		Standard Dilution*	
Protein	30.0	g	15.0	g
(Lactoglobulin and Lactalbumin 60%, Casein 40%)				
Fat	72.6	g	36.3	g
Carbohydrate	144.6	g	72.3	g
Minerals (Ash)	6.8	g	3.4	g
Calcium	800	mg	400	mg
Phosphorus	600	mg	300	mg
Magnesium	100	mg	50	mg
Iron	24	mg	12	mg
Iodine	200	mcg	100	mcg
Zinc	10	mg	5.0	mg
Copper	1.2	mg	0.60	mg
Manganese	68	mcg	34	mcg
Sodium	460	mg	230	mg
Potassium	1500	mg	750	mg
Chloride	860	mg	430	mg
Water	806	g	902	g
Crude fiber	0	g		
Calories per fl oz	40		20	
Calories per liter	1352		676	

Vitamins Per Liter (Standard Dilution*):

Vitamin A	2000	I.U.
Vitamin D	400	I.U.
Vitamin E	20	I.U.
Vitamin K_1	55	mcg
Vitamin C	55	mg
Thiamine (Vit. B_1)	0.65	mg
Riboflavin (Vit. B_2)	1.0	mg
Vitamin B_6	0.40	mg
Vitamin B_{12}	1.5	mcg
Niacin	7.0	mg
Folic Acid	100	mcg
Pantothenic Acid	3.0	mg
Biotin	11	mcg

*Standard dilution is equal amounts Similac With Whey + Iron Concentrated Liquid and water. (FAN 341-01)

Composition: Ready To Feed
Ingredients: Ⓤ-D Water, nonfat milk, lactose, soy oil, coconut oil, whey protein concentrate, minerals (calcium phosphate tribasic, sodium chloride, potassium citrate, ferrous sulfate, magnesium chloride, zinc sulfate, cupric sulfate, manganese sulfate), soy lecithin, mono- and diglycerides, vitamins (ascorbic acid, alpha-tocopheryl acetate, niacinamide, calcium pantothenate, vitamin A palmitate, thiamine chloride hydrochloride, riboflavin, pyridoxine hydrochloride, folic acid, phylloquinone, vitamin D_3, biotin, cyanocobalamin), carrageenan and taurine.

Nutrients (wt/liter):

Protein	15.0	g
(Lactoglobulin and Lactalbumin 60%, Casein 40%)		
Fat	36.3	g
Carbohydrate	72.3	g
Minerals (Ash)	3.4	g
Calcium	400	mg
Phosphorus	300	mg
Magnesium	50	mg
Iron	12	mg
Iodine	100	mcg
Zinc	5.0	mg
Copper	0.60	mg
Manganese	34	mcg
Sodium	230	mg
Potassium	750	mg
Chloride	430	mg
Water	902	g
Crude Fiber	0	g
Calories per fl oz	20	
Calories per liter	676	

Vitamins Per Liter:

Vitamin A	2000	I.U.
Vitamin D	400	I.U.
Vitamin E	20	I.U.
Vitamin K_1	55	mcg
Vitamin C	55	mg
Thiamine (Vit. B_1)	0.65	mg
Riboflavin (Vit. B_2)	1.0	mg
Vitamin B_6	0.40	mg
Vitamin B_{12}	1.5	mcg
Niacin	7.0	mg
Folic Acid	100	mcg
Pantothenic Acid	3.0	mg
Biotin	11	mcg

The addition of iron to this formula conforms to the recommendation of the Committee on Nutrition of the American Academy of Pediatrics. (FAN 341-01)

TRONOLANE®
Cream:
(pramoxine hydrochloride 1%)
Suppositories:
(pramoxine 1% as pramoxine and pramoxine HCl)

Description: Tronolane contains a topical anesthetic agent (pramoxine HCl), chemically unrelated to the benzoate esters of the "caine" type, which is chemically designated as a 4-n-butoxyphenyl gammamorpholinopropylether hydrochloride. The cream contains the following inactive ingredients: Beeswax, cetyl alcohol, cetyl esters wax, glycerin, methylparaben, propylparaben, sodium lauryl sulfate and water. The suppository contains the following inactive ingredient: Hydrogenated cocoa glycerides.

Indications: Tronolane is a topical anesthetic indicated for the temporary relief of the pain, burning, itching and discomfort that accompanies hemorrhoids. It has a soothing, lubricant action on mucous membranes.
Tronolane contains a rapidly acting topical anesthetic producing analgesia that lasts up to 5 hours. Because the drug is chemically unrelated to other anesthetics, cross-sensitization is unlikely. Patients who are already sensitized to the "caine" anesthetics can generally use Tronolane.
The emollient/emulsion base of Tronolane cream provides soothing lubrication making bowel movements more comfortable. Tronolane cream is in a nondrying base that is nongreasy and nonstaining to undergarments.

Warnings: If bleeding is present, consult physician. Certain persons can develop allergic reactions to ingredients in this product. During treatment, if condition worsens or persists 7 days, consult physician. For children under 12 years, use only as directed by physician. As with any drug, if you are pregnant or nursing a baby, we recommend that you seek the advice of a health professional before using this product.

Dosage and Administration: CREAM: Apply up to five times daily, especially morning, night, and after bowel movements, or as directed by physician.
External—Apply liberally to affected area. *Intrarectal*—Remove cap from tube and attach clean applicator. Remove protective cover from clean applicator. Squeeze tube to fill applicator and lubricate tip with cream. Gently insert applicator into rectum and squeeze tube again. Thoroughly cleanse applicator after use.

Dosage and Administration: SUPPOSITORIES: Use up to five times daily, especially morning, night, and after bowel movements, or as directed by physician. Detach one suppository from pack. Tear notch at pointed end and remove wrapper before insertion. Insert suppository into the rectum, pointed end first.

How Supplied: Tronolane is available in 1-oz, 2-oz cream tubes and 10 and 20 count suppository boxes.
Shown in Product Identification Section, page 426

If desired, additional information on any Ross Product will be provided upon request to Ross Laboratories.

Rowell Laboratories, Inc.
210 MAIN STREET W.
BAUDETTE, MN 56623

BALNEOL®
Perianal cleansing lotion

Composition: Contains water, mineral oil, propylene glycol, glyceryl stearate/PEG-100 stearate, PEG-40 stearate, laureth-4, PEG-4 dilaurate, lanolin oil, sodium acetate, carbomer-934, triethanolamine, methylparaben, dioctyl sodium sulfosuccinate, fragrance, acetic acid.

Action and Uses: BALNEOL is a soothing, emollient cleanser for hygienic cleansing of irritated perianal and external vaginal areas. It helps relieve itching and other discomforts, helps stop irritation due to toilet tissue. BALNEOL gently yet thoroughly cleanses and provides a soothing, protecting film.

Administration and Dosage: For cleansing without discomfort after each bowel movement, a small amount of BALNEOL is spread on tissue or cotton and used to wipe the perianal area. Also used between bowel movements and at bedtime for additional comfort. For cleansing and soothing the external vaginal area: to be used on clean tissue or cotton as often as necessary.

Caution: In all cases of rectal bleeding, consult physician promptly. If irritation persists or increases, discontinue use and consult physician.

How Supplied: 4 oz plastic bottle.

HYDROCIL® INSTANT

Description: A concentrated hydrophilic mucilloid containing 95% psyllium. Hydrocil Instant mixes instantly, is sugar-free, low in potassium and contains less than 10 mg. of sodium per dose.

Indications: Hydrocil Instant is a natural bulk forming fiber useful in the treatment of constipation and other conditions as directed by a physician.

Directions: The usual adult dose is one packet or scoopful poured into an 8 oz. glass. Add water, fruit juices or other liquid and stir. It mixes instantly. Drink immediately. Take in the morning and night or as directed by a physician. Follow each dose with another glass of liquid.

How Supplied: In unit-dose packets of 3.7 grams that are available in boxes of 30's or 500's. Also in 250 gram jars with a measuring scoop. Each packet or scoopful, 3.7 grams, contains one usual adult dose of psyllium hydrophilic mucilloid, 3.5 grams.

Rydelle Laboratories, Inc.
Subsidiary of S. C. Johnson & Son, Inc.
1525 HOWE STREET
RACINE, WI 53403

FIBERALL™ Natural Flavor

Description: Fiberall is a bulk forming nonirritant laxative which contains no sugar. The active ingredient is refined hydrophilic mucilloid, a recognized dietary fiber, extracted from the seed husk of blond psyllium seed (Plantago ovata). The smooth gelatinous bulk formed by Fiberall encourages peristaltic activity and a more normal elimination of the bowel contents.
The recommended dose of one slightly rounded teaspoonful (5g) contains 3.4g of psyllium hydrophilic mucilloid, wheat bran, less than 10mg of sodium, less than 60mg of potassium, and provides less than 6 calories.

Indications: Fiberall is indicated for the management of chronic constipation, temporary constipation caused by illness or pregnancy, in irritable bowel syndrome, and for constipation related to duodenal ulcer or diverticulosis. Fiberall is also indicated for stool softening in patients with hemorrhoids after anorectal surgery.

Actions: The homogenous, high fiber formula of Fiberall is readily dispersed in liquids and acts without irritants or stimulants in the gastrointestinal tract.

Dosage and Administration: The recommended daily dosage for adults is one slightly rounded teaspoonful (5g) stirred into an 8 oz. glass of cool water or other liquid and taken orally one to three times daily according to the individual response. An additional glass of liquid is recommended and generally provides optimal response. Maximum benefits are usually obtained after two or three days of regular use of Fiberall.

Contraindications: fecal impaction or intestinal obstruction.

How Supplied: Powder, in 5, 10 and 15 oz. containers.
Shown in Product Identification Section, page 426

FIBERALL™ Orange Flavor

Description: Fiberall is a bulk forming nonirritant laxative which contains no sugar. The active ingredient is refined hydrophilic mucilloid, a recognized dietary fiber, extracted from the seed husk of blond psyllium seed (Plantago ovata). The smooth gelatinous bulk formed by Fiberall encourages peristaltic activity

Continued on next page

Rydelle—Cont.

and a more normal elimination of the bowel contents.

The recommended dose of one rounded teaspoonful (5.9g) contains 3.4g of psyllium hydrophilic mucilloid, wheat bran, natural and artificial flavor, less than 40mg of saccharin, citric acid, yellow #6 Lake and beta-carotene (coloring agents) less than 10mg of sodium, less than 60mg potassium, and provides less than 10 calories.

Indications: Fiberall is indicated for the management of chronic constipation, temporary constipation caused by illness or pregnancy, in irritable bowel syndrome, and for constipation related to duodenal ulcer or diverticulosis. Fiberall is also indicated for stool softening in patients with hemorrhoids after anorectal surgery.

Actions: The homogenous, high fiber formula of Fiberall is readily dispersed in liquids and acts without irritants or stimulants in the gastrointestinal tract.

Dosage and Administration: The recommended daily dosage for adults is one slightly rounded teaspoonful (5.9g) stirred into an 8 oz. glass of cool water or other liquid and taken orally one to three times daily according to the individual response. An additional glass of liquid is recommended and generally provides optimal response. Maximum benefits are usually obtained after two or three days of regular use of Fiberall.

Contraindications: fecal impaction or intestinal obstruction.

How Supplied: Powder, in 5, 10 and 15 oz. containers.

Shown in Product Identification Section, page 426

Scherer Laboratories, Inc.
14335 GILLIS ROAD
DALLAS, TEXAS 75244

HuMIST
Humidifying Saline Nasal Mist

Composition: Sodium chloride 0.65% with 0.35% chlorabutanol (as a preservative) in a soothing, buffered, isotonic solution that is physiologically compatable with nasal membranes.

Actions and Uses: HuMIST, saline nasal mist, provides immediate safe relief from the discomfort of dry nasal mucosa, with no danger from continuous use. HuMIST is an ideal moisturizer for adjunctive use with systemic nasal decongestants, and whenever nasal dryness is caused by lack of humidity, dusty or air conditioned atmospheres, drug therapy, or overuse of decongestant sprays and inhalers. HuMIST also alleviates "crusting" following nosebleeds, surgery, and/or cauterization.

Dosage and Administration: Spray twice into each nostril. May also be used as drops. Use as often as needed.

How Supplied: 45 cc plastic squeeze bottle.

XERO-LUBE
Saliva Substitute–Oral Lubricant

XERO-LUBE has been accepted by the Council on Dental Therapeutics of the American Dental Association.

Composition: XERO-LUBE closely resembles normal human saliva in electrolyte content, viscosity, and pH. XERO-LUBE is pleasantly flavored and the fluoride concentration is 2 parts per million.

Actions and Uses: XERO-LUBE provides immediate effective safe relief of dry mouth (Xerostomia) symptoms. The moistening and lubricating actions are sustained because of the saliva-like viscosity.

Warnings: Keep this and all medicines out of children's reach.

Dosage and Administration: Aim and depress plunger to spray directly into mouth. May be used as often as needed to moisten the oral cavity. XERO-LUBE may be swallowed or expectorated.

How Supplied: XERO-LUBE is available in a 6 fluid ounce plastic bottle with a pump-spray top.

Schering Corporation
GALLOPING HILL ROAD
KENILWORTH, NJ 07033

A and D Ointment
REG. T.M.

Description: An ointment containing the emollients, anhydrous lanolin and petrolatum.

Indications: *Diaper rash*—**A and D Ointment** provides prompt, soothing relief for diaper rash and helps heal baby's tender skin; forms a moisture-proof shield that helps protect against urine and detergent irritants; comforts baby's skin and helps prevent chafing. *Chafed Skin*—**A and D Ointment** helps skin retain its vital natural moisture; quickly soothes chafed skin in adults and children and helps prevent abnormal dryness. *Abrasions and Minor Burns*—**A and D Ointment** soothes and helps relieve the smarting and pain of abrasions and minor burns, encourages healing and prevents dressings from sticking to the injured area.

Warning: Keep this and all drugs out of the reach of children.

Overdosage: In case of accidental ingestion, seek professional assistance or contact a poison control center immediately.

Dosage and Administration: *Diaper Rash*—Simply apply a thin coating of **A and D Ointment** at each diaper change. A modest amount is all that is needed to provide protective and healing action. *Chafed Skin*—Gently smooth a small quantity of **A and D Ointment** over the area to be treated. *Abrasions, Minor Burns*—Wash with lukewarm water and mild soap. When dry, apply **A and D Ointment** liberally. When a sterile dressing is used, change the dressing daily and apply fresh **A and D Ointment**. If no improvement occurs after 48 to 72 hours or if condition worsens, consult your physician.

How Supplied: A and D Ointment is available in 1½-ounce (42.5 g) and 4-ounce (113 g) tubes and 1-pound (454 g) jars.

Store away from heat.

Copyright© 1973, 1977, Schering Corporation. All rights reserved.

Shown in Product Identification Section, page 426

AFRIN®
Nasal Spray 0.05%
Menthol Nasal Spray 0.05%
Nose Drops 0.05%
Pediatric Nose Drops 0.025%

Description: AFRIN products contain oxymetazoline hydrochloride, the longest acting topical nasal decongestant available. Each ml of AFRIN Nasal Spray and Nose Drops contains oxymetazoline hydrochloride, USP 0.5 mg (0.05%); aminoacetic acid 3.8 mg; sorbitol solution, USP 57.1 mg; phenylmercuric acetate 0.02 mg; benzalkonium chloride 0.2 mg; sodium hydroxide to adjust the pH to a weak acid solution (5.5-6.5); and purified water, q.s. 1 ml.
Each ml of AFRIN Pediatric Nose Drops contains oxymetazoline hydrochloride, USP 0.25 mg (0.025%); aminoacetic acid 3.8 mg; sorbitol solution, USP 57.1 mg; phenylmercuric acetate 0.02 mg; benzalkonium chloride 0.2 mg; hydrochloric acid to adjust the pH to a weak acid solution (4.0-5.0); and purified water, q.s. 1 ml.
AFRIN Menthol Nasal Spray contains cooling aromatic vapors of menthol, eucalyptol and camphor in addition to the ingredients of AFRIN Nasal Spray.

Indications: For temporary relief of nasal congestion "associated with" colds, hay fever and sinusitis.

Actions: The sympathomimetic action of AFRIN products constrict the smaller arterioles of the nasal passages, producing a prolonged, gentle and predictable decongesting effect. In just a few minutes a single dose, as directed, provides prompt, temporary relief of nasal congestion that lasts up to 12 hours. AFRIN products last up to 3 or 4 times longer than most ordinary nasal sprays.
AFRIN products used at bedtime help restore freer nasal breathing through the night.

Warnings: Do not exceed recommended dosage because symptoms may occur, such as burning, stinging, sneezing or increase of nasal discharge. Do not use these products for more than 3 days. If symptoms persist, consult a physician. The use of the dispensers by more than one person may spread infection. Keep these and all medicines out of the reach of children.

Overdosage: In case of accidental ingestion, seek professional assistance or contact a Poison Control Center immediately.

Dosage and Administration: Because AFRIN has a long duration of action, twice-a-day administration—in the morning and at bedtime—is usually adequate.
AFRIN Nasal Spray and Menthol Nasal Spray, 0.05%—For adults and children 6 years of age and over: With head upright, spray 2 or 3 times into each nostril twice daily—morning and evening. To spray, squeeze bottle quickly and firmly and sniff briskly. Not recommended for children under six.
AFRIN Nose Drops—For adults and children 6 years of age and over: Tilt head back, apply 2 or 3 drops into each nostril twice daily—morning and evening. Immediately bend head forward toward knees. Hold a few seconds, then return to upright position. Not recommended for children under six.
AFRIN Pediatric Nose Drops—Children 2 through 5 years of age: Tilt head back, apply 2 or 3 drops into each nostril twice daily—morning and evening. Promptly move head forward toward knees. Hold a few seconds, then return child to upright position. For children under 2 years, use only as directed by a physician.
How Supplied: AFRIN Nasal Spray 0.05% (1:2000), 15 ml and 30 ml plastic squeeze bottles.
AFRIN Menthol Nasal Spray 0.05% (1:2000), 15 ml plastic squeeze bottle.
AFRIN Nose Drops, 0.05% (1:2000), 20 ml dropper bottle.
AFRIN Pediatric Nose Drops, 0.025% (1:4000), 20 ml dropper bottle.
Store all nasal sprays and nose drops between 2° and 30°C (36° and 86°F).
Shown in Product Identification Section, page 426

AFRINOL®
Repetabs® Tablets
Long-Acting Nasal Decongestant

Active Ingredients: Each Repetabs Tablet contains: 120 mg pseudoephedrine sulfate. Half the dose (60 mg) is released after the tablet is swallowed and the other half is released hours later; continuous relief is provided for up to 12 hours . . . without drowsiness.

Indications: For temporary relief of nasal congestion due to the common cold, hay fever or other upper respiratory allergies, and nasal congestion associated with sinusitis.

Actions: Promotes nasal and/or sinus drainage, helps decongest sinus openings, sinus passages.

Warnings: Do not exceed recommended dosage because at higher doses nervousness, dizziness or sleeplessness may occur. Do not take this preparation if you have high blood pressure, heart disease, diabetes, or thyroid disease, except under the advice and supervision of a physician. If symptoms do not improve within 7 days or are accompanied by high fever, consult a physician before continuing use. Keep this and all drugs out of the reach of children.
As with any drug, if you are pregnant or nursing a baby, seek the advice of a health professional before using this product.

Drug Interactions: Do not take this product if you are presently taking a prescription antihypertensive or antidepressant drug containing a monoamine oxidase inhibitor, except under the advice and supervision of a physician.

Overdosage: In case of accidental overdose, seek professional assistance or contact a poison control center immediately.

Dosage and Administration: Adults and children 12 years and over—One tablet every 12 hours. AFRINOL is not recommended for children under 12 years of age.

How Supplied: AFRINOL Repetabs Tablets—Boxes of 12 and bottles of 100. Store between 2° and 30°C (36° and 86° F) Protect from excessive moisture.
Shown in Product Identification Section, page 426

CHLOR-TRIMETON®
Allergy Syrup
Allergy Tablets 4 mg
Long Acting Allergy REPETABS®
Tablets 8 mg and 12 mg.

Active Ingredients: Each Allergy Tablet contains: 4 mg CHLOR-TRIMETON (brand of chlorpheniramine maleate, USP); Each REPETABS® Tablet contains: 8 mg or 12 mg CHLOR-TRIMETON (brand of chlorpheniramine maleate). Half the dose is released after the tablet is swallowed, and the other half is released hours later; continuous relief is provided for up to 12 hours.
Each teaspoonful (5 ml) of Allergy Syrup contains: 2 mg CHLOR-TRIMETON (brand of chlorpheniramine maleate) in a pleasant-tasting syrup containing approximately 7% alcohol.

Indications: For temporary relief of hay fever symptoms: sneezing; running nose; watery, itchy eyes, itching of the nose or throat.

Actions: The active ingredient in CHLOR-TRIMETON is an antihistamine with anticholinergic (drying) and sedative side effects. Antihistamines appear to compete with histamine for cell receptor sites on effector cells.

Warnings: May cause drowsiness. May cause excitability especially in children. Do not take these products if you have asthma, glaucoma or difficulty in urination due to enlargement of the prostate

gland, or give the REPETABS Tablets to children under 12 years, or the Allergy Syrup and Tablets to children under 6 years, except under the advice and supervision of a physician. Keep these and all drugs out of the reach of children.
As with any drug, if you are pregnant or nursing a baby, seek the advice of a health professional before using this product.

Precautions: Avoid driving a motor vehicle or operating heavy machinery. Avoid alcoholic beverages while taking these products.

Overdosage: In case of accidental overdose, seek professional assistance or contact a Poison Control Center immediately.

Dosage and Administration: Allergy Syrup—Adults and Children 12 years and over: Two teaspoonfuls (4 mg) every 4 to 6 hours, not to exceed 12 teaspoonfuls in 24 hours; Children 6 through 11 years: one teaspoonful (2 mg) every 4 to 6 hours, not to exceed 6 teaspoonfuls in 24 hours; For children under 6 years, consult a physician.
Allergy Tablets—Adults and Children 12 years and over: One tablet (4 mg) every 4 to 6 hours, not to exceed 6 tablets in 24 hours. Children 6 through 11 years: One half the adult dose (break tablet in half) every 4 to 6 hours, not to exceed 3 whole tablets in 24 hours. For children under 6 years, consult a physician.
Allergy REPETABS Tablets—Adults and Children 12 years and over: One tablet in the morning and one tablet in the evening, not to exceed 24 mg (3 tablets of 8 mg; 2 tablets of 12 mg.) in 24 hours. For children under 12 years, consult a physician.

Professional Labeling: Dosage—Allergy Syrup: Children 2 through 5 years: ½ teaspoonful (1 mg) every 4 to 6 hours; Allergy Tablets: Children 2 through 5 years: one-quarter tablet (1 mg) every 4 to 6 hours.
Allergy REPETABS Tablets—Children 6 to 12 years: One tablet (8 mg) at bedtime or during the day, as indicated.

How Supplied: CHLOR-TRIMETON Allergy Tablets, 4 mg, yellow compressed, scored tablets impressed with the Schering trademark and product identification letters, TW or numbers, 080; box of 24, bottles of 100 and 1000.
CHLOR-TRIMETON Allergy Syrup: 2 mg per 5 ml, blue-green-colored liquid; 4-fluid ounce (118 ml). Protect from light; however, if color fades potency will not be affected.
CHLOR-TRIMETON Allergy REPETABS Tablets, 8 mg, sugar-coated, yellow tablets branded in red with the Schering trademark and product identification letters, CC or numbers, 374; boxes of 24, 48, bottles of 100 and 1000.

Continued on next page

Information on Schering products appearing on these pages is effective as of January 1, 1985.

Schering—Cont.

CHLOR-TRIMETON REPETABS Tablets, 12 mg, sugar coated orange tablets branded in black with Schering trademark and product identification letters AAE or numbers 009; boxes of 12 and 24, bottles of 100 and 1000.
Store the tablets and syrup between 2° and 30°C (36° and 86°F).

*Shown in Product Identification
Section, page 426*

CHLOR–TRIMETON® Decongestant Tablets
Long Acting CHLOR–TRIMETON® Decongestant REPETABS® Tablets

Active Ingredients: Each tablet contains: 4 mg. CHLOR-TRIMETON (brand of chlorpheniramine maleate, USP) and 60 mg. pseudoephedrine sulfate.
Each REPETABS Tablet contains: 8 mg CHLOR-TRIMETON (brand of chlorpheniramine maleate) and 120 mg pseudoephedrine sulfate. Half the dose of each ingredient is released after the tablet is swallowed and the other half is released hours later providing continuous long-lasting relief up to 12 hours.

Indications: For temporary relief of nasal congestion due to hay fever and associated with sinusitis.

Actions: The antihistamine, chlorpheniramine maleate, provides temporary relief of running nose, sneezing, itching of the nose or throat, and itchy and watery eyes as may occur in allergic rhinitis (such as hayfever). The decongestant, pseudoephedrine sulfate reduces swelling of nasal passages; shrinks swollen membranes; and temporarily restores freer breathing through the nose.

Warnings: If symptoms do not improve within seven days or are accompanied by high fever, consult your physician before continuing use. May cause drowsiness. May cause excitability especially in children. Do not exceed recommended dosage because at higher doses nervousness, dizziness or sleeplessness may occur. Do not give the Decongestant Tablets to children under 6 years or the REPETABS Tablets to children under 12 years except under the advice and supervision of a physician. Do not take these products if you have asthma, glaucoma, difficulty in urination due to enlargement of the prostate gland, high blood pressure, heart disease, diabetes or thyroid disease, except under the advice and supervision of a physician.
As with any drug, if you are pregnant or nursing a baby, seek the advice of a health professional before using this product.

Drug Interaction: Do not take this product if you are presently taking a prescription antihypertensive or antidepressant medication containing a monoamine oxidase inhibitor, except under the advice and supervision of a physician.

Precautions: Avoid driving a motor vehicle or operating heavy machinery. Avoid alcoholic beverages while taking this product. Keep these and all drugs out of the reach of children.

Overdosage: In case of accidental overdose, seek professional assistance or contact a Poison Control Center immediately.

Dosage and Administration: Tablets —ADULTS AND CHILDREN 12 YEARS AND OVER: One tablet every 4 to 6 hours, not to exceed 4 tablets in 24 hours. CHILDREN 6 THROUGH 11 YEARS —One half the adult dose (break tablet in half) every 4 to 6 hours not to exceed 2 whole tablets in 24 hours. For children under 6 years, consult a physician. REPETABS Tablets—ADULTS AND CHILDREN 12 YEARS AND OVER: one tablet every 12 hours.

Professional Labeling: Tablets— Children 2-5 years—one quarter the adult dose every 4 hours, not to exceed 1 tablet in 24 hours.

How Supplied: CHLOR-TRIMETON Decongestant Tablets—boxes of 24 and 48. Long Acting CHLOR-TRIMETON Decongestant REPETABS Tablets boxes of 12 and 36.
Store these CHLOR-TRIMETON Products between 2° and 30°C (36° & 86°F); and protect from excessive moisture.

*Shown in Product Identification
Section, page 426*

COD LIVER OIL CONCENTRATE
Tablets
Capsules
Tablets with Vitamin C

Active Ingredients: Tablets—A pleasantly flavored concentrate of cod liver oil with Vitamins A & D added. Each tasty, chewable tablet provides: 4000 IU of vitamin A and 200 IU of vitamin D.
Capsules—A concentrate of cod liver oil with Vitamins A and D added. Each capsule provides: 10,000 IU of vitamin A and 400 IU of vitamin D.
Tablets with Vitamin C—A pleasantly-flavored concentrate of cod liver oil with Vitamins A, D and C added. Each tablet provides, 4000 IU of Vitamin A, 200 IU of Vitamin D and 50 mg of Vitamin C.
Tablets may be chewed or swallowed.

Indications: Cod Liver Oil Concentrate Tablets and Capsules are recommended for prevention and treatment of diseases due to deficiencies in Vitamins A and D. The tablets with Vitamin C are recommended for prevention and treatment of diseases due to deficiencies of Vitamins A, D and C.

Warnings: Keep these and all drugs out of the reach of children.
As with any drug, if you are pregnant or nursing a baby, seek the advice of a health professional before using these products.

Precautions: Cod Liver Oil Concentrate Tablets and Tablets with Vitamin C

contain FD&C Yellow No. 5 (tartrazine) as a color additive.
Persons sensitive to tartrazine or aspirin should consult a physician.

Overdosage: In case of accidental overdose, seek professional assistance or contact a Poison Control Center immediately.

Dosage and Administration: Tablets: Two tablets daily, or as prescribed by a physician, taken preferably before meals.
Capsules: One capsule daily, or as prescribed by a physician, taken preferably before meals.
Tablets with Vitamin C: Two tablets daily, taken preferably before meals.

How Supplied: Cod Liver Oil Concentrate Tablets: bottles of 100 and 240. Cod Liver Oil Concentrate Capsules: bottles of 40 and 100. Cod Liver Oil Concentrate Tablets with Vitamin C: bottles of 100 tablets.

*Shown in Product Identification
Section, page 427*

CORICIDIN® Tablets
CORICIDIN 'D'® Decongestant Tablets
CORICIDIN® Cough Syrup
CORICIDIN® Decongestant Nasal Mist

Active Ingredients: CORICIDIN Tablets—2 mg CHLOR-TRIMETON® (brand of chlorpheniramine maleate, USP); 325 mg (5gr) aspirin, USP.
CORICIDIN 'D' Decongestant Tablets—2 mg chlorpheniramine maleate, USP; 12.5 mg phenylpropanolamine hydrochloride, USP; 325 mg (5 gr) aspirin, USP.
CORICIDIN Cough Syrup—Each teaspoonful (5 ml) of fruit-flavored syrup contains 10 mg dextromethorphan hydrobromide; 12.5 mg phenylpropanolamine hydrochloride, USP; 100 mg guaifenesin and less than 0.5% alcohol.
CORICIDIN Decongestant Nasal Mist—0.5% phenylephrine hydrochloride, USP.

Indications: CORICIDIN Tablets—For effective, temporary relief of cold and flu symptoms.
CORICIDIN 'D' Decongestant Tablets— For effective, temporary relief of congested cold, flu and sinus symptoms.
CORICIDIN Cough Syrup—For temporary relief of coughs and stuffy noses.
CORICIDIN Decongestant Nasal Mist— For temporary relief of nasal congestion associated with the common cold, hay fever or sinusitis.

Actions: CORICIDIN Tablets relieve annoying cold and flu symptoms such as minor aches and pains, fever, sneezing, running nose and watery/itchy eyes.
CORICIDIN 'D' Tablets relieve the same annoying cold and flu symptoms as well as stuffy nose, nasal membrane swelling and sinus headache.
CORICIDIN Cough Syrup helps loosen the phlegm in a non-productive cough, temporarily soothes irritated throat

membranes, suppresses annoying coughs and helps relieve stuffy noses.

CORICIDIN Decongestant Nasal Mist is "symptom specific" and designed to shrink swollen nasal membranes promptly and help restore freer breathing through the nose.

Warnings: CORICIDIN Tablets—Drink a full glass of water with each dose. Adults should not take this product for more than 10 days; children 6 through 11 not more than 5 days. If fever persists or recurs, neither adults nor children should use for more than 3 days. If symptoms persist or new ones occur, consult your physician. May cause drowsiness. May cause excitability, especially in children. This product contains aspirin. Do not take this product if you are allergic to aspirin or if you have asthma, glaucoma, difficulty in urination due to enlargement of the prostate gland, stomach distress, ulcers or bleeding problems, or give this product to children under 6 years, except under the advice and supervision of a physician. Stop taking this product if ringing in the ears or other symptoms occur. Keep this and all drugs out of the reach of children. As with any drug, if you are pregnant or nursing a baby, seek the advice of a health professional before using this product.

CORICIDIN 'D' Decongestant Tablets—Drink a full glass of water with each dose. Adults should not take this product for more than 7 days; children 6 through 11 not more than 5 days. If fever persists or recurs, neither adults nor children should use for more than 3 days. If symptoms persist or new ones occur, consult your physician. May cause drowsiness. May cause excitability especially in children. Do not exceed recommended dosage because at higher doses nervousness, dizziness, elevation of blood pressure, or sleeplessness may occur. This product contains aspirin. Do not take this product if you are allergic to aspirin or if you have asthma, glaucoma, difficulty in urination due to enlargement of the prostate gland, stomach distress, ulcers or bleeding problems, high blood pressure, heart disease, diabetes or thyroid disease, or give this product to children under 6 years, except under the advice and supervision of a physician. Stop taking this product if ringing in the ears or other symptoms occur. Keep this and all drugs out of the reach of children. As with any drug, if you are pregnant or nursing a baby, seek the advice of a health professional before using this product.

CORICIDIN Cough Syrup—Do not exceed recommended dosage because at higher doses nervousness, dizziness or sleeplessness are more likely to occur. This product should not, except under the direction of a physician, be used for persistent or chronic cough such as occurs with smoking, asthma or emphysema or where cough is accompanied by excessive secretions. CORICIDIN Cough Syrup should not be used in children under 2 years of age or by persons with high blood pressure, heart disease, diabetes or thyroid disease, except under the advice

and supervision of a physician. Keep this and all drugs out of the reach of children. As with any drug, if you are pregnant or nursing a baby, seek the advice of a health professional before using this product.

CORICIDIN Decongestant Nasal Mist—Do not exceed recommended dosage because symptoms may occur such as burning, stinging, sneezing, or increase of nasal discharge. Do not use this product for more than 3 days. If symptoms persist, consult a physician. The use of this dispenser by more than one person may spread infection. For adult use only. Do not give this product to children under 12 years of age except under the advice and supervision of a physician. Keep this and all medicines out of the reach of children.

Drug Interactions: CORICIDIN Tablets—Do not take this product if you are presently taking a prescription drug for anticoagulation (thinning of the blood), diabetes, gout or arthritis, except under the advice and supervision of a physician.

CORICIDIN 'D' Decongestant Tablets—Do not take this product if you are presently taking a prescription antihypertensive or antidepressant medication containing a monoamine oxidase inhibitor or a prescription drug for anticoagulation (thinning of the blood), diabetes, gout or arthritis, except under the advice and supervision of a physician.

CORICIDIN Cough Syrup—Do not take this product if you are presently taking a prescription antihypertensive or antidepressant medication containing a monoamine oxidase inhibitor, except under the advice and supervision of a physician.

Precautions: CORICIDIN Tablets and CORICIDIN 'D' Decongestant Tablets—Avoid alcoholic beverages while taking these products. Also avoid driving a motor vehicle or operating heavy machinery.

CORICIDIN Cough Syrup—A persistent cough may be a sign of a serious condition. If cough or other symptoms persist for more than one week, tend to recur or are accompanied by high fever, rash or persistent headache, consult a physician before continuing use.

Overdosage: In case of accidental overdose of the tablets or syrup or accidental ingestion of the nasal mist, seek professional assistance or contact a Poison Control Center immediately.

Dosage and Administration: CORICIDIN Tablets—Adults and children 12 years and over—2 tablets every 4 hours not to exceed 12 tablets in 24 hours. Children 6 through 11 years: 1 tablet every 4 hours not to exceed 5 tablets in 24 hours.

CORICIDIN 'D' Decongestant Tablets—Adults and children 12 years and over: 2 tablets every 4 hours not to exceed 12 tablets in 24 hours. Children 6 through 11 years: 1 tablet every 4 hours not to exceed 5 tablets in 24 hours.

CORICIDIN Cough Syrup—Adults and children 12 years and over: 2 teaspoon-

fuls every 4 hours. Children 6–11 years: 1 teaspoonful every 4 hours. Children 2–5 years: ½ teaspoonful every 4 hours. Do not exceed 6 doses per day.

CORICIDIN Decongestant Nasal Mist—For adults and children 12 years of age and over: With head upright spray two or three times in each nostril, not more frequently than every four hours.

How Supplied: CORICIDIN Tablets—bottles of 12, 24, 60, 100 and 1000. Dispensing Package, box of 100 packets, 4 tablets in each packet.

CORICIDIN 'D' Decongestant Tablets—bottles of 12, 24, 50, and 100. Dispensing Package, box of 100 packets, 4 tablets in each packet.

CORICIDIN Cough Syrup—bottles of 4 oz. (118 ml).

CORICIDIN Decongestant Nasal Mist—Plastic squeeze bottles of ⅔ fl. oz. (20 ml).

Store the tablets, nasal mist, and syrup between 2° and 30°C (36° and 86°F). Protect the tablets from excessive moisture.

Shown in Product Identification Section, page 427

CORICIDIN® MEDILETS® Tablets for Children
CORICIDIN® DEMILETS® Tablets for Children

Active Ingredients: CORICIDIN MEDILETS Tablets—1.0 mg CHLOR-TRIMETON® (brand of chlorpheniramine maleate, USP); phenylpropanolamine hydrochloride, USP, 6.25 mg.

CORICIDIN DEMILETS Tablets—1.0 mg chlorpheniramine maleate, USP; 80 mg acetaminophen, USP; 6.25 mg phenylpropanolamine hydrochloride, USP.

Indications: CORICIDIN MEDILETS Tablets—For temporary relief of congested cold and sinus symptoms in children. CORICIDIN DEMILETS Tablets—For temporary relief of children's congested cold, flu and sinus symptoms.

Actions: CORICIDIN MEDILETS Tablets provide relief of annoying cold and sinus symptoms: running nose, sneezing and watery/itchy eyes.

CORICIDIN DEMILETS Tablets provide relief of annoying cold, flu and sinus symptoms: running nose, stuffy nose, sneezing, watery/itchy eyes, minor aches, pains and fever.

Warnings: CORICIDIN MEDILETS Tablets—If symptoms do not improve within 7 days or are accompanied by high fever, consult a physician before continuing use. This product may cause drowsiness; therefore, driving a motor vehicle or operating heavy machinery must be avoided while taking it. Alcoholic beverages must also be avoided while taking this product. It may cause excitability, especially in children. Do not exceed recommended dosage because at higher

Continued on next page

Schering—Cont.

doses nervousness, dizziness, elevation of blood pressure, or sleeplessness are more likely to occur. Do not give this product to persons who have asthma, glaucoma, difficulty in urination due to enlargement of the prostate gland, high blood pressure, heart disease, diabetes, or thyroid disease, or to children less than 6 years old, except under the advice and supervision of a physician. Keep this and all drugs out of the reach of children. As with any drug, if you are pregnant or nursing a baby, seek the advice of a health professional before using this product.

CORICIDIN DEMILETS Tablets—Give water with each dose. Do not give this product for more than 5 days, but if fever is present, persists or recurs, limit dosage to 3 days; if symptoms persist or new ones occur, consult a physician. This product may cause drowsiness, therefore, driving a motor vehicle or operating heavy machinery must be avoided while taking it. Alcoholic beverages must also be avoided while taking this product. It may cause excitability, especially in children. Do not exceed recommended dosage because at higher doses severe liver damage, nervousness, dizziness, elevation of blood pressure or sleeplessness are more likely to occur. Do not administer this product to persons who have asthma, glaucoma, difficulty in urination due to enlargement of the prostate gland, high blood pressure, heart disease, diabetes or thyroid disease, or give this product to children less than 6 years old, except under the advice and supervision of a physician. Keep this and all drugs out of the reach of children. As with any drug, if you are pregnant or nursing a baby, seek the advice of a health professional before using this product.

Drug Interactions: CORICIDIN MEDILETS and DEMILETS Tablets—Do not give this product to persons who are presently taking a prescription antihypertensive or antidepressant medication containing a monoamine oxidase inhibitor or an appetite-controlling medication containing phenylpropanolamine except under the advice and supervision of a physician.

Overdosage: In case of accidental overdose, seek professional assistance or contact a Poison Control Center immediately.

Dosage and Administration: CORICIDIN MEDILETS Tablets—Under 6 years: As directed by a physician. Children 6 through 11 years: Two MEDILETS Tablets every 4 hours not to exceed 12 tablets in a 24-hour period, or as directed by a physician.
CORICIDIN DEMILETS Tablets—Under 6 years: As directed by a physician. 6 through 11 years: Two DEMILETS Tablets every 4 hours not to exceed 12 tablets in a 24-hour period, or as directed by a physician.

How Supplied: CORICIDIN MEDILETS Tablets—boxes of 24 and 36, indi-

vidually wrapped in a child's protective pack.
CORICIDIN DEMILETS Tablets—boxes of 24 and 36, individually wrapped in a child's protective pack.
Store the tablets between 2° and 30°C (36° and 86°F). Protect from excessive moisture.

Shown in Product Identification Section, page 427

CORICIDIN® Extra Strength Sinus Headache Tablets

Active Ingredients: Each tablet contains: acetaminophen 500 mg (500 mg is a non-standard extra strength tablet of acetaminophen, as compared to the standard of 325 mg); CHLOR-TRIMETON (brand of chlorpheniramine maleate) 2 mg; phenylpropanolamine hydrochloride 12.5 mg.

Indications: For temporary relief of sinus headache and congestion.

Actions: CORICIDIN Sinus Headache Tablets have been formulated with an antihistamine for temporary relief of the running nose that often accompanies upper respiratory allergies and sinusitis; a non-aspirin pain reliever for temporary relief of sinus headache pain and a decongestant for temporary relief of nasal membrane swelling, thus promoting freer breathing.

Warnings: Consult your physician: if symptoms persist, do not improve within 7 days, if new symptoms occur, or if fever persists for more than 3 days (72 hours) or recurs. May cause drowsiness. May cause excitability, especially in children. Do not exceed recommended dosage because severe liver damage may occur and at higher doses nervousness, dizziness, elevation of blood pressure, or sleeplessness are more likely to occur. Except under the advice and supervision of a physician, this product should not be used in children less than 12 years old or by persons with high blood pressure, heart disease, diabetes or thyroid disease, asthma, glaucoma or difficulty in urination due to enlargement of the prostate gland. Keep this and all drugs out of the reach of children. As with any drug, if you are pregnant or nursing a baby, seek the advice of a health professional before using this product.

Drug Interactions: Do not take this product if you are presently taking a prescription antihypertensive or antidepressant medication containing a monoamine oxidase inhibitor, except under the advice and supervision of a physician.

Precautions: Avoid alcoholic beverages while taking this product. Also, avoid driving a motor vehicle or operating heavy machinery.

Overdosage: In case of accidental overdose, seek professional assistance or contact a poison control center immediately.

Dosage and Administration: Adults and children 12 years and older: 2 tablets every 6 hours not to exceed 8 tablets in a

24-hour period, or as directed by a physician. Swallow one tablet at a time.
Store between 2° and 30°C (36° and 86°F). Protect from excessive moisture.

How Supplied: Box of 24.

DEMAZIN®
Decongestant-Antihistamine
REPETABS® Tablets
Syrup

Active Ingredients: Each REPETABS® Tablet contains: 20 mg. phenylephrine and 4 mg CHLOR-TRIMETON® (brand of chlorpheniramine maleate, USP). Half the dose is in the outside coating for rapid absorption and prompt effect. The other half is in the inner core coated for repeat action.
Each teaspoonful (5 ml.) of syrup contains 2.5 mg. phenylephrine hydrochloride, USP and 1 mg. CHLOR-TRIMETON® (brand of chlorpheniramine maleate, USP) in a pleasant-tasting syrup containing approximately 7.5% alcohol.

Indications: For temporary relief of nasal congestion, watery eyes, running nose, and sneezing associated with hay fever, sinus congestion and the common cold.

Actions: Phenylephrine hydrochloride is a sympathomimetic agent which acts as an upper respiratory and pulmonary decongestant and mild bronchodilator. It exerts desirable sympathomimetic action with relatively little central nervous system excitation, so that wakefulness and nervousness are reduced to a minimum. Chlorpheniramine maleate antagonizes many of the characteristic effects of histamine. It is of value clinically in the prevention and relief of many allergic manifestations.
The oral administration of phenylephrine hydrochloride with chlorpheniramine maleate produces a complementary action on congestive conditions of the upper respiratory tract, thus often obviating the need for topical nasal therapy.

Warnings: If symptoms do not improve within 7 days or are accompanied by high fever consult a physician before continuing use. May cause drowsiness. May cause excitability especially in children. Do not exceed recommended dosage because at higher doses nervousness, dizziness or sleeplessness are more likely to occur. Except under the advice and supervision of a physician, these products should not be used in children under 6 years of age or by persons with high blood pressure, heart disease, diabetes, thyroid disease, asthma, glaucoma or difficulty in urination due to enlargement of the prostate gland.
Keep these and all drugs out of the reach of children.
As with any drug, if you are pregnant or nursing a baby, seek the advice of a health professional before using this product.

Drug Interaction: Do not take this product if you are presently taking a prescription antihypertensive or antidepressant drug containing a monoamine oxidase inhibitor, except under the advice and supervision of a physician.

Precautions: Avoid alcoholic beverages while taking these products. Also avoid driving a motor vehicle or operating heavy machinery. Contains FD&C yellow #5 (tartrazine) as a color additive. Persons sensitive to tartrazine or aspirin should consult a physician.

Overdosage: In case of accidental overdose, seek professional assistance or contact a Poison Control Center immediately.

Dosage and Administration: Tablets —Adults and children 12 years and over: One tablet morning and evening. Children under 12 years, consult a physician. Syrup—Adults: Two teaspoonfuls four times daily or as directed by a physician. Children 6 to 12 years: One teaspoonful four times daily or as directed by a physician. For children under 6 years, consult a physician. Not more than 4 doses every 24 hours.

Professional Labeling: Dosage: Syrup—Children 2 to 5 years: 1 teaspoonful, four times daily.

How Supplied: DEMAZIN REPETABS Tablets, blue, sugar-coated tablets branded in red with the Schering trademark and either product identification letters, ADD or numbers, 133; box of 24 tablets and bottles of 100 and 1000. DEMAZIN Syrup, blue-colored liquid, bottles of 4 fluid ounces (118 ml). Store the syrup between 2° and 25°C (36° and 77°F).

Shown in Product Identification Section, page 427

DERMOLATE® Anti-Itch Cream
DERMOLATE® Anti-Itch Spray
DERMOLATE® Anal-Itch Ointment
DERMOLATE® Scalp-Itch Lotion

Active Ingredients: DERMOLATE Anti-Itch Cream contains hydrocortisone 0.5% in a greaseless, vanishing cream. DERMOLATE Anti-Itch Spray contains hydrocortisone 0.5% in a clear, cooling, fast-drying spray. Alcohol content 24%. DERMOLATE Anal-Itch Ointment contains hydrocortisone 0.5% in a soothing, lubricating ointment. DERMOLATE Scalp-Itch Lotion contains hydrocortisone 0.5% in a clear, non-greasy liquid that dries in minutes. Isopropyl alcohol content 47%.

Indications: DERMOLATE Anti-Itch Cream and Spray—For the temporary relief of minor skin irritations, itching and rashes due to eczema, dermatitis, insect bites, poison ivy, poison oak, poison sumac, soaps, detergents, cosmetics and jewelry. DERMOLATE Anal-Itch Ointment—For the temporary relief of itchy anal areas. Also for minor skin irritations and itching due to eczema and dermatitis. DERMOLATE Scalp-Itch Lotion—For temporary relief of itching and minor scalp irritation due to scalp dermatitis.

Actions: DERMOLATE Anti-Itch Cream and Spray provide temporary relief of itching and minor skin irritation. DERMOLATE Anal-Itch Ointment provides temporary relief of anal itching, minor skin irritations and itching due to eczema and dermatitis. DERMOLATE Scalp-Itch Lotion provides temporary relief of itching and minor scalp irritation due to scalp dermatitis.

Warnings: All DERMOLATE forms are for external use only. Avoid contact with the eyes. Discontinue use and consult a physician if condition worsens or if symptoms persist for more than seven days. Do not use on children under 2 years of age except under the advice and supervision of physician. Keep these and all drugs out of the reach of children.

Overdosage: In case of accidental ingestion, seek professional assistance or contact a Poison Control Center immediately.

Dosage and Administration: DERMOLATE Anti-Itch Cream—*For adults and children 2 years of age and older:* Gently massage into affected skin area not more than 3 or 4 times daily. *For children under 2 years of age,* there is no recommended dosage except under the advice and supervision of a physician. DERMOLATE Anti-Itch Spray—*For adults and children 2 years of age and older:* Spray on affected skin area not more than 3 or 4 times daily. *For children under 2 years of age,* there is no recommended dosage except under the advice and supervision of a physician. DERMOLATE Anal-Itch Ointment— *Adults and children 2 years of age and older:* Apply to affected area not more than 3 to 4 times daily. *For children under 2 years of age,* there is no recommended dosage except under the advice and supervision of a physician. DERMOLATE Scalp-Itch Lotion—*For adults and children 2 years of age and older:* Part the hair and apply directly to the scalp by squeezing a small amount onto affected areas. Massage into the scalp and repeat this process until desired coverage is achieved. Maintain normal hair care but do not wash out DERMOLATE Lotion immediately after application. Apply to affected scalp areas not more than 3 to 4 times daily. *For children under 2 years of age,* there is no recommended dosage except under the advice and supervision of a physician.

How Supplied: DERMOLATE Anti-Itch Cream—30 g (1.0 oz.) tube, and 15 g (½ oz) tubes and institutional package, 50 × 2g (1/15 oz) tubes. DERMOLATE Anti-Itch Spray—45 ml (1.5 fl. oz.) pump spray bottle. DERMOLATE Anal-Itch Ointment—30 g (1.0 fl. oz.) tube. DERMOLATE Scalp-Itch Lotion—30 ml (1 fl. oz.) plastic squeeze bottle. Store all forms between 2° and 30°C (36° and 86°F). Protect the spray from freezing.

Shown in Product Identification Section, page 427

DISOPHROL® Chronotab® Sustained–Action Tablets

Active Ingredients: EACH DISOPHROL Chronotab SUSTAINED-ACTION TABLET CONTAINS: 120 mg of pseudoephedrine sulfate and 6 mg of dexbrompheniramine maleate. Half of the medication is released after the tablet is swallowed and the remaining amount of medication is released hours later providing continuous long-lasting relief for 12 hours.

Indications: For temporary relief of nasal congestion due to the common cold, hay fever, or other upper respiratory allergies, and associated with sinusitis. Helps decongest sinus openings, sinus passages. Reduces swelling of nasal passages; shrinks swollen membranes; and temporarily restores freer breathing through the nose. Alleviates running nose, sneezing, itching of the nose or throat, and itchy and watery eyes as may occur in allergic rhinitis (such as hay fever).

Warnings: If symptoms do not improve within 7 days or are accompanied by high fever, consult a physician before continuing use. May cause drowsiness. May cause excitability especially in children. Do not exceed recommended dosage because at higher doses nervousness, dizziness, or sleeplessness may occur. Do not give this product to children under 12 years except under the advice and supervision of a physician. Do not take this product if you have asthma, glaucoma, difficulty in urination due to enlargement of the prostate gland, high blood pressure, heart disease, diabetes, or thyroid disease except under the advice and supervision of a physician. As with any drug, if you are pregnant or nursing a baby, seek the advice of a health professional before using this product.

Drug Interaction: Do not take this product if you are presently taking a prescription antihypertensive or antidepressant drug containing a monoamine oxidase inhibitor except under the advice and supervision of a physician.

Precaution: Avoid driving a motor vehicle or operating heavy machinery. Avoid alcoholic beverages while taking this product. Keep this and all drugs out of the reach of children.

Overdosage: In case of accidental overdose, seek professional assistance or contact a Poison Control Center immediately.

Dosage and Administration: ADULTS AND CHILDREN 12 YEARS AND OVER—one tablet every 12 hours. Do not exceed two tablets in 24 hours.

Continued on next page

Information on Schering products appearing on these pages is effective as of January 1, 1985.

Schering—Cont.

How Supplied: DISOPHROL Chronotab Sustained-Action Tablets, sugar-coated, cherry-red tablets branded in black with either the product identification code 85-WMH or one of the Schering trademarks and the numbers, 231; bottle of 100.

Store between 2° and 30°C (36° and 86°F).
© 1982, Schering Corporation.

DRIXORAL®
Sustained-Action Tablets

Active Ingredients: EACH DRIXORAL SUSTAINED-ACTION TABLET CONTAINS: 120 mg of pseudoephedrine sulfate and 6 mg of dexbrompheniramine maleate. Half of the medication is released after the tablet is swallowed and the remaining amount of medication is released hours later providing continuous long-lasting relief for 12 hours.

Indications: For temporary relief of nasal congestion due to the common cold, hay fever, or other upper respiratory allergies, and associated with sinusitis. Helps decongest sinus openings, sinus passages. Reduces swelling of nasal passages; shrinks swollen membranes; and temporarily restores freer breathing through the nose. Alleviates running nose, sneezing, itching of the nose or throat, and itchy and watery eyes as may occur in allergic rhinitis (such as hay fever).

Actions: The antihistamine, dexbrompheniramine maleate, provides temporary relief of sneezing; watery, itchy eyes; running nose due to hay fever and other upper respiratory allergies. The decongestant, pseudoephedrine sulfate, temporarily restores freer breathing through the nose and promotes sinus drainage.

Warnings: If symptoms do not improve within 7 days or are accompanied by high fever, consult a physician before continuing use. May cause drowsiness. May cause excitability especially in children. Do not exceed recommended dosage because at higher doses nervousness, dizziness, or sleeplessness may occur. Do not give this product to children under 12 years except under the advice and supervision of a physician. Do not take this product if you have asthma, glaucoma, difficulty in urination due to enlargement of the prostate gland, high blood pressure, heart disease, diabetes, or thyroid disease except under the advice and supervision of a physician.
As with any drug, if you are pregnant or nursing a baby, seek the advice of a health professional before using this product.

Drug Interaction: Do not take this product if you are presently taking a prescription antihypertensive or antidepressant drug containing a monoamine oxidase inhibitor except under the advice and supervision of a physician.

Precaution: Avoid driving a motor vehicle or operting heavy machinery. Avoid alcoholic beverages while taking this product.
Keep this and all drugs out of the reach of children.

Overdosage: In case of accidental overdose, seek professional assistance or contact a Poison Control Center immediately.

Dosage and Administration: ADULTS AND CHILDREN 12 YEARS AND OVER—one tablet every 12 hours. Do not exceed two tablets in 24 hours.

How Supplied: DRIXORAL Sustained-Action Tablets, green, sugar-coated tablets branded in black with the product name, boxes of 10, 20, and 40, bottle of 100.
Store between 2° and 30°C (36° and 86°F).
© 1982, Schering Corporation.
Shown in Product Identification Section, page 427

EMKO® BECAUSE®
Vaginal Contraceptive Foam

Description: A non-hormonal, non-scented aerosol foam contraceptive in a portable applicator/foam unit containing six applications of an 8.0% concentration of the spermicide nonoxynol-9.

Indications: Vaginal contraceptive intended for the prevention of pregnancy. BECAUSE Foam provides effective protection alone or it may be used instead of spermicidal jelly or cream to give added protection with a diaphragm.
BECAUSE Foam also may be used to give added protection to other methods of contraception: with a condom; as a backup to the IUD or oral contraceptives during the first month of use; in the event more than one oral contraceptive pill is forgotten and extra protection is needed during that menstrual cycle.

Actions: Each applicatorful of BECAUSE Foam provides the correct amount of nonoxynol-9, the most widely used spermicide, to prevent pregnancy effectively. The foam covers the inside of the vagina and forms a layer of spermicidal material between the sperm and the cervix. The powerful spermicide prevents pregnancy by killing sperm after contact. BECAUSE Foam is effective immediately upon insertion. No waiting period is needed for effervescing or melting to take place since BECAUSE is introduced into the vagina as a foam.

Warnings: If vaginal or penile irritation occurs and continues, a physician should be consulted. Not effective orally. Where pregnancy is contraindicated, further individualization of the contraceptive program may be needed. Do not burn, incinerate or puncture container. Keep this and all drugs out of the reach of children and in case of accidental ingestion, call a Poison Control Center, emergency medical facility, or a doctor.

Dosage and Administration: Although no contraceptive can guarantee 100% effectiveness, for reliable protection against pregnancy follow directions. One applicatorful of BECAUSE Contraceptive Foam must be inserted before each act of sexual intercourse. BECAUSE Foam can be inserted immediately or up to one hour before intercourse. If more than one hour has passed before intercourse or if intercourse is repeated, another applicatorful of BECAUSE Foam must be inserted.

Directions for Use: The BECAUSE CONTRACEPTOR has a foam container attached to an applicator barrel.
With the container pushed all the way into the barrel, shake well. Pull the container upward until it stops. Tilt container to side to release foam into barrel. Allow foam to fill barrel to about one inch from end and return container to straight position. Foam will expand to fill remainder of barrel.
Hold contraceptor at top of the barrel part and gently insert applicator barrel deep into the vagina (close to the cervix). For ease of insertion, lie on your back with knees bent. With applicator barrel in place, push container all the way into the barrel. This deposits the foam properly. Remove the Contraceptor with the container still pushed all the way in the applicator barrel to avoid withdrawing any of the foam. No waiting period is needed before intercourse. BECAUSE Contraceptive Foam is effective immediately after proper insertion.
As with other vaginal contraceptive foam, cream and jelly products, douching is *not* recommended after using BECAUSE Foam. However, if douching is desired for cleansing purposes, you *must* wait at least six hours following your last act of sexual intercourse to allow BECAUSE Foam's full spermicidal activity to take place. Refer to package insert directions and diagrams for further details and applicator cleansing instructions.
How to Use the BECAUSE CONTRACEPTOR with a Diaphragm.
Insert one applicatorful of BECAUSE Foam directly into the vagina according to above directions and then insert diaphragm. After insertion, BECAUSE Foam is effective immediately and remains effective up to one hour before intercourse. If more than one hour has passed or you are going to repeat intercourse, insert another applicatorful of BECAUSE Foam *without removing your diaphragm.*

Storage: Contents under pressure. Do not burn, incinerate, or puncture the applicator. Store at normal room temperature. Do not expose to extreme heat or open flame or store at temperatures above 120°F. If stored at temperatures below 60°F, warm to room temperature before using.

How Supplied: Disposable 10 gm CONTRACEPTOR containing six applications of BECAUSE Contraceptive Foam. This foam is also available in two other forms, PRE-FIL® Foam with the "fill-in-advance" applicator and EMKO® Foam with the regular applicator.

Shown in Product Identification Section, page 427

EMKO®
Vaginal Contraceptive Foam

Description: A non-hormonal, non-scented aerosol foam contraceptive containing an 8.0% concentration of the spermicide nonoxynol-9.

Indications: Vaginal contraceptive intended for the prevention of pregnancy. EMKO Foam provides effective protection alone or it may be used instead of spermicidal jelly or cream to give added protection with a diaphragm.
EMKO Foam also may be used to give added protection to other methods of contraception: with a condom; as a backup to the IUD or oral contraceptives during the first month of use; in the event more than one oral contraceptive pill is forgotten and extra protection is needed during that menstrual cycle.

Actions: Each applicatorful of EMKO Foam provides the correct amount of nonoxynol-9, the most widely used spermicide, to prevent pregnancy effectively. The foam covers the inside of the vagina and forms a layer of spermicidal material between the sperm and the cervix. The powerful spermicide prevents pregnancy by killing sperm after contact. EMKO Foam is effective immediately upon insertion. No waiting period is needed for effervescing or melting to take place since EMKO is introduced into the vagina as a foam.

Warnings: If vaginal or penile irritation occurs and continues, a physician should be consulted. Where pregnancy is contraindicated, further individualization of the contraceptive program may be needed. Do not burn, incinerate or puncture can. Keep this and all drugs out of the reach of children and in case of accidental ingestion, call a Poison Control Center, emergency medical facility, or a doctor.

Dosage and Administration: Although no contraceptive can guarantee 100% effectiveness, for reliable protection against pregnancy read and follow directions carefully. One applicatorful of EMKO Contraceptive Foam must be inserted before each act of sexual intercourse. EMKO Foam can be inserted immediately or up to one hour before intercourse. If more than one hour has passed before intercourse or if intercourse is repeated, another applicatorful of EMKO Foam must be inserted.

Directions for Use:
Check Foam Supply with Weigh Cap.
With the cap on the can, hold the can in midair by the white button. As long as the black is showing, a full dose of foam is available. When the black begins to disappear, purchase a new can of EMKO Foam. USE *only if black is showing* to assure a full application. SHAKE CAN WELL before filling applicator. *Remove cap and place the can in an upright position on a level surface.* Place the EMKO regular applicator in an upright position

over valve on top of can. Press down on the applicator gently. Allow foam to fill to the ridge in applicator barrel. The plunger will rise up as the foam fills the applicator. Remove the filled applicator from the can to stop flow. Hold the filled applicator by the barrel and gently insert deep into the vagina (close to the cervix). For ease of insertion, lie on your back with knees bent. With the applicator in place, push plunger into applicator until it stops. This deposits the foam properly. Remove the applicator with the plunger still pushed all the way in to avoid withdrawing any of the foam. No waiting period is needed before intercourse. EMKO Contraceptive Foam is effective immediately after proper insertion. As with other vaginal contraceptive foam, cream, and jelly products, douching is *not* recommended after using EMKO Foam. However, if douching is desired for cleansing purposes, you *must* wait at least six hours following your last act of sexual intercourse to allow EMKO Foam's full spermicidal activity to take place. Refer to package insert directions and diagrams for further details and applicator cleansing instructions.
How to Use EMKO with a Diaphragm.
Insert one applicatorful of EMKO Foam directly into the vagina according to above directions and then insert your diaphragm. After insertion, EMKO Foam is effective immediately and remains effective up to one hour before intercourse. If more than one hour has passed or you are going to repeat intercourse, insert another applicatorful of EMKO Foam *without removing your diaphragm.*

Storage: Contents under pressure. Do not burn, incinerate or puncture can. Store at normal room temperature. Do not expose to extreme heat or open flame or store at temperatures above 120°F. If stored at temperatures below 60°F, warm to room temperature before using.

How Supplied: EMKO Contraceptive Foam, 40 gm can with applicator and storage purse. Refill cans without applicator and purse available in 40 gm and 90 gm sizes. All sizes feature a unique weighing cap that indicates when a new foam supply is needed. EMKO Foam also comes in two other forms, PRE-FIL® with the "fill-in-advance" applicator and BECAUSE® CONTRACEPTOR®, the portable six-use, combination foam/applicator unit.

Shown in Product Identification Section, page 427

EMKO® PRE-FIL®
Vaginal Contraceptive Foam

Description: A non-hormonal, non-scented aerosol foam contraceptive, for use with the "fill-in-advance" applicator, containing an 8.0% concentration of the spermicide nonoxynol-9.

Indications: Vaginal contraceptive intended for the prevention of pregnancy. PRE-FIL Foam provides effective protection alone or it may be used instead of

spermicidal jelly or cream to give added protection with a diaphragm.
PRE-FIL Foam also may be used to give added protection to other methods of contraception: with a condom; as a backup to the IUD or oral contraceptives during the first month of use; in the event more than one oral contraceptive pill is forgotten and extra protection is needed during that menstrual cycle.

Actions: Each applicatorful of PRE-FIL Foam provides the correct amount of nonoxynol-9, the most widely used spermicide, to prevent pregnancy effectively. The foam covers the inside of the vagina and forms a layer of spermicidal material between the sperm and the cervix. The powerful spermicide prevents pregnancy by killing sperm after contact. PRE-FIL Foam is effective immediately upon insertion. No waiting period is needed for effervescing or melting to take place since PRE-FIL is introduced into the vagina as a foam.

Warnings: If vaginal or penile irritation occurs and continues, a physician should be consulted. Where pregnancy is contraindicated, further individualization of the contraceptive program may be needed. Do not burn, incinerate or puncture can. Keep this and all drugs out of the reach of children and in case of accidental ingestion, call a Poison Control Center, emergency medical facility, or a doctor.

Dosage and Administration: Although no contraceptive can guarantee 100% effectiveness, for reliable protection against pregnancy read and follow directions carefully. One applicatorful of PRE-FIL Contraceptive Foam must be inserted before each act of sexual intercourse. PRE-FIL Foam can be inserted immediately or up to one hour before intercourse. If more than one hour has passed before intercourse or if intercourse is repeated, another applicatorful of PRE-FIL Foam must be inserted.

Directions for Use:
Check Foam Supply with Weigh Cap.
With the cap on the can, hold the can in midair by the white button. As long as the black is showing, a full dose of foam is available. When the black begins to disappear, purchase a new can of PRE-FIL FOAM. USE *only if black is showing* to assure a full application. SHAKE CAN GENTLY before filling applicator.
Remove cap and place the can in an upright position on a level surface.
PRE-FIL Foam can only be used with the special "fill-in-advance" applicator. The PRE-FIL applicator has two parts: an inner tube and an outer barrel. Remove inner tube from outer barrel. Place *inner* tube in upright position over valve on top of can and press down until pink plunger stops rising. Continue to press for a few seconds before removing inner tube from

Continued on next page

Information on Schering products appearing on these pages is effective as of January 1, 1985.

Schering—Cont.

can. To be sure inner tube is completely filled, press pink plunger. If it can be depressed, inner tube is not full—repeat filling procedure.

Place inner tube into outer barrel. *The foam can only be released when the inner tube is inside the outer barrel.* Gently insert applicator deep into the vagina (close to the cervix). For ease of insertion, lie on your back with knees bent. With the applicator in place, push pink plunger back into applicator until it stops. This deposits the foam properly. Remove the applicator with the plunger still pushed all the way in to avoid withdrawing any of the foam. No waiting period is needed before intercourse. PRE-FIL Contraceptive Foam is effective immediately after proper insertion.

PRE-FIL's "fill-in-advance" applicator can be filled and stored, ready for use either immediately or up to seven days.

As with other vaginal contraceptive foam, cream and jelly products, douching is *not* recommended after using PRE-FIL Foam. However, if douching is desired for cleansing purposes, you *must* wait at least six hours following your last act of sexual intercourse to allow PRE-FIL Foam's full spermicidal activity to take place. Refer to package insert directions and diagrams for further details and applicator cleansing instructions.

How to Use PRE-FIL with a Diaphragm Insert one applicatorful of PRE-FIL Foam directly into the vagina according to above directions and then insert diaphragm. After insertion, PRE-FIL Foam is effective immediately and remains effective up to one hour before intercourse. If more than one hour has passed or you are going to repeat intercourse, insert another applicatorful of PRE-FIL Foam *without removing your diaphragm.*

Storage: Contents under pressure. Do not burn, incinerate, or puncture can or filled applicator. Store at normal room temperature. Do not expose to extreme heat or open flame or store at temperatures above 120°F. If stored at temperatures below 60°F, warm to room temperature before using. Prefilled applicator may be stored up to seven days.

How Supplied: EMKO PRE-FIL Contraceptive Foam, 30 gm can with applicator and purse. Refill can without applicator and purse in 60 gm size. Both sizes feature a unique weighing cap that indicates when a new supply of foam is needed. This foam also comes in two other forms, EMKO® Foam with the regular applicator and BECAUSE® CONTRACEPTOR®, the portable six-use, combination foam/applicator unit.

Shown in Product Identification Section, page 427

MOL–IRON®
Tablets
CHRONOSULE® Capsules
Tablets with Vitamin C

Active Ingredients: MOL-IRON products contain a specially processed preparation of ferrous sulfate. They are highly effective and unusually well tolerated even by children and pregnant women. Tablets: Each tablet contains 195 mg ferrous sulfate, USP (39 mg elemental iron). CHRONOSULE Capsules: Each capsule contains 390 mg ferrous sulfate, USP (78 mg elemental iron) in sustained release form.

Tablets with Vitamin C: Each tablet contains 195 mg ferrous sulfate (39 mg elemental iron) and 75 mg ascorbic acid.

Indications: For the prevention and treatment of iron-deficiency anemias. The CHRONOSULE capsules supply adequate amounts of iron in the form of specially coated beadlets, fabricated to disintegrate gradually over a 6 to 8 hour period, effecting a continued release of absorbable ferrous iron while traversing the stomach and small intestine.
Unpleasant side effects are minimized.

Warnings: Keep these and all drugs out of the reach of children. In case of accidental overdose, seek professional assistance or contact a Poison Control Center immediately. As with any drug, if you are pregnant or nursing a baby, seek the advice of a health professional before using this product.

Precautions: MOL-IRON Tablets, Tablets with Vitamin C, and CHRONO-SULE capsules contain FD&C Yellow No. 5 (tartrazine) as a color additive. Persons sensitive to tartrazine or aspirin should consult a physician.

Dosage and Administration: Tablets—(Taken preferably after meals): Adults and Children 12 years and older—1 or 2 tablets 3 times daily; Children 6 through 11 years—1 tablet 3 times daily; or as prescribed by a physician. CHRONOSULE Capsules—(Taken preferably after meals): Adults and Children 12 years and older—1 CHRONOSULE capsule once or twice daily; Children 6 through 11 years—1 capsule daily; or as prescribed by a physician. Tablets with Vitamin C—(Taken preferably after meals): Adults and Children 12 years and older—1 or 2 tablets 3 times daily; Children 6 through 11 years—1 tablet 3 times daily; or as prescribed by a physician.

How Supplied: MOL-IRON Tablets—brownish colored tablets, bottles of 100; MOL-IRON CHRONOSULE Capsules—bottles of 30 and 250; MOL-IRON Tablets with Vitamin C—bottles of 100.
Store the tablet and capsule forms between 2° and 30°C (36° and 86°F).

Shown in Product Identification Section, page 427

SUNRIL® Premenstrual Capsules

Active Ingredients: Each capsule contains: Acetaminophen 300 mg, an effective analgesic. Pamabrom 50 mg (2-amino- 2-methyl- 1-propanol- 8-bromotheophyllinate), a mild, effective diuretic. Pyrilamine maleate 25 mg, a mild antihistamine.

Indications: For relief of premenstrual tension, edema and related pain.

Warning: Keep out of reach of children. As with any drug, if you are pregnant or nursing a baby, seek the advice of a health professional before using this product.

Precautions: Do not drive or operate machinery while taking this medication as this preparation may cause drowsiness. Limit dosage to no more than 10 consecutive days unless recommended by your physician. Should not be used by anyone with a known sensitivity to any one of the ingredients.

Overdosage: In case of accidental overdose, seek professional assistance or contact a Poison Control Center immediately.

Dosage and Administration: 1 capsule every 3 to 4 hours. Do not exceed 4 capsules within a 24 hour period. Start using at first sign of discomfort, usually 4 to 7 days before onset of menstruation.

How Supplied: SUNRIL® Premenstrual Capsules are pink and lavender capsules; available in bottles of 100. Store at room temperature.

TINACTIN® Antifungal
Cream 1%
Solution 1%
Powder 1%
Powder (1%) Aerosol
Liquid (1%) Aerosol
Jock Itch Cream 1%
Jock Itch Spray Powder 1%

Description: TINACTIN Cream 1% is a white homogeneous, nonaqueous preparation containing the highly active synthetic fungicidal agent, tolnaftate. Each gram contains 10 mg tolnaftate solubilized in polyethylene glycol-400 and propylene glycol with carboxypolymethylene, monoamylamine, titanium dioxide, and butylated hydroxytoluene.

TINACTIN Jock Itch Cream 1% is a smooth white homogeneous cream containing the highly active synthetic fungicidal agent, tolnaftate. Each gram contains 10 mg tolnaftate finely dispersed in a water-washable emulsion containing white petrolatum, propylene glycol, cetearyl alcohol, mineral oil, polyethylene glycol 1000 monocetyl ether, sodium phosphate monobasic monohydrate and chlorocresol. Phosphoric acid and sodium hydroxide used to adjust pH.

TINACTIN Solution 1% contains in each ml tolnaftate, 10 mg and butylated hydroxytoluene, 1 mg in a nonaqueous, homogeneous vehicle of polyethylene glycol-400. The solution solidifies at low temperatures but liquefies readily when warmed, retaining its potency.

TINACTIN Liquid Aerosol contains 91 mg tolnaftate in a vehicle of butylated hydroxytoluene and polyethylene-polypropylene glycol monobutyl ether. It also contains 36% denatured alcohol w/w and sufficient inert propellant of isobutane to make 113 g. The spray deposits solution containing a concentration of 1% tolnaftate.

Each gram of TINACTIN Powder 1% contains tolnaftate 10 mg in a vehicle of corn starch and talc.

TINACTIN Powder Aerosol contains 91 mg tolnaftate in a vehicle of butylated hydroxytoluene, talc, and polyethylene-polypropylene glycol monobutyl ether. It also contains 14% denatured alcohol and sufficient inert propellant of isobutane to make 100 grams. The spray deposits a white clinging powder containing a concentration of 1% tolnaftate.

TINACTIN Jock Itch Spray Powder contains 91 mg tolnaftate in a vehicle of butylated hydroxytoluene, talc, and polyethylene-polypropylene glycol monobutyl ether. It also contains 14% denatured alcohol and sufficient inert propellant of isobutane to make 100 grams. The spray deposits a white clinging powder containing a concentration of 1% tolnaftate.

Indications: TINACTIN Cream, Solution, Liquid Aerosol and TINACTIN Jock Itch Cream are highly active antifungal agents that are effective in killing superficial fungi of the skin which cause tinea pedis (athlete's foot), tinea cruris (jock itch) and tinea corporis (body ringworm). TINACTIN Powder, Powder Aerosol and TINACTIN Jock Itch Spray Powder are effective in killing superficial fungi of the skin which cause tinea cruris (jock itch) and tinea pedis (athlete's foot). All forms begin to relieve burning, itching and soreness within 24 hours. The powder and powder aerosol forms aid the drying of naturally moist areas.

Actions: The active ingredient in TINACTIN, tolnaftate, is a highly active synthetic fungicidal agent that is effective in the treatment of superficial fungous infections of the skin. It is inactive systemically, virtually nonsensitizing, and does not ordinarily sting or irritate intact or broken skin, even in the presence of acute inflammatory reactions. TINACTIN products are odorless, greaseless, and do not stain or discolor the skin, hair, or nails.

Warnings: Keep these and all drugs out of the reach of children. Do not use in children under 2 years of age except under the advice and supervision of a physician.

TINACTIN Powder Aerosol and Liquid Aerosol: Avoid spraying in eyes. Contents under pressure. Do not puncture or incinerate. Flammable mixture, do not use or store near heat or open flame. Exposure to temperatures above 120°F may cause bursting. Never throw container into fire or incinerator. Use only as directed. Intentional misuse by deliberately concentrating and inhaling the contents can be harmful or fatal.

Precautions: If irritation occurs or symptoms do not improve within 10 days, discontinue use and consult your physician or podiatrist.

TINACTIN products are for external use only. Keep out of eyes.

TINACTIN is not effective on nail or scalp infections.

Overdosage: In case of accidental ingestion, seek professional assistance or contact a Poison Control Center immediately.

Dosage and Administration: Children under 12 years of age should be supervised in the use of TINACTIN.

TINACTIN Cream and TINACTIN Jock Itch Cream—Wash and dry infected area. Then apply one-half inch ribbon of cream and rub gently on infected area morning and evening or as directed by a doctor. Spread evenly. Best results in athlete's foot and body ringworm are usually obtained with 4 weeks' use of this product and in jock itch, with 2 weeks' use. To help prevent recurrence of athlete's foot, continue treatment for two weeks after disappearance of all symptoms.

TINACTIN Solution—Wash and dry infected area. Then apply two or three drops morning and evening or as directed by a doctor, and massage gently to cover the infected area. Best results in athlete's foot and body ringworm are usually obtained with 4 weeks' use of this product and in jock itch, with 2 weeks' use. To help prevent recurrence of athlete's foot, continue treatment for two weeks after disappearance of all symptoms.

TINACTIN Liquid Aerosol—Wash and dry infected area. Spray from a distance of 6 to 10 inches morning and evening or as directed by a doctor. For athlete's foot, spray between toes and on feet. For jock itch, spray infected area. Best results in athlete's foot are usually obtained with 4 weeks' use of this product and in jock itch, with 2 weeks' use. Continue treatment for two weeks after symptoms disappear. To help prevent reinfection of athlete's foot, bathe daily, dry carefully and apply TINACTIN Powder daily.

TINACTIN Powder—Wash and dry infected area. Sprinkle powder liberally on all areas of infection and in shoes or socks morning and evening or as directed by a doctor. Best results in athlete's foot are usually obtained with 4 weeks' use of this product and in jock itch, with 2 weeks' use. Continue treatment for two weeks after symptoms disappear. To prevent recurrence of athlete's foot, bathe daily, dry carefully and apply TINACTIN Powder.

TINACTIN Powder Aerosol and TINACTIN Jock Itch Spray Powder—Wash and dry infected area. Shake container well before using. Spray liberally from a distance of 6 to 10 inches onto affected area morning and night or as directed by a doctor. Best results in athlete's foot are usually obtained with 4 weeks' use of this product and in jock itch, with 2 weeks' use. To help prevent recurrence of athlete's foot, bathe daily, dry carefully and apply TINACTIN Powder Aerosol.

How Supplied: TINACTIN Antifungal Cream 1%, 15 g (½ oz) collapsible tube with dispensing tip. TINACTIN Antifungal Solution 1%, 10 ml (⅓ oz) plastic squeeze bottle. TINACTIN Antifungal

Liquid (1%) Aerosol, 113 g (4 oz) spray can. TINACTIN Antifungal Powder 1%, 45 g (1.5 oz) plastic container. TINACTIN Antifungal Powder (1%) Aerosol, 100 g (3.5 oz) spray can. TINACTIN Antifungal Jock Itch Cream 1%, 15 g (½ oz) collapsible tube with dispensing tip. TINACTIN Antifungal Jock Itch Spray Powder (1%), 100 g (3.5 oz) spray can.

Store TINACTIN products between 36° and 86°F (2° and 30°C).

© 1984, Schering Corporation, Kenilworth NJ 07033

Shown in Product Identification Section, page 427 & 428

Information on Schering products appearing on these pages is effective as of January 1, 1985.

Searle Consumer Products
Division of G. D. Searle & Co.
BOX 5110
CHICAGO, IL 60680

**DRAMAMINE® Liquid
(dimenhydrinate syrup USP)
DRAMAMINE® Tablets
(dimenhydrinate USP)**

Description: Dimenhydrinate is the chlorotheophylline salt of the antihistaminic agent diphenhydramine. Dimenhydrinate contains not less than 53% and not more than 56% of diphenhydramine, and not less than 44% and not more than 47% of 8-chlorotheophylline, calculated on the dried basis.

Actions: While the precise mode of action of dimenhydrinate is not known, it has a depressant action on hyperstimulated labyrinthine function.

Indications: Dramamine is indicated for the prevention and treatment of the nausea, vomiting or vertigo of motion sickness. Such an illness may arise from the motion of ships, planes, trains, automobiles, buses, swings, or even amusement park rides. Regardless of the cause of motion sickness, Dramamine has been found to be effective in its prevention or treatment.

Warnings: Caution should be used when Dramamine is taken in conjunction with certain antibiotics that may cause ototoxicity, since Dramamine is capable of masking ototoxic symptoms and an irreversible state may be reached. As with any drug, pregnant or nursing women should seek the advice of a health professional before using this product.

Precautions: Drowsiness may be experienced, especially with high dosages, although this action frequently is not undesirable in some conditions for which the drug is used. However, because of possible drowsiness, patients taking Dramamine should be cautioned against operating automobiles or dangerous ma-

Continued on next page

Searle Consumer—Cont.

chinery. Avoid alcoholic beverages while taking medication. Dramamine should not be used in the presence of asthma, glaucoma, or enlargement of the prostate gland, except on advice of a physician.

Dosage and Administration

Dramamine Tablets: To prevent motion sickness, the first dose should be taken ½ to 1 hour before starting the activity. Additional medication depends on travel conditions. *Adults:* Nausea or vomiting may be expected to be controlled for approximately 4 hours with 50 mg of Dramamine (dimenhydrinate), and prevented by a similar dose every 4 hours. Its administration may be attended by some degree of drowsiness in some patients, and 100 mg every 4 hours may be given in conditions in which drowsiness is not objectionable or is even desirable. The usual adult dosage is 1 to 2 tablets every 4 to 6 hours, not to exceed 8 tablets in 24 hours. *Children 6 to 12 years:* ½ to 1 tablet every 6 to 8 hours, not to exceed 3 tablets in 24 hours. *Children 2 to 6 years:* Up to ½ tablet every 6 to 8 hours, not to exceed 1½ tablets in 24 hours. Children may also be given Dramamine cherry-flavored liquid in accordance with directions for use. Not for frequent or prolonged use except on advice of a physician. Do not exceed recommended dosage.

Dramamine Liquid: To prevent motion sickness, the first dose should be taken ½ to 1 hour before starting the activity. Additional medication depends on travel conditions. *Adults:* 4 to 8 teaspoonfuls (4 ml per teaspoonful) every 4 to 6 hours, not to exceed 32 teaspoonfuls in 24 hours. *Children 6 to 12 years:* 2 to 4 teaspoonfuls every 6 to 8 hours, not to exceed 12 teaspoonfuls in 24 hours. *Children 2 to 6 years:* 1 to 2 teaspoonfuls every 6 to 8 hours, not to exceed 6 teaspoonfuls in 24 hours. *Children under 2 years:* Only on advice of a physician.

Not for frequent or prolonged use except on advice of a physician. Do not exceed recommended dosage. Use of a measuring device is recommended for all liquid medication.

How Supplied: *Tablets*—scored, white tablets of 50 mg, with SEARLE debossed on one side and 1701 on the other side, in packets of 12 and bottles of 36 and 100 (OTC); also available in single-dose packets of 100 and in bottles of 1,000. *Liquid*—12.5 mg per 4 ml, ethyl alcohol 5%, bottles of 3 fl oz (OTC); also available in pint bottles.

Shown in Product Identification Section, page 428

EQUAL® Packets
EQUAL® Sweet-Tabs
(low-calorie sweetener)

Description: Equal contains Nutra-Sweet® brand of aspartame (L-aspartyl-L-phenylalanine methyl ester), a sweetening agent made from protein components such as those found naturally in many foods. One packet equals the sweetness of 2 teaspoons of sugar; one Sweet-Tab equals the sweetness of 1 teaspoon of sugar.

Actions: Equal dissolves quickly in hot or cold beverages with minimal stirring. It can also be used to sweeten other foods, such as fruits and cereal.

Usage: Equal is a low-calorie sweetener for persons who want to or must restrict their intake of sugar. It contains no sucrose or saccharin and is sodium free. Each packet contains approximately 1 g of carbohydrate and provides 4 calories. Each tablet provides less than half a calorie. Equal tablets are not for use in cooking or baking, but Equal powder can be added to some recipes immediately after cooking.

Warning: Phenylketonurics should be aware that Equal contains phenylalanine.

How Supplied: Packets are available in cartons of 50, 100 and 200; Sweet-Tabs are available in dispensers of 100.

Shown in Product Identification Section, page 428

ICY HOT® Balm
(topical analgesic balm)
ICY HOT® Rub
(topical analgesic cream)

Active Ingredients: Icy Hot Balm contains methyl salicylate 29%, menthol 7.6%. Icy Hot Rub contains methyl salicylate 12%, menthol 9%.

Description: Icy Hot Balm and Icy Hot Rub are topically applied analgesics containing two active ingredients, methyl salicylate and menthol. It is the particular concentration of these ingredients, in combination with inert ingredients, that results in the distinct, combined heating/cooling sensation of Icy Hot.

Actions: Icy Hot is classified as a counterirritant which, when rubbed into the intact skin, provides relief of deep-seated pain through a counterirritant action rather than through a direct analgesic effect. In acting as a counterirritant, Icy Hot replaces the perception of pain with another sensation that blocks deep pain temporarily by its action on or near the skin surface.

Indications: Icy Hot helps bring temporary relief from minor arthritis pain and its stiffness, helps temporarily block minor pain from simple backache, and helps soothe sore muscles.

Warnings: For external use only as directed. Keep away from children to avoid accidental poisoning. If swallowed, induce vomiting and call a physician immediately. For children under 12, consult a physician before use. Avoid contact with eyes, mouth, genitalia, and mucous membranes. Do not apply to wounds or to damaged or very sensitive skin. Diabetics and people with impaired circulation should use Icy Hot only upon the advice of a physician. Do not wrap, bandage or apply external heat or hot water. If condition worsens, or if symptoms persist for more than 7 days or clear up and occur again within a few days, discontinue use of this product and consult a physician.

Adverse Reactions: The most common adverse reactions that may occur with Icy Hot use are skin irritation and blistering. The most serious adverse reaction is severe toxicity that occurs if the product is ingested.

Dosage and Administration: Apply Icy Hot to the painful area; massage until Icy Hot is completely absorbed. Repeat as necessary up to four times daily.

How Supplied: Icy Hot Balm is available in jars in two sizes—3½ oz and 7 oz. Icy Hot Rub is available in tubes in two sizes—1¼ oz and 3 oz.

Shown in Product Identification Section, page 428

Regular Flavor
METAMUCIL® Powder
(psyllium hydrophilic mucilloid)

Description: Regular Flavor Metamucil is a bulk laxative containing refined hydrophilic mucilloid, a highly efficient dietary fiber derived from the husk of the psyllium seed (*Plantago ovata*). An equal amount of dextrose, a carbohydrate, is added as a dispersing agent. Each dose contains about 1 mg of sodium, 31 mg of potassium, and 14 calories. Carbohydrate content is approximately 3.5 g; psyllium mucilloid content is 3.4 g.

Actions: Metamucil provides a bland, nonirritating bulk and promotes normal elimination. It is uniform, instantly miscible, palatable, and nonirritative in the gastrointestinal tract.

Indications: Metamucil is indicated in the management of chronic constipation, in irritable bowel syndrome, as adjunctive therapy in the constipation of duodenal ulcer and diverticular disease, in the bowel management of patients with hemorrhoids, and for constipation during pregnancy, convalescence, and senility.

Contraindications: Intestinal obstruction, fecal impaction.

Dosage and Administration: The usual adult dosage is one rounded teaspoonful (7 g) stirred into a standard 8-oz glass of cool water or other suitable liquid and taken orally one to three times a day, depending on the need and response. It may require continuing use for 2 or 3 days to provide optimal benefit. Best results are observed if each dose is followed by an additional glass of liquid.

How Supplied: Powder, containers of 7 oz, 14 oz, and 21 oz (OTC); also available in cartons of 100 single-dose (7 g) packets.

Shown in Product Identification Section, page 428

Sugar Free Regular Flavor
METAMUCIL® Powder
(psyllium hydrophilic mucilloid)

Description: Sugar Free Regular Flavor Metamucil is a bulk laxative containing refined hydrophilic mucilloid, a highly efficient dietary fiber derived from the husk of the psyllium seed (*Plantago ovata*), which has been sweetened with NutraSweet® brand of aspartame. It contains no chemical stimulants or sugar. Each dose contains 3.4 g of psyllium mucilloid, less than 0.01 g of sodium, 0.006 g of phenylalanine, and about 1 calorie.

Actions: Metamucil provides a bland, nonirritating bulk and promotes normal elimination. It is uniform, instantly miscible, palatable, and nonirritative in the gastrointestinal tract.

Indications: Metamucil is indicated in the management of chronic constipation, in irritable bowel syndrome, as adjunctive therapy in the constipation of duodenal ulcer and diverticular disease, in the bowel management of patients with hemorrhoids, and for constipation during pregnancy, convalescence, and senility.

Contraindications: Intestinal obstruction, fecal impaction.

Warning: Phenylketonurics should be aware that Sugar Free Metamucil contains phenylalanine.

Dosage and Administration: The usual adult dosage is one rounded teaspoonful (3.7 g) stirred into a standard 8-oz glass of cool water or other suitable liquid and taken orally one to three times a day, depending on the need and response. It may require continuing use for 2 or 3 days to provide optimal benefit. Best results are observed if each dose is followed by an additional glass of liquid.

How Supplied: Powder, containers of 3.7 oz, 7.4 oz, and 11.1 oz (OTC); also available in cartons of 100 single-dose (3.7 g) packets.
Shown in Product Identification Section, page 428

Orange Flavor
METAMUCIL® Powder
Strawberry Flavor
METAMUCIL® Powder
(psyllium hydrophilic mucilloid)

Description: Orange Flavor and Strawberry Flavor Metamucil are bulk laxatives containing refined hydrophilic mucilloid, a highly efficient dietary fiber derived from the husk of the psyllium seed (*Plantago ovata*), with sucrose (a carbohydrate) as a dispersing agent, citric acid, flavoring, and coloring. Each dose contains about 1 mg of sodium, 31 mg of potassium, and 28 calories. Carbohydrate content is approximately 7.1 g; psyllium mucilloid content is 3.4 g.

Actions: Metamucil provides a bland, nonirritating bulk and promotes normal elimination. It is uniform, instantly mis-

cible, palatable, and nonirritative in the gastrointestinal tract.

Indications: Metamucil is indicated in the management of chronic constipation, in irritable bowel syndrome, as adjunctive therapy in the constipation of duodenal ulcer and diverticular disease, in the bowel management of patients with hemorrhoids, and for constipation during pregnancy, convalescence, and senility.

Contraindications: Intestinal obstruction, fecal impaction.

Dosage and Administration: The usual adult dosage is one rounded tablespoonful (11 g) stirred into a standard 8-oz glass of cool water and taken orally one to three times a day, depending on the need and response. It may require continuing use for 2 or 3 days to provide optimal benefit. Best results are observed if each dose is followed by an additional glass of liquid.

How Supplied: Powder, containers of 7 oz, 14 oz, and 21 oz.
Shown in Product Identification Section, page 428

Regular Flavor
INSTANT MIX METAMUCIL®
(psyllium hydrophilic mucilloid)

Description: Regular Flavor Instant Mix Metamucil is a bulk laxative containing refined hydrophilic mucilloid, a highly efficient dietary fiber derived from the husk of the psyllium seed (*Plantago ovata*), together with citric acid, sucrose (a carbohydrate), potassium bicarbonate, calcium carbonate, flavoring, and sodium bicarbonate. Each dose contains approximately 7 mg of sodium, 60 mg of calcium, 280 mg of potassium, and less than 4 calories. Carbohydrate content is about 0.9 g: psyllium mucilloid content is 3.6 g.

Actions: Instant Mix Metamucil provides a bland, nonirritating bulk and promotes normal elimination. It is effervescent and requires no stirring, and it is uniform, instantly miscible, palatable, and nonirritative in the gastrointestinal tract.

Indications: Instant Mix Metamucil is indicated in the management of chronic constipation, in irritable bowel syndrome, as adjunctive therapy in the constipation of duodenal ulcer and diverticular disease, in the bowel management of patients with hemorrhoids, and for constipation during pregnancy, convalescence, and senility.

Contraindications: Intestinal obstruction, fecal impaction.

Dosage and Administration: The usual adult dosage is the contents of one packet (6.4 g) taken one to three times daily as follows: (1) Entire contents of a packet are poured into a standard 8-oz water glass. (2) The glass is slowly filled with cool water. (3) Entire contents are to be drunk immediately. (An additional

glass of water may be taken for best results.)

How Supplied: Cartons of 16 and 30 single-dose (6.4 g) packets (OTC); also available in cartons of 100 single-dose (6.4 g) packets.
Shown in Product Identification Section, page 428

Orange Flavor
INSTANT MIX METAMUCIL®
(psyllium hydrophilic mucilloid)

Description: Orange Flavor Instant Mix Metamucil is a bulk laxative containing refined hydrophilic mucilloid, a highly efficient dietary fiber derived from the husk of the psyllium seed (*Plantago ovata),* together with sucrose (a carbohydrate), citric acid, potassium bicarbonate, flavoring, coloring, and sodium bicarbonate. Each dose contains approximately 6 mg of sodium, 307 mg of potassium, and 4½ calories. Carbohydrate content is about 1.1 g; psyllium mucilloid content is 3.6 g.

Actions: Instant Mix Metamucil provides a bland, nonirritating bulk and promotes normal elimination. It is effervescent and requires no stirring, and it is uniform, instantly miscible, palatable, and nonirritative in the gastrointestinal tract.

Indications: Instant Mix Metamucil is indicated in the management of chronic constipation, in irritable bowel syndrome, as adjunctive therapy in the constipation of duodenal ulcer and diverticular disease, in the bowel management of patients with hemorrhoids, and for constipation during pregnancy, convalescence, and senility.

Contraindications: Intestinal obstruction, fecal impaction.

Dosage and Administration: The usual adult dosage is the contents of one packet (6.4 g) taken one to three times daily as follows: (1) Entire contents of a packet are poured into a standard 8-oz water glass. (2) The glass is slowly filled with cool water. (3) Entire contents are to be drunk immediately. (An additional glass of water may be taken for best results.)

How Supplied: Cartons of 16 and 30 single-dose (6.4 g) packets.
Shown in Product Identification Section, page 428

PROMPT®
(psyllium hydrophilic mucilloid with sennosides)

Description: Prompt combines a natural-source stimulant laxative with bulk-producing dietary fiber for gentle overnight relief from constipation. Prompt contains no artificial chemicals. Each individual-dose packet or one rounded teaspoonful of bulk powder (6.5 g) contains psyllium hydrophilic mucilloid 3.5 g, and sennosides 12.4 mg, with sucrose.

Continued on next page

Searle Consumer—Cont.

Actions: Prompt provides gentle, effective stimulation to the colon, and additionally provides bland, nonirritating bulk to encourage normal elimination. The bulk in the bowel aids in the prevention of rebound constipation, thus helping to avoid a laxative habit.

Indication: Prompt is indicated for short-term relief of constipation. Onset of action is generally within 8 to 10 hours.

Contraindications: Intestinal obstruction, fecal impaction.

Warnings: Prompt or any laxative should not be taken when nausea, vomiting, or abdominal pain is present. Habitual use of laxatives may result in dependence on them. As with any drug, pregnant or nursing women should seek the advice of a health professional before using this product.

Drug Interactions: None known.

Symptoms and Treatment of Oral Overdosage: Treat symptomatically; there is no specific antidote.

Dosage and Administration: *Adults:* A single daily dose is usually taken at bedtime. Stir the contents of one to two packets, or one to two rounded teaspoonfuls of bulk powder, into an 8-oz glass of cold juice or water and drink immediately. *Children 6 to 12 years:* Use one-half of the adult dose.

How Supplied: Powder, containers of 2½ oz and 5 oz; single-dose packets, cartons of 12 (OTC); also available in cartons of 100 single-dose (6.5 g) packets.
Shown in Product Identification Section, page 428

The preceding prescribing information for Searle Consumer Products was current as of February 1, 1985.

Solgar Company, Inc.
410 OCEAN AVENUE
LYNBROOK, NY 11563

STRESS FORMULA
B–COMPLEX WITH C

Provides dietary supplementation for Vitamin C and B-Complex.

Supplied: Bottles of 100, 250 and 500 tablets.

BETA CAROTENE CAPSULES
(PROVITAMIN A)

Each capsule provides: Natural Beta Carotene (Provitamin A) sufficient to convert to 11,000 IU of Vitamin A.

Supplied: Bottles of 50 and 100 capsules.

BIOTIN TABLETS
300 mcg, 600 mcg (VITAMIN H)

Supplied: Bottles of 100 and 250 tablets.

CALCIUM 600
From Oyster Shells

Two tablets provide 1200 mg of calcium (calcium carbonate) with 400 IU of vitamin D.

Supplied: Bottles of 60 and 120 tablets.

CHEWS–EZE TABLETS
NATURAL CHILDREN'S CHEWABLE VITAMIN SUPPLEMENT WITH BEE POLLEN AND ORANGE JUICE CRYSTALS. SALT AND STARCH FREE
• VEGETARIAN FORMULA

Provides essential multi-vitamins for children under 4 years of age. Chew or allow to dissolve in the mouth. May be crushed and sprinkled over cereal or dissolved in milk or other liquids.
Each Tablet Provides:

Vitamin A	5000 IU
Vitamin D	400 IU
Vitamin B-1	3 mg
Vitamin B-2	6 mg
Niacinamide	1.71 mg
Vitamin C	100 mg
Vitamin B-12	5 mcg
Vitamin E	5 IU

Supplied: Bottles of 30, 90, 180 tablets.

CHOLINE/INOSITOL TABLETS
250/250 mg

A dietary supplement containing Choline and Inositol, members of the B-Complex family.

Supplied: Bottles of 100 and 250 tablets.

FORMULA B–50 CAPSULES
HIGH POTENCY B-COMPLEX FORMULA

A balanced proportion of all the recognized B-Complex factors.
Each Capsule Provides:

Vitamin B-1	50 mg
Vitamin B-2	50 mg
Vitamin B-6	50 mg
Vitamin B-12	50 mcg
Niacinamide	50 mg
Folic Acid	400 mcg
Pantothenic Acid	50 mg
Para Aminobenzoic Acid	50 mg
Choline Bitartrate	50 mg
Inositol	50 mg
Biotin	50 mcg

Supplied: Bottles of 50, 100 and 250 capsules.

FORMULA VM–75 TABLETS
EXTRA HIGH POTENCY— BALANCED B-COMPLEX WITH CHELATED MINERALS

Each Tablet Daily Provides:

Vitamin C (with Rose Hips)	250 mg
Vitamin E (d-Alpha Tocopherol)	150 IU
Vitamin A (Palmitate)	25,000 IU
Vitamin D	1,000 IU
Vitamin B-1 (Thiamine)	75 mg
Vitamin B-2 (Riboflavin)	75 mg
Vitamin B-6 (Pyridoxine)	75 mg
Vitamin B-12	75 mcg
Niacinamde	75 mg
Choline Bitartrate	75 mg
Inositol	75 mg
Para Aminobenzoic Acid	75 mg
Pantothenic Acid	75 mg
Biotin	75 mcg
Folic Acid	400 mcg
Rutin	25 mg
Citrus Bioflavonoid Complex	25 mg
Hesperidin Complex	5 mg
Betaine HCl	25 mg
Glutamic Acid	25 mg
Iodine (Kelp)	150 mcg
Calcium Amino Acid Chelate	50 mg
Potassium Amino Acid Complex	10 mg
Iron Amino Acid Chelate	10 mg
Magnesium Amino Acid Chelate	7.2 mg
Manganese Amino Acid Chelate	6.1 mg
Zinc Amino Acid Chelate	15 mg
Selenium	10 mcg

Supplied: Bottles of 30, 60, 90 and 180 tablets.
Shown in Product Identification Section, page 428

HY–C TABLETS
HIGH POTENCY VITAMIN C SUPPLEMENT

Vitamin C with Rose Hips and Citrus Bioflavonoid Complex, Rutin and Hesperidin Complex.
Each Tablet Contains:

Vitamin C	600 mg
Citrus Bioflavonoid Complex	100 mg
Rutin	50 mg
Hesperidin Complex	25 mg

Supplied: Bottles of 50, 100, 250, 500 and 1000 tablets.

LIVER TABLETS
11 GRAINS

Natural Desiccated and Defatted Argentinian Liver fortified with Vitamin B-12 and Red Bone Marrow. Provides the naturally occurring B-Complex Factors and Amino Acids found in Dried Beef Liver.

Supplied: Bottles of 100, 250, 500 and 1000 tablets.

L–TRYPTOPHAN CAPSULES
500 mg

Supplied: Bottles of 30, 60 and 90 capsules.

VITAMIN B-1 TABLETS (Thiamine)
25 mg, 50 mg, 100 mg and 500 mg

Supplied: Bottles of 100, 250 and 500 tablets.

VITAMIN B-2 TABLETS (Riboflavin)
10 mg, 25 mg, 50 mg and 100 mg

Supplied: Bottles of 100, 250 and 500 tablets.

VITAMIN B-6 TABLETS (Pyridoxine)
25 mg, 50 mg, 100 mg and 500 mg

Supplied: Bottles of 100, 250 and 500 tablets.

VITAMIN B-12 TABLETS
50 mcg, 100 mcg, 250 mcg, 500 mcg and 1000 mcg

Supplied: Bottles of 100, 250 and 500 tablets.

VITAMIN C TABLETS (Ascorbic Acid)
500 mg

Supplied: Bottles of 100, 250 and 500 tablets or capsules.

VITAMIN E CAPSULES
100 IU, 200 IU, 400 IU and 1000 IU D-ALPHA TOCOPHEROL plus MIXED TOCOPHEROLS

Supplied: Bottles of 50, 100, 250, 500 and 1000 capsules.

ZINC "50" TABLETS

Each Tablet Provides:
Zinc Gluconate (Organically
  Complexed)..................................409 mg
providing elemental Zinc ....50 mg

Supplied: Bottles of 100, 250 and 500 tablets.

E. R. Squibb & Sons, Inc.
GENERAL OFFICES
P.O. BOX 4000
PRINCETON, NJ 08540

E.T. THE EXTRA-TERRESTRIAL™
Children's Chewable Vitamins

E.T. Vitamins come in the 4 fruity flavors most preferred by children.

Each tablet contains:

		percent US RDA* ages 4-12
Vitamin A	5,000 IU	100
Vitamin D	400 IU	100
Vitamin E	30 IU	100
Vitamin C	60 mg	100
Folic Acid	0.4 mg	100
Thiamine	1.5 mg	100
Riboflavin	1.7 mg	100
Niacin	20 mg	100
Vitamin B$_6$	2 mg	100
Vitamin B$_{12}$	6 mcg	100

*US Recommended Daily Allowances

Usage: For 12 year olds and under—chew one tablet daily.

How Supplied: Bottles of 60.

Storage: Store at room temperature; avoid excessive heat.

KEEP OUT OF THE REACH OF CHILDREN.

E.T. THE EXTRA-TERRESTRIAL™
Children's Chewable Vitamins
With Iron

E.T. Vitamins come in the 4 fruity flavors most preferred by children.

Each tablet contains:

		percent US RDA* ages 4-12
Vitamin A	5,000 IU	100
Vitamin D	400 IU	100
Vitamin E	30 IU	100
Vitamin C	60 mg	100
Folic Acid	0.4 mg	100
Thiamine	1.5 mg	100
Riboflavin	1.7 mg	100
Niacin	20 mg	100
Vitamin B$_6$	2 mg	100
Vitamin B$_{12}$	6 mcg	100
Iron	18 mg	100

*US Recommended Daily Allowances

Usage: For 12 year olds and under—chew one tablet daily.

How Supplied: Bottles of 60.

Storage: Store at room temperature; avoid excessive heat.

KEEP OUT OF THE REACH OF CHILDREN.

THERAGRAN® LIQUID
(High Potency Vitamin Supplement)

Each 5 ml. teaspoonful contains:

		Percent US RDA*
Vitamin A	10,000 IU	200
Vitamin D	400 IU	100
Vitamin C	200 mg	333
Thiamine	10 mg	667
Riboflavin	10 mg	588
Niacin	100 mg	500
Vitamin B$_6$	4.1 mg	205
Vitamin B$_{12}$	5 mcg	83
Pantothenic Acid	21.4 mg	214

*US Recommended Daily Allowance

Usage: For 12 year olds and older—1 teaspoonful daily.

How Supplied: In bottles of 4 fl. oz.

Storage: Store at room temperature; avoid excessive heat.

ADVANCED FORMULA THERAGRAN® TABLETS
(High Potency Multivitamin Formula)

Each tablet contains:

		Percent US RDA*
Vitamin A (as Palmitate)	5,500 IU	110
Vitamin C (Ascorbic Acid)	120 mg	200
Vitamin B$_1$ (as Thiamine Mononitrate)	3 mg	200
Vitamin B$_2$ (Riboflavin)	3.4 mg	200
Niacin (as Niacinamide)	30 mg	150
Vitamin B$_6$ (as Pyridoxine Hydrochloride)	3 mg	150
Vitamin B$_{12}$ (Cyanocobalamin)	9 mcg	150
Vitamin D (Ergocalciferol)	400 IU	100
Vitamin E (dl-α-Tocopheryl Acetate)	30 IU	100
Pantothenic Acid (as Calcium Pantothenate)	10 mg	100
Folic Acid	0.4 mg	100
Biotin	15 mcg	5

*US Recommended Daily Allowance

Usage: For 12 year olds and older—1 tablet daily.

How Supplied: Bottles of 1000; Packs of 30, 100, and 180; and Unimatic® cartons of 100.
Storage: Store at room temperature; avoid excessive heat.

ADVANCED FORMULA THERAGRAN-M® TABLETS
(High Potency Multivitamin Formula with Minerals)

Each tablet contains:

VITAMINS		Percent US RDA*
Vitamin A (as Palmitate)	5,500 IU	110
Vitamin C (Ascorbic Acid)	120 mg	200
Vitamin B$_1$ (as Thiamine Mononitrate)	3 mg	200
Vitamin B$_2$ (Riboflavin)	3.4 mg	200
Niacin (as Niacinamide)	30 mg	150
Vitamin B$_6$ (as Pyridoxine Hydrochloride)	3 mg	150
Vitamin B$_{12}$ (Cyanocobalamin)	9 mcg	150
Vitamin D (Ergocalciferol)	400 IU	100
Vitamin E (dl-α-Tocopheryl Acetate)	30 IU	100
Pantothenic Acid (as Calcium Pantothenate)	10 mg	100
Folic Acid	0.4 mg	100
Biotin	15 mcg	5
MINERALS		
Iodine (as Potassium Iodide)	150 mcg	100
Iron (as Ferrous Fumarate)	27 mg	150
Magnesium (as Magnesium Oxide)	100 mg	25

Continued on next page

Squibb—Cont.

Copper (as Cupric Sulfate)	2 mg	100
Zinc (as Zinc Sulfate)	15 mg	100
Manganese (as Manganese Sulfate)	5 mg	**
Chromium (from Processed Yeast)	15 mcg	**
Selenium (from Processed Yeast)	10 mcg	**
Molybdenum (from Processed Yeast)	15 mcg	**

ELECTROLYTES

Potassium (as Potassium Salts)	7.5 mg	**
Chloride (as Potassium Chloride)	7.5 mg	**

*US Recommended Daily Allowance
**US RDA not established

Usage: For 12 year olds and older—1 tablet daily.

How Supplied: Bottles of 1000; Packs of 30, 60, 100, and 180; and Unimatic® cartons of 100.

Storage: Store at room temperature; avoid excessive heat.

Shown in Product Identification Section, page 428

THERAGRAN® STRESS FORMULA
(High Potency Multivitamin Formula with Iron and Biotin)

Each FILMLOK® tablet contains:		Percent US RDA*
Vitamin E (dl-α- Tocopheryl Acetate)	30 IU	100
Vitamin C (Ascorbic Acid)	600 mg	1000
B VITAMINS		
Folic Acid	400 mcg	100
Vitamin B$_1$ (as Thiamine Mononitrate)	15 mg	1000
Vitamin B$_2$ (Riboflavin)	15 mg	882
Niacin (as Niacinamide)	100 mg	500
Vitamin B$_6$ (as Pyridoxine Hydrochloride)	25 mg	1250
Vitamin B$_{12}$ (Cyanocobalamin)	12 mcg	200
Biotin	45 mcg	15
Pantothenic Acid (as Calcium Pantothenate)	20 mg	200
Iron (as Ferrous Fumarate)	27 mg	150

*US Recommended Daily Allowance for Adults

Usage: For adults—1 tablet daily or as directed by physician.

How Supplied: Bottles of 75.

Storage: Store at room temperature; avoid excessive heat.

FILMLOK is a Squibb trademark for veneer-coated tablets.

Shown in Product Identification Section, page 428

Stellar Pharmacal Corp.
Div./Star Pharmaceuticals, Inc.
1990 N.W. 44TH STREET
R.R. 2, BOX 904J
POMPANO BEACH, FL
33067-9802

STAR–OTIC®
Antibacterial, Antifungal,
Nonaqueous Ear Solution
For Prevention of "Swimmer's Ear"

Active Ingredients: Acetic acid 1.0% nonaqueous, Burow's solution 10%, Boric acid 1.0%, in a propylene glycol vehicle, with an acid pH and a low surface tension.

Indications: For the prevention of otitis externa, commonly called "Swimmer's Ear".

Actions: Star-Otic is antibacterial, antifungal, hydrophilic, has an acid pH and a low surface tension. Acetic acid and boric acid inhibit the rapid multiplication of microorganisms and help maintain the lining mantle of the ear canal in its normal acid state. Burow's solution (aluminum acetate) is a mild astringent. Propylene glycol reduces moisture in the ear canal.

Warning: Do not use in ear if tympanic membrane (ear drum) is perforated or punctured.

Drug Interaction Precaution: No known drug interaction. Virtually non-sensitizing and safe to use as directed.

Symptoms and Treatment of Overdosage: Discontinue use if undue irritation or sensitivity occurs.

Dosage and Administration: Adults and Children: For the prevention of otitis externa (Swimmer's Ear) instill 2-3 drops of Star-Otic in each ear before and after swimming or bathing in susceptible persons, or as directed by physician.

Professional Labeling: Same as those outlined under Indications.

How Supplied: Available in 15 cc measured drop, safety tip, plastic bottle.
Shown in Product Identification Section, page 428

Stuart Pharmaceuticals
Div. of ICI Americas Inc.
WILMINGTON, DE 19897

All Stuart products are packaged with tamper-resistant features as required by applicable Federal Regulations.

ALternaGEL®
Liquid
High-Potency Aluminum Hydroxide Antacid

Composition: ALternaGEL is available as a white, pleasant-tasting, low sodium, high-potency aluminum hydroxide liquid antacid.

Each 5 ml. teaspoonful contains 600 mg. aluminum hydroxide (equivalent to dried gel, USP) providing 16 milliequivalents (mEq) of acid-neutralizing capacity (ANC), and less than 2.5 mg. (0.109 mEq) of sodium per teaspoonful.

Indications: ALternaGEL is indicated for the symptomatic relief of hyperacidity associated with peptic ulcer, gastritis, peptic esophagitis, gastric hyperacidity, hiatal hernia, and heartburn.
ALternaGEL will be of special value to those patients for whom magnesium-containing antacids are undesirable, such as patients with renal insufficiency, patients requiring control of attendant G.I. complications resulting from steroid or other drug therapy, and patients experiencing the laxation which may result from magnesium or combination antacid regimens.

Directions for Use: One or two teaspoonfuls, as needed, between meals and at bedtime, or as directed by a physician. May be followed by a sip of water if desired.

Patient Warnings: Keep this and all drugs out of the reach of children.
ALternaGEL may cause constipation. Except under the advice and supervision of a physician, more than 18 teaspoonfuls should not be taken in a 24-hour period, or the maximum recommended dosage taken for more than two weeks.

Drug Interaction Precaution: ALternaGEL should not be taken concurrently with an antibiotic containing any form of tetracycline.

How Supplied: ALternaGEL is available in bottles of 12 and 5 fluid ounces and 1 fluid ounce hospital unit-dose bottles.
NDC 0038-0860.
Shown in Product Identification Section, page 428

DIALOSE® Capsules
Stool Softener

Composition: Each capsule contains docusate potassium, 100 mg.

Action and Uses: DIALOSE is indicated for treating constipation due to hardness, or lack of moisture in the intestinal contents. DIALOSE is an effective stool softener, whose gentle action will help to restore normal bowel function gradually, without griping or discomfort.

Warning: As with any drug, if you are pregnant or nursing a baby, seek the advice of a health professional before using this product.
Keep this and all drugs out of the reach of children.

Dosage and Administration:
Adults: Initially, one capsule three times a day.
Children, 6 years and over: One capsule at bedtime, or as directed by physician.
Children, under 6 years: As directed by physician.
It is helpful to increase the daily intake of fluids by taking a glass of water with

All Stuart products are packaged with tamper-resistant features as required by applicable Federal Regulations.

---

each dose. When adequate laxation is obtained, the dose may be adjusted to meet individual needs.

How Supplied: Bottles of 36, 100, and 500 pink capsules, identified "STUART 470". Also available in 100 capsule unit dose boxes (10 strips of 10 capsules each). NDC 0038-0470.

Shown in Product Identification Section, page 429

DIALOSE® PLUS Capsules
Stool Softener
plus Peristaltic Activator

Composition: Each capsule contains: docusate potassium, 100 mg. and casanthranol, 30 mg.

Action and Uses: DIALOSE PLUS Is indicated for the treatment of constipation generally associated with any of the following: hardness, or lack of moisture in the intestinal contents, or decreased intestinal motility.

DIALOSE PLUS combines the advantages of the stool softener, docusate potassium, with the peristaltic activating effect of casanthranol.

Warning: As with any drug, if you are pregnant or nursing a baby, seek the advice of a health professional before using this product. And, as with any laxative, DIALOSE PLUS should not be used when abdominal pain, nausea, or vomiting are present. Frequent or prolonged use may result in dependence on laxatives.

Keep this and all drugs out of the reach of children.

Dosage and Administration:
Adults: Initially, one capsule two times a day.
Children: As directed by physician. When adequate laxation is obtained the dose may be adjusted to meet individual needs.

It is helpful to increase the daily intake of fluids by taking a glass of water with each dose.

How Supplied: Bottles of 36, 100, and 500 yellow capsules, identified "STUART 475". Also available in 100 capsule unit dose boxes (10 strips of 10 capsules each).
NDC 0038-0475.

Shown in Product Identification Section, page 429

EFFERSYLLIUM® Instant Mix
Natural Fiber Bulking Agent

Composition: Each rounded teaspoonful, or individual packet (7 g.) contains psyllium hydrocolloid, 3 g.

Actions and Uses: EFFERSYLLIUM produces a soft, lubricating bulk which promotes natural elimination. EFFERSYLLIUM is not a one-dose, fast-acting bowel regulator. Administration

---

for several days may be needed to establish regularity.

Effersyllium contains less than 5 mg. sodium per rounded teaspoonful and is considered dietetically sodium-free.

Indications: EFFERSYLLIUM is indicated to restore normal bowel habits in chronic constipation, to promote normal elimination in irritable bowel syndrome, and to ease passage of stools in presence of anorectal disorders.

Dosage and Administration:
Adults: One rounded teaspoonful, or one packet, in a glass of water one to three times a day, or as directed by physician.
Children, 6 years and over: One level teaspoonful, or one-half packet (3.5 g.) in one-half glass of water at bedtime, or as directed by physician. *Children, under 6 years:* As directed by physician.
Note: To avoid caking, always use a dry spoon to remove EFFERSYLLIUM from its container. Dosage should be placed in a dry glass. Add water, stir and drink immediately. REPLACE CAP TIGHTLY. KEEP IN A DRY PLACE.

Warning: Keep this and all drugs out of the reach of children. CAUTION: People sensitive to psyllium powder should avoid inhalation as it may cause an allergic reaction such as wheezing.

How Supplied: Bottles of 9 oz. and 16 oz. tan, granular powder. Convenience packets, 7 g. per packet in boxes of 12 or 24. NDC 0038-0440.

Shown in Product Identification Section, page 428

FERANCEE®
Chewable Tablets

Composition: Each tablet contains: iron (from 200 mg. ferrous fumarate), 67 mg. and Vitamin C (as ascorbic acid, 49 mg. and sodium ascorbate, 114 mg.), 150 mg. Contains FD&C Yellow #5 (tartrazine) as a color additive.

Action and Uses: A pleasant-tasting hematinic for iron-deficiency anemias, well-tolerated FERANCEE is particularly useful when chronic blood loss, onset of menses, or pregnancy create additional demands for iron supplementation. The peach-cherry flavored chewable tablets dissolve quickly in the mouth and may be either chewed or swallowed.

Dosage and Administration:
Adults: Two tablets daily, or as directed by physician.
Children over 6 years of age: One tablet daily, or as directed by physician.
Children under 6 years of age: As directed by physician.

Warning: As with any drug, if you are pregnant or nursing a baby, seek the advice of a health professional before using this product.

How Supplied: Bottles of 100 brown and yellow, two-layer tablets identified "STUART 650" on brown layer.

Note: A childproof cap is standard on each bottle as a safeguard against accidental ingestion by children.
NDC 0038-0650.

FERANCEE®–HP Tablets
High Potency Hematinic

Composition: Each tablet contains: iron (from 330 mg. ferrous fumarate), 110 mg.; Vitamin C (as ascorbic acid, 350 mg. and sodium ascorbate, 281 mg.), 600 mg.

Action and Uses: FERANCEE-HP is a high potency formulation of iron and Vitamin C and is intended for use as either:
(1) a maintenance hematinic for those patients needing a daily iron supplement to maintain normal hemoglobin levels, or
(2) intensive therapy for the acute and/or severe iron deficiency anemia where a high intake of elemental iron is required.
The use of well-tolerated ferrous fumarate provides high levels of elemental iron with a low incidence of gastric distress. The inclusion of 600 mg. of Vitamin C per tablet serves to maintain more of the iron in the absorbable ferrous state.

Precautions: Because FERANCEE-HP contains 110 mg. of elemental iron per tablet, it is recommended that its use be limited to adults, i.e. over age 12 years. As with all medication, FERANCEE-HP should be kept out of the reach of children.

Dosage and Administration:
For maintenance: One tablet-a-day should be sufficient to maintain normal hemoglobin levels in most patients with a history of recurring iron deficiency anemia.
For acute and/or severe iron deficiency anemia, one tablet taken two or three times per day after meals. (Each tablet provides 110 mg. elemental iron.)

How Supplied: FERANCEE-HP is supplied in bottles of 60 red, film coated, oval shaped tablets.
NDC 0038-0863.
Note: A childproof safety cap is standard on each bottle as a safeguard against accidental ingestion by children.
Shown in Product Identification Section, page 429

HIBICLENS®
Antiseptic Antimicrobial Skin Cleanser
(chlorhexidine gluconate)

Description: HIBICLENS is an antiseptic antimicrobial skin cleanser possessing bactericidal activities. HIBICLENS contains 4% chlorhexidine gluconate, a chemically unique hexamethylenebis biguanide with 4% isopropyl alcohol, in a mild, sudsing base adjusted to pH 5.0–6.5 for optimal activity and stability as well as compatability with the normal pH of the skin.

Continued on next page

Stuart—Cont.

All Stuart products are packaged with tamper-resistant features as required by applicable Federal Regulations.

Action: HIBICLENS is bactericidal on contact. It has antiseptic activity and a persistent antimicrobial effect against a wide range of microorganisms, including gram-positive bacteria, and gram-negative bacteria such as *Pseudomonas aeruginosa.* The effectiveness of HIBICLENS is not significantly reduced by the presence of organic matter, such as pus or blood.[1]

In a study[2] simulating surgical use, the immediate bactericidal effect of HIBICLENS after a single six-minute scrub resulted in a 99.9% reduction in resident bacterial flora, with a reduction of 99.98% after the eleventh scrub. Reductions on surgically gloved hands were maintained over the six-hour test period.

HIBICLENS displays persistent antimicrobial action. In one study[2], 93% of a radiolabeled formulation of HIBICLENS remained present on uncovered skin after five hours.

HIBICLENS prevents skin infection thereby reducing the risk of cross-infection.

Indications: HIBICLENS is indicated for use as a surgical scrub, as a health-care personnel handwash, for preoperative showering and bathing, as a patient preoperative skin preparation, and as a skin wound cleanser and general skin cleanser.

Safety: The extensive use of chlorhexidine gluconate for over 20 years outside the United States has produced no evidence of absorption of the compound through intact skin. The potential for producing skin reactions is extremely low. HIBICLENS can be used many times a day without causing irritation, dryness, or discomfort. When used for cleaning superficial wounds, HIBICLENS will neither cause additional tissue injury nor delay healing.

Precautions: HIBICLENS is for topical use only. The sudsing formulation may be irritating to the eyes. If HIBICLENS should get into the eyes, rinse out promptly and thoroughly with water. Keep out of ears. Chlorhexidine gluconate, like various other antimicrobial agents, has been reported to cause deafness when instilled in the middle ear. In the presence of a perforated eardrum particular care should be taken to prevent exposure of inner ear tissues to HIBICLENS.

HIBICLENS should not be used by persons with sensitivity to any of its components. Adverse reactions, including dermatitis and photosensitivity, are rare, but if they do occur, discontinue use. Keep this and all drugs out of the reach of children. AVOID EXCESSIVE HEAT. (Do not exceed 104°F.)

HIBICLENS is nonstaining but hypochlorite bleaches may react with HIBICLENS to cause brown stains in linens or clothing. Soiled fabrics which have come in contact with HIBICLENS should be laundered without bleach or only with an oxidizing bleach such as sodium perborate. An initial flush operation of linen exposed to HIBICLENS will also be helpful in avoiding stains.

Directions for Use:
Skin wound and general skin cleansing
Thoroughly rinse area to be cleansed with water. Apply sufficient HIBICLENS and wash gently. Rinse again thoroughly.

Patient preoperative skin preparation:
Apply HIBICLENS liberally to surgical site and swab for at least two minutes. Dry with a sterile towel. Repeat procedure for an additional two minutes and dry with a sterile towel.

Health-care personnel use
SURGICAL HAND SCRUB
Wet hands and forearms with water. Scrub for 3 minutes with about 5 ml. of HIBICLENS and a wet brush, paying particular attention to the nails, cuticles, and interdigital spaces. A separate nail cleaner may be used. Rinse thoroughly. Wash for an additional 3 minutes with 5 ml. of HIBICLENS and rinse under running water. Dry thoroughly.

Directions for use of HIBICLENS™ Sponge/Brush: Open package and remove nail cleaner. Wet hands. Use nail cleaner under fingernails and to clean cuticles. Wet hands and forearms to the elbow with warm water. (Avoid using very cold or very hot water.) Wet sponge side of sponge/brush. Squeeze and pump immediately to work up adequate lather. Apply lather to hands and forearms using sponge side of the product. Start 3 minute scrub by using the brush side of the product to scrub only nails, cuticles, and interdigital areas. Use sponge side for scrubbing hands and forearms. (Avoid using brush on these more sensitive areas.) Rinse thoroughly with warm water. Scrub for an additional 3 minutes using sponge side only. To produce additional lather, add a small amount of water and pump the sponge. (While scrubbing, do not use excessive pressure to produce lather—a small amount of lather is all that is required to adequately cleanse skin with HIBICLENS.) Rinse and dry thoroughly, blotting hands and forearms with a soft sterile towel.

HAND WASH
Wet hands with water. Dispense about 5 ml. of HIBICLENS into cupped hands and wash in a vigorous manner for 15 seconds. Rinse and dry thoroughly.

How Supplied: For general handwashing locations: disposable, unit-of-use 22 ml. impregnated Sponge/Brushes with Nail Picks; pocket-size, 15 ml. foil Packettes; plastic disposable bottles of 4 oz. and 8 oz. with dispenser caps; and 16 oz. filled globes.

For surgical scrub areas: disposable, unit-of-use 22 ml. impregnated Sponge/Brushes with Nail Picks; plastic disposable bottles of 32 oz. and 1 gal.

The 32 oz. bottle is designed for a special foot-operated wall dispenser. A hand operated wall dispenser is available for the 16 oz. globe. Hand pumps are available for 16 oz., 32 oz., and 1 gal. sizes NDC 0038-0575.

References:
1. Lowbury EJL, and Lilly HA: The effect of blood on disinfection of surgeons' hands, Brit. J. Surg. 61:19–21 (Jan.) 1974.
2. Peterson AF, Rosenberg A, Alatary SD: Comparative evaluation of surgical scrub preparations, Surg Gynecol. Obstet. 146:63–65 (Jan. 1978.

Shown in Product Identification Section, page 429

HIBISTAT®
(chlorhexidine gluconate)
Germicidal Hand Rinse

Description: HIBISTAT is a germicidal hand rinse effective against a wide range of microorganisms. HIBISTAT is a clear colorless liquid containing 0.5% w/v chlorhexidine gluconate in 70% isopropyl alcohol with emollients.

Actions and Uses: HIBISTAT is indicated for health-care personnel use as a germicidal hand rinse. HIBISTAT is for hand hygiene on physically clean hands. It is used in those situations where hands are physically clean, but in need of degerming, when routine handwashing is not convenient or desirable. HIBISTAT provides rapid germicidal action and has a persistent effect.

HIBISTAT should be used in-between patients and procedures where there are no sinks available or continued return to the sink area is inconvenient or time-consuming. HIBISTAT can be used as an alternative to detergent-based products when hands are physically clean. Also HIBISTAT is an effective germicidal hand rinse following a soap and water handwash.

Cautions: Keep out of eyes and ears. If HIBISTAT should get into eyes or ears rinse out promptly and thoroughly with water. Chlorhexidine gluconate has been reported to cause deafness when instilled in the middle ear through perforated ear drums. Irritation or other adverse reactions, such as dermatitis or photosensitivity are rare, but if they do occur, discontinue use. Keep this and all drugs out of the reach of children.
AVOID EXCESSIVE HEAT. (Do not exceed 104°F.)

Directions for Use: Dispense about a ml. of HIBISTAT into cupped hands and rub vigorously until dry (about 15 seconds), paying particular attention to nails and interdigital spaces. HIBISTAT dries rapidly in use. No water or toweling are necessary.

How Supplied: In plastic disposable bottles of 4 oz. and 8 oz. with flip-top cap. NDC 0038-0585.

KASOF® Capsules
High Strength Stool Softener

Composition: Each KASOF capsule contains docusate potassium, 240 mg.

All Stuart products are packaged with tamper-resistant features as required by applicable Federal Regulations.

Action and Uses: KASOF provides a highly efficient wetting action to restore moisture to the bowel, thus softening the stool to prevent straining. KASOF is especially valuable for the severely constipated, as well as patients with anorectal disorders, such as hemorrhoids and anal fissures. KASOF is ideal for patients with any condition that can be complicated by straining at stool, for example, cardiac patients. The action of KASOF does not interfere with normal peristalsis and generally does not cause griping or extreme sensations of urgency. KASOF is sodium-free, containing a unique potassium formulation, without the problems associated with sodium intake. The simple, one-a-day dosage helps assure patient compliance in maintaining normal bowel function.

Warning: As with any drug, if you are pregnant or nursing a baby, seek the advice of a health professional before using this product. Keep this and all drugs out of the reach of children.

Dosage and Administration: Adults: 1 KASOF capsule daily for several days, or until bowel movements are normal and gentle. It is helpful to increase the daily intake of fluids by drinking a glass of water with each dose.

How Supplied: KASOF is available in bottles of 30 and 60 brown, gelatin capsules, identified "Stuart 380". NDC 0038-0380.

Shown in Product Identification Section, page 429

MYLANTA®
Liquid and Tablets
Antacid/Antiflatulent

Composition: Each chewable tablet or each 5 ml. (one teaspoonful) of liquid contains:

Aluminum hydroxide
(Dried Gel, USP in tablet and equiv. to Dried Gel, USP in liquid)........200 mg.
Magnesium hydroxide ....200 mg.
Simethicone......................................20 mg.

Sodium Content: MYLANTA contains an insignificant amount of sodium per daily dose and is considered dietetically sodium free. Typical values are 0.68 mg. (0.03 mEq) sodium per 5 ml. teaspoonful of liquid; 0.77 mg. (0.03 mEq) per tablet.

Acid Neutralizing Capacity: Each teaspoonful of MYLANTA liquid will neutralize 12.7 mEq of acid. Each MYLANTA tablet will neutralize 11.5 mEq.

Indications: MYLANTA, a well-balanced combination of two antacids and simethicone, provides consistently dependable relief of symptoms associated with gastric hyperacidity, and mucus-entrapped air or "gas". These indications include:

Common heartburn (pyrosis)
Hiatal hernia
Peptic esophagitis
Gastritis
Peptic ulcer

The soft, easy-to-chew tablets and exceptionally pleasant tasting liquid encourage patients' acceptance, thereby minimizing the skipping of prescribed doses. MYLANTA is appropriate whenever there is a need for effective relief of temporary gastric hyperacidity and mucus-entrapped gas.

Directions for Use: One or two teaspoonfuls of liquid or one or two tablets, well-chewed, every two to four hours between meals and at bedtime, or as directed by physician.

Patient Warnings: Keep this and all drugs out of the reach of children. Except under the advice and supervision of a physician: Do not take more than 24 teaspoonfuls or 24 tablets in a 24 hour period or use the maximum dose for more than two weeks. Do not use this product if you have kidney disease.

Drug Interaction Precaution: Do not use with patients who are presently taking a prescription antibiotic containing any form of tetracycline.

How Supplied: MYLANTA is available as a white, pleasant tasting liquid suspension, and as a two-layer yellow and white chewable tablet, identified on yellow layer "STUART 620". Liquid supplied in bottles of 5 oz. and 12 oz. Tablets supplied in boxes of individually wrapped 40's and 100's, economy size bottles of 180, and consumer convenience pocket packs of 48. Also available for hospital use in liquid unit doses of 1 oz., and bottles of 5 oz.
NDC 0038-0610 (liquid). NDC 0038-0620 (tablets).

Shown in Product Identification Section, page 429

MYLANTA®-II
Liquid and Tablets
Double-Strength
Antacid/Antiflatulent

Composition: Each chewable tablet or each 5 ml. (one teaspoonful) of liquid contains:

Aluminum hydroxide
(Dried Gel, USP in tablet and equiv. to Dried Gel, USP in liquid) 400 mg.
Magnesium hydroxide 400 mg.
Simethicone 30 mg.

Sodium Content: MYLANTA-II contains an insignificant amount of sodium per daily dose and is considered dietetically sodium free. Typical values are 1.14 mg. (0.05 mEq) sodium per 5 ml. teaspoonful of liquid; 1.3 mg. (0.06 mEq) per tablet.

Acid Neutralizing Capacity: Each teaspoonful of MYLANTA-II liquid will neutralize 25.4 mEq of acid. Each MYLANTA-II tablet will neutralize 23.0 mEq.

Indications: MYLANTA-II is a double-strength antacid with an antiflatulent. The soft, easy-to-chew tablets and exceptionally pleasant tasting liquid encourage patient acceptance, thereby minimizing the skipping of prescribed doses. MYLANTA-II provides consistently dependable relief of the symptoms of peptic ulcer and other problems related to acid hypersecretion. The high potency of MYLANTA-II is achieved through its concentration of noncalcium antacid ingredients. Thus MYLANTA-II can produce both rapid and long-lasting neutralization without the acid rebound associated with calcium carbonate. The balanced formula of aluminum and magnesium hydroxides minimizes undesirable bowel effects. Simethicone is effective for the relief of concomitant distress caused by mucus-entrapped gas and swallowed air.

Directions for Use: One or two teaspoonfuls of liquid, or one or two tablets, well-chewed, between meals and at bedtime, or as directed by physician. Because patients with peptic ulcer vary greatly in both acid output and gastric emptying time, the amount and schedule of dosages should be varied accordingly.

Patient Warnings: Keep this and all drugs out of the reach of children. Except under the advice and supervision of a physician: Do not take more than 12 teaspoonfuls or 12 tablets in a 24 hour period or use the maximum dose for more than two weeks. Do not use this product if you have kidney disease.

Drug Interaction Precaution: Do not use with patients who are presently taking a prescription antibiotic containing any form of tetracycline.

How Supplied: MYLANTA-II is available as a white, pleasant tasting liquid suspension, and a two-layer green and white chewable tablet, identified on green layer "STUART 851". Liquid supplied in 12 oz. and 5 oz. bottles. Tablets supplied in boxes of 60 individually wrapped chewable tablets and consumer convenience pocket packs of 24. Also available for hospital use in liquid unit doses of 1 oz., and bottles of 5 oz.
NDC 0038-0852 (liquid). NDC 0038-0851 (tablets).

Shown in Product Identification Section, page 429

MYLICON® Tablets and Drops
Antiflatulent

Composition: Each tablet or 0.6 ml. of drops contains simethicone, 40 mg.

Action and Uses: For relief of the painful symptoms of excess gas in the digestive tract. MYLICON is a valuable adjunct in the treatment of many conditions in which the retention of gas may be a problem, such as: postoperative gaseous distention, air swallowing, functional dyspepsia, peptic ___ or irritable colon, divert___ The defoaming acti___ lieves flatulence ___ venting the f___ rounded gas ___ nal tract. M___ and intes___ sion of ___ alesce; ___ nated mor___ flatus.

Stuart—Cont.

All Stuart products are packaged with tamper-resistant features as required by applicable Federal Regulations.

Dosage and Administration:
Tablets—One or two tablets four times daily after meals and at bedtime. May also be taken as needed up to 12 tablets daily or as directed by a physician. TABLETS SHOULD BE CHEWED THOROUGHLY.
Drops—0.6 ml. four times daily after meals and at bedtime. May also be taken as needed up to 500 mg. daily or as directed by a physician. Shake well before using.
Keep this and all drugs out of the reach of children.

How Supplied: Bottles of 100 and 500 white, scored, chewable tablets, identified front "STUART", reverse "450," and dropper bottles of 30 ml. (1 fl. oz.) pink, pleasant tasting liquid. Also available in 100 tablet unit dose boxes (10 strips of 10 tablets each).
NDC 0038-0450 (tablets).
NDC 0038-0630 (drops).
Shown in Product Identification Section, page 429

MYLICON®–80 Tablets
High-Capacity Antiflatulent

Composition: Each tablet contains simethicone, 80 mg.

Action and Uses: For relief of the painful symptoms of excess gas in the digestive tract. MYLICON-80 is a high capacity antiflatulent for adjunctive treatment of many conditions in which the retention of gas may be a problem, such as the following: air swallowing, functional dyspepsia, postoperative gaseous distension, peptic ulcer, spastic or irritable colon, diverticulitis.
MYLICON-80 has a defoaming action that relieves flatulence by dispersing and preventing the formation of mucus-surrounded gas pockets in the gastrointestinal tract. MYLICON-80 acts in the stomach and intestines to change the surface tension of gas bubbles enabling them to coalesce; thus, the gas is freed and is eliminated more easily by belching or passing flatus.

Dosage and Administration: One tab-[...] four times daily after meals and at [...] time. May also be taken as needed up [...] ablets daily or as directed by a phy-[...] TABLETS SHOULD BE [...]ED THOROUGHLY.
[...]is and all drugs out of the reach [...]en.

[...]plied: Economical bottles of [...]venience packages of individ-[...]ed 12 and 48 pink, scored, [...]blets identified "STUART [...]vailable in 100 tablet unit [...]strips of 10 tablets each).

NDC 0038-0858.
Shown in Product Identification Section, page 429

OREXIN® SOFTAB® Tablets

Composition: Each tablet contains: thiamine mononitrate, 10 mg.; Vitamin B$_6$ (as pyridoxine hydrochloride), 5 mg.; and Vitamin B$_{12}$ (cyanocobalamin), 25 mcg.

Action and Uses: OREXIN is a high-potency vitamin supplement providing thiamine mononitrate and Vitamins B$_6$ and B$_{12}$.
OREXIN SOFTAB tablets are specially formulated to dissolve quickly in the mouth. They may be chewed or swallowed. Dissolve tablet in a teaspoonful of water or fruit juice if liquid is preferred.

Dosage and Administration: One tablet daily, or as directed by physician.

How Supplied: Bottles of 100 pale pink SOFTAB tablets, identified "STUART". NDC 0038-0280.
Shown in Product Identification Section, page 429

PROBEC®–T Tablets

Composition: Each tablet contains: Vitamin C (as ascorbic acid, 67 mg. and sodium ascorbate, 600 mg.), 600 mg.; thiamine mononitrate, 15 mg.; riboflavin, 10 mg.; Vitamin B$_6$ (as pyridoxine hydrochloride), 5 mg.; Vitamin B$_{12}$ (cyanocobalamin), 5 mcg.; niacinamide, 100 mg.; calcium pantothenate, 20 mg.

Actions and Uses: PROBEC-T is a high-potency B complex supplement with 600 mg. of Vitamin C in easy to swallow odorless tablets.

Dosage and Administration: One tablet a day with a meal, or as directed by physician.

How Supplied: Bottles of 60, salmon colored, capsule-shaped tablets.
NDC 0038-0840.
Shown in Product Identification Section, page 429

THE STUART FORMULA® Tablets

Composition: Each tablet contains:
Vitamins: Vitamin A (as palmitate), 5000 I.U.; Vitamin D (ergocalciferol), 400 I.U.; Vitamin E (as dl-alpha tocopheryl acetate), 15 I.U.; Vitamin C (as ascorbic acid), 60 mg.; folic acid, 0.4 mg.; thiamine (as thiamine mononitrate), 1.5 mg.; riboflavin, 1.7 mg.; niacin (as niacinamide), 20 mg.; Vitamin B$_6$ (as pyridoxine hydrochloride), 2 mg.; Vitamin B$_{12}$ (cyanocobalamin), 6 mcg.
Minerals: calcium 160 mg.; phosphorus, 125 mg.; iodine, 150 mcg.; iron (from 54 mg. ferrous fumarate) 18 mg.; magnesium, 100 mg.

Actions and Uses: The STUART FORMULA tablet provides a well-balanced multivitamin/multimineral formula intended for use as a daily dietary supplement for adults and children over age four.

Dosage and Administration: One tablet daily or as directed by a physician.

How Supplied: Bottles of 100 and 250 white round tablets. Childproof safety caps are standard on both bottles as a safeguard against accidental ingestion by children.
NDC 0038-0866.
Shown in Product Identification Section, page 429

STUART PRENATAL® Tablets

Composition: Each tablet contains:

Vitamins:	% U.S. RDA*	
A (as acetate)	100%	8,000 I.U.
D (ergocalciferol)	100%	400 I.U.
E (as dl-alpha tocopheryl acetate)	100%	30 I.U.
C (ascorbic acid)	100%	60 mg.
Folic Acid	100%	0.8 mg.
Thiamine (as thiamine mononitrate)	100%	1.7 mg.
Riboflavin	100%	2 mg.
Niacin (as niacinamide)	100%	20 mg.
B$_6$ (as pyridoxine hydrochloride)	160%	4 mg.
B$_{12}$ (cyanocobalamin)	100%	8 mcg.
Minerals:		
Calcium (from 679 mg. calcium sulfate anhydrous)	15%	200 mg.
Iodine (from potassium iodide)	100%	150 mcg.
Iron (from 182 mg. ferrous fumarate)	333%	60 mg.
Magnesium (from magnesium oxide)	22%	100 mg.

* Recommended Daily Allowance

Action and Uses: STUART PRENATAL is a multivitamin/multimineral supplement for pregnant and lactating women. It provides vitamins equal to 100% or more of the U.S. RDA for pregnant and lactating women, plus essential minerals, including 60 mg. of elemental iron as well-tolerated ferrous fumarate, and 200 mg. of elemental calcium (non-alkalizing and phosphorus-free). Stuart Prenatal also contains .8 mg. folic acid.

Dosage and Administration: During and after pregnancy, one tablet daily after a meal, or as directed by a physician.

How Supplied: Bottles of 100 and 500 pink capsule-shaped tablets. A childproof safety cap is standard on 100 tablet bottles as a safeguard against accidental ingestion by children.
NDC 0038-0270.
Shown in Product Identification Section, page 429

STUARTINIC® Tablets

Composition: Each tablet contains: iron (from 300 mg. ferrous fumarate), 100 mg.; Vitamin C (as ascorbic acid, 300 mg. and sodium ascorbate, 225 mg.), 500 mg.; Vitamin B$_{12}$ (cyanocobalamin), 25 mcg.; thiamine mononitrate, 6 mg.; riboflavin, 6 mg.; Vitamin B$_6$ (as pyridoxine hydrochloride), 1 mg.; niacinamide, 20 mg.; calcium pantothenate, 10 mg.

Action and Uses: STUARTINIC is a complete hematinic for patients with history of iron deficiency anemia who also lack proper amounts of B-complex vitamins due to inadequate diet.

The use of well-tolerated ferrous fumarate in STUARTINIC provides a high level of elemental iron with a low incidence of gastric distress. The inclusion of 100 mg. of Vitamin C per tablet serves to maintain more of the iron in the absorbable ferrous state. The B-complex vitamins improve nutrition where B-complex deficient diets contribute to the anemia.

Precautions: Because STUARTINIC contains 100 mg. of elemental iron per tablet, use should be confined to adults, i.e. over age 12 years. Keep this and all drugs out of the reach of children.

Warning: If you are pregnant or nursing a baby, seek the advice of a health professional before using this product.

Dosage and Administration: One tablet daily taken after a meal to maintain normal hemoglobin levels in most patients with chronic iron deficiency anemia resulting from inadequate diet. Higher doses of STUARTINIC can be taken as directed by the physician.

How Supplied: STUARTINIC is supplied in bottles of 60 film coated, oval shaped tablets. NDC 0038-0862.
Note: A childproof safety cap is standard on each 60 tablet bottle as a safeguard against accidental ingestion by children.

Shown in Product Identification Section, page 429

All Stuart products are packaged with tamper-resistant features as required by applicable Federal Regulations.

Sunrise & Rainbow
9526 W. PICO BLVD.
LOS ANGELES, CA 90035

NURSAMIL™
breastfeeding formula
Powdered whole-food mix fortified with vitamins and minerals.

Description: A nutritious formulation of milk, barley, and egg designed to provide breastfeeding women with at least 100% of the U.S. Recommended Daily Allowances (U.S. RDA) of vitamins and minerals in two servings a day.
Nursamil also provides 80% of the U.S. RDA for protein for nursing women in two servings a day.

Ingredients: Total milk protein, barley malt, dicalcium phosphate, whey solids, lecithin, egg white solids, magnesium oxide, ascorbic acid, d-alpha tocophyl, ferrous fumarate, zinc oxide, niacinimide, vitamin A palmitate, calcium pantothenate, copper sulfate, pyridoxine hydrochloride, thiamine hydro-

chloride, riboflavin, folic acid, biotin, vitamin D, potassium iodide and cyanocobalamin.
Enjoy Nursamil by itself, or blended with your favorite fruit or natural flavoring to add variety.
Nursamil IS NOT A SOLE FOOD.

How Supplied: Cans of 16 oz (1 lb). Twenty-two (22) servings per can.

NUTRIMIL™
weaning formula
Powdered whole-food supplement with vitamins and minerals.

Description: A nutritious formulation of whole milk, barley, and maple syrup designed for supplemental feeding of babies and small children up to the age of four (4) years. Can be served in a bottle, cup, glass or over cereal.

Ingredients: Dry whole milk powder, barley malt, pure maple syrup granules, soybean oil, lecithin, calcium carbonate, magnesium carbonate, calcium ascorbate, ferrous gluconate, inositol, zinc gluconate, low alpha type mixed tocopherol concentrate, d-alpha tocopheryl acetate, niacin, copper gluconate, calcium pantothenate, vitamin A palmitate, thiamine mononitrate, pyridoxine hydrochloride, riboflavin, potassium iodide, phylloquinone, folic acid, biotin, cholecalciferol, cyanocobalamin.
Nutrimil IS NOT A SOLE FOOD.

Nutrients:	(32 grams) Powder	100Kcal (20 grams) Powder
Calories	160	100
Protein	5 G	3.11 G
Carbohydrate	16 G	10.142 G
Fat	8 G	5 G
Linoleic Acid	1.8 G	1.12 G

Serving Size:	per 8-ounce serving 4 level Tbsp. (32 grams)	per 100Kcal (20 grams)
Vitamin A	560 I.U.	350 I.U.
Vitamin C (Ascorbic Acid)	24 mg	15 mg
Thiamine (Vitamin B1)	192 mcg	120 mcg
Riboflavin (Vitamin B2)	224 mcg	140 mcg
Niacin	2.2 mg	1.35 mg
Calcium	201.6 mg	126 mg
Iron	1.6 mg	1 mg
Vitamin D	96 I.U.	60 I.U.
Vitamin E	5.6 I.U.	3.5 I.U.
Vitamin B6	112 mcg	70 mcg
Folic Acid (Folacin)	24 mcg	15 mcg
Vitamin B12	0.48 mcg	0.3 mcg
Phosphorous	144 mg	90 mg
Iodine	17.6 mcg	11 mcg
Magnesium	28.8 mg	18 mg
Zinc	1.36 mg	0.85 mg
Copper	136 mcg	85 mcg
Biotin	12.8 mcg	8 mcg
Pantothenic Acid	800 mcg	500 mcg
Choline	25.6 mg	16 mg
Inositol	17.6 mg	11 mg
Vitamin K	20.8 mcg	13 mcg
Manganese	272 mcg	170 mcg
Sodium	56 mg	35 mg
Potassium	235.2 mg	147 mg
Chloride	147.2 mg	92 mg

The carbohydrates of Nutrimil are supplied from a combination of barley, maple, and milk (lactose) rather than lactose alone. Lactose is only approximately 20% of this total formlation.

Preparation: Standard dilution is 2 fluid ounces of warm water for every (1) one level tablespoon of powder. (20 cal/fluid ounce).

How Supplied: Cans of 16 oz (1 lb) 14—8 ounce servings.
Shown in Product Identification Section, page 429

PRENATAMIL™
pregnancy formula
Powdered whole-food mix fortified with vitamins and minerals.

Description: A nutritious formulation of milk, barley, and egg designed to provide pregnant women with at least 100% of the U.S. Recommended Daily Allowance (U.S. RDA) of vitamins and minerals in two servings a day.
Also provides 80% of the U.S. RDA for protein for pregnant women in two servings a day.

Ingredients: Total milk protein, barley malt, dicalcium phosphate, whey solids, lecithin, egg white solids, magnesium oxide, ascorbic acid, d-alpha tocopheryl, ferrous fumarate, zinc oxide, niacinimide, vitamin A palmitate, calcium pantothenate, copper sulfate, pyridoxine hydrochloride, thiamine hydrochloride, riboflavin, folic acid, biotin, vitamin D, potassium iodide and cyanocobalamin.
Enjoy Prenatamil by itself, or blended with your favorite fruit or natural flavoring to add variety.
Prenatamil IS NOT A SOLE FOOD.

How Supplied: Cans of 16 oz (1 lb). Twenty-two (22) servings per can.

Syntex Laboratories, Inc
3401 HILLVIEW AVENUE
PALO ALTO, CA 94304

CARMOL® 10
10% urea lotion
for total body
dry skin care.

Active Ingredient: Urea 10% in a blend of purified water, stearic acid, isopropyl palmitate, propylene glycol dipelargonate, PEG-8 dioleate, propylene glycol, PEG-8 distearate, cetyl alcohol, sodium laureth sulfate, trolamine, carbomer 940, xanthan gum; scented with hypoallergenic fragrance.

Indications: For total body dry skin care.

Actions: Keratolytic CARMOL 10 is non-occlusive, contains no mineral oil or petrolatum. CARMOL 10 is hypoaller-

Continued on next page

Syntex—Cont.

genic; contains no lanolin, parabens or other preservatives.

Precautions: For external use only. Discontinue use if irritation occurs. Keep out of the reach of children. In case of accidental ingestion, seek professional assistance or contact a poison control center immediately.

Dosage and Administration: Rub in gently on hands, face or body. Repeat as necessary.

How Supplied: 6 fl. oz. bottle.

CARMOL® 20
20% Urea Cream
Extra strength for
rough, dry skin

Active Ingredients: Urea 20% in a non-lipid vanishing cream containing purified water, isopropyl myristate, isopropyl palmitate, stearic acid, propylene glycol, trolamine, sodium laureth sulfate, carbomer 940, hypoallergenic fragrance, xanthan gum.

Indications: Especially useful on rough, dry skin of hands, elbows, knees and feet.

Actions: Keratolytic. Contains no parabens, lanolin or mineral oil.

Precautions: For external use only. Keep away from eyes. Use with caution on face or broken or inflamed skin; transient stinging may occur. Discontinue use if irritation occurs. Keep out of the reach of children. In case of accidental ingestion, seek professional assistance or contact a poison control center immediately.

Dosage and Administration: Apply once or twice daily or as directed. Rub in well.

How Supplied: 3 oz. tubes, 1 lb. jars.

Thompson Medical Company, Inc.
919 THIRD AVENUE
NEW YORK, NY 10022

MAXIMUM STRENGTH
APPEDRINE®
Appetite Suppressant for Weight Loss

Each tablet contains:

Phenylpropanolamine HCl	25 mg

Each three tablets contain:

Vitamin A	5000 IU
Vitamin D	400 IU
Vitamin E	30 IU
Vitamin C (Ascorbic Acid)	60 mg
Folic Acid	0.4 mg
Vitamin B_1 (Thiamine HCl)	1.5 mg
Vitamin B_2 (Riboflavin)	1.7 mg
Niacinamide	20 mg
Vitamin B_6 (Pyridoxine HCl)	2 mg
Vitamin B_{12} (Cyanocobalamin)	6 mcg
d-Calcium Pantothenate	10 mg
Iodine (as Potassium Iodide)	150 mcg
Iron (as Ferrous Sulfate)	12 mg
Copper (as Cupric Sulfate)	2 mg
Zinc (as Zinc Oxide)	15 mg

Description: The daily dosage contains phenylpropanolamine HCl, an appetite suppressant, and 100% of the recommended daily adult requirement of major vitamins which may be inadvertently omitted from a low calorie diet. The active ingredient in MAXIMUM STRENGTH APPEDRINE is clinically proven effective for appetite control and weight loss.

Indications: MAXIMUM STRENGTH APPEDRINE is indicated as adjunctive therapy in the treatment of weight reduction based on caloric restriction.

Caution: Read Before Using. For adult use only. Do not give this product to children under 12 years of age. Persons between the age of 12 and 18 or over 60 are advised to consult their physician or pharmacist before using this or any drug. As with this or any drug, unwanted symptoms such as headaches, nervousness, rapid pulse, dizziness, sleeplessness, palpitations or other symptoms have occasionally been reported. Should any occur, discontinue use and consult your physician.

Warning: Do Not Exceed Recommended Dosage. Taking more of this or any drug than is recommended can cause untoward health complications. It is sensible to check your blood pressure regularly. Do not use if you have high blood pressure, diabetes, heart, thyroid, kidney, or other disease or are being treated for high blood pressure or depression except under the advice and supervision of a physician. As with any drug if you are pregnant or nursing a baby, seek the advice of a health professional before using this product. When you have attained your desired weight loss or are able to control your appetite naturally, use Appedrine only as needed.

Drug Interaction Precaution: Do not take if you are presently taking another medication containing phenylpropanolamine, or any type of nasal decongestant or a prescription antihypertensive or antidepressant drug containing a monoamine oxidase inhibitor, or any other type of prescription medication except under the advice and supervision of a physician.

Dosage and Administration: Adults: One tablet 30 minutes before each meal three times a day with one or two full glasses of water. Each tablet keeps working 4 hours.

How Supplied: Maximum Strength APPEDRINE® packages of 30 and 60 tablets packaged with 1200 calorie Maximum Strength Appedrine Diet Plan.

References: Silverman, H.I., D.Sc., Kreger, B., M.D., Lewis, G., M.D., et al, Lack of Side Effects From Orally Administered Phenylpropanolamine with Caffeine: A Controlled Three-Phase Study, Current

Therapeutic Research 28, 2:18, 180 (Aug.).
Shown in Product Identification Section, page 430

AQUA–BAN® Tablets
Each tablet contains:

Ammonium Chloride	325 mg
Caffeine	100 mg
Enteric coated	

MAXIMUM STRENGTH
AQUA–BAN® PLUS Tablets
Each tablet contains:

Ammonium Chloride	650 mg
Caffeine	200 mg
Ferrous Sulfate	6 mg
Enteric Coated	

Description: Clinically proven AQUA BAN and AQUA-BAN PLUS "water pills" work fast, effectively to help eliminate excess water.

Cautions: For occasional use only. Do not exceed recommended dose since side effects may occur which include nervousness, anxiety, irritability, palpitations or difficulty in falling asleep (if taken within 4 hours of bedtime). If fatigue or drowsiness persists continuously for more than 2 weeks, consult a physician. Do not give to children under 12 years of age. The recommended dose of this product contains about as much caffeine as two cups of coffee. Take this product with caution while taking caffeine-containing beverages because large doses of caffeine may cause side effects as cautioned above.

Warnings: Do not use if you have kidney disease, liver disease or pulmonary insufficiency. Discontinue use if nausea vomiting or gastrointestinal distress occur. As with any drug, if you are pregnant or nursing a baby, seek the advice of a health professional before using this product. KEEP THIS AND ALL MEDICATION OUT OF THE REACH OF CHILDREN. In case of accidental overdose seek professional assistance or contact a poison control center immediately.

Dosage and Administration: AQUA BAN Tablets: 2 tablets, 3 times a day after meals starting 5 or 6 days before expected menstrual period. Discontinue at onset of period. Do not take for longer than 6 days in any one month. MAXIMUM STRENGTH AQUA-BAN PLUS Tablets: 1 tablet, 3 times a day, after meals starting 5 or 6 days before expected menstrual period. Discontinue at onset of period. Do not take for longer than 6 days in any one month.

How Supplied: AQUA-BAN Tablets: Packages of 60 tablets (2 month supply). MAXIMUM STRENGTH AQUA-BAN PLUS Tablets: Packages of 30 tablets (1 month supply).

Reference: Hoffman, Jerome, J., M.D., A Double-Blind Crossover Clinical Trial of an Over the Counter Diuretic in the Treatment of Premenstrual Tension and Weight Gain, Current Therapeutic Research, 26, 5-575, 1979 (Nov.)
Shown in Product Identification Section, page 430

ASPERCREME™
External Analgesic Rub

Description: 10% Trolamine Salicylate in a lotion and odorless creme. ASPERCREME is a clinically proven rub that relieves pain effectively without stomach upset aspirin may cause.

Actions: External analgesic with rapid penetration and absorption.

Indications: An effective salicylate analgesic for temporary relief from minor pains of arthritis, rheumatism and muscular aches.

Warnings: Use only as directed. If prone to aspirin or salicylate allergic reaction, consult physician before using. If redness is present or condition worsens, or if pain persists for more than 7 days, discontinue use and consult a physician. Do not use on children under 10 years of age. Do not apply if skin is irritated or if irritation develops. As with any drug, if you are pregnant or nursing a baby, seek the advice of a health professional before using this product. For external use only. Avoid contact with eyes. Keep this and all medicines out of the reach of children.

Precautions: Occasionally where this product has been used extensively, moderate peeling of the skin may occur. This is a normal reaction to salicylates on the skin, and should not warrant discontinuing use of the product.

Dosage and Administration: Apply generously. Massage into painful area until thoroughly absorbed into skin, 3 or 4 times daily, especially before retiring. Relief lasts for hours.

How Supplied: Lotion; 6 oz. plastic bottle. Cream; 1¼ oz., 3 oz., and 5 oz. plastic tubes.

References: Golden, Emanuel L., M.D., A Double-Blind Comparison of Orally Ingested Aspirin and a Topically Applied Salicylate Cream in the Relief of Rheumatic Pain, Current Therapeutic Research, 24, 5:524, 1978 (Sept.). Rabinowitz, J. L., M.D., "Comparative Tissue Absorption of Oral 14C Aspirin and Topical Triethanolamine 14C-Salicylate in Human and Canine Knee Joints," Journal of Clinical Pharmacology 1982, 22:42–48.
Shown in Product Identification Section, page 430

CONTROL Capsules
Prolonged action anorectic for weight control containing phenylpropanolamine HCl 75 mg

Description: Phenylpropanolamine HCl is a sympathomimetic, related to ephedrine but with no untoward CNS stimulation. Useful as an anorexiant.

Indication: CONTROL is indicated as adjunctive therapy in a regimen of weight reduction based on caloric restriction in the management and control of simple exogenous obesity. In controlled clinical studies comparing PPA to placebo, patients lost an average of 1.2 lbs per week using PPA.

Caution: For Adults use only. Do not exceed recommended dose. If nervousness, dizziness, sleeplessness, rapid pulse, palpitations or other symptoms occur discontinue medication and consult your physician. It is sensible to check your blood pressure regularly. If you have or are being treated for high blood pressure, heart, diabetes, thyroid or other disease, or while pregnant, or nursing or under the age of 18 do not take this drug except under the advice of a physician. Keep this and all drugs out of the reach of children. In case of accidental overdose seek professional assistance or contact a Poison Control Center immediately.

Precaution: Avoid use if taking prescription, anti-hypertensive and antidepressive drugs containing monoamine oxidase inhibitors or other medication containing sympathomimetic amines. When you have attained your desired weight loss or are able to control your weight naturally, use only as needed.

Adverse Reactions: Side effects are rare when taken as directed. Nausea or nasal dryness may occasionally occur.

Dosage and Administration: One capsule with a full glass of water once a day at mid-morning (10:00 A.M.).

How Supplied: CONTROL Capsules—Packages of 14, 28 and 56 capsules, packaged with 1200 Calorie CONTROL Diet Plan.

References: Silverman, H. I., D.Sc., Kreger, B., M.D., Lewis, G., M.D., et al. Lack of Side Effects from Orally Administered Phenylpropanolamine and Phenylpropanolamine With Caffeine: A Controlled Three Phase Study, Current Therapeutic Research 28, 2:18, 1980 (Aug.).
Shown in Product Identification Section, page 430

CORTIZONE-5

Active Ingredient: 0.5% Hydrocortisone in an odorless creme.

Indications: For the temporary relief of minor skin irritations, itching and rashes due to eczema, dermatitis, poison ivy, oak, sumac, insect bites, soap, cosmetics, detergents, jewelry and itchy genital and anal areas.

Warnings: For external use only. Avoid contact with the eyes. In case of accidental ingestion, get professional assistance or contact a Poison Control Center immediately. Do not use on children under two years of age unless under the administration and supervision of a physician. If condition worsens or symptoms persist for more than seven days, discontinue use and contact a physician.

Dosage and Administration: For adults and children two years of age and older. Apply to affected area, not more than three or four times daily.

How Supplied: Available in 1 oz. tubes, creme or ointment.
Shown in Product Identification Section, page 430

DEXATRIM® Capsules
Prolonged action anorectic for weight control contains
phenylpropanolamine HCl 50 mg
DEXATRIM® Extra Strength Capsules w/Vitamin C
phenylpropanolamine 75 mg
Vitamin C 180 mg
(immediate release)
DEXATRIM® Caffeine-Free Extra Strength
phenylpropanolamine 75 mg
DEXATRIM® Extra Strength Plus Vitamins
phenylpropanolamine 75 mg

Each capsule also contains:
(immediate release)
Vitamin C (as Ascorbic Acid) ....60 mg
Folic Acid (as Folacin) ....400 mcg
Vitamin B1 (as Thiamine Mononitrate) ....1.5 mg
Vitamin B2 (as Riboflavin) ....1.7 mg
Niacinamide ....20 mg
Vitamin B6 (as Pyridoxine hydrochloride) ....2 mg
Vitamin B12 (as Cyanocobalamin) 6 mcg
Biotin ....30 mcg
Pantothenic Acid (as Calcium Pantothenate) ....10 mg
Iodine (as Potassium Iodide) .....150 mcg
Iron (as Ferrous Sulfate) ....7.5 mg
Copper (as Cupric Sulfate) ....2 mg
Zinc (as Zinc Oxide) ....15 mg
Manganese ....3 mg
Chromium ....50 mcg

Description: Phenylpropanolamine hydrochloride is a sympathomimetic, related to ephedrine but with no untoward CNS stimulation. Useful as an anorexiant. Extra Strength Dexatrim Plus Vitamins contains 100% of the RDA requirement.

Indication: DEXATRIM, Extra Strength Dexatrim w/Vitamin C, Caffeine-Free Extra Strength Dexatrim and Extra Strength Dexatrim Plus Vitamins are indicated as adjunctive therapy in a regimen of weight reduction based on caloric restriction in the management and control of simple exogenous obesity.

Caution: Read Before Using. For adult use only. Do not give this product to children under 12 years of age. Persons between the ages of 12 and 18 or over 60 are advised to consult their physician or pharmacist before using this or any drug. As with this or any drug, unwanted symptoms such as headaches, nervousness, rapid pulse, dizziness, sleeplessness, palpitations or other symptoms have occasionally been reported. Should any occur, discontinue use and consult your physician.

Warning: Do Not Exceed Recommended Dosage. Taking more of this or any drug than is recommended can cause untoward health complications. It is sensible to check your blood pressure regularly. Do not use if you have high blood
Continued on next page

Thompson—Cont.

pressure, diabetes, heart, thyroid, kidney, or other disease or are being treated for high blood pressure or depression except under the advice and supervision of a physician. As with any drug if you are pregnant or nursing a baby, seek the advice of a health professional before using this product. When you have attained your desired weight loss or are able to control your appetite naturally, use Dexatrim only as needed.

Drug Interaction Precaution: Do not take if you are presently taking another medication containing phenylpropanolamine, or any type of nasal decongestant or a prescription antihypertensive or antidepressant drug containing a monoamine oxidase inhibitor, or any other type of prescription medication except under the advice and supervision of a physician.
KEEP THIS AND ALL MEDICATION OUT OF THE REACH OF CHILDREN. In case of accidental overdose seek professional assistance or contact a poison control center immediately.

Adverse Reactions: Side effects are rare when taken as directed. Nausea or nasal dryness may occasionally occur.

Dosage and Administration:
DEXATRIM® Capsules: One capsule with a full glass of water mid-morning (10:00 AM)

How Supplied:
DEXATRIM® Capsules: Packages of 28 or 56 with 1250 calorie DEXATRIM Diet Plan
Extra Strength DEXATRIM® w/Vitamin C and Caffeine Free Extra Strength Dexatrim Capsules: Packages of 20 and 40 with 1250 calorie DEXATRIM Diet Plan.
Extra Strength DEXATRIM® Plus Vitamins Capsules: Packages of 16's and 32's, with 1250 calorie DEXATRIM diet plan.

References: Silverman, H. I., D.Sc., Kreger, B., M.D., Lewis, G., M.D., et al., Lack of Side Effects From Orally Administered Phenylpropanolamine and Phenylpropanolamine with Caffeine: A Controlled Three-Phase Study, Current Therapeutic Research 28, 2:18, 1980 (Aug.).

Shown in Product Identification Section, page 430

ENCARE®
Vaginal Contraceptive Suppositories

Description: Encare is an effective contraceptive in vaginal suppository form.

Active Ingredient: Each suppository contains 2.27% nonoxynol 9, the most widely used non-prescription spermicide.

Actions: Encare dissolves in the vagina and gently effervesces, protecting against pregnancy in two ways: (1) It creates a physical barrier preventing sperm from entering the cervical opening; (2) It provides a direct spermicidal or sperm immobilizing action.

Indications: Encare is effective in the prevention of pregnancy when used as directed.
Encare may also be used in conjunction with a diaphragm in place of a second application of cream or jelly. In addition, there is clinical evidence that vaginal spermicides may offer women protection against gonorrhea and other venereal disease.[1]
Encare is easy to insert and requires no applicator. At least 10 minutes before intercourse, place one Encare insert with your forefinger as far as possible into the vagina, towards the small of your back. Best protection will occur when Encare is placed deep in the vagina. You may feel a pleasant sensation of warmth. This is Encare beginning to effervesce and distribute nonoxynol 9 within the vagina. For best results, follow package instructions.
Primary Use: When oral contraceptives or the IUD are contraindicated; for patients concerned about hormonal or mechanical side effects; when sexual activity is infrequent or intermittent.
Temporary Use: During the first few months on pills and the first three months after IUD insertion; when doctors recommend temporary rest from oral contraceptives; before trying to get pregnant, after giving birth, before surgery.
In Combination With Other Methods: For added protection with condoms; as backup protection in case pills are forgotten; for extra midcycle protection with the IUD.

Precautions: As with all spermicides, some users experience irritation in using the product. If either partner experiences irritation, discontinue use. If irritation persists, consult a physician.
Do not take orally.
Keep out of reach of children.
If your doctor has told you that you should not become pregnant, consult with your doctor to determine the best contraceptive program for you. Encare is approximately as effective as vaginal foam contraceptives in actual use, but is not as effective as the pill or IUD.

Dosage and Administration: For best protection against pregnancy, it is essential to follow package instructions. It is essential that you insert Encare at least 10 minutes before intercourse. Protection lasts during the period from ten minutes to one hour following insertion. A new Encare must be inserted each time intercourse is repeated. Encare can be used safely as frequently as needed. If a douche is desired, wait at least 6 hours following intercourse. When used as directed, Encare provides effective contraceptive protection. However no contraceptive product can provide an absolute guarantee against pregnancy.
Distributed by Thompson Medical Company.

How Supplied: Boxes of 12 and 24 inserts. Encare should be stored at a temperature below 86° F (30° C).

References
[1] *Vaginal Spermicides and Gonorrhea,* Hershel Jick, M.D.; Marian T. Hannan, M.P.H.; Andy Stergachis, PhD; Fred Heidrich, M.D.; David R. Perera, M.D.; Kenneth J. Rothman, D.P.H., Journal of the American Medical Association, October 1, 1982, Vol. 248, No. 13, pages 1619–1621.

Rev. 12/82
Shown in Product Identification Section, page 430

MAXIMUM STRENGTH PROLAMINE™ Capsules
Continuous Action Appetite Suppressant for Weight Loss

Each capsule contains:
Phenylpropanolamine HCl   37.5 mg

Description: Each capsule contains phenylpropanolamine hydrochloride an appetite suppressant. PROLAMINE is a two a day appetite suppressant. One capsule in the morning helps reduce appetite at lunch and in the afternoon the second capsule before dinner helps control appetite at dinner time and throughout the evening.

Indications: MAXIMUM STRENGTH PROLAMINE is indicated as adjunctive therapy in the regimen of weight reduction based on caloric restriction. In a six-week double-blind study of 70 obese patients comparing phenylpropanolamine HCl to a placebo, 35% of the subjects taking phenylpropanolamine HCl experienced a weight loss of 8 pounds or more. Only 9% of the subjects taking placebo lost that amount of weight. Results were statistically significant at the 0.05 probability level.[1]

Caution: Read Before Using. For adult use only. Do not give this product to children under 12 years of age. Persons between the age of 12 and 18 or over 60 are advised to consult their physician or pharmacist before using this or any drug. As with this or any drug, unwanted symptoms such as headaches, nervousness, rapid pulse, dizziness, sleeplessness, palpitations or other symptoms have occasionally been reported. Should any occur, discontinue use and consult your physician.

Warning: Do Not Exceed Recommended Dosage. Taking more of this or any drug than is recommended can cause untoward health complications. It is sensible to check your blood pressure regularly. Do not use if you have high blood pressure, diabetes, heart, thyroid, kidney, or other disease or are being treated for high blood pressure or depression except under the advice and supervision of a physician. As with any drug if you are pregnant or nursing a baby, seek the advice of a health professional before using this product. When you have attained your desired weight loss or are able to control your appetite natually, use Prolamine only as needed.

Drug Interaction Precaution: Do not take if you are presently taking another medication containing phenylpropanolamine, or any type of nasal decongestant or a prescription antihypertensive or anidepressant drug containing a monoamine oxidase inhibitor, or any other type of prescription medication except under the advice and supervision of a physician.

KEEP THIS AND ALL MEDICATION OUT OF THE REACH OF CHILDREN. In case of accidental overdose, seek professional assistance or contact a poison control center immediately.

Dosage and Administration: Take one capsule at 10:00 A.M. and 1 capsule at 4 P.M. Take each capsule with a full glass of water.

How Supplied: Maximum Strength PROLAMINE™ Capsules: Packages of 20 and 50 packaged with 1200 Calorie PROLAMINE Diet Plan.
1. Report on file, Professional Services, Thompson Medical Company, Inc.

Reference: Silverman, H. I., D.Sc., Kreger, B., M.D., Lewis, G., M.D., et al. Lack of Side Effects from Orally Administered Phenylpropanolamine and Phenylpropanolamine With Caffeine: A Controlled Three-Phase Study, Current Therapeutic Research 28, 2:18, 1980 (Aug.).
Altschuler, S., M.D., Conte, A., M.D., Sebok, M., M.D., Marlin, R.L., Ph.D., Winick, C., Ph.D., Three controlled trials of weight loss with phenylpropanolamine, International Journal of Obesity (1982) 6, 549–556.
Shown in Product Identification Section, page 430

MAXIMUM STRENGTH SLEEPINAL™
Night-Time Sleep-Aid Capsules

Description: Just one Maximum Strength Sleepinal capsule taken before bedtime helps to reduce the difficulty of falling asleep and you fall asleep faster. With Sleepinal capsules, you'll wake up feeling well rested.
Sleepinal has a non-narcotic formula and has been clinically proven safe and effective when taken as directed. So, for the relief of occasional sleeplessness, take Maximum Strength Sleepinal.

Ingredients: Each capsule contains 50 mg. diphenhydramine HCl.

Direction: Take 1 capsule 20 minutes before going to bed, or as directed by a physician.

Warnings: Do not exceed recommended dosage. Do not give to children under 12 years of age. Do not use if you are taking any other type of medication without first consulting a physician or pharmacist. Take this product with caution if alcohol is being consumed.
If sleeplessness persists continuously for more than 2 weeks, consult a physican since insomnia may be a sign of serious underlying medical illness.

As with any drug, if you are pregnant or nursing a baby, seek the advice of health professional before using this product.
DO NOT TAKE THIS PRODUCT IF YOU HAVE ASTHMA, GLAUCOMA OR ENLARGEMENT OF THE PROSTATE GLAND EXCEPT UNDER THE ADVICE AND SUPERVISION OF A PHYSICIAN.
KEEP THIS AND ALL MEDICATIONS OUT OF THE REACH OF CHILDREN. In case of accidental overdose, contact a physician immediately.
SLEEPINAL™ Capsules are individually sealed in tamper resistant bubble strips. Do not use if plastic bubbles or foil backing is torn, punctured, cut or visibly tampered with.

How Supplied: SLEEPINAL™ Capsules: Packages of 16 and 32 capsules. Store capsules in a dry place at controlled temperature 60°–86°F (15°–30°C).
Shown in Product Identification Section, page 430

SLIM–FAST™

Description: Losing weight on the Slim-Fast Diet Plan can be a fast, pleasant and satisfying experience. Each 3 glasses of Slim Fast provides 100% of the U.S. recommended daily allowances of 11 essential vitamins, 7 important minerals; plus natural protein, fiber, bran and potassium. When taken as directed Slim Fast acts as a well balanced, nutritious meal substitute offering a high degree of taste, pleasure and satisfaction. Slim-Fast tastes delicious, it's easy to lose weight, because it counts the calories for you.

Ingredients: Nonfat Dry Milk, Sucrose, Whey Powder, Dextrose, Dutch Processed Cocoa, Calcium Caseinate, Microcrystalline Cellulose, Fructose, Bran Fiber, Malto-Dextrins, Natural and Artificial Flavors, Lecithin, Carrageenan, and the following Vitamins and Minerals: Magnesium Oxide, Tricalcium Phosphate, Potassium Citrate, Ferric Orthophosphate, Vitamin E Acetate, Ascorbic Acid, Niacinamide, Vitamin A Palmitate, Zinc Oxide, Copper Gluconate, Calcium Pantothenate, Manganese Sulfate, Vitamin B12, Pyridoxine Hydrochloride, Vitamin D2, Thiamine Mononitrate, Riboflavin, Biotin, Folic Acid, Potassium Iodide.

Nutritional Information:
Serving Size: 1 oz.
Servings per container: 16

Each Serving Provides:	One Serving	One Serving with 8 oz. protein fortified skim milk
Calories	90	190
Protein	5 grams	15 grams
Carbohydrate	18 grams	32 grams
Fat	less than 1 gram	1 gram
Fiber	2 grams	2 grams

PERCENTAGE OF ADULT U.S. RECOMMENDED DAILY ALLOWANCE (U.S. RDA)

	One Serving	With 8 oz. skim milk
Protein	10%	35%
Vitamin A	25%	35%
Vitamin C (Ascorbic Acid)	30%	35%
Thiamine (Vitamin B1)	30%	35%
Riboflavin (Vitamin B2)	10%	35%
Niacin	35%	35%
Calcium	15%	50%
Iron	35%	35%
Vitamin D	10%	35%
Vitamin E	35%	35%
Vitamin B6	30%	35%
Folic Acid	20%	25%
Vitamin B12	20%	35%
Phosphorous	15%	40%
Iodine	35%	35%
Magnesium	25%	35%
Zinc	30%	35%
Copper	35%	35%
Biotin	35%	35%
Pantothenic Acid	25%	35%
Manganese	1 mg*	1 mg*
Potassium	240 mg*	680 mg*

*No U.S. RDA established

Directions: Simply add 1 rounded measuring scoop (included in can) or 2 rounded tablespoons (1 oz.) of Slim-Fast powder to 8 fluid ounces of protein fortified skim milk. Stir and serve (if you prefer use a shaker).
Slim-Fast mixes instantly into a delicious nutritionally satisfying diet meal replacement.

For Fast Weight Loss: Enjoy Slim-Fast twice daily in place of breakfast and lunch. For dinner eat a well balanced meal as specified in the enclosed diet plan.

For Faster Weight Loss: Enjoy Slim-Fast as a total program of 4 meals a day for no more than 2 weeks out of 4 or 3 days each week. Be sure to also drink 4 to 5 (8 oz.) glasses of water each day.

For Weight Maintenance: Enjoy Slim-Fast once daily in place of either breakfast or lunch and for the other two meals, follow a nutritionally balanced eating program.

Caution: Anyone with high blood pressure, diabetes, heart, liver, kidney, thyroid, pernicious anemia or other disease or during pregnancy, while nursing or anyone under the age of 18, should consult a physician before starting any weight loss program.

How Supplied: SLIM-FAST Natural Beverage Powder—Chocolate, 16 oz. cans and 8-1 oz. packets; Vanilla, 16 oz. cans; Strawberry, 16 oz. cans; Chocolate Malt, 16 oz. cans.
Also Available: SLIM-FAST Chocolate Pudding, 16 oz. cans. SLIM-FAST Hot Cocoa Mix, 16 oz. cans.
Shown in Product Identification Section, page 430

Products are cross-indexed by generic and chemical names in the **YELLOW SECTION**

Ulmer Pharmacal
A Krelitz Industries Company
2440 FERNBROOK LANE
MINNEAPOLIS, MN 55441

CLINITAR™ CREAM

Uses: Helps control subacute and chronic psoriasis and eczema.

Contains: Stantar 2%, a special extract, equivalent to 2% crude coal tar in a cosmetically elegant oil in water based cream virtually odor free and inconspicuous.

Directions: Apply to the affected areas once or twice daily or as directed by a physician.

Caution: For External Use Only. If undue irritation develops, discontinue use and consult a physician. Use cautiously in the sun. Coal tar can sensitize the skin to sunlight.
KEEP OUT OF THE REACH OF CHILDREN.

How Supplied: 4 fl. oz. (120 ml.) tubes, NDC 0127-2145-06.

CLINITAR™ SHAMPOO

Uses: Clinitar shampoo helps control dandruff, psoriasis and seborrhea of the scalp.

Contains: Stantar 2%, a special extract, equivalent to 2% crude coal tar as a clear amber shampoo with a clean fragrance. Leaves no residual tar odor on the hair. Leaves the hair clean and manageable.

Directions: Wet the hair and apply sufficient to obtain a good lather. Rub into the hair and scalp. Rinse and repeat the application. Leave the lather for 5 minutes and then rinse thoroughly. Use 1–3 times a week or as directed by a physician.

Caution: For External Use Only. Do not apply to acutely inflamed or broken skin. If irritation develops discontinue use and consult a physician. Temporary discoloration of blond, bleached or tinted hair can occur when using products containing tar. Do not store in direct sunlight. Avoid contact with the eyes.
KEEP OUT OF THE REACH OF CHILDREN.

How Supplied: 4 fl. oz. (120 ml.) tubes, NDC 0127-2135-06.

CLINITAR™ STICK

The mechanism of coal tar effect is still not fully known. Several qualities, though, have been ascribed to coal tar for many years. Some of these qualities overlap each other, including: antiseptic, antipruritic, anti-inflammatory, bacteriostatic and keratoplastic.

Description: CLINITAR™ Stick 5% contains: coal tar 5%. in a wax base containing Peanut Oil, Cetyl Palmitate, White Wax, Cocoa Butter, Lanolin Alcohol and BHT.

Clinical Pharmacology: When coal tar is used topically for therapeutic purposes, it is used either as crude coal tar or in medical preparations containing 1–5% coal tar. In the treatment of eczemas, the coal tar preparation usually is used as the sole medication, while in the treatment of psoriasis, coal tar application is combined with irradiation with long-waved ultraviolet light (UVB). Different modifications of Goeckerman's treatment have been developed, but in the original treatment, the patient is exposed to UVB irradiation 24 hours after application of the coal tar. In one of the Goeckerman modifications, the tar preparation is left on the skin only 2 hours before irradiation.

Indications: CLINITAR™ is indicated to help control subacute and chronic psoriasis and eczemas, e.g. atopic dermatitis, neurodermatitis and contact dermatitis in the chronic phases of the diseases.

Contraindications: CLINITAR™ is contraindicated in:
1. Patients allergic to coal tar or other ingredients contained in this product.
2. Patients suffering from generalized pustular psoriasis and skin infections.
3. Patients being treated with the Goeckerman regimen simultaneously with systemic drugs which act as photosensitizers, e.g. sulfonamides, fentiazides and tetracyclines.

Warnings:
1. CLINITAR™ should not be applied to broken, inflamed or infected skin areas, except on the advice of a physician.
2. Avoid eye contact. If this occurs, rinse eyes thoroughly with water.
3. Skin treated with CLINITAR™ should not be exposed to UV or direct sunlight for 24 hours, unless otherwise directed by a physician.
4. CLINITAR™ should not be used by patients suffering from immunological or systemic diseases, unless otherwise directed by a physician.
5. If condition does not improve after use as directed, discontinue use and contact a physician.
6. Staining of clothing may occur which is normally removed by standard laundering methods.
7. Do not use on children under 2 years of age except as directed by a doctor.
8. Do not use this product in or around the rectum or in genital area or groin except on the advice of a doctor.

Precautions:
1. All patients should be advised of the photosensitizing effects of coal tar preparations.
2. There has been proven no casual connection between the therapeutic use of coal tar in the treatment of dermatological diseases and skin cancer. In a recent retrospective study, Stern et.al. (1980), recommends careful surveillance for early tumor detection among patients suffering from psoriasis who receive long-term therapy combining coal tar and ultraviolet irradiation.

3. It is not known if CLINITAR™ can cause fetal harm when used on pregnant women. CLINITAR™ should be used on pregnant women only upon the advice of a physician.
4. CLINITAR™ has not been evaluated for absorption in nursing mothers and should be used only upon the advice of a physician.

Adverse Reactions: Systemic toxicity has been noted in very rare cases and only where the patient is suffering from immunological or systemic diseases. Use of CLINITAR™ and UVA-light irradiation may cause stinging and pain at the irradiation sights due the photosensitizing effects.

Dosage: Apply lightly, once or twice daily, or as directed by a physician. Normally, in the Goeckerman regimen, application of CLINITAR™ is followed by exposure to UVB light after 24 hours.
Note: Excess residue must be carefully removed prior to irradiation.

Overdoses: In case of accidential ingestion, seek professional assistance or contact a Poison Control Center immediately.

Shelf-Life: CLINITAR™ can be stored up to 3 years when kept in a cool, dry place at 8–15°C.

How Supplied:
NDC 0127-2130-82, 20 ml. stick.
KEEP THIS AND ALL DRUGS OUT OF THE REACH OF CHILDREN.
FOR EXTERNAL USE ONLY.

LOBANA® BATH OIL

Contains: Mineral Oil, Octyl Hydroxystearate, Lanolin Oil, PEG-4 Dilaurate, Wheat Germ Glycerides, Fragrance and Coloring.

Description: A fragrant bath supplement that is readily dispersible in water.

Actions: Conditions as it soothes and softens dry, itching skin. Helps maintain natural skin moisture and increase moisture penetration.

Warnings: For External Use Only. In presence of an open wound or infection, consult a physician for proper treatment.

Directions:
BATH: Add one or two capfuls directly to water in tub or whirlpool. Allow bathing for at least ten minutes. Pat dry with towel.
SHOWER: Apply, then rub onto wet skin. Rinse. Pat dry with towel.

Supplied:

4 fl. oz.	NDC 0127-3036-06
8 fl. oz.	NDC 0127-3036-12

LOBANA® BODY LOTION

Contains: Deionized Water, Mineral Oil, Triethanolamine Stearate, Stearic Acid, Lanolin, Cetyl Alcohol, Potassium Stearate, Propylene Glycol, Methylparaben, Propylparaben and Fragrance.

Description: Greaseless, rapid absorption and the absence of residual sticky film assures easy application for hand and body massage.

Actions: Lanolin rich to help keep the skin soft. Contains no evaporating alcohol which dries the skin. Protected by a preservative system which guards against microbial contamination.

Warnings: For External Use Only. If sensitivity occurs, discontinue use.

Supplied:
4 fl. oz. bottle   Catalog No. 1540-06
8 fl. oz. bottle   Catalog No. 1540-12

LOBANA® BODY POWDER

Contains: Corn Starch, Sodium Bicarbonate, Silica and Methylbenzethonium Chloride

Description: Helps to protect the skin from symptoms of chafing, rubbing and friction while minimizing body odor.

Actions: Absorbs moisture, perspiration and noxious secretions as it lubricates those surfaces that are in continuous contact. Provides effective deodorant action.

Warning: For External Use Only.

Directions: For routine use after a bed linen or diaper change, bath or massage.

Supplied:
8 ounce shaker bottle
                         Catalog No. 1538-88

LOBANA® BODY SHAMPOO

Contains: Chloroxylenol (a broad-spectrum antimicrobial agent) in a mild, sudsing base with conditioners and emollients.

Description: A pH balanced body and hair cleanser.

Actions: Conditions while it cleans, while providing bacteriostatic and fungistatic activity. Gives a desirable "after feel". Extra rich in emollients to keep the skin soft.

Warning: For External Use Only.

Directions: Apply to a moistened washcloth, directly to the skin or to moistened hair. Bathe/shampoo and rinse in normal manner.

Supplied:
8 fl. oz   NDC 0127-2411-12

LOBANA® CONDITIONING SHAMPOO

Contains: Deionized Water, TEA Lauryl Sulfate, Cocamidopropyl Betaine, Cocamide DEA, Quaternium 33, Ethyl Hexanediol, Sodium Chloride, Citric Acid, Fragrance, Quaternium 15 and Coloring.

Description: A pH balanced shampoo that conditions as it cleans the hair.

Actions: Adds fullness and body to the hair. Leaves conditioned hair feeling soft and manageable.

Supplied:
8 fl. oz. bottle   Catalog No. 2080-12
gallon   Catalog No. 2080-16

LOBANA® DERM-ADE CREAM

Contains: Vitamins A, D and E in a vanishing cream base with moisturizers, emollients and Silicone.

Description: Provides relief from diaper rash, minor burns, sunburn and other minor skin irritations—including those associated with ileostomy and colostomy drainage on the skin.

Actions: Soothes and softens irritated skin and promotes healing. Forms a protective film against urine and other irritants. Helps to retain natural skin moisture.

Warnings: For external use only. If infection or other signs develop, discontinue use and consult a physician.

Directions: Apply liberally as required. If necessary, clean the affected area prior to application.

How Supplied:
2 oz. jar   NDC 0127-1722-77
8 oz. jar   NDC 0127-1722-88

LOBANA® LIQUID HAND SOAP

Contains: Chloroxylenol, a broad-spectrum antimicrobial agent.

Description: A pH balanced, pearlescent, pleasantly scented Health-care Personnel Handwash with conditioners and emollients.

Warning: For External Use Only.

Directions: Wet skin and spread soap on hands and forearms. Scrub well and rinse thoroughly after washing.

Supplied:
14 fl. oz. portable dispenser
                   NDC 0127-3220-08

LOBANA® PERI-GARD

Contains: Vitamins A & D in an emollient ointment base with Chloroxylenol.

Actions: A water-resistant ointment recommended for the perineal area that protects the skin from irritation caused by urine, feces or drainage.

Warning: Should infection be present, consult a physician for proper treatment.

Directions: Apply directly to the perineal area.

Supplied:
2 oz. jar   NDC 0127-1365-77
8 oz. jar   NDC 0127-1365-88

LOBANA® PERINEAL CLEANSE

Contains: Quaternium 12 in a mild, sudsing base with conditioners and emollients.

Description: For routine use to remove feces, urine and vomit and destroy their odors.

Actions: Eliminates source of skin irritation as it destroys odors. The perineal area is left fresh, clean and soft.

Warnings: For external use only. If infections or other signs develop, discontinue use and consult a physician.

Directions: Spray on patient problem areas, and soiled linen. Wipe with cloth or underpad. Spray on a wet cloth and use to gently wash the affected skin area. Then wipe with a clean, wet cloth.

Supplied:
4 oz. sprayer   NDC 0127-1085-06
8 oz. sprayer   NDC 0127-1085-12
gallon   NDC 0127-1085-16
5-gallon   NDC 0127-1085-07

VERUCID™ GEL

Composition: Salicylic Acid 11%, Lactic Acid 4%, Copper (II) Acetate (corresponding to 1.1 mg of copper per 100 g.) in a gel consisting of Collodion, Rosin, Alcohol and Venice Turpentine.

Indications: Topical treatment of common, juvenile, plantar, mosaic warts, corns and callouses. Most warts will disappear after 12 weeks of treatment with Verucid™, providing instructions are carefully and consistently followed.

Contraindications: VERUCID™ GEL is contraindicated in diabetics or patients with poor blood circulation. Not to be used on moles, birthmarks, warts with hair growing from them, genital warts, or warts on the face or mucous membrane.

Warning: For External Use Only. Highly flammable. Do not apply to facial or anogenital warts. Avoid contact with the eyes.

Caution: Excessive abrasion will cause stinging when Verucid™ is applied. Warts are contagious and any person suffering from warts should always use their own towel.

Directions:
1. Every night soak the wart in hot water for 5 minutes.
2. Dry thoroughly.
3. Apply a thin layer of Verucid™ to the wart and allow to spread. Within a few minutes a protective film will form. This film is insoluble in water and makes a bandage unnecessary.
4. In the morning, remove elastic film, rub away the wart surface carefully with the Verucid™ abrasive, soak the wart in hot water for 5 minutes and reapply.
5. Follow the instructions described above or as directed by your physician.
6. If no improvement is seen after 12 weeks consult your physician.

How Supplied: NDC 0127-3003-81 5 g. tube
NDC 0127-3003-93 Kit—5 g. tube with pumice.

Continued on next page

Ulmer—Cont.

VLEMINCKX' Solution
(Topical Acne Treatment and Scabicide)

Composition: A saturated solution of Calcium Polysulfides, principally Calcium Pentasulfide and Calcium Thiosulfate.

Indications: For treatment of certain resistant types of non-inflammatory dermatoses such as cystic and papular types of acne vulgaris and other dermatoses which may respond to sulfur treatment including control and treatment of scabies. Vleminckx' has a mild desquamation action.

Directions For Use: For treatment of acne and other responding dermatoses, wash affected area thoroughly with hot water and soap and apply Vleminckx' Solution diluted with hot water 1:32 to 1:9 as hot compresses one or two times daily. Frequency of use and dilution may vary as directed by physician. For scabies use as above using 1:9 dilution for three days or as directed by physician.

Warning: If any irritation appears, stop treatment immediately and consult your physician. Keep away from eyes. In case of contact, flush eyes thoroughly. Avoid contact with non-stainless metals. Keep Out of Reach of Children. FOR EXTERNAL USE ONLY.

How Supplied:
Catalog No. NDC 0127-3350-02
One Pint Bottles

The Upjohn Company
KALAMAZOO, MI 49001

BACIGUENT® Antibiotic Ointment

Active Ingredient: Each gram contains 500 units of bacitracin.

Indications: *Baciguent* is a first aid ointment to help prevent infection and aid in the healing of minor cuts, burns and abrasions.

How Supplied: Available in ½ oz, 1 oz and 4 oz tubes.

CHERACOL D® Cough Formula

Active Ingredients: Each teaspoonful (5 ml) contains dextromethorphan hydrobromide, 10 mg, and guaifenesin, 100 mg, in a pleasant-tasting vehicle. Contains 4.75% alcohol.

Indications: *Cheracol D* Cough Formula helps quiet dry, hacking coughs, and helps loosen phlegm and mucus. Recommended for adults and children 2 years of age and older.

Dosage and Administration: Adults: 2 teaspoonfuls. Children 2 to 6 years: ½ teaspoonful. These doses may be repeated every four hours if necessary.

How Supplied: Available in 2 oz, 4 oz and 6 oz bottles.

Shown in Product Identification Section, page 430

CHERACOL PLUS®
Head Cold/Cough Formula

Active Ingredients: Each tablespoonful (15 ml) contains phenylpropanolamine hydrochloride, 25 mg, dextromethorphan hydrobromide, 20 mg, and chlorpheniramine maleate, 4 mg. Contains 8% alcohol.

Indications: *Cheracol Plus* syrup is an effective 3-ingredient, maximum strength formula for the temporary relief of head cold symptoms and cough (without narcotic side effects).

Dosage and Administration: Adults and children over 12 years of age: 1 tablespoonful every 4 hours or as directed by a physician. Do not take more than 6 tablespoonfuls in a 24-hour period. Do not administer to children under 12 years of age.

How Supplied: Available in 4 oz and 6 oz bottles.
Shown in Product Identification Section, page 430

CITROCARBONATE® Antacid

Active Ingredients: When dissolved, each 3.9 grams (1 teaspoonful) contains sodium bicarbonate, 0.78 gram and sodium citrate, 1.82 grams. Each teaspoonful contains 30.46 mEq (700.6 mg) of sodium.

Indications: For the relief of heartburn, acid indigestion, and sour stomach; and upset stomach associated with these symptoms.

Dosage and Administration: Adults: 1 to 2 teaspoonfuls (not to exceed 5 teaspoonfuls per day) in a glass of cold water after meals. Children 6 to 12 years: ¼ to ½ adult dose. For children under 6 years: Consult physician. Persons 60 years or older: ½ to 1 teaspoonful after meals.

How Supplied: Available in 4 oz and 8 oz bottles.

CORTAID® Cream
CORTAID® Ointment
CORTAID® Lotion
(hydrocortisone acetate)
CORTAID® Spray
(hydrocortisone)
Antipruritic

Description: *Cortaid* Cream contains hydrocortisone acetate (equivalent to 0.5% hydrocortisone) in a greaseless, odorless, vanishing cream that leaves no residue. *Cortaid* Ointment contains hydrocortisone acetate (equivalent to 0.5% hydrocortisone) in a soothing, lubricating ointment. *Cortaid* Lotion contains hydrocortisone acetate (equivalent to 0.5% hydrocortisone) in a greaseless, odorless, vanishing lotion. *Cortaid* Spray contains 0.5% hydrocortisone in a quick drying, non-staining, non-aerosol, vanishing liquid spray; alcohol content 46%.

Indications: All *Cortaid* forms are indicated for the temporary relief of minor itchy skin irritations, inflammation, and rashes due to eczema, dermatitis, insect bites, poison ivy, poison oak, poison sumac, soaps, detergents, cosmetics, and jewelry, and with the exception of *Cortaid* Spray, for external genital and anal itching.

Uses: The vanishing action of *Cortaid* Cream makes it cosmetically acceptable when the skin rash treated is on an exposed part of the body such as the hands or arms. *Cortaid* Ointment is best used where protection, lubrication and soothing of dry and scaly lesions is required; the ointment is also preferred for treating itchy genital and anal areas. *Cortaid* Lotion is thinner than the cream and is especially suitable for hairy body areas such as the scalp or arms. *Cortaid* Spray is a quick drying, non-staining formulation suitable for covering large areas of the skin.

Warnings: All *Cortaid* formulations are for external use only. Avoid contact with the eyes. If condition worsens or if symptoms persist for more than 7 days, discontinue use of this product and consult a physician. Do not use on children under 2 years of age except under the advice and supervision of a physician. Keep this and all drugs out of the reach of children. In case of accidental ingestion, seek professional assistance or contact a poison control center immediately.

Dosage and Administration: For adults and children 2 years of age and older, apply as follows: *Cortaid* Cream, *Cortaid* Ointment or *Cortaid* Lotion: gently massage into the affected area not more than 3 to 4 times daily. *Cortaid* Spray: spray on affected area not more than 3 to 4 times daily.

How Supplied: *Cortaid* formulations (hydrocortisone acetate) are available in: Cream ½ oz and 1 oz tubes; Ointment ½ oz and 1 oz tubes; Lotion 1 oz and 2 oz bottles. *Cortaid* Spray (hydrocortisone) is available in 1.5 fluid oz pump spray bottles.

Shown in Product Identification Section, page 430

CORTEF® Feminine Itch Cream
(hydrocortisone acetate)
Antipruritic

Description: *Cortef* Feminine Itch Cream contains hydrocortisone acetate (equivalent to hydrocortisone 0.5%) in an odorless, vanishing cream base that quickly disappears into the skin to avoid staining of clothing.

Indications: For effective temporary relief of minor skin irritations and external genital itching. It relieves the itch and takes the redness out of the skin to break the annoying itch/scratch cycle.

Warnings: For external use only. Avoid contact with the eyes. If condition worsens, or if symptoms persist for more than 7 days, discontinue use of this product and consult a physician. Do not use on children under 2 years of age except under the advice and supervision of a physician. Keep this and all drugs out of the reach of children. In case of accidental ingestion, seek professional assistance or contact a poison control center immediately.

Dosage and Administration: Apply to affected area not more than 3 to 4 times daily.

How Supplied: *Cortef* Feminine Itch Cream (hydrocortisone acetate) is available in ½ oz tubes.

KAOPECTATE®
Anti-Diarrhea Medicine

Active Ingredients: Each fluid ounce (2 tablespoonfuls) contains kaolin, 90 grains; pectin, 2 grains, in a pleasant-tasting liquid. Contains no alcohol.

Indications: For the relief of diarrhea. Relieves diarrhea within 24 hours without constipating.

Dosage and Administration: For best results, take full recommended dose at first sign of diarrhea and after each bowel movement or as needed. Adults: 4 to 8 tablespoonfuls. Children over 12 years: 4 tablespoonfuls. Children 6 to 12 years: 2 to 4 tablespoonfuls. Children 3 to 6 years: 1 to 2 tablespoonfuls. Infants and children under 3 years old: only as directed by a physician.

How Supplied: Available in 3 oz unit-dose, 8 oz, 12 oz, 16 oz, and gallon bottles; bilingual labeling in Spanish and English available for 8 oz and 12 oz bottles.
Shown in Product Identification Section, page 430

KAOPECTATE CONCENTRATE®
Anti-Diarrhea Medicine

Active Ingredients: Each fluid ounce (2 tablespoonfuls) contains kaolin, 135 grains; pectin, 3 grains, in a peppermint-flavored liquid. Contains no alcohol.

Indications: For the relief of diarrhea. Relieves diarrhea within 24 hours without constipating.

Dosage and Administration: For best results, take full recommended dose at first sign of diarrhea and after each bowel movement or as needed. Adults: 3 to 6 tablespoonfuls. Children over 12 years: 3 tablespoonfuls. Children 6 to 12 years: 2 tablespoonfuls. Children 3 to 6 years: 1 tablespoonful. Infants and children under 3 years: only as directed by a physician.

How Supplied: Available in 3 oz unit-dose, 8 oz and 12 oz bottles.
Shown in Product Identification Section, page 430

KAOPECTATE® Tablet Formula
Attapulgite Formula Anti-Diarrhea Medicine

Active Ingredients: Each tablet contains 600 mg attapulgite.

Indications: For the relief of diarrhea. Relieves diarrhea and the cramps and pain that accompany it within 24 hours without constipating.

Dosage and Administration: Swallow whole tablets with water; do not chew. For best results, take full recommended dose at first sign of diarrhea and after each bowel movement or as needed. Adults: 2 tablets, not to exceed 14 tablets in 24 hours.
Children 6-12 years: 1 tablet, not to exceed 7 tablets in 24 hours.
Children under 6 years of age: Use liquid *Kaopectate* or *Kaopectate Concentrate®* Anti-Diarrhea Medicine.

How Supplied: Available in 12 tablet and 20 tablet packages.
Shown in Product Identification Section, page 431

MYCIGUENT® Antibiotic Ointment

Active Ingredient: Each gram contains 5 mg of neomycin sulfate (equivalent to 3.5 mg neomycin).

Indications: *Myciguent* is a first aid ointment to help prevent infection and aid in the healing of minor cuts, burns and abrasions.

How Supplied: Available in ½ oz, 1 oz and 4 oz tubes.

MYCITRACIN® Triple Antibiotic Ointment

Active Ingredients: Each gram contains 500 units of bacitracin, 5 mg of neomycin sulfate (equivalent to 3.5 mg neomycin) and 5000 units of polymyxin B sulfate.

Indications: *Mycitracin* is a first aid ointment to help prevent infection and aid in the healing of minor cuts, burns and abrasions.

How Supplied: Available in ½₃₂ oz unit-dose, ½ oz and 1 oz tubes.
Shown in Product Identification Section, page 431

PYRROXATE® Capsules
Nasal Decongestant/Antihistamine/Analgesic Capsules

Description: *Pyrroxate* provides single-capsule, multisymptom relief for colds, allergies, nasal/sinus congestion, runny nose, sneezing, and watery eyes. Because it contains the non-aspirin analgesic **acetaminophen,** *Pyrroxate* gives temporary relief of occasional minor aches, pains, headache, and helps in the reduction of fever. *Pyrroxate* is caffeine and aspirin-free.

Ingredients: Each *Pyrroxate* capsule contains: chlorpheniramine maleate, 4 mg; phenylpropanolamine HCl, 25 mg; acetaminophen, 500 mg. The 500 mg (7.69 gr) strength of acetaminophen per capsule is non-standard, as compared to the established standard of 325 mg (5 gr) acetaminophen per capsule.

Indications: *Pyrroxate* Capsules are for the temporary relief of runny nose, sneezing, itching of the nose or throat; for the temporary relief of nasal congestion due to the common cold, allergies (hay fever), and sinus congestion; for the temporary relief of occasional aches, pains, and headache; and for the reduction of fever.

Actions: Chlorpheniramine maleate is an antihistamine effective in controlling runny nose, sneezing, watery eyes, and itching of the nose and throat. Phenylpropanolamine HCl is an oral nasal decongestant effective in relieving nasal/sinus congestion due to the common cold or allergies (hay fever). Acetaminophen is a clinically effective analgesic and antipyretic without aspirin side effects.

Warnings: Do not take this product for more than 7 days. If symptoms persist, do not improve, or new ones occur, or if fever persists for more than 3 days, discontinue use and consult your physician. Do not take this product if you have asthma, glaucoma, difficulty in urination due to the enlargement of the prostate gland, high blood pressure, diabetes, thyroid disease, or if you are presently taking a prescription antihypertensive or antidepressant drug containing a monamine oxidase inhibitor, except under the advice and supervision of a physician. Do not exceed recommended dosage because severe liver damage may occur and at higher doses, nervousness, dizziness or sleeplessness may occur. Do not take this product for the treatment of arthritis except under the advice and supervision of a physician.

Cautions: Avoid alcoholic beverages, driving a motor vehicle, or operating heavy machinery while taking this product. This product may cause drowsiness or excitability, especially in children. Keep this and all drugs out of the reach of children. In case of accidental overdose, seek professional assistance or contact a poison control center immediately.

Dosage and Administration: Take 1 capsule every 4 hours or as directed by a physician. Do not take more than 6 capsules in a 24-hour period. Do not administer to children under 12 years of age.

How Supplied: Black/yellow capsules available in blister packages of 24 and bottles of 500.
Shown in Product Identification Section, page 431

UNICAP® Capsules/Tablets
Multivitamin Supplement in Original Capsule Form
Sugar and Sodium Free Tablet

Indications: Dietary multivitamin supplement of ten essential vitamins in easy to swallow capsule or tablet form for adults and children 4 or more years of age.

Continued on next page

Upjohn—Cont.

Each capsule (or tablet) contains:

		% U.S. RDA*
Vitamin A	5000 Int. Units	100
Vitamin D	400 Int. Units	100
Vitamin E	15 Int. Units	50
Vitamin C	60 mg	100
Folic Acid	400 mcg	100
Thiamine	1.5 mg	100
Riboflavin	1.7 mg	100
Niacin	20 mg	100
Vitamin B$_6$	2 mg	100
Vitamin B$_{12}$	6 mcg	100

*Percentage of U.S. Recommended Daily Allowances

Recommended Dosage: 1 capsule or tablet daily

How Supplied: Available in bottles of 90, 120 (90 + 30 free), 240 and 1000 capsules; bottles of 90 and 120 (90 + 30 free) tablets.
Shown in Product Identification Section, page 431

UNICAP JR™ Chewable Tablets

Indications: Dietary multivitamin supplement with essential vitamins in an orange-flavored tablet . For **children** 4 or more years of age.

		% U.S. RDA*
Vitamin A	5000 Int. Units	100
Vitamin D	400 Int. Units	100
Vitamin E	15 Int. Units	50
Vitamin C	60 mg	100
Folic Acid	400 mcg	100
Thiamine	1.5 mg	100
Riboflavin	1.7 mg	100
Niacin	20 mg	100
Vitamin B$_6$	2 mg	100
Vitamin B$_{12}$	6 mcg	100

* ·Percentage of U.S. Recommended Daily Allowances

Recommended Dosage: 1 tablet daily

How Supplied: Available in bottles of 90 and 120 (90 + 30 free) tablets.
Shown in Product Identification Section, page 431

UNICAP M® Tablets
Multivitamins and Minerals
Sugar Free and Sodium Free

Indications: Dietary supplement of essential vitamins and minerals including iron and calcium for persons 12 or more years of age.

		% U.S. RDA
Vitamin A	5000 Int. Units	100
Vitamin D	400 Int. Units	100
Vitamin E	30 Int. Units	100
Vitamin C	60 mg	100
Folic Acid	400 mcg	100
Thiamine	1.5 mg	100
Riboflavin	1.7 mg	100
Niacin	20 mg	100
Vitamin B$_6$	2 mg	100
Vitamin B$_{12}$	6 mcg	100
Pantothenic Acid	10 mg	100
Iodine	150 mcg	100
Iron	18 mg	100
Copper	2 mg	100
Zinc	15 mg	100
Calcium	60 mg	6
Phosphorus	45 mg	5
Manganese	1 mg	+
Potassium	5 mg	+

+ Recognized as essential in human nutrition, but no U.S. Recommended Daily Allowance (U.S. RDA) has been established.

Recommended Dosage: 1 tablet daily

How Supplied: Available in bottles of 30, 90, 120 (90 + 30 free), 180 and 500 tablets.
Shown in Product Identification Section, page 431

UNICAP® Plus Iron Tablets
Multivitamin Supplement with 100% of the U.S. RDA for Iron
Low in Sodium

Indications: Dietary multivitamin supplement with essential vitamins plus iron for persons 12 or more years of age.

		% U.S. RDA*
Vitamin A	5000 Int. Units	100
Vitamin D	400 Int. Units	100
Vitamin E	15 Int. Units	50
Vitamin C	60 mg	100
Folic Acid	400 mcg	100
Thiamine	1.5 mg	100
Riboflavin	1.7 mg	100
Niacin	20 mg	100
Vitamin B$_6$	2 mg	100
Vitamin B$_{12}$	6 mcg	100
Pantothenic Acid	10 mg	100
Iron	18 mg	100

* Percentage of U.S. Recommended Daily Allowances.

Recommended Dosage: 1 tablet daily

How Supplied: Available in bottles of 90 and 120 (90 + 30 free) tablets.
Shown in Product Identification Section, page 431

UNICAP® Senior Tablets
Multivitamins and Minerals including Calcium
Sugar Free and Sodium Free

Indications: Dietary supplement of essential vitamins and minerals especially formulated for people 50 years and over to reflect the recommendations of the National Academy of Sciences—National Research Council.

		% U.S. RDA
Vitamin A	5000 Int. Units	100
(includes 200 IU Beta-Carotene)		
Vitamin D	200 Int. Units	50
Vitamin E	15 Int. Units	50
Vitamin C	60 mg	100
Folic Acid	400 mcg	100
Thiamine	1.2 mg	80
Riboflavin	1.4 mg	70
Niacin	16 mg	80
Vitamin B$_6$	2.2 mg	110
Vitamin B$_{12}$	3 mcg	50
Pantothenic Acid	10 mg	100
Iodine	150 mcg	100
Iron	10 mg	56
Copper	2 mg	100
Zinc	15 mg	100
Calcium	100 mg	10
Phosphorus	77 mg	8
Magnesium	30 mg	8
Manganese	1 mg	+
Potassium	5 mg	+

+ Recognized as essential in human nutrition, but no U.S. Recommended Daily Allowance (U.S. RDA) has been established.

Recommended Dosage: 1 tablet daily

How Supplied: Available in bottles of 90 and 120 (90 + 30 free) tablets.
Shown in Product Identification Section, page 431

UNICAP T® Tablets
Stress Formula
High Potency
Vitamin-Mineral Supplement with Zinc and Selenium
Sugar Free and Sodium Free

Indications: High potency dietary supplement of essential vitamins and minerals for persons 12 or more years of age.

		% U.S. RDA
Vitamin A	5000 Int. Units	100
Vitamin D	400 Int. Units	100
Vitamin E	30 Int. Units	100
Vitamin C	500 mg	833
Folic Acid	400 mcg	100
Thiamine	10 mg	667
Riboflavin	10 mg	588
Niacin	100 mg	500
Vitamin B$_6$	6 mg	300
Vitamin B$_{12}$	18 mcg	300
Pantothenic Acid	25 mg	250
Iodine	150 mcg	100
Iron	18 mg	100
Copper	2 mg	100
Zinc	15 mg	100
Manganese	1 mg	+
Potassium	5 mg	+
Selenium	10 mcg	+

+ Recognized as essential in human nutrition, but no U.S. Recommended Daily Allowance (U.S. RDA) has been established.

Recommended Dosage: 1 tablet daily

How Supplied: Available in bottles of 60 and 500 tablets.
Shown in Product Identification Section, page 431

Products are cross-indexed
by product classifications
in the
BLUE SECTION

Upsher-Smith Laboratories, Inc.
14905 23RD AVE., NORTH
MINNEAPOLIS, MN 55441

LUBRIN™ INSERTS

Description: Lubrin™ is a vaginal lubricating insert specifically formulated and designed for women when lack of sufficient vaginal lubrication is interfering with sexual intercourse. Gynecologist-tested, Lubrin™ Inserts are easy-to-use inserts that are unscented, colorless and water soluble. Because Lubrin™ liquefies within the vagina, it can be conveniently and discreetly inserted prior to intercourse to simulate the body's lubrication. **Lubrin™ Inserts are non-medicated and are not a contraceptive.**

Ingredients: PEG-6-32, PEG-20, caprylic/capric tryglyceride, glycerin, laureth-23, and PEG-40 stearate.

Indication For Use: Lubrin™ Inserts are specifically designed to provide prolonged vaginal lubrication for sexual intercourse. Lubrin™ Inserts can be particularly beneficial for women who may experience lack of vaginal lubrication due to factors such as everyday stress, anxiety or as a side effect of certain medications. In addition, lack of vaginal lubrication is a common problem following childbirth, menopause, hysterectomy and/or oophorectomy.

Dosage and Administration: Remove Lubrin™ Inserts from wrapper just prior to insertion. Before intercourse, place one insert into the vagina using the index finger and push as far as possible toward the small of the back. A Lubrin™ Insert may be inserted from five minutes to thirty minutes before intercourse. Five to ten minutes usually provides ample time for the insert to begin to dissolve and lubricate the walls of the vagina. The lubricating action will last for several hours.

How Supplied: Lubrin™ Inserts are available in packages of five.
Shown in Product Identification Section, page 431

The Vale Chemical Co., Inc.
1201 LIBERTY ST.
ALLENTOWN, PA 18102

GLYCOTUSS
(Guaifenesin)

Description: GLYCOTUSS (guaifenesin) is an orally effective expectorant to help loosen phlegm (sputum) and bronchial secretions.
Each tablet (or teaspoonful of syrup) contains:
Guaifenesin ....100 mg.

Indications and Usage: GLYCOTUSS (guaifenesin) is useful for the symptomatic relief of respiratory conditions associated with dry, unproductive cough, and in the presence of mucus in the respiratory tract. Its long action and effective stimulation of respiratory secretions make it a valuable aid in removing the cause of the cough instead of merely suppressing it. It is useful in the relief of the dry cough associated with the common cold, pertussis, measles and influenza.

Warning: Persons with a high fever or persistent cough should not use this preparation unless directed by a physician.
As with any drug, if you are pregnant or nursing a baby, seek the advice of a health professional before using this product.

Dosage and Administration: Tablets: Adult, 2 tablets every 4 hours, not to exceed 12 tablets in a 24 hour period. Children (age 6 to under 12 years), 1 tablet every 4 hours, not to exceed 6 tablets in a 24 hour period. Children (age 2 to under 6 years), ½ tablet every 4 hours not to exceed 3 tablets in a 24 hour period, or as directed by a physician. Do not administer to children under 2 years of age unless directed by a physician.
Syrup: Same as for tablets; 1 teaspoonful is equivalent to 1 tablet.

How Supplied: GYLCOTUSS Tablets are available in bottles of 100, 500 and 1000 tablets. GLYCOTUSS Syrup is available in one dozen 3 oz. bottles, 1 pint, and 1 gallon.

Vera Products, Inc.
601 W. JACKSON
HARLINGEN, TX 78550

LILY OF THE DESERT
Aloe Vera Gelly

Active Ingredient: 97% Aloe Vera Gel.

Description: ALOE VERA GELLY is a clear, smooth gel formulated with 97% pure Aloe Vera, which is a natural derivative of the Aloe Vera plant.

Indications: ALOE VERA GELLY contains 97% pure Aloe Vera Gel for topical relief of minor cuts, burns, insect bites, chafing, cold sores, skin irritations, sunburn, and other problems related to the skin and tissues. Also useful as a skin moisturizer.

Directions For Use: Cleanse area thoroughly. Apply ALOE VERA GELLY topically to affected area. Repeat application as required.

How Supplied: 4 oz (120 ml) tube.
Shown in Product Identification Section, page 431

LILY OF THE DESERT
ALOE VERA JUICE

Active Ingredient: 99.8% Aloe Vera Gel.

Description: ALOE VERA JUICE contains 99.8% pure Aloe Vera and is derived from the Aloe Vera plant. ALOE VERA JUICE is generally believed to be a digestive supplement. Many people have reported to feel more energetic after consuming ALOE VERA JUICE.

Directions For Use: Considered to be a food supplement as well as a tonic, suggested use is 1 to 2 oz. per day. Can be consumed as is or mixed with fruit juices.
Shown in Product Identification Section, page 431

Vicks Health Care Division
RICHARDSON-VICKS INC.
TEN WESTPORT ROAD
WILTON, CT 06897

DAYCARE® LIQUID
DAYCARE® CAPSULES
Multi-Symptom Colds Medicine

Active Ingredients: LIQUID — per fluid ounce (2 tbs.) or **CAPSULE** — per two capsules, contains Acetaminophen 650mg., Dextromethorphan HBr 20mg., pseudoephedrine hydrochloride 60mg. DAYCARE LIQUID also contains Alcohol 10%.

Indications: For temporary relief of major colds symptoms as follows:
Nasal congestion, coughing, aches and pains, fever, and cough irritated throat of a cold or flu without drowsy side effects.

Actions: VICKS DAYCARE is a decongestant, antitussive, analgesic and antipyretic. It helps clear stuffy nose, congested sinus openings. Calms, quiets coughing. Eases headache pain and the ache-all-over feeling. Reduces fever due to colds and flu. It relieves these symptoms without drowsiness. DAYCARE LIQUID is also a demulcent and soothes a cough irritated throat.

Warning: Do not administer the liquid to children under 2 and the capsules to children under 6 years of age unless directed by a physician. Do not exceed recommended dosage because at higher doses, nervousness, dizziness, or sleeplessness may occur. If symptoms do not improve within seven days or are accompanied by high fever, consult a physician before continuing use. Persons with high fever or persistent cough, or high blood pressure, diabetes, heart or thyroid disease should not use this preparation unless directed by a physician. Do not use more than 10 days (adults), 5 days (children under 12 years).

Drug Interaction Precaution: Do not take this product if you are presently taking a prescription antihypertensive or antidepressant drug containing MAO inhibitor except under the advice and supervision of a physician.

Overdosage: In case of accidental overdose, seek professional assistance or contact a Poison Control Center immediately.

Continued on next page

Vicks Health Care—Cont.

Dosage:
ADULTS one fluid ounce (2 tbs.) LIQ-UID, or 2 CAPSULES.
CHILDREN (6 to 12 years) One-half ounce (1 tbs.) LIQUID, or 1 CAPSULE every 4 hours. Maximum 4 doses per day.
CHILDREN (2 to 6 years) 1½ tsp LIQ-UID

How Supplied: Available in: **LIQUID** with child resistant cap—6 and 10 fl. oz. plastic bottles; **CAPSULES** in child resistant packages—20 and 36.
Shown in Product Identification Section, page 431

FORMULA 44® COUGH CONTROL DISCS

Active Ingredients per disc: Dextromethorphan (equivalent to Dextromethorphan Hydrobromide) 5 mg., Benzocaine 1.25 mg., Special Vicks Medication (menthol, anethole, peppermint oil) 0.35% in a dark brown sugar base.

Indications: Provides temporary relief from coughs and relieves throat irritation caused by colds, flu, bronchitis.

Actions: VICKS FORMULA 44 COUGH CONTROL DISCS are antitussive, local anesthetic and demulcent cough drops. They calm, quiet coughs and help coat and soothe irritated throats.

Warning: Do not exceed recommended dosage. Do not administer to children under 4 unless directed by physician. Persistent cough may indicate presence of a serious condition. Persons with high fever or persistent cough should not use this preparation unless directed by physician. As with all medication, keep out of reach of children. As with any drug, if you are pregnant or nursing a baby, seek the advice of health professional before using this product.

Overdosage: In case of accidental overdose, seek professional assistance or contact a Poison Control Center immediately.

Dosage:
ADULTS (12 years and over) 2 discs. Dissolve in mouth. Two additional discs every three hours as needed.
CHILDREN (4 to 12 years) 1 disc. Dissolve in mouth. One additional disc every three hours as needed.

How Supplied: Available as individual foil wrapped portable packets in boxes of 24.

FORMULA 44® COUGH MIXTURE

Active Ingredients per 2 tsp. (10 ml.): Dextromethorphan Hydrobromide 30 mg., Doxylamine Succinate 7.5 mg. in a pleasant tasting, dark brown syrup base. Also contains Alcohol 10%.
Indications: For the temporary relief of coughs due to colds, flu, bronchitis.

Actions: VICKS FORMULA 44 COUGH MIXTURE is an antitussive, antihistamine and demulcent. Calms and quiets coughs. Reduces sneezing and sniffling. Coats, soothes irritated throat.

Warning: Do not exceed recommended dosage unless directed by a physician. Do not administer to children under 6 years of age unless directed by a physician. Persistent cough may indicate the presence of a serious condition. Persons with a high fever or persistent cough should not use the product unless directed by a physician. FORMULA 44 may cause drowsiness. Do not drive or operate machinery while taking the product. If relief does not occur within three days, discontinue use and consult a physician. As with all medication, keep out of reach of children. As with any drug, if you are pregnant or nursing a baby, seek the advice of a health professional before using this product.

Overdosage: In case of accidental overdose, seek professional assistance or contact a Poison Control Center immediately.

Dosage:
Adults: 12 years and over—2 teaspoonfuls
Children: 6 to 12 years: 1 teaspoonful
Repeat every 4 hours as needed.
No more than 4 doses per day.
How Supplied: Available in 3 fl. oz., 6 fl. oz. and 8 fl. oz. bottles.
Shown in Product Identification Section, page 431

FORMULA 44D® DECONGESTANT COUGH MIXTURE

Active Ingredients per 3 tsp. (15 ml.): Dextromethorphan Hydrobromide 30 mg., Phenylpropanolamine Hydrochloride 37.5 mg., Guaifenesin (Glyceryl Guaiacolate) 300 mg. in a red, cherry-flavored, cooling syrup. Also contains alcohol 10%.

Indications: Relieves coughs, decongests nasal passages and loosens upper chest congestion due to colds, flu, bronchitis.

Actions: VICKS FORMULA 44D is an antitussive, nasal decongestant, expectorant and demulcent. It calms, quiets coughs; relieves nasal congestion; loosens phlegm, mucus; and coats, soothes an irritated throat.

Warning: Do not exceed recommended dosage unless directed by physician. Do not administer to children under 2 years of age unless directed by physician. Persistent cough may indicate the presence of a serious condition. Persons with a high fever or persistent cough or with high blood pressure, diabetes, heart or thyroid disease should not use this preparation unless directed by physician. As with all medication, keep out of reach of children. As with any drug, if you are pregnant or nursing a baby, seek the ad-

vice of a health professional before using this product.

Overdosage: In case of accidental overdose, seek professional assistance or contact a Poison Control Center immediately.

Dosage:

> MAXIMUM STRENGTH DOSE: ADULT DOSE 12 years and over—3 teaspoonfuls, every 6 hours as needed. No more than 4 doses per day.

REGULAR STRENGTH DOSE:
Repeat every 4 hours as needed. No more than 6 doses per day.
ADULT DOSE 12 years and over—
2 teaspoonfuls
CHILD DOSE 6–12 years—
1 teaspoonful
2–6 years—
½ teaspoonful.

How Supplied: Available in 3 fl. oz., 6 fl. oz. and 8 fl. oz. bottles.
Shown in Product Identification Section, page 431

FORMULA 44M® MULTI-SYMPTOM COUGH MIXTURE

Active Ingredients: per 4 tsp. (20 ml.): Dextromethorphan Hydrobromide 30 mg., Pseudoephedrine Hydrochloride 60 mg., Guaifenesin 200 mg., Acetaminophen 500 mg. in a bluish-red fruit flavored syrup. Also contains alcohol 20%.

Indications: Relieves coughs, decongests nasal passages, loosens upper chest congestion, and eases pain of a cough-irritated throat due to cold, bronchitis, or flu-like conditions.

Actions: VICKS FORMULA 44M is an antitussive, nasal decongestant, expectorant demulcent and analgesic. It calms, quiets coughs; relieves nasal congestion; loosens phlegm, mucus; and coats, soothes and eases the pain of an irritated throat.

Warning: Severe or persistent cough or sore throat, or sore throat accompanied by high fever, headache, nausea and vomiting may be serious. If you have the above symptoms, do not use more than 2 days and consult physician promptly. Do not exceed recommended dosage because with higher doses, nervousness, dizziness or sleeplessness may occur. If symptoms of congestion do not improve within seven days or are accompanied by high fever, consult a physician before continuing use. Persons with a high fever, persistent cough or with high blood pressure, diabetes, heart or thyroid disease should not use this preparation unless directed by physician. As with any drug, if you are pregnant or nursing a baby, seek the advice of a health professional before using this preparation. Do not administer to children under 6 years of age.

Drug Interaction Precaution: Do not take this product if you are presently taking a prescription antihypertensive or antidepressant drug containing and MAO Inhibitor except under the advice and supervision of a physician.

Overdosage: In case of accidental overdose, seek professional assistance or contact a Poison Control Center immediately.

Dosage: 12 years and over—4 teaspoonfuls (20 ml)
6–12 years—2 teaspoonfuls (10 ml)
Repeat every 6 hours as needed. No more than 4 doses per day.

How Supplied: Available in 4 fl. oz. and 8 fl. oz. bottles.
Shown in Product Identification Section, page 431

HEADWAY® CAPSULES
HEADWAY® TABLETS
For colds, sinus, allergy.

Active Ingredients per two capsules or tablets: Acetaminophen 650mg., Phenylpropanolamine HCl 37.5mg., Chlorpheniramine Maleate 4mg.

Indications: Relieves nasal congestion, runny nose, sneezing, itchy watery eyes, aches and pains caused by a cold, sinus or allergy problem.

Actions: HEADWAY is a nasal decongestant, antihistamine, analgesic and antipyretic. It provides hours of effective relief from symptoms of head colds, sinus and nasal allergies.

Warning: This preparation may cause excitability, especially in children. This medication may cause drowsiness. Avoid alcoholic beverages, driving a motor vehicle, and operating heavy machinery while taking this medication. Do not give to children under 6 years of age or exceed the recommended dosage unless directed by a physician. Persons having asthma, glaucoma, high blood pressure, heart disease, diabetes, thyroid disease, high fever, or difficulty in urination due to enlargement of the prostate gland should not use this product except under the advice and supervision of a physician. Do not use for more than 10 days unless directed by physician. As with any drug, if you are pregnant or nursing a baby, seek the advice of a health professional before using this product.

Overdosage: In case of accidental overdose, seek professional assistance or contact a Poison Control Center immediately.

Dosage:
ADULTS—2 capsules or tablets
CHILDREN (6–12 years) 1 capsule or tablet
Dose every 4 hours, not to exceed 4 doses per day.

How Supplied: Child-resistant sealed packets. Available in 16 and 36 sizes for Capsules and 20 and 40 sizes for tablets.
Shown in Product Identification Section, page 431

NYQUIL®
Nighttime Colds Medicine in oral liquid form.

Active Ingredients per fluid oz. (2 tbs.): Acetaminophen 1000 mg., Doxylamine Succinate 7.5 mg., Pseudoephedrine HCl 60 mg, and Dextromethorphan Hydrobromide 30 mg. Also contains Alcohol 25%, and FD&C Yellow No. 5 (tartrazine).

Indications: For the temporary relief of major cold and flu-like symptoms, as follows: nasal & sinus congestion, coughing, sneezing, minor sore throat pain, aches and pains, runny nose, headache, fever.

Actions: Decongestant, antipyretic, antihistaminic, antitussive, analgesic. Helps decongest nasal passages and sinus openings, relieves sniffles and sneezing, eases aches and pains, reduces fever, soothes headache, minor sore throat pain, and quiets coughing due to a cold. By relieving these symptoms, also helps patient to sleep and get the rest he needs.

Warning: Do not exceed recommended dosage because at higher doses nervousness, dizziness or sleepnessness may occur. If symptoms do not improve in 3 days, or are accompanied by high fever, consult physician before continuing use. Do not take if you have high blood pressure, heart disease, diabetes or thyroid disease except under advice and supervision of a physician. This preparation may cause drowsiness. Do not drive or operate machinery while taking this medication. Do not give to children under 12 years of age. Do not use for more than 10 days. As with any drug, if you are pregnant or nursing a baby, seek the advice of a health professional before using this product.

Drug Interaction Precaution: Do not take this product if you are presently taking a prescription antihypertensive or antidepressant drug containing MAO inhibitor except under the advice and supervision of a physician.

KEEP OUT OF REACH OF CHILDREN

Overdosage: In case of accidental overdose, seek professional assistance or contact a Poison Control Center immediately.

Dosage and Dosage Form: A green, anise-flavored oral liquid (syrup). A plastic measuring cup with 1 and 2 tablespoonful gradations is supplied.
ADULTS (12 and over): One fluid ounce (2 tablespoonfuls) at bedtime.
Not recommended for children.
If confined to bed or at home, a total of 4 doses may be taken per day, each 6 hours apart.

How Supplied: Available in 6, 10, and 14 fl. oz. plastic bottles.
Shown in Product Identification Section, page 432

SINEX™
Decongestant Nasal Spray

Active Ingredients: Phenylephrine Hydrochloride 0.5%, Cetylpyridinium Chloride 0.04%, Special Vicks Blend of Aromatics (menthol, eucalyptol, camphor, methyl salicylate). Also contains Thimerosol 0.001% as a preservative.

Indications: For prompt, temporary relief of nasal congestion due to head colds, hay fever, allergies, and sinusitis.

Actions: VICKS SINEX is a decongestant nasal spray. The product shrinks swollen membranes to restore freer breathing; gives fast relief of nasal stuffiness and congested sinus openings; allows congested sinuses to drain; and instantly cools irritated nasal passages.

Warning: Do not exceed recommended dosage. Follow directions for use carefully. For children under 6 years, consult your physician. If condition persists consult physician. As with all medication, keep out of reach of children.

Overdosage: In case of accidental ingestion, seek professional assistance or contact a Poison Control Center immediately.

Directions For Use: Keep head and dispenser upright. May be used every 4 hours as needed.
ADULTS: Spray quickly, firmly 2 times up each nostril, sniffing the spray upward.
CHILDREN 6 to 12 years: Spray 1 time up each nostril.

How Supplied: Available in ½ fl. oz. and 1 fl. oz. plastic spray bottles.
Shown in Product Identification Section, page 432

SINEX™ LONG-ACTING
Decongestant Nasal Spray

Active Ingredient: Oxymetazoline Hydrochloride 0.05% in an aqueous solution containing mentholated vapors. Also contains thimerosal 0.001% as a preservative.

Indications: For prompt, temporary relief of nasal congestion due to colds, hay fever, allergies, and sinusitis.

Actions: Oxymetazoline constricts the arterioles of the nasal passages—resulting in a nasal decongestant effect which lasts up to twelve hours, restoring freer breathing through the nose. SINEX LONG-ACTING helps decongest sinus openings and sinus passages thus promoting sinus drainage.

Warning: Do not exceed recommended dosage because symptoms may occur such as burning, stinging, sneezing or increase of nasal discharge. Do not use the product for more than three days. If symptoms persist, consult a physician. The use of this dispenser by more than one person may spread infection.

Overdosage: In case of accidental ingestion, seek professional assistance or

Continued on next page

Vicks Health Care—Cont.

contact a Poison Control Center immediately. As with all medication, keep out of reach of children.

Dosage and Aministration: With head upright, spray 2 or 3 times in each nostril twice daily (morning and evening) or as directed by a physician. Squeeze quickly, firmly, and sniff deeply. Not recommended for children under 6 years of age.

How Supplied: Available in ½ fl. oz. and 1 fl. oz. plastic spray bottles.

Shown in Product Identification Section, page 432

TEMPO®
Antacid with Antigas Action

Description: Each soft drop contains Calcium Carbonate 414 mg., Aluminum Hydroxide 133 mg., Magnesium Hydroxide 81 mg., Simethicone 20 mg.
—Acid consuming capacity: 14 mEq per drop
—Sodium content: 2.5 mg (0.11 mEq) per drop

Indications: Dissolves quickly as you chew to afford rapid relief from symptoms of acid indigestion; heartburn, sour eructations, belching, and associated gas symptoms.

Actions: TEMPO® is an antacid and antiflatulent in a pleasant tasting, spearmint flavored, soft drop, which dissolves quickly as it is chewed, providing rapid action. It has no chalky or gritty taste.

Directions for Use: Chew one TEMPO® antacid every two or three hours as symptoms occur or as directed by a physician.

Warning: Do not take more than 12 units in a 24-hour period or use the maximum dosage for more than two weeks except under the advice and supervision of a physician. Keep this and all drugs out of reach of children.

Drug Interaction Precaution: All aluminum-containing antacids, including TEMPO®, may prevent proper absorption of tetracycline. Do not take this product if you are presently taking any form of tetracycline.

How Supplied: Foil wrapped in cartons of 10, 30 or 60 drops. Each drop is individually wrapped and enclosed in a foil-lined pouch containing 5 drops.

Shown in Product Identification Section, page 432

VAPOSTEAM®
Liquid Medication for Hot Steam Vaporizers.

Active Ingredients: Polyoxyethylene Dodecanol 1.6%, Aromatics (eucalyptus oil 1.7%, camphor 6.2%, menthol 3.2%, Tincture of Benzoin 5%, in a liquid vehicle. Also contains Alcohol 55%.

Indications: For the symptomatic relief of colds, coughs, chest congestion.

Actions: VAPOSTEAM increases the action of steam to help relieve colds symptoms in the following ways: relieves coughs of colds, even croupy coughs, eases stuffy nasal congestion, loosens phlegmy chest congestion, and moistens dry, irritated breathing passages.

Caution: For steam medication only. Not to be taken by mouth. Persistent coughing may indicate the presence of a serious condition. If symptoms persist, discontinue use and consult physician. Persons with high fever or persistent cough should not use this preparation except as directed by a physician. Keep away from open flame or extreme heat. Do not direct steam from vaporizer towards face.

KEEP OUT OF REACH OF CHILDREN.

Overdosage: In case of accidental overdose, seek professional assistance or contact a Poison Control Center immediately.

Dosage and Administration: In a hot steam vaporizer: Use one tablespoonful of VAPOSTEAM with each quart of water added to the vaporizer. In an open bowl: Simply add VAPOSTEAM to any ordinary bowl of hot water—2 teaspoonfuls for each pint of water—and breathe in the medicated vapors.

How Supplied: Available in 4 fl. oz. and 6 fl. oz. bottles.

VATRONOL®
Nose Drops

Active Ingredients: Ephedrine Sulfate 0.5%, Special Vicks Aromatic Blend (menthol, eucalyptol, camphor, methyl salicylate) 0.06% in an aqueous base. Also contains Thimerosal 0.001% as a preservative.

Indications: Relieves nasal congestion caused by head colds and hay fever.

Actions: VICKS VATRONOL is a decongestant nose drop. It helps restore freer breathing by relieving nasal stuffiness and congested sinus openings. VATRONOL also cools irritated nasal passages.

Warning: Do not exceed recommended dosage. Overdosage may cause nervousness, restlessness, or sleeplessness. Do not use for more than 4 consecutive days or administer to children under 6, unless directed by a physician. As with all medication, keep out of reach of children.

Overdosage: In case of accidental overdose, seek professional assistance or contact a Poison Control Center immediately.

Dosage:
ADULTS: Fill dropper to upper mark.
CHILDREN (6–12 years): Fill dropper to lower mark.
Apply up one nostril, repeat in other nostril.

Repeat every 4 hours as needed.

How Supplied: Available in ½ fl. oz. and 1 fl. oz. dropper bottles.

VICKS® COUGH SILENCERS
Cough Drops

Active Ingredients per lozenge: Dextromethorphan (expressed as Dextromethorphan Hydrobromide) 2.5 mg., Benzocaine 1 mg., Special Vicks Medication (menthol, anethole, peppermint oil) 0.35% in a cooling green, sugar base. Contains FD&C Yellow No. 5 (tartrazine) as a color additive.

Indications: Provides all-day relief from coughs of colds, excessive smoking, dry or irritated throats when used as directed.

Actions: VICKS COUGH SILENCERS are antitussive, local anesthetic and demulcent throat lozenges.

Warning: Do not administer to children under 4 years of age unless directed by a physician. Severe or persistent cough, sore throat, or sore throat accompanied by fever, headache, nausea and vomiting may be serious. Consult physician promptly. Persons with a high fever or persistent cough should not use this preparation unless directed by a physician. As with all medication, keep out of reach of children. As with any drug, if you are pregnant or nursing a baby, seek the advice of a health professional before using this product.

Overdosage: In case of accidental overdose, seek professional assistance of contact a Poison Control Center immediately.

Dosage: Age 12 and over, 2 drops, dissolve in mouth one at a time, then 1 or 2 each hour as needed. Ages 4 to 12, 1 drop, dissolve in mouth then 1 drop each hour as needed. Do not exceed recommended dosage.

How Supplied: Available in boxes of 14's.

VICKS® CHILDREN'S COUGH SYRUP
Expectorant, Antitussive Cough Syrup

Active Ingredients per tsp. (5 ml.): Dextromethorphan Hydrobromide 3.5 mg., Guaifenesin 25 mg., in a red, cherry-flavored, syrup base. Also contains Alcohol 5%.

Indications: Provides temporary relief of coughs due to colds, helps loosen phlegm and rid passageways of bothersome mucus, and soothes a cough-irritated throat.

Actions: VICKS COUGH SYRUP is an antitussive, expectorant and demulcent. It calms, quiets coughs of colds, flu and bronchitis; loosens phlegm, promotes drainage of bronchial tubes; and coats and soothes a cough irritated throat.

Warning: Do not exceed recommended dosage. Do not administer to children under 2 years of age unless directed by a physician. Persistent cough may indicate the presence of a serious condition. Persons with a high fever or persistent cough should not use this preparation unless directed by a physician. As with all medication, keep out of reach of children. As with any drug, if you are pregnant or nursing a baby, seek the advice of a health professional before using this product.

Overdosage: In case of accidental overdose seek professional assistance or contact a Poison Control Center immediately.

Dosage:
12 years and over: 3 teaspoonfuls
6–12 years: 2 teaspoonfuls
2–6 years: 1 teaspoonful
Repeat every 4 hours as needed.

How Supplied: Available in 3 fl. oz. and 6 fl. oz. bottles.

VICKS® INHALER
with decongestant action

Active Ingredients per inhaler: l-Desoxyephedrine 50 mg., Special Vicks Medication (menthol, camphor, methyl salicylate, bornyl acetate) 150 mg.

Indications: Provides temporary relief of nasal congestion of colds and hay fever. Decongests sinus openings.

Actions: VICKS INHALER is an intranasal inhaled decongestant. It shrinks swollen membranes and provides fast relief from a stuffy nose.

Warning: As with all medication, keep out of reach of children.

Overdosage: In case of accidental overdose, seek professional assistance or contact a Poison Control Center immediately.

Directions For Use: Inhale medicated vapor through each nostril while blocking off other nostril. Use as often as needed.
VICKS INHALER is medically effective for 3 months after first use.

How Supplied: Available as a cylindrical plastic nasal inhaler (net wt. 0.007 oz.).

VICKS® THROAT LOZENGES

Active Ingredients per lozenge: Benzocaine 5 mg., Cetylpyridinium Chloride 1.66 mg., Special Vicks Medication (menthol, camphor, eucalyptus oil) in a red cooling sugar base.

Indications: For fast-acting temporary relief of minor sore throat pain, and minor coughs due to colds.

Actions: VICKS THROAT LOZENGES are local anesthetic and demulcent cough drops. They temporarily soothe minor sore throat irritations—ease pain—and relieve irritation and dryness of mouth and throat.

Warning: Do not exceed recommended dosage. Severe or persistent cough, sore throat, or sore throat accompanied by high fever, headache, nausea, and vomiting may be serious. Consult physician promptly. Do not use more than 2 days or administer to children under 3 years of age unless directed by physician. As with all medication, keep out of reach of children.

Overdosage: In case of accidental overdosage, seek professional assistance or contact a Poison Control Center immediately.

Dosage: ADULTS AND CHILDREN 3 years and over: allow one lozenge to dissolve slowly in mouth. Repeat hourly as needed.

How Supplied: Box of 12's.

VICKS® VAPORUB®
Decongestant Vaporizing Ointment

For use as a rub or in steam.

Active Ingredients: Special Vicks Medication (menthol 2.6%, camphor 4.73%, eucalyptus oil 1.2%, spirits of turpentine 4.5%) in a petrolatum base.

Indications: For the symptomatic relief of nasal congestion (up to 8 hours), bronchial mucous congestion, coughs, laryngitis and huskiness, muscular tightness and muscular aches and pains due to colds. Also for chapped hands.

Actions: The inhaled vapors of VICKS VAPORUB have a decongestant and antitussive effect. Applied externally, the medication acts as a local analgesic. The ointment is soothing to chapped hands and skin.

Warning: For external application and use in steam only. Do not swallow or place in nostrils. If fever is present or cough or other symptoms persist, see your doctor. In case of illness in very young children, it is wise to consult your physician. To avoid possibility of fire, never expose VAPORUB to flame or place VAPORUB in any container in which you are heating water. Do not direct steam from vaporizer toward face. As with all medication, keep out of reach of children.

Overdosage: In case of accidental overdosage, seek professional assistance or contact a Poison Control Center immediately.

Dosage:
AS A RUB: For relief of head and chest cold symptoms and coughs due to colds. Rub on throat, chest and back. Cover with a dry warm cloth if desired. Repeat as needed, especially at bedtime for continuous breathing relief.
For relief of muscle tightness, apply hot, moist towel to affected area. Remove towel, then massage well with VAPORUB. Cover with a dry, warm cloth if desired.
For chapped hands and skin, apply liberally as a dressing.
IN STEAM: Fill medicine cup of vaporizer with VICKS VAPORUB and follow directions of vaporizer manufacturer. VAPORUB may also be used in a steam bowl. Fill a bowl ¾ full with steaming water and add 2 teaspoonfuls of VAPORUB (after removing from heat). Then inhale steaming vapors. Add extra steaming water as steam decreases.

How Supplied: Available in 1.5 oz., 3.0 oz. and 6.0 oz. plastic jars.
Shown in Product Identification Section, page 432

Vicks Pharmacy Products Division
RICHARDSON-VICKS INC.
TEN WESTPORT ROAD
WILTON, CT 06897

CREMACOAT™ 1
Throat Coating Cough Medicine

Active Ingredients: Each 15 ml (3 teaspoonfuls) contains:
Dextromethorphan
Hydrobromide .... 30 mg.
In a red, cherry-flavored, creamy liquid. Also contains Alcohol 10%.

Indications: CREMACOAT 1 calms, quiets coughs due to colds.

Actions: CREMACOAT 1 is a nonnarcotic antitussive and demulcent formulation. Dextromethorphan acts centrally to calm coughs while the thick and creamy demulcent formula of CREMACOAT 1 soothes cough-irritated throats and shields sensitive cough receptors in the mucosa of the oropharynx and hypopharynx where coughs due to colds frequently begin.

Warning: Do not exceed recommended dosage. Do not administer to children under 2 years of age unless directed by a physician. Persistent cough may indicate the presence of a serious condition. Persons with a high fever or persistent cough should not use this preparation unless directed by a physician. As with any drug, if pregnant or nursing a baby, seek the advice of a health professional before using this product. Keep this and all drugs out of the reach of children.

Overdosage: In case of accidental overdose, seek professional assistance or contact a Poison Control Center immediately.

Dosage:
ADULTS
(12 years and older) ... 3 teaspoonfuls
CHILDREN
(6 to 12 years) .... 1½ teaspoonfuls
CHILDREN
(2 to 6 years) .... ¾ teaspoonfuls
No more than 4 doses per day. Repeat every 6 hours as needed.

How Supplied: Available in 3 fl. oz. and 6 fl. oz. bottles.

CREMACOAT™ 2
Throat Coating Cough Medicine

Active Ingredient: Each 15 ml (3 teaspoonfuls) contains:

Continued on next page

Vicks Pharmacy—Cont.

Guaifenesin
(Glyceryl Guaiacolate)..............200 mg.
In a orange-colored, orange-flavored creamy liquid. Also contains Alcohol 10%.

Indications: CREMACOAT 2 relieves coughs due to colds.

Actions: CREMACOAT 2 is an expectorant and demulcent formulation. Guaifenesin loosens phlegm in upper chest and makes coughs due to colds more productive. In addition, the thick, creamy formulation soothes cough-irritated throats and shields sensitive cough receptors in the mucosa of the oropharynx and hypopharynx where coughs frequently begin.

Warning: Do not exceed recommended dosage. Do not administer to children under 2 years of age unless directed by a physician. Persistent cough may indicate the presence of a serious condition. Persons with a high fever or cough which persists for more than 1 week should not use this preparation unless directed by a physician. As with any drug, if pregnant or nursing a baby, seek the advice of a health professional before using this product. Keep this and all drugs out of the reach of children.

Overdosage: In case of accidental overdose, seek professional assistance or contact a Poison Control Center immediately.

Dosage:
ADULTS
(12 years and older) ... 3 teaspoonfuls
CHILDREN
(6 to 12 years) .... 1½ teaspoonfuls
CHILDREN
(2 to 6 years) .... ¾ teaspoonful
No more than 6 doses per day. Repeat every 4 hours as needed.

How Supplied: Available in 3 fl. oz. and 6 fl. oz. bottles.

CREMACOAT™ 3
Throat Coating Cough Medicine

Active Ingredients: Each 15 ml (3 teaspoonfuls) contains:
Dextromethorphan
Hydrobromide..............................20 mg.
Phenylpropanolamine
Hydrochloride............................37.5 mg.
Guaifenesin
(Glyceryl Guaiacolate)..............200 mg.
In a bluish-red, raspberry-flavored creamy liquid. Also contains Alcohol 10%.

Indications: CREMACOAT 3 calms, quiets coughs, loosens phlegm and mucus in upper chest, and relieves nasal congestion due to colds.

Actions: CREMACOAT 3 is a nonnarcotic antitussive, nasal decongestant, expectorant, and demulcent formulation. Guaifenesin loosens phlegm and mucus in upper chest. Phenylpropanolamine hydrochloride relieves nasal congestion. Dextromethorphan acts cen-

trally to calm coughs, while the thick, creamy formulation soothes cough-irritated throats and shields sensitive cough receptors in the mucosa of the oropharynx and hypopharynx where coughs due to colds frequently begin.

Warning: Do not exceed recommended dosage. Do not administer to children under 2 years of age unless directed by a physician. Persistent cough may indicate the presence of a serious condition. Persons with a high fever or persistent cough or with high blood pressure, diabetes, heart or thyroid disease should not use this preparation unless directed by a physician. As with any drug, if pregnant or nursing a baby, seek the advice of a health professional before using this product. Keep this and all drugs out of the reach of children.

Overdosage: In case of accidental overdose, seek professional assistance or contact a Poison Control Center immediately.

Dosage:
ADULTS
(12 years and older) ... 3 teaspoonfuls
CHILDREN
(6 to 12 years) .... 1½ teaspoonfuls
CHILDREN
(2 to 6 years) .... ¾ teaspoonful
No more than 4 doses per day. Repeat every 4 hours as needed.

How Supplied: Available in 3 fl. oz. and 6 fl. oz. bottles.

CREMACOAT™ 4
Throat Coating Cough Medicine

Active Ingredients: Each 15 ml (3 teaspoonfuls) contain:
Dextromethorphan
Hydrobromide .... 20 mg.
Phenylpropanolamine
Hydrochloride .... 37.5 mg.
Doxylamine Succinate .... 7.5 mg.
In a pink, black cherry-flavored creamy liquid. Also contains Alcohol 10%.

Indications: CREMACOAT 4 quiets coughs, relieves nasal congestion, dries nasal drip due to colds.

Actions: CREMACOAT 4 is a nonnarcotic antitussive, nasal decongestant, antihistiminic and demulcent formulation. Phenylpropanolamine hydrochloride relieves nasal congestion. Doxylamine succinate relieves sneezing and dries nasal drip. The dextromethorphan hydrobromide acts centrally to calm coughs, while the thick, creamy formulation soothes cough-irritated throats and shields sensitive cough receptors in the mucosa of the oropharynx and hypopharynx where coughs due to colds frequently begin.

Warning: Do not exceed recommended dosage. Do not administer to children under 6 years of age unless directed by a physician. Persistent cough may indicate the presence of a serious condition. Persons with a high fever or cough or with high blood pressure, diabetes, heart or thyroid disease should not use this preparation unless directed by a physician.

This preparation may cause drowsiness. Do not drive or operate machinery while taking this medication. If relief does not occur within 3 days, discontinue use and see a physician. As with any drug, if pregnant or nursing a baby, seek the advice of a health professional before using this product. Keep this and all drugs out of the reach of children.

Overdosage: In case of accidental overdose, seek professional assistance or call a Poison Control Center immediately.

Dosage:
ADULT
(12 years and older) ......3 teaspoonfuls
CHILDREN
(6 to 12 years).............1½ teaspoonfuls
No more than 4 doses per day. Repeat every 4 hours as needed.

How Supplied: Available in 3 fl. oz. and 6 fl. oz. bottles.

PERCOGESIC®
Analgesic Tablets

Description: Each tablet contains:
Acetaminophen ....325 mg
Phenyltoloxamine citrate ....30 mg

Indications: For relief of pain and discomfort due to headache, for temporary relief of pain associated with muscle and joint soreness, neuralgia, sinusitis, minor menstrual cramps, the common cold, toothache, and minor aches and pains of rheumatism and arthritis.

Warning: If arthritic or rheumatic pain persists for more than 10 days; in the presence of redness or swelling; or in arthritic or rheumatic conditions affecting children under 12 years of age, consult a physician immediately. When used for temporary, symptomatic relief of colds, do not use for more than 3 days, except as directed by a physician. This preparation may cause drowsiness. Do not drive or operate machinery while taking this medication. Do not administer to children under 6 years of age or exceed recommended dosage unless directed by a physician. Keep this and all drugs out of the reach of children. As with any drug, if you are pregnant or nursing a baby, seek the advice of a health professional before using this product.

Overdosage: In case of overdosage, seek professional assistance or contact a poison control center immediately.

Dosage and Administration:
ADULTS (12 years and over)—1 or 2 tablets every four hours. Maximum daily dose—8 tablets
CHILDREN (6–12 years)—one-half adult dose. Maximum daily dose—4 tablets
Do not use for more than 12 days unless directed by a physician.

How Supplied: Child-resistant sealed packets of 24 tablets and bottles of 50 and 90 tablets.
Shown in Product Identification Section, page 432

Vidal Sassoon, Inc.
2049 CENTURY PARK EAST
LOS ANGELES, CA 90067

SASSOON D™ SHAMPOO

Description: A unique drug free shampoo system formulated to remove loose dandruff flakes and to help moisturize dry scalp.

Composition: A pleasantly scented, high foaming yet gentle shampoo base containing ampholytic and anionic surfactants, collagen derived proteins, substantive conditioners, herbal extracts, and panthenol.

Indications and Actions: Sassoon D was specifically developed for those individuals who do not require nor desire the effect of harsh or medicated shampoos to remove loose dandruff flakes. Clinical studies show that Sassoon D removes loose dandruff flakes and moisturizes dry scalp.

Consumer Precautions: For External Use Only. Keep out of children's reach. Avoid getting shampoo in eyes—if this occurs, thoroughly rinse eyes with water.

Dosage and Administration: Gentle enough to use on a daily basis. Apply to damp hair. Lather. Leave on 60 seconds. Rinse well. Repeat.

How Supplied: Available in 8 oz. and 12 oz. plastic bottles. Scientifically formulated to work with Sassoon D Scalp and Hair Conditioner.
Samples available. Request for samples must be in written form, no phone requests.
Send to: Vidal Sassoon, Inc.
Research & Development
Dept.-PDR
2049 Century Park East
Los Angeles, CA 90067
*Shown in Product Identification
Section, page 432*

Wakunaga of America Co., Ltd.
Subsidiary of Wakunaga
Pharmaceutical Co., Ltd.
23510 TELO AVENUE
SUITE 5
TORRANCE, CA 90505

KYOLIC®
Odor Modified Garlic

Active Ingredient: Aged Garlic Extract.

Indications: Dietary Supplement.

Suggested Use: Average serving, four capsules or tablets a day during or after meals.

How Supplied: Liquid—Kyolic-Aged Garlic Extract Flavor and Odor Modified Enriched with Vitamin B₁(and empty gelatine capsules) 2 fl oz (62 capsules) and 4 fl oz (124 capsules). Kyolic-Aged Garlic Extract Flavor and Odor Modified

Plain (and empty gelatine capsules) 2 fl oz (62 capsules) and 4 fl oz (124 capsules).
Tablets and Capsules—Kyolic-Formula 101 Tablets: Aged Garlic Extract Powder (270 mg) blended with Brewers Yeast (27 mg), Kelp (9 mg) and Algin (9 mg) bottles of 100 and 200 tablets. Kyolic-Formula 101 Capsules: Aged Garlic Extract Powder (270 mg) blended with Brewers Yeast (27 mg), Kelp (9 mg) and Algin (9 mg) bottles of 100 and 200 capsules. Kyolic-Formula 103 Capsules: Aged Garlic Extract Powder (220 mg) blended with Calcium Lactate (200 mg), and Vitamin C (100 mg) bottles of 100 capsules. Kyolic-Super Formula 100 Tablets: Aged Garlic Extract Powder (270 mg) blended with natural vegetable sources: Cellulose and Algin, bottles of 100 and 200 tablets.
*Shown in Product Identification
Section, page 432*

Walker, Corp & Co., Inc.
P.O. BOX 1320
EASTHAMPTON PL. &
N. COLLINGWOOD AVE.
SYRACUSE, NY 13201

EVAC–U–GEN®

Description: Evac-U-Gen® is available as purple scored tablets, each containing 97.2 mg. of yellow phenolphthalein.

Action and Uses: For temporary relief of occasional constipation and to help restore a normal pattern of evacuation. A mild, non-griping, stimulant laxative in chewable, anise-flavored form, Evac-U-Gen provides gentle, overnight relief by softening of the feces through selective action on the intramural nerve plexus of intestinal smooth muscle, and increases the propulsive peristaltic activity of the colon. It is frequently helpful in preparing the bowel for diagnostic procedures.

Indications: Because of its gentle and non-toxic nature, Evac-U-Gen is suitable in pregnancy, in the presence of hemorrhoids, for children and the elderly. Safe for nursing mothers, it does not affect the infant. It may be especially useful when straining at the stool is a hazard, as in hernia, cardiac or hypertensive patients.

Contraindications: Contraindicated in patients with a history of sensitivity to phenolphthalein. Evac-U-Gen should not be used when abdominal pain, nausea, vomiting, or other symptoms of appendicitis are present.

Side Effects: If skin rash appears, use of Evac-U-Gen or other preparations containing phenolphthalein should be discontinued. May cause coloration of feces or urine if such are sufficiently alkaline.

Warning: Frequent or prolonged use may result in dependence on laxatives. Keep this and all medication out of reach of children.

Administration and Dosage: Adults: chew one or two tablets night or morn-

ing. **Children:** Over 6, chew ½ tablet daily. Intensity of action is proportional to dosage, but individually effective doses vary. Evac-U-Gen is usually active 6 to 8 hours after administration, but residual action may last 3 to 4 days.

How Supplied: Evac-U-Gen is available in bottles of 35, 100, 500, 1000 and 6000 tablets.

Walker Pharmacal Company
4200 LACLEDE AVENUE
ST. LOUIS, MO 63108

PRID SALVE
(Smile's PRID Salve)
Drawing Salve and Anti-infectant

Active Ingredients: Ichthammol (Ammonium Ichthosulfonate) Phenol (Carbolic Acid) Lead Oleate, Rosin, Bees Wax, Lard.

Description: PRID has a very stiff consistency and is almost black in color.

Indication: PRID is an anti-infective salve, which also serves as a skin protective ointment. As a drawing salve, PRID softens the skin around the foreign body, and assists the natural rejection. PRID also helps to prevent the spread of infection. PRID aids in relieving the discomfort of minor skin irritations, superficial cuts, scratches and wounds. PRID is also helpful in the treatment of boils and carbuncles. PRID has been used with some success in the treatment of acne and furunculosis as well as other skin disorders.

Warning: When applied to fingers or toes, do not use a bandage; use loose gauze so as to not interfere with circulation. Apply according to directions for use and in no case to large areas of the body without a physician's direction. Keep out of eyes.

Caution: If PRID salve is not effective in 10 days, see your physician.

Directions For Use: Wash affected parts thoroughly with hot water; dry and apply PRID at least twice daily on a clean bandage or gauze. After irritation subsides, repeat application once a day for several days. DO NOT irritate by squeezing or pressing skin area.

How Supplied: PRID is packaged in a telescoping orange metal can containing 20 grams of PRID salve.

Products are cross-indexed by
generic and chemical names
in the
YELLOW SECTION

Wallace Laboratories
HALF ACRE ROAD
CRANBURY, NJ 08512

MALTSUPEX®
(malt soup extract)
Powder, Liquid, Tablets

Composition: 'Maltsupex' is a nondiastatic extract from barley malt, which is available in powder, liquid, and tablet form. 'Maltsupex' has a gentle laxative action and promotes soft, easily passed stools. Each **Tablet** contains 750 mg of 'Maltsupex' and approximately 0.15 to 0.25 mEq of potassium. Each tablespoonful (0.5 fl oz) of **Liquid** and each heaping tablespoonful of **Powder** contains approximately 16 grams of Malt Soup Extract and 3.1 to 5.5 mEq of potassium.

Indications: 'Maltsupex' is indicated for the dietary management and treatment of functional constipation in infants and children. It is also useful in treating constipation in adults, including those with laxative dependence.

Warnings: Do not use when abdominal pain, nausea or vomiting are present. If constipation persists, consult a physician. Keep this and all medications out of the reach of children.
'Maltsupex' Powder and Liquid only—Do not use these products except under the advice and supervision of a physician if you have kidney disease.
As with any drug, if you are pregnant or nursing a baby, seek the advice of a health professional before using this product.

Precautions: In patients with diabetes, allow for carbohydrate content of approximately 14 grams per tablespoonful of **Liquid** (56 calories), 13 grams per tablespoonful of **Powder** (52 calories), and 0.6 grams per Tablet (3 calories).
Tablets only: This product contains FD&C Yellow No. 5 (tartrazine) which may cause allergic-type reactions (including bronchial asthma) in certain susceptible individuals. Although the overall incidence of FD&C Yellow No. 5 (tartrazine) sensitivity in the general population is low, it is frequently seen in patients who also have aspirin hypersensitivity.

Dosage and Administration: General—The recommended daily dosage of 'Maltsupex' may vary from 6 to 32 grams for infants (2 years or less) and 12 to 64 grams for children and adults, accompanied by adequate fluid intake with each dose. Use the smallest dose that is effective and lower dosage as improvement occurs. Use heaping measures of the **Powder.** 'Maltsupex' **Liquid** mixes more easily if stirred first in one or two ounces of warm water.
Powder and Liquid (Usual Dosage)—
Adults: 2 tablespoonfuls (32 g) twice daily for 3 or 4 days, or until relief is noted, then 1 to 2 tablespoonfuls at bedtime for maintenance, as needed. Drink a full glass (8 oz) of liquid with each dose.
Children: 1 or 2 tablespoonfuls in 8 ounces of liquid once or twice daily (with

cereal, milk or preferred beverage). **Bottle-Fed Infants (over 1 month):** ½ to 2 tablespoonfuls in the day's total formula, or 1 to 2 teaspoonfuls in a single feeding to correct constipation. To prevent constipation (as when switching to whole milk) add 1 to 2 teaspoonfuls to the day's formula or 1 teaspoonful to every second feeding. **Breast-Fed Infants (over one month):** 1 to 2 teaspoonfuls in 2 to 4 ounces of water or fruit juice once or twice daily.
Tablets—**Adults:** Start with 4 tablets (3 g) four times daily (with meals and bedtime) and adjust dosage according to response. Drink a full glass (8 oz) of liquid with each dose.

How Supplied: 'Maltsupex' is supplied in 8 ounce (NDC 0037-9101-12) and 16 ounce (NDC 0037-9101-08) jars of 'Maltsupex' Powder; 8 fluid ounce (NDC 0037-9001-12) and 1 pint (NDC 0037-9001-08) bottles of 'Maltsupex' Liquid; and in bottles of 100 'Maltsupex' Tablets (NDC 0037-9201-01).
'Maltsupex' **Powder** and **Liquid** are Distributed by
WALLACE LABORATORIES
Division of
CARTER-WALLACE, INC.
Cranbury, New Jersey 08512
*Shown in Product Identification
Section, page 432*
'Maltsupex' **Tablets** are Manufactured by
WALLACE LABORATORIES
Division of
CARTER-WALLACE, INC.
Cranbury, New Jersey 08512
Rev. 1/83

RYNA™
(Liquid)
RYNA–C®
(Liquid)
RYNA–CX®
(Liquid)

Description:
Each 5 ml (one teaspoonful) of **RYNA Liquid** contains:
Chlorpheniramine maleate ....2 mg
Pseudoephedrine hydrochloride ..30 mg
in a clear, slightly yellow colored, lemon-vanilla flavored demulcent base containing no sugar, dyes, or alcohol.
Each 5 ml (one teaspoonful) of **RYNA-C Liquid** contains, in addition:
Codeine phosphate ....10 mg
　(WARNING: May be habit-forming)
in a clear, colorless to slightly yellow, cinnamon-flavored, demulcent base containing no sugar, dyes, or alcohol.
Each 5 ml (one teaspoonful) of **RYNA-CX Liquid** contains:
Codeine phosphate ....10 mg
　(WARNING: May be habit-forming)
Pseudoephedrine hydrochloride ..30 mg
Guaifenesin ....100 mg
in a clear, colorless, cherry-vanilla-menthol flavored demulcent base containing no sugar, dyes, or alcohol.

Actions:
Chlorpheniramine maleate in RYNA and RYNA-C is an antihistamine that antagonizes the effects of histamine.

Codeine Phosphate in RYNA-C and RYNA-CX is a centrally-acting antitussive that relieves cough.
Pseudoephedrine hydrochloride in RYNA, RYNA-C and RYNA-CX is a sympathomimetic nasal decongestant that acts to shrink swollen mucosa of the respiratory tract.
Guaifenesin in RYNA-CX is an expectorant that increases mucus flow to help prevent dryness and relieve irritated respiratory tract membranes.

Indications:
RYNA is indicated for the temporary relief of the concurrent symptoms of nasal congestion, sneezing, itchy and watery eyes, and running nose as occurs with the common cold or allergic rhinitis.
RYNA-C is indicated for the above when cough is also a concurrent symptom.
RYNA-CX is indicated for the temporary relief of the concurrent symptoms of dry, nonproductive cough and nasal congestion.

Directions:
Adults: 2 teaspoonfuls every 6 hours.
Children 6–under 12 years: 1 teaspoonful every 6 hours.
Children 2–under 6 years: ½ teaspoonful every 6 hours (see WARNINGS).
Do not exceed 4 doses in 24 hours.

Warnings:
Do not give these products to children taking other medications. Do not give RYNA or RYNA-C to children under 6 years, nor RYNA-CX to children under 2 years except under the advice and supervision of a physician. Do not exceed recommended dosage unless directed by a physician because nervousness, dizziness, or sleeplessness may occur at higher doses. If symptoms do not improve within 3 days or are accompanied by high fever, discontinue use and consult a physician.
As with any drug, if you are pregnant or nursing a baby, seek the advice of a health professional before using this product.
For RYNA-C and RYNA-CX only: Codeine may cause or aggravate constipation. A persistent cough may be a sign of a serious condition.
Do not take these products except under the advice and supervision of a physician if you have any of the following symptoms or conditions: cough that persists more than 3 days or tends to recur; chronic cough, such as occurs with smoking, asthma, or emphysema; cough accompanied by excessive secretions, high fever, rash, or persistent headache; chronic pulmonary disease or shortness of breath; high blood pressure; thyroid disease or diabetes.
For RYNA and RYNA-C only: Do not take these products except under the advice and supervision of a physician if you have asthma, glaucoma, or difficulty in urination due to enlargement of the prostate. Both products contain an antihistamine which may cause excitability, especially in children, or drowsiness or which may impair mental alertness. Combined

with alcohol, sedatives, or other depressants may have an additive effect. Do not drive motor vehicles, operate machinery, or drink alcoholic beverages while taking these products.
KEEP THIS AND ALL DRUGS OUT OF THE REACH OF CHILDREN. IN CASE OF ACCIDENTAL OVERDOSE, SEEK PROFESSIONAL ASSISTANCE OR CONTACT A POISON CONTROL CENTER IMMEDIATELY.

Caution: If pregnant or nursing a baby, consult your physician or pharmacist before using these products.

Drug Interaction Precaution: Do not take these products if you are presently taking a prescription antihypertensive or antidepressant drug containing a monoamine oxidase inhibitor, except under the advice and supervision of a physician.

How Supplied:
RYNA: bottles of 4 fl oz (NDC 0037-0638-66) and one pint (NDC 0037-0638-68).
RYNA-C: bottles of 4 fl oz (NDC 0037-0522-66) and one pint (NDC 0037-0522-68).
RYNA-CX: bottles of 4 fl oz (NDC 0037-0801-66) and one pint (NDC 0037-0801-68).

WALLACE LABORATORIES
Division of
CARTER-WALLACE, Inc.
Cranbury, New Jersey 08512
Rev. 6/82
*Shown in Product Identification
Section, page 432*

SYLLACT®
(Powdered Psyllium Seed Husks)

Description: Each rounded teaspoonful of fruit-flavored **'Syllact'** contains approximately 3.3 g of powdered psyllium seed husks and an equal amount of dextrose as a dispersing agent, and provides about 14 calories. Potassium sorbate, methyl and propylparaben are added as preservatives.

Actions: The active ingredient in 'Syllact' is hydrophilic mucilloid, non-absorbable dietary fiber derived from the powdered husks of natural psyllium seed, which acts by increasing the water content and bulk volume of stools. It gives 'Syllact' a bland, non-irritating, laxative action and promotes physiologic evacuation of the bowel.

Indications: 'Syllact' is indicated for the treatment of constipation and, when recommended by a physician, in other disorders where the effect of additional bulk and fiber is desired.

Warnings: Do not swallow dry. Drink a full glass (8 oz) of water or other liquid with each dose. If constipation persists, consult a physician. Do not use if fecal impaction, intestinal obstruction, or abdominal pain, nausea or vomiting are present. Keep this and all medications out of the reach of children.
As with any drug, if you are pregnant or nursing a baby, seek the advice of a

health professional before using this product.

Dosage and Administration: The actual daily dosage depends on the need and response of the patient. Adults may take up to 9 teaspoonfuls daily, in divided doses, for several days to provide optimum benefit when constipation is chronic or severe. Lower the dosage as improvement occurs. Use a dry spoon to measure powder. Tighten lid to keep out moisture.
Usual Adult Dosage—One rounded teaspoonful of 'Syllact' in a full glass (8 oz) of cool water or other beverage taken orally one to three times daily. If desired, an additional glass of liquid may be taken after each dose.
Children's Dosage—6 years and older—Half the adult dosage with the same fluid intake requirement.

How Supplied: 'Syllact' Powder—in 10 oz jars (NDC 0037-9501-13).
Rev. 1/83
WALLACE LABORATORIES
Division of
CARTER-WALLACE, INC.
Cranbury, New Jersey 08512
*Shown in Product Identification
Section, page 432*

Warner-Lambert Company
**201 TABOR ROAD
MORRIS PLAINS, NJ 07950**

Warner-Lambert Inc.
SANTURCE, P.R. 00911

HALLS® MENTHO–LYPTUS®
Cough Tablets

Active Ingredients: Each tablet contains eucalyptus oil and menthol.

Indications: For temporary relief of minor throat irritation and cough due to colds and to allergies. Makes nasal passages feel clearer.

Warning: Persistent cough may indicate presence of a serious condition. Persons with high fever or persistent cough should use this preparation only as directed by a physician.

Dosage: Allow to dissolve slowly in mouth. Repeat as often as necessary.

How Supplied: Halls Mentho-Lyptus Cough Tablets are available in single sticks of 9 tablets each, in 3-stick packs, and in bags of 30 tablets. They are available in four flavors: Regular, Cherry, Honey-Lemon and Ice Blue. There is also a Sugar Free Regular flavor available in single sticks of 5 tablets each.
*Shown in Product Identification
Section, page 433*

LISTERINE® Antiseptic

Active Ingredients: Thymol, Eucalyptol, Methyl Salicylate and Menthol. Also

contains: Water, Alcohol 26.9%, Benzoic Acid, Poloxamer 407 and Caramel.

Indications: For general oral hygiene, plaque inhibition, bad breath, minor cuts, scratches, insect bites, infectious dandruff.

Actions: Listerine Antiseptic, a unique combination of aromatic oils in a hydroalcoholic vehicle, provides long lasting oral deodorant activity. Its antibacterial action against odor causing bacteria and dental plaque, its odor-masking properties, and its low surface tension which aids in the removal of oral debris, account for its efficacy as an oral mouthwash and gargle.

Warnings: Do not administer to children under three years of age. Keep this and all drugs out of the reach of children. Not for ingestion.

Directions: For bad breath, plaque reduction and general oral hygiene—Rinse full strength for 30 seconds with ⅔ ounce (4 teaspoonfuls) morning and night.
For minor cuts, scratches and insect bites—apply directly to injury.
For infectious dandruff symptoms—massage on scalp.

Storage: Cold weather may cloud Listerine. Its antiseptic properties are not affected.

How Supplied: Listerine Antiseptic is supplied in 3, 6, 12, 18, 24 and 32 fl. oz. bottles.
*Shown in Product Identification
Section, page 433*

MAXIMUM STRENGTH LISTERINE ANTISEPTIC THROAT LOZENGES

Active Ingredients: Each lozenge contains: Hexylresorcinol 4.0 mg.

Indications: For fast temporary relief of minor sore throat pain.

Actions: When allowed to dissolve slowly in the mouth Listerine Lozenges bathes the throat with the soothing pain relieving action of Hexylresorcinol a safe and effective topical anesthetic. Listerine Lozenges provide fast temporary relief from minor sore throat pain of colds, smoking and mouth irritations.

Warnings: Severe or persistent sore throat, or sore throat accompanied by high fever, headache, nausea and vomiting, may be serious. Consult physician promptly. Do not use more than 2 days or administer to children under 3 years of age unless directed by a physician. Keep this and all drugs out of the reach of children.

Dosage: 1 lozenge every 2 hours as needed.

Storage: Store at room temperature.

How Supplied: 24 count packages

Also Available: Regular Strength Listerine Lozenges (Hexylresorcinol 2.4

Continued on next page

Warner-Lambert—Cont.

mg.) in Cherry, Lemon-Mint and Regular flavors.

LISTERMINT® with Fluoride Anticavity Dental Rinse and Mouthwash

Active Ingredient: Sodium Fluoride (0.02%). Also contains: Water, SD alcohol 38-B (6.65%), glycerin, poloxamer 407, sodium lauryl sulfate, sodium citrate, flavoring, sodium saccharin, zinc chloride, citric acid, D&C Yellow No. 10, FD&C Green No. 3.

Indications: Aids in prevention of dental cavities.

Directions: Adults and children 6 years of age and older: Use twice a day after brushing teeth with toothpaste. Vigorously swish 10 ml. (2 teaspoonfuls) of rinse between teeth for 1 minute and spit out. Do not swallow the rinse. Do not eat or drink for 30 minutes after rinsing.

Warnings: Children under 12 years of age should be supervised in the use of this product. Consult a dentist or physician for use in children under 6 years of age. Developing teeth of children under 6 years of age may become permanently discolored if excessive amounts of fluoride are repeatedly swallowed. This is not a dentifrice and should not be used as a substitute for regular toothbrushing. Keep this and all drugs out of reach of children.

How Supplied: Listermint with Fluoride is supplied to consumers in 6, 12, 18, 24 and 32 fl. oz. bottles.

*Shown in Product Identification
Section, page 433*

LUBRIDERM® CREAM
Dry Skin Cream

Composition:
Scented: Contains Water, Mineral Oil, Petrolatum, Glycerin, Glyceryl Stearate, PEG-100 Stearate, Squalane, Lanolin, Lanolin Alcohol, Lanolin Oil, Cetyl Alcohol, Sorbitan Laurate, Fragrance, Methylparaben, Butylparaben, Propylparaben, Quaternium-15.
Unscented: Contains Water, Mineral Oil, Petrolatum, Glycerin, Glyceryl Stearate, PEG-100 Stearate, Squalane, Lanolin, Lanolin Alcohol, Lanolin Oil, Cetyl Alcohol, Sorbitan Laurate, Methylparaben, Butylparaben, Propylparaben, Quaternium-15.

Actions and Uses: Lubriderm Cream is an emollient cream indicated for relieving extremely dry, chapped skin. The formula contains emollients which help restore and maintain the skin's normal suppleness while smoothing, soothing and softening.

Administration and Dosage: Apply several times daily.

Precautions: For external use only.

How Supplied: Available in 4 oz. tubes.

LUBRIDERM® LOTION
Skin Lubricant Moisturizer

Composition:
Scented—Contains Water, Mineral Oil, Petrolatum, Sorbitol, Lanolin, Lanolin Alcohol, Stearic Acid, Triethanolamine, Cetyl Alcohol, Fragrance, Butylparaben, Methylparaben, Propylparaben, Sodium Chloride.
Unscented—Contains Water, Mineral Oil, Petrolatum, Sorbitol, Lanolin, Lanolin Alcohol, Stearic Acid, Triethanolamine, Cetyl Alcohol, Butylparaben, Methylparaben, Propylparaben, Sodium Chloride.

Actions and Uses: Lubriderm Lotion is an oil-in-water emulsion indicated for use in softening, soothing and moisturizing dry chapped skin. Lubriderm relieves the roughness, tightness and discomfort associated with dry or chapped skin and helps protect the skin from further drying.
Lubriderm's extra rich formula smoothes easily into skin without leaving a sticky film.

Administration and Dosage: Apply as often as needed to hands, face and body for skin protection.

Precautions: For external use only.

How Supplied:
Scented: Available in 1, 4, 8 and 16 fl. oz. plastic bottles.
Unscented: Available in 8 and 16 fl. oz. plastic bottles.

*Shown in Product Identification
Section, page 433*

LUBRIDERM LUBATH®
BATH–SHOWER OIL

Composition: Contains mineral oil, PPG-15 Stearyl Ether, Oleth-2, Nonoxynol-5, Fragrance, D&C Green No. 6.

Actions and Uses: Lubriderm Lubath Bath-Shower Oil is a lanolin-free, mineral oil based, bath oil designed for softening and soothing dry skin during the bath. The formula disperses into countless droplets of oil that coat the skin and help lubricate and soften. It is equally effective in hard or soft water and provides an excellent way to moisturize the skin.

Administration and Dosage: One to two capfuls (16 oz. size) or two to four capfuls (8 oz. size) in bath, or apply with moistened cloth in shower and rinse. For use as a skin cleanser, rub into wet skin and rinse.

Precautions: Avoid getting in eyes, if this occurs, flush with clear water. When using any bath oil, take precautions against slipping. For external use only.

How Supplied: Available in 8 and 16 fl. oz. plastic bottles.

*Shown in Product Identification
Section, page 433*

MEDIQUELL Chewy Cough Squares

Active Ingredient: Each square contains dextromethorphan hydrobromide 15 mg.

Indications: Mediquell is a pleasant tasting cough medicine concentrated into soft chewable squares for relief of coughs due to colds, flu, bronchial irritations. Each dose relieves coughs for up to eight hours. Mediquell is non-narcotic and is safe for children and adults.

Actions: Non-narcotic, non-alcoholic cough suppressant formulation effective for up to 8 hours. Dextromethorphan acts centrally to elevate the cough threshold without the side effects associated with narcotic antitussives.

Warnings: Do not use if cough persists or high fever is present since these may indicate the presence of a serious condition. As with any drug, if you are pregnant or nursing a baby, seek the advice of a health professional before using this product.
Do not take this product for persistent or chronic cough such as occurs with smoking, asthma or emphysema or where cough is accompanied by excessive secretions except under the advice and supervision of a physician. Keep this and all medicines out of the reach of children.

Directions for Use: Chew and swallow Mediquell according to the following dose indications:
Adult Dose:
  12 years and over—2 squares
Child Dose:
  6–12 years—1 square
  2–6 years—½ square
  Under 2 years: use only as directed by a physician
Repeat every 6 to 8 hours as needed. Do not exceed 4 doses per day.

How Supplied: Available in 12 and 24 tablet packages.

*Shown in Product Identification
Section, page 433*

ROLAIDS®

Active Ingredient: Dihydroxyaluminum Sodium Carbonate. 334 mg. contains 53 mg. sodium per tablet.

Indications: For the relief of heartburn, sour stomach or acid indigestion and upset stomach associated with these symptoms.

Actions: Rolaids® provides rapid neutralization of stomach acid accompanied by the release of carbon dioxide. Each tablet has acid neutralizing capacity of 75–80 ml. of 0.1N hydrochloric acid and the ability to maintain the pH of the stomach contents close to 3.5 for a significant period of time—the pH never reaching into the alkaline region.
Due to the relatively low solubility and other physical and chemical properties of dihydroxyaluminum sodium carbonate (DASC), it is for the most part nonabsorbed.
Although sodium is present in DASC, the sodium is available for absorption only

when the antacid reacts with stomach acid. When Rolaids are consumed in excess of the amount of acid present in the stomach, this sodium is unavailable for absorption and the active ingredient is passed through the digestive system unchanged, with no sodium released.

Warnings: Keep this and all drugs out of the reach of children. Do not take more than 24 tablets in a 24 hour period, nor use the maximum dosage of this product for more than two weeks, nor use this product if you are on a sodium restricted diet, except under the advice and supervision of a physician.

Drug Interaction Precaution: Do not take this product if you are presently taking a prescription antibiotic drug containing any form of tetracycline.

Dosage and Administration: Chew 1 or 2 tablets as symptoms occur. Repeat hourly if symptoms return or as directed by a physician.

How Supplied: One roll contains 12 tablets; 3-Pack contains three 12-tablet rolls; One bottle contains 75 tablets; one bottle contains 150 tablets.

Shown in Product Identification Section, page 433

SINUTAB® Tablets*
*Product of Warner-Lambert Inc.

Active Ingredients: Each tablet contains:
Acetaminophen ....325 mg.
Pseudoephedrine HCl ....30 mg.
Chlorpheniramine Maleate ....2 mg.

Indications: For temporary relief of sinus headache, congestion and running nose.

Actions: Sinutab® contains an analgesic (acetaminophen) to relieve pain, a decongestant (pseudoephedrine HCl) to reduce congestion of the nasopharyngeal mucosa, and an antihistamine (chlorpheniramine maleate) to help control allergic symptoms.
Acetaminophen is both analgesic and antipyretic. Because acetaminophen is not a salicylate, Sinutab® can be used by patients who are allergic to aspirin. Pseudoephedrine HCl, a sympathomimetic drug, provides vasoconstriction of the nasopharyngeal mucosa resulting in a nasal decongestant effect.
Chlorpheniramine maleate is an antihistamine to provide relief of running nose, sneezing, itching of the nose or throat, and itchy and watery eyes as may occur in allergic rhinitis.

Warnings: Do not give to children under 6 years of age or use for more than 10 days unless directed by a physician. Keep this and all drugs out of the reach of children.

Caution: Do not exceed recommended dosage. Individuals with high blood pressure, heart disease, diabetes, thyroid disease, or those using monoamine oxidase inhibitors, should use only as directed by physician. This preparation may cause

drowsiness. Do not drive or operate machinery while taking this medication.

Dosage: Adults: 2 tablets every 4 hours. Do not exceed 8 tablets in 24 hours. Otherwise, as directed by a physician. Children (6–12 years): one-half the adult dosage.

Storage: Store at room temperature.

How Supplied: Sinutab® tablets are pink, uncoated and scored so that tablets may be split in half. They are supplied in safety-capped bottles of 100 tablets, in child-resistant blister packs in boxes of 12 tablets and in easy-to-open (exempt) blister packs of 30 tablets.

Shown in Product Identification Section, page 433

SINUTAB® Maximum Strength Formula*
Tablets and Capsules
*Product of Warner-Lambert Inc.

Active Ingredients: Each tablet/capsule contains:
Acetaminophen ....500 mg.
Pseudoephedrine HCl ....30 mg.
Chlorpheniramine Maleate ....2 mg.

Indications: For temporary relief of sinus headache and congestion, to promote nasal and sinus drainage, and to alleviate running nose as may occur in allergic rhinitis (such as hay fever).

Actions: Sinutab® Maximum Strength Formula contains an analgesic (acetaminophen) to relieve pain, a decongestant (pseudoephedrine HCl) to reduce congestion of the nasopharyngeal mucosa, and an antihistamine (chlorpheniramine maleate) to help control allergic symptoms.
Acetaminophen is both analgesic and antipyretic. Because acetaminophen is not a salicylate, Sinutab® Maximum Strength Formula can be used by patients who are allergic to aspirin. Pseudoephedrine HCl, a sympathomimetic drug, provides vasoconstriction of the nasopharyngeal mucosa resulting in a nasal decongestant effect.
Chlorpheniramine maleate is an antihistamine incorporated to provide relief of running nose, sneezing, itching of the nose or throat, and itchy and watery eyes as may occur in allergic rhinitis.

Warnings: Do not give this product to children under 12 years of age except under the advice and supervision of a physician. May cause drowsiness. May cause excitability especially in children. Except under the advice and supervision of a physician, do not take this product if you have asthma, glaucoma, difficulty in urination due to enlargement of the prostate gland, high blood pressure, heart disease, diabetes, or thyroid disease. Do not exceed recommended dosage because at higher dosage nervousness, dizziness, sleeplessness, or severe liver damage may occur. If symptoms persist, do not improve within 7 days, or are accompanied by high fever, or if new symptoms occur, consult a physician before con-

tinuing use. Do not take this product for more than 10 days.
Keep this and all drugs out of the reach of children. In case of accidental overdose, seek professional assistance or contact a Poison Control Center immediately.

Drug Interaction Precaution: Do not take this product if you are presently taking a prescription antihypertensive or antidepressant drug containing a monoamine oxidase inhibitor except under the advice and supervision of a physician.

Caution: Avoid driving a motor vehicle or operating heavy machinery, and avoid alcoholic beverages while taking this product.

Dosage: Adults: 2 tablets/capsules every 6 hours, not to exceed 8 tablets/capsules in 24 hours. Otherwise, as directed by a physician.

Storage: Store at room temperature.

How Supplied: Sinutab® Maximum Strength Formula capsules are red and yellow. The tablets are yellow and uncoated. They are supplied in child-resistant blister packs in boxes of 24 tablets/capsules.

Shown in Product Identification Section, page 433

SINUTAB II® Maximum Strength No Drowsiness Formula
Tablets and Capsules*
*Product of Warner-Lambert Inc.

Active Ingredients: Each tablet/capsule contains:
Acetaminophen ....500 mg.
Pseudoephedrine HCl ....30 mg.

Indications: For temporary relief of sinus headache and to promote nasal and sinus drainage.

Actions: Sinutab II® Maximum Strength No Drowsiness Formula tablets and capsules contain: an analgesic (Acetaminophen) to relieve pain, and a decongestant (Pseudoephedrine HCl) to reduce congestion of the nasopharyngeal mucosa.
Acetaminophen is both analgesic and antipyretic. Because Acetaminophen is not a salicylate Sinutab II® Maximum Strength No Drowsiness Formula can be used by patients who are allergic to aspirin.
Pseudoephedrine HCl, a sympathomimetic drug, provides vaso-constriction of the nasopharyngeal mucosa resulting in a nasal decongestant effect.
The absence of antihistimine in the formula provides the added benefit of reduced likelihood of drowsiness side effects.

Warnings: Do not give this product to children under 12 years of age except under the advice and supervision of a physician. Do not exceed recommended dosage because at higher doses nervousness, dizziness, sleeplessness, or severe liver damage may occur. Do not take this medica-

Continued on next page

Warner-Lambert—Cont.

tion if you have high blood pressure, heart disease, diabetes, or thyroid disease except under the advice and supervision of a physician. If symptoms persist, do not improve within 7 days, or are accompanied by high fever, or if new symptoms occur, consult a physician before continuing use. Do not take this product for more than 10 days. As with any drug, if you are pregnant or nursing a baby, seek professional advice before using this product. Keep this and all drugs out of the reach of children. In case of accidental overdose, seek professional assistance or contact a poison control center immediately.

Drug Interaction Precaution: Do not take this product if you are presently taking a prescription antihypertensive or antidepressant drug containing a monoamine oxidase inhibitor except under the advice and supervision of a physician.

Dosage: 2 tablets/capsules every 6 hours, not to exceed 8 tablets/capsules in 24 hours. Otherwise, as directed by a physician.

Storage: Store at room temperature.

How Supplied: Sinutab II® Maximum Strength No Drowsiness Formula tablets are light orange and uncoated. The capsules are orange and white. They are supplied in child-resistant blister packs in boxes of 24 tablets/capsules.
Shown in Product Identification Section, page 433

Westwood Pharmaceuticals Inc.
100 FOREST AVENUE
BUFFALO, NY 14213

ALPHA KERI®
Therapeutic Shower and Bath Oil

Composition: Contains mineral oil, Hydroloc™ brand of Westwood's PEG-4 dilaurate, lanolin oil, fragrance, benzophenone-3, D&C green 6.

Action and Uses: ALPHA KERI is a water-dispersible, antipruritic oil for the care of dry skin. ALPHA KERI effectively deposits a thin, uniform, emulsified film of oil over the skin. This film helps relieve itching, lubricates and softens the skin. ALPHA KERI Shower and Bath Oil is an all-over skin moisturizer. Only Alpha Keri contains Hydroloc™—the unique emulsifier that provides a more uniform distribution of the therapeutic oils to moisturize dry skin. ALPHA KERI is valuable as an aid in the treatment of dry, pruritic skin and mild skin irritations such as chronic atopic dermatitis; pruritus senilis and hiemalis; contact dermatitis; "bath-itch"; xerosis or asteatosis; ichthyosis; soap dermatitis; psoriasis.

Administration and Dosage: AL-PHA KERI *should always be used with*

water, either added to water or rubbed on to wet skin. Because of its inherent cleansing properties it is not necessary to use soap when ALPHA KERI is being used.
For exact dosage, label directions should be followed.
BATH: Added as directed to bathtub of water. For optimum relief: 10 to 20 minutes soak.
SHOWER: Dispense a small amount into hand and rub on to wet skin. Rinse as desired and pat dry.
SPONGE BATH: Added as directed to a basin of warm water then rubbed over entire body with washcloth.
SITZ BATH: Added as directed to tub water. Soak should last for 10 to 20 minutes.
INFANT BATH: Added as directed to basin or bathinette of water.
SKIN CLEANSING OTHER THAN BATH OR SHOWER: A small amount is rubbed on to wet skin. Rinse. Pat dry.

Precaution: The patient should be warned to guard against slipping in tub or shower.

How Supplied: 4 fl. oz. (NDC 0072-3600-04), 8 fl. oz. (NDC 0072-3600-08; NSN 6505-00-890-2027) and 16 fl. oz. (NDC 0072-3600-16) plastic bottles. Also available for patients who prefer to shower—ALPHA KERI SPRAY—5 oz. (NDC 0072-3600-05) aerosol container.
Shown in Product Identification Section, page 433

FOSTEX® MEDICATED CLEANSING BAR
Acne Skin Cleanser

Composition: Contains 2% sulfur, 2% salicylic acid, plus a combination of soapless cleansers and wetting agents.

Action and Uses: FOSTEX MEDICATED CLEANSING BAR is a surface-active, penetrating anti-seborrheic cleanser for therapeutic washing of the skin in the local treatment of acne and other skin conditions characterized by excessive oiliness. Degreases, dries and mildly desquamates.

Dosage and Administration: Use FOSTEX MEDICATED CLEANSING BAR instead of soap. Wash entire affected area 2 or 3 times daily, or as physician directs. Rinse well. The desired degree of dryness and peeling may be obtained by regulating frequency of use.

Caution: Avoid contact with eyes. In case of contact, flush with water. If undue skin irritation develops or increases, discontinue use and consult physician. For external use only.

How Supplied: 3¾ oz. (NDC 0072-3000-01; NSN 6505-00-116-1315) bar.
Shown in Product Identification Section, page 433

FOSTEX® 5% BENZOYL PEROXIDE GEL
Antibacterial Acne Gel

Composition: Contains 5% benzoyl peroxide.

Action and Uses: FOSTEX 5% BENZOYL PEROXIDE GEL is a penetrating, disappearing gel which helps kill bacteria that can cause acne. Helps prevent new pimples before they appear. Drying action promotes gentle peeling to help clear acne skin.

Indications: A topical aid for the control of acne vulgaria.

Dosage and Administration: After washing, rub FOSTEX 5% BPO into affected areas twice daily. In fair-skinned individuals or in excessively dry climates start with only one application daily. The desired degree of dryness and peeling may be obtained by regulating frequency of use.

Caution: Avoid contact with eyes, lips and mucous membranes. In case of contact, flush with water. Persons with very sensitive skin or a known allergy to benzoyl peroxide should not use this medication. If itching, redness, burning or swelling occurs, discontinue use. For external use only. May bleach dyed fabrics. Keep this and all drugs out of reach of children. Store at controlled room temperature (59°–86°F).

How Supplied: 1.5 oz (NDC 0072-3300-02) plastic tube.
Shown in Product Identification Section, page 433

FOSTEX 10% BENZOYL PEROXIDE CLEANSING BAR
Antibacterial Acne Cleanser

Composition: 10% Benzoyl peroxide.

Action and Uses: FOSTEX 10% BENZOYL PEROXIDE CLEANSING BAR helps kill bacteria that can cause acne. Helps prevent new pimples before they appear. Drying action promotes gentle peeling to help clear your skin.

Indications: A topical aid for the control of acne vulgaris.

Dosage and Administration: Use FOSTEX 10% BENZOYL PEROXIDE CLEANSING BAR instead of soap. For best results, wash entire affected area gently with fingertips for 1 to 2 minutes, 2 to 3 times daily, or as physician directs. Rinse well. The desired degree of dryness and peeling may be obtained by regulating frequency of use.

Caution: Avoid contact with eyes, lips and mucous membranes. In case of contact, flush with water. Persons with very sensitive skin or a known allergy to benzoyl peroxide should not use this medication. If itching, redness, burning or swelling occurs, discontinue use. If symptoms persist, consult a physician. For external use only. May bleach hair and dyed fabrics. Store at controlled room temperature (59°–86°F).

How Supplied: 3¾ oz. (NDC 0072-2900-03) bar.

Shown in Product Identification Section, page 433

FOSTEX® 10% BENZOYL PEROXIDE GEL
Antibacterial Acne Gel

Composition: Contains 10% benzoyl peroxide.

Action and Uses: FOSTEX 10% BENZOYL PEROXIDE GEL provides super strong protection against acne with 10% benzoyl peroxide... the strongest concentration of the most effective acne fighter you can buy without a prescription. Penetrates to kill bacteria that can cause acne. Helps prevent new pimples before they appear. Drying action promotes peeling to help clear skin. Wear day and night for invisible acne treatment.

Dosage and Administration: Before applying Fostex 10% Benzoyl Peroxide Gel, start fresh with a Fostex cleanser—to clean skin effectively. After washing, rub Fostex 10% Benzoyl Peroxide Gel into entire affected area twice daily, or as physician directs. In fair-skinned individuals or in excessively dry climates, start with only one application daily. The desired degree of dryness and peeling may be obtained by regulating frequency of use.

Caution: Avoid contact with eyes, lips and mucous membranes. In case of contact, flush with water. Persons with very sensitive skin or a known allergy to benzoyl peroxide should not use this medication. If itching, redness, burning or swelling occurs, discontinue use. If symptoms persist, consult a physician. For external use only. May bleach dyed fabrics. Keep this and all drugs out of the reach of children.

How Supplied: 1.5 oz (NDC 0072-4300-01) plastic tube.

Shown in Product Identification Section, page 433

FOSTEX 10% BENZOYL PEROXIDE TINTED CREAM
Antibacterial Acne Cream

Composition: 10% Benzoyl Peroxide

Action and Uses: Fostex 10% Benzoyl Peroxide Tinted Cream provides super-strong protection against acne with 10% benzoyl peroxide ... the strongest concentration of the most effective acne fighter you can buy without a prescription. Conceals as it helps heal. Helps prevent new pimples. Drying action promotes peeling to help clear skin. Wear this skin-tone acne medication day and night.

Dosage and Administration: Start fresh with a Fostex cleanser to clean skin effectively. After washing, rub Fostex 10% Benzoyl Peroxide Tinted Cream to entire affected area twice daily, or as a physician directs. In fair-skinned individuals or in excessively dry climates,

start with only one application daily. The desired degree of dryness and peeling may be obtained by regulating frequency of use.

Caution: Avoid contact with eyes, lips and mucous membranes. In case of contact, flush with water. Persons with very sensitive skin or a known allergy to benzoyl peroxide should not use this medication. If itching, redness, burning or swelling occurs, discontinue use. If symptoms persist consult a physician. For external use only. May bleach dyed fabrics. Keep this and all drugs out of reach of children. Store at controlled room temperature (59–86°F).

How Supplied: 1½ oz. (NDC 0072-4002-01).

Shown in Product Identification Section, page 433

FOSTEX 10% BENZOYL PEROXIDE WASH
Antibacterial Acne Wash

Composition: 10% Benzoyl peroxide.

Action and Uses: FOSTEX 10% BENZOYL PEROXIDE WASH helps kill bacteria that can cause acne. Helps prevent new pimples before they appear. Drying action promotes gentle peeling to help clear your acne.

Indications: A topical aid for the control of acne vulgaris.

Dosage and Administration: Shake well. Wet skin; wash entire affected are with FOSTEX 10% BENZOYL PEROXIDE WASH instead of soap. Wash gently for 1 to 2 minutes, 2 to 3 times daily, or as physician directs. The desired degree of dryness and peeling may be obtained by regulating frequency of use.

Caution: Avoid contact with eyes, lips and mucous membranes. In case of contact, flush with water. Persons with very sensitive skin or a known allergy to benzoyl peroxide should not use this medication. If itching, redness, burning or swelling occurs, discontinue use. If symptoms persist, consult a physician. May bleach dyed fabrics. Store at controlled room temperature (59°–86°F).

How Supplied: 5 oz. (NDC 0072-3100-05) plastic bottles.

Shown in Product Identification Section, page 433

KERI® LOTION
Skin Lubricant—Moisturizer

Composition: Contains mineral oil in a base of water, propylene glycol, glyceryl stearate/PEG-100 stearate, PEG-40 stearate, PEG-4 dilaurate, laureth-4, lanolin oil, methylparaben, propylparaben, fragrance, carbomer-934, triethanolamine, dioctyl sodium sulfosuccinate, quaternium-15. Freshly-scented: FD&C blue 1, D&C yellow 10.

Action and Uses: KERI LOTION lubricates and helps hydrate the skin, making it soft and smooth. It relieves itching, helps maintain a normal mois-

ture balance and supplements the protective action of skin lipids. Indicated for generalized dryness and itching; detergent hands; chapped or chafed skin; sunburn; "winter-itch"; aging, dry skin; diaper rash; heat rash.

Dosage and Administration: Apply as often as needed. Use particularly after bathing and exposure to sun, water, soaps and detergents.

How Supplied: 6½ oz. (NDC 0072-4600-56; NSN 6505-01-009-2897), 13 oz. (NDC 0072-4600-63) and 20 oz. (NDC 0072-4600-70) plastic bottles. Also available as KERI LOTION FRESHLY SCENTED—6½ oz. (NDC 0072-4500-56), 13 oz. (NDC 0072-4500-63), and 20 oz. (NDC 0072-4500-70) plastic bottles.

Shown in Product Identification Section, page 433

PRESUN® 15 SUNSCREEN LOTION
Ultra Sunscreen Protection

Composition: 5% Aminobenzoic acid (PABA), 5% Padimate O (octyl dimethyl PABA) 3% oxybenzone, 58% SD alcohol 40.

Actions and Uses: PRESUN 15, a clear PABA formula, provides 15 times an individual's natural protection. Liberal and regular use may reduce the chance of premature aging of the skin and skin cancer from overexposure to the sun. PRESUN 15 provides the highest degree of sunburn protection.

Dosage and Administration: Shake well. Apply liberally and evenly to **dry skin** before exposure; let dry before dressing. Reapply to dry skin after swimming or excessive perspiration, or after towel drying. Repeated applications during prolonged exposure are recommended. If used, cosmetics or emollients may be applied after PRESUN.

Warnings: For external use only. Do not use if sensitive to p-aminobenzoic acid (PABA), or related compounds (such as benzocaine, sulfonamides, aniline dyes or PABA esters). Discontinue use if irritation or rash appars. Transient facial stinging may occur in hot, humid weather. Avoid contact with eyes. In case of contact, flush eyes with water. Avoid flame. Avoid contact with fabric or other materials as staining may result. Keep out of the reach of children.

How Supplied: 4 oz. (NDC 0072-8800-04) plastic bottle, NSN 6505-01-121-2335.

Shown in Product Identification Section, page 433

PRESUN® 15 CREAMY SUNSCREEN
Ultra Sunscreen Protection

Composition: 8% Padimate O (Octyl dimethyl PABA), 3% oxybenzone.

Action and Uses: PRESUN 15 CREAMY, a water-resistant, non-staining moisturizing formula, provides 15 times an individual's natural protection.

Continued on next page

Westwood—Cont.

Liberal and regular use may help reduce the chance of premature aging of the skin and skin cancer from overexposure to the sun. PRESUN 15 CREAMY permits limited tanning while reducing the chance of sunburn. PRESUN 15 CREAMY maintains its degree of protection even after 40 minutes in the water.

Dosage and Administration: Shake well. Gently smooth liberal amount evenly onto **dry skin** before sun exposure. Do not rub in. Reapply to dry skin after prolonged swimming or excessive perspiration, or after towel drying. Repeated applications during prolonged sun exposure are recommended.

Warnings: For external use only. Do not use if sensitive to p-aminobenzoic acid (PABA), or related compounds (such as benzocaine, sulfonamides, aniline dyes, or PABA esters). Discontinue use if irritation or rash appears. Avoid contact with eyes. In case of contact, flush eyes with water. Keep out of the reach of children.

How Supplied: 4 oz. (NDC 0072-8904-04) plastic bottle, NSN 6505-01-121-2336.
Shown in Product Identification Section, page 433

SEBULEX® and SEBULEX® CREAM
Antiseborrheic Treatment Shampoo

Composition: Contains 2% sulfur and 2% salicylic acid in SEBULYTIC® brand of surface-active cleansers and wetting agents.

Action and Uses: A penetrating therapeutic shampoo for the temporary relief of itchy scalp and the scaling of dandruff, SEBULEX helps relieve itching, remove dandruff, excess oil. It penetrates and softens the crusty, matted layers of scales adhering to the scalp, and leaves the hair soft and manageable.

Dosage and Administration: SEBULEX liquid should be shaken before being used. SEBULEX or SEBULEX CREAM is massaged into wet scalp. Lather should be allowed to remain on scalp for about 5 minutes and then rinsed. Application is repeated, followed by a thorough rinse. Initially, SEBULEX or SEBULEX CREAM can be used daily, or every other day, or as directed, depending on the condition. Once symptoms are under control, one or two treatments a week usually will maintain control of itching, oiliness and scaling.

Caution: If undue skin irritation develops or increases, discontinue use. For external use only. Contact with eyes should be avoided. In case of contact, flush eyes thoroughly with water.

How Supplied: SEBULEX in 4 oz. (NDC 0072-2700-04), NSN 6508-00-116-1362 and 8 oz. (NDC 0072-2700-08) plastic bottles. SEBULEX CREAM in 4 oz. (NDC 0072-2800-04) plastic tube.
Shown in Product Identification Section, page 433

SEBULON® DANDRUFF SHAMPOO
Antiseborrheic Treatment and Conditioning Shampoo

Composition: 2% Zinc pyrithione. Also contains: Water, TEA-lauryl sulfate, disodium oleamido PEG-2 sulfosuccinate, cocamide DEA, acetamide MEA, magnesium aluminum silicate, dydroxpropyl guar, fragrance, FD & D green 3 and D & C green 5.

Action and Uses: Sebulon Shampoo—specially formulated to relieve the itching and flaking of dandruff and seborrheic dermatitis. Leaves hair clean and manageable.

Dosage and Administration: Shake well before using. For best results use at least twice a week. Can be used daily, if desired. Wet hair, apply to scalp and massage vigorously. Rinse and repeat.

Caution: For external use only. If condition worsens or does not improve after regular use of this product as directed, discontinue use. Avoid contact with the eyes—if this occurs, rinse thoroughly with water.

How Supplied: 4 oz. (0072-2500-04) and 8 oz. (0072-2500-08) plastic bottles.
Shown in Product Identification Section, page 433

Whitehall Laboratories Inc.
Division of American Home Products Corporation
685 THIRD AVENUE
NEW YORK, NY 10017

ADVIL™
Ibuprofen Tablets, USP
Pain Reliever/Fever Reducer

Warning: ASPIRIN SENSITIVE PATIENTS. Do not take this product if you have had a severe allergic reaction to aspirin, e.g.—asthma, swelling, shock or hives, because even though this product contains no aspirin or salicylates cross-reactions may occur in patients allergic to aspirin.

Active Ingredient: Each tablet contains ibuprofen 200 mg.

Indications: For the temporary relief of minor aches and pains associated with the common cold, headache, toothache, muscular aches, backache, for the minor pain of arthritis, for the pain of menstrual cramps, and for reduction of fever.

Dosage and Administration: Adults: Take one tablet every 4 to 6 hours while symptoms persist. If pain or fever does not respond to one tablet, two tablets may be used but do not exceed six tablets in 24 hours unless directed by a doctor. The smallest effective dose should be used. Take with food or milk if occasional and mild heartburn, upset stomach, or stomach pain occurs with use. Consult a

doctor if these symptoms are more than mild or if they persist. Children: Do not give this product to children under 12 except under the advice and supervision of a doctor. Keep this and all drugs out of the reach of children. In case of accidental overdose, seek professional assistance or contact a poison control center immediately.

Warnings: Do not take for pain for more than 10 days or for fever for more than 3 days unless directed by a doctor. If pain or fever persists or gets worse, if new symptoms occur, or if the painful area is red or swollen, consult a doctor. These could be signs of serious illness. If you are under a doctor's care for any serious condition, consult a doctor before taking this product. As with aspirin and acetaminophen, if you have any condition which requires you to take prescription drugs or if you have had any problems or serious side effects from taking any non-prescription pain reliever, do not take this product without first discussing it with your doctor. If you experience any symptoms which are unusual or seem unrelated to the condition for which you took ibuprofen, consult a doctor before taking any more of it. Although ibuprofen is indicated for the same conditions as aspirin and acetaminophen, it should not be taken with them except under a doctor's direction. Before using any drug, including this product, you should seek the advice of a health professional if you are pregnant or nursing a baby. IT IS ESPECIALLY IMPORTANT NOT TO USE IBUPROFEN DURING THE LAST 3 MONTHS OF PREGNANCY UNLESS SPECIFICALLY DIRECTED TO DO SO BY A DOCTOR BECAUSE IT MAY CAUSE PROBLEMS IN THE UNBORN CHILD OR COMPLICATIONS DURING DELIVERY.

Professional Labeling: Same as stated under Indications.

How Supplied: Coated tablets in bottles of 8, 24, 50, and 100.

Storage: Store at room temperature; avoid excessive heat (40°C, 104°F).
Shown in Product Identification Section, page 434

ANACIN®
Analgesic Tablets and Capsules

Active Ingredients: Each tablet or capsule contains: Aspirin 400 mg., Caffeine 32 mg.

Indications and Actions: Anacin relieves pain of headache, neuralgia, neuritis, sprains, muscular aches, discomforts and fever of colds, pain caused by tooth extraction and toothache, menstrual discomfort. Anacin also temporarily relieves the minor aches and pains of arthritis and rheumatism.

Warnings: As with any drug, if you are pregnant or nursing a baby, seek the advice of a health professional before using this product. Keep this and all medicines out of children's reach. In case of accidental overdose, contact a physician immediately.

Precautions: If pain persists for more than 10 days, or redness is present, or in arthritic or rheumatic conditions affecting children under 12 years of age, consult a physician immediately.

Dosage: Two tablets or capsules with water every 4 hours, as needed. Do not exceed 10 tablets or 10 capsules daily. For children 6–12, half the adult dosage.

Professional Labeling: Same as those outlined under Indications.

How Supplied: Tablets: In tins of 12's and bottles of 30's, 50's, 100's, 200's and 300's. Capsules: In bottles of 20's, 40's and 75's. Professional Samples: Available upon request. Write Whitehall Laboratories, PDR Dept., New York, N.Y. 10017.

Shown in Product Identification Section, page 434

MAXIMUM STRENGTH ANACIN®
Analgesic Tablets and Capsules

Active Ingredients: Each tablet or capsule contains: Aspirin 500 mg., Caffeine 32 mg.

Indications and Actions: Maximum Strength Anacin provides fast, effective, temporary relief of headaches, minor aches, pains and fever . . . temporary relief of minor aches and pains of arthritis and rheumatism . . . discomforts and fever of colds or "flu" . . . pain caused by tooth extraction and discomfort associated with normal menstrual periods.

Precautions: If pain persists for more than 10 days, or redness is present, or in arthritic or rheumatic conditions affecting children under 12 years of age, consult a physician immediately.

Warnings: As with any drug, if you are pregnant or nursing a baby, seek the advice of a health professional before using this product. Keep this and all medicines out of children's reach. In case of accidental overdose, contact a physician immediately.

Dosage: Adults: 2 tablets or capsules with water 3 or 4 times a day. Do not exceed 8 tablets or capsules in any 24 hour period. Not recommended for children under 12 years of age.

How Supplied: Tablets: Tins of 12's and bottles of 20's, 40's, 75's, and 150's. Capsules: bottles of 30's and 60's.

Children's ANACIN–3®
Acetaminophen
Chewable Tablets, Liquid, Drops

Description: Each Children's Anacin-3 Chewable Tablet contains 80 mg. acetaminophen in a cherry flavored tablet. Children's Anacin-3 acetaminophen Liquid is stable, cherry flavored, red in color and contains 7% alcohol. Infants' Anacin-3 Drops are stable, fruit flavored, red in color and contain 7% alcohol. Children's Anacin-3 Liquid: Each 5 ml. contains 160 mg. acetaminophen.

Infants' Anacin-3 Drops: Each 0.8 ml. (one calibrated dropperful) contains 80 mg. acetaminophen.

Indications and Actions: Children's Anacin-3 Chewable Tablets, Liquid and Infants' Anacin-3 Drops are safe and effective 100% aspirin free products designed for treatment of infants and children with conditions requiring reduction of fever or relief of pain—such as mild upper respiratory infections (tonsillitis, common cold, "grippe"), headache, myalgia, post-immunization reactions, post-tonsillectomy discomfort and gastroenteritis. In conjunction with antibiotics or sulfonamides, Anacin-3 acetaminophen is useful as an analgesic and antipyretic in many bacterial or viral infections, such as bronchitis, pharyngitis, tracheobronchitis, sinusitis, pneumonia, otitis media, and cervical adenitis.

Caution: If fever persists for more than 3 days or recurs, or if pain continues for more than 5 days, consult your physician immediately.
Phenylketonurics: tablets contain Phenylalanine.

Warnings: Keep this and all medicines out of the reach of children. In case of accidental overdose contact a physician immediately.

Precautions and Adverse Reactions: A-3 acetaminophen has rarely been found to produce an any side effects. If a rare sensitivity reaction occurs, the drug should be stopped. It is usually well tolerated by aspirin-sensitive patients.

Dosage: All dosages may be repeated every 4 hours. Do not exceed 5 dosages in any 24 hour period.
Children's Anacin-3 Chewable Tablets: 1–2 years, 18 to 23 lbs: one and one half tablets. 2–3 years, 24 to 35 lbs: two tablets. 4–5 years, 36 to 47 lbs: three tablets. 6–8 years, 48–59 lbs: four tablets. 9–10 years, 60 to 71 lbs: five tablets. 11–12 years, 72 to 95 lbs: six tablets.
Children's Anacin-3 Liquid: (Special cup for measuring dosage is provided) 4–11 months, 12 to 17 lbs: one-half teaspoon. 12–23 months, 18 to 23 lbs: three-quarters teaspoon. 2–3 years, 24 to 35 lbs: one teaspoon. 4–5 years, 36 to 47 lbs: one and one-half teaspoons. 6–8 years, 48 to 59 lbs: two teaspoons. 9–10 years, 60 to 71 lbs: two and one-half teaspoons. 11–12 years, 72 to 95 lbs: three teaspoons.
Infants' Anacin-3 Drops: 0–3 months, 6 to 11 lbs: one-half dropperful. 4–11 months, 12 to 17 lbs: one dropperful. 12–23 months, 18 to 23 lbs: one and one-half dropperful. 2–3 years, 24 to 35 lbs: 2 dropperful. 4–5 years, 36 to 47 lbs: 3 dropperful.

Overdosage: Acetaminophen in massive overdosage may cause hepatic toxicity in some patients. In all cases of suspected overdose, immediately call your regional poison center or the Rocky Mountain Poison Center for assistance in diagnosis and for directions in the use of N-acetylcysteine as an antidote, a use currently restricted to investigational status. The occurence of acetaminophen

overdose toxicity is uncommon in the pediatric age group. Even with large overdoses, children appear to be less vulnerable than adults to developing hepatotoxicity. This may be due to age-related differences that have been demonstrated in the metabolism of acetaminophen. Despite these differences, the measures outlined below should be immediately initiated in any child suspected of having ingested an overdose of acetaminophen.
Early symptoms following a potentially hepatotoxic overdose may include: nausea, vomiting, diaphoresis and general malaise. Clinical and laboratory evidence of hepatic toxicity may not be apparent until 48 to 72 hours post-ingestion. The stomach should be emptied promptly by lavage or by induction of emesis with syrup of ipecac. If an acute dose of 150 mg/kg body weight or greated was ingested, or if the dose cannot be accurately determined, a serum acetaminophen assay should be obtained as early as possible, but no sooner than four hours post-ingestion. Liver function studies should be obtained and repeated at 24-hour intervals. The antidote N-acetylcysteine should be administered as early as possible, and within 16 hours of the overdose ingestion for optimal results. Following recovery there are no residual, structural or functional hepatic abnormalities.

How Supplied: Chewable Tablets (colored pink, scored, imprinted "Children A–3")—Bottles of 30. Liquid (colored red)—bottles of 2 and 4 fl. oz. Drops (colored red)—bottles of ½ oz. (15 ml.) with calibrated plastic dropper.
All packages listed above have child-resistant safety caps and tamper resistant packaging.

Shown in Product Identification Section, page 434

Maximum Strength
ANACIN-3®
Acetaminophen Tablets and Capsules

Regular Strength
ANACIN-3®
Acetaminophen Tablets

Active Ingredients: Maximum Strength: Each tablet or capsule contains acetaminophen 500 mg. Regular Strength: Each tablet contains acetaminophen 325 mg. Both Maximum Strength and Regular Strength tablets are coated with a thin water soluble coating for easy swallowing. This inert coating is not an enteric coating and will not slow the onset of action.

Indications and Actions: Anacin-3 is a safe and effective 100% aspirin-free analgesic and antipyretic that acts fast to provide temporary relief from pain of headache, colds or "flu", sinusitis, muscle aches, bursitis, sprains, overexertion, backache, and menstrual discomfort. Also for temporary relief of minor arthritis pain, toothaches and to reduce fever. Anacin-3 is particularly well suited in

Continued on next page

Whitehall—Cont.

the presence of aspirin sensitivity, upper gastrointestinal disorders, and anticoagulant therapy. It is usually well tolerated by aspirin-sensitive patients.

Warnings: Keep this and all medicines out of reach of children. In case of accidental overdose, contact a physician immediately. As with any drug, if you are pregnant or nursing a baby, seek the advice of a health professional before using this product.

Caution: If pain persists for more than 10 days or redness is present or in arthritic or rheumatic conditions affecting children under 12, consult a physician immediately.

Dosage and Administration: Maximum Strength: Adults: Two tablets or capsules 3 or 4 times a day. Do not exceed 8 tablets or capsules in any 24-hour period. Regular Strength: Adults: Two to three tablets every 4 hours not to exceed 12 tablets in any 24 hour period. Children (6–12): ½ to 1 tablet 3 to 4 times daily. Consult a physician for use by children under 6 or for use longer than 10 days.

Overdosage: Acetaminophen in massive overdosage may cause hepatic toxicity in some patients. In all cases of suspected overdose, immediately call your regional poison control center, or the Rocky Mountain Poison Control Center, for assistance in diagnosis and for directioins in the use of N-acetylcysteine as an antidote, a use currently restricted to investigational status. In adults, hepatic toxicity has rarely been reported with acute overdoses of less than 10 grams and fatalities with less than 15 grams. Importantly, young children seem to be more resistant than adults to the hepatotoxic effect of an acetaminphen overdose. Despite this, the measures outined below should be initiated in any adult or child suspected of having ingested an acetaminophen overdose.
Early symptoms following a potentially hepatoxic overdose may include: nausea, vomiting, diaphoresis and general malaise. Clinical and laboratory evidence of hepatic toxicity may not be apparent until 48 to 72 hours post ingestion. The stomach should be emptied promptly by lavage or by induction of emesis with syrup of ipecac. Patients' estimates of the quantity of a drug ingested are notoriously unreliable. Therefore, if an acetaminophen overdose is suspected, a serum acetaminophen assay should be obtained as early as possible, but no sooner than four hours following ingestion. Liver function studies should be obtained initially and at 24 hour intervals. The antidote, N-acetylcysteine, should be administered as early as possible, and within 16 hours of the overdose ingestion for optimal results. Following recovery, there is no residual, structural or functional hepatic abnormalities.

Professional Labeling: Same as those outlined under Indications.

How Supplied: Maximum Strength: Tablets (colored white, imprinted "A-3" and "500")—tins of 12 and bottles of 30, 60, and 100; Capsules (colored blue and white, imprinted "Anacin-3")—bottles of 24, 50, and 72. Regular Strength: Tablets (colored white, scored, imprinted "A-3") in bottles of 24, 50, and 100.
Shown in Product Identification Section, page 434

ANBESOL® Liquid and Gel Antiseptic Anesthetic

Description: Anbesol is a safe and effective antiseptic-anesthetic that can be used by all family members for the temporary relief of minor mouth pain such as toothache, teething, sore gums, and denture irritation. Anbesol Liquid also soothes, relieves the pain and helps dry cold sores and fever blisters.
Anbesol is also an excellent first-aid measure that provides fast, temporary pain relief and helps prevent infection from minor cuts, scrapes, and burns.

Active Ingredients: Liquid: Benzocaine (6.3% w/v), Phenol (0.5% w/v), Povidone-Iodine (Yields 0.04% Iodine), Alcohol (70%). Gel: Benzocaine (6.3% w/v), Phenol (0.5% w/v), Alcohol (70%).

Indications: For fast temporary pain relief of toothache, teething, denture irritation, minor mouth irritations, cold sores, fever blisters, minor cuts, scrapes, and burns.

Actions: Temporarily deadens sensations of nerve endings to provide relief of pain and discomfort; reduces oral bacterial flora temporarily as an aid in oral hygiene.

Warnings: Flammable. Keep away from fire or flame. Avoid smoking during application and until product has dried. Do not use near eyes. Keep this and all medicines out of the reach of children.

Precautions: Not for prolonged use. If the condition persists or irritation develops, discontinue use and consult your physician or dentist. Anbesol Gel not for use under dental work.

Dosage and Administration: Apply topically to the affected area within the mouth on or around the lips. Wipe Liquid on with cotton, cotton swab or finger tip.

For Denture Irritation: Anbesol Gel —Apply thin layer to affected area and do not reinsert dental work until irritation/pain is relieved. Rinse mouth before reinserting. If irritation/pain persists, contact your physician.

Professional Labeling: Same as outlined under Indications.

How Supplied: Liquid in two sizes— .31 fl. oz. (9 ml.) and .74 fl. oz. (22 ml.) bottles. Clear Gel in .25 oz. (7.2 gram) tube.
Shown in Product Identification Section, page 434

ARTHRITIS PAIN FORMULA
By the Makers of Anacin® Analgesic Tablets

Active Ingredients: Each tablet contains 7½ grains microfined aspirin. Also contains two buffers, 20 mg. dried Aluminum Hydroxide Gel and 60 mg. Magnesium Hydroxide.

Indications and Actions: Arthritis Pain Formula provides fast, temporary relief from minor aches and pain of arthritis and rheumatism and low back pain. Also relieves the pain of headache, neuralgia, neuritis, sprains, muscular aches, discomforts and fever of colds, pain caused by tooth extraction and toothache, and menstrual discomfort.

Warnings: Keep this and all medications out of children's reach. In case of accidental overdose, contact a physician immediately. As with any drug, if you are pregnant or nursing a baby, seek the advice of a health professional before using this product.

Caution: In arthritic or rheumatic conditions, if pain persists for more than 10 days, or redness is present, consult a physician immediately.

Dosage and Administration: Adult Dosage: 2 tablets, 3 or 4 times a day. Do not exceed 8 tablets in any 24 hour period. For children under 12, consult your physician.

Professional Labeling: Same as stated under "Indications".

How Supplied: In plastic bottles of 40, 100 and 175 tablets.
Shown in Product Identification Section, page 434

SAFETY COATED APF®
ARTHRITIS PAIN FORMULA™
By the makers of Anacin® Analgesic Tablets

Active Ingredients: Each tablet contains 500 mg. aspirin with a special enteric safety coating.

Indications: Safety Coated APF provides hours of temporary relief from minor aches and pains of arthritis and rheumatism. It also helps relieve low back pain and the pain of neuralgia, neuritis and muscular aches.

Actions: Safety Coated APF contains 500 mg. aspirin and is maximum strength. Its special safety coating is designed to dissolve in the small intestine, not in the stomach, for maximum stomach protection.

Warning: Discontinue use if ringing in the ears or other symptoms occur. Keep this and all medications out of children's reach. In case of accidental overdose, consult a physician immediately. As with any drug, if you are pregnant or nursing a baby, seek the advice of a health professional before using this product.

Caution: In arthritic or rheumatic conditions, if pain persists for more than 10 days or redness is present, consult a physician immediately.

Dosage and Administration: Adult Dosage: 2 tablets every 6 hours with water. Do not exceed 8 tablets in any 24 hour period. In children under 12, consult your physician.

Professional Labeling: Same as those outlined under Indications.

How Supplied: In plastic bottles of 24, 60 and 125 tablets.

Shown in Product Identification Section, page 434

COMPOUND W®
Liquid and Gel

Active Ingredients: Liquid: Salicylic Acid 17% w/w, in a flexible collodion vehicle, Ether 63.5%. Gel: Salicylic Acid 17% w/w, in a flexible collodion vehicle, Alcohol 67.5% by volume.

Indications: Removes common warts quickly—painlessly.

Actions: Warts are common benign skin lesions caused by an infectious virus which stimulates mitosis in the basal cell layer resulting in the production of elevated epithelial growths. The keratolytic action of salicylic acids in a flexible collodion vehicle causes the cornified epithelium to swell, soften, macerate and then desquamate.

Warnings: Do not use on face, genitals, or on mucous membranes. If you are a diabetic, or have impaired circulation, do not use as it may cause serious complications. Do not use on moles, birthmarks, or on areas that do not have the typical appearance of the common wart. Flammable—keep away from fire or flame. Avoid smoking during application and until product has dried. For external use only. In case of accidental ingestion, seek professional assistance or contact a poison control center immediately. Keep this and all medicines out of the reach of children. Store at room temperature. Replace cap tightly.

Dosage and Administration: Use twice daily—morning and night. Soak the affected area in hot water for at least five minutes. If any tissue has been loosened, remove by rubbing with a washcloth or soft brush. Dry thoroughly. Using the glass rod provided with the liquid or by squeezing the tube of Gel, completely cover the wart only with solution. To avoid irritating the skin surrounding the wart, confine the solution to the wart only. Allow to dry, then re-apply. The area covered with the medicine will appear white. Follow this procedure twice daily for the next 6 to 7 days. Most warts should clear within this time period. However, if the wart still remains, continue the treatment for up to another seven days. If redness and irritation occur, discontinue using for a couple of days and then try again.

Professional Labeling: Same as those outlined under Indications.

How Supplied: Compound W is available in .31 fluid oz. clear bottles with glass applicators. Compound W Gel is available in .25 oz. tubes.

DENOREX®
Medicated Shampoo
DENOREX®
Mountain Fresh Herbal Scent
Medicated Shampoo
DENOREX®
Medicated Shampoo and Conditioner

Active Ingredients:
Lotion: Coal Tar Solution 9.0%, Menthol 1.5%, Alcohol 7.5%. Also contains TEA-Lauryl Sulfate, Water, Lauramide DEA, Stearic Acid, Chloroxylenol.
Shampoo and Conditioner: Coal Tar Solution 9.0%, Menthol 1.5%, Alcohol 7.5%. Also contains TEA-Lauryl Sulfate, Water, Lauramide DEA, PEG-27 Lanolin, Quaternium 23, Fragrance, Chloroxylenol, Hydroxypropyl Methylcellulose, Citric Acid.
Gel: Coal Tar Solution 9.0%, Menthol 1.5%, Alcohol 7.5%. Also contains TEA-Lauryl Sulfate, Water, Hydroxypropyl Methylcellulose, Chloroxylenol.

Indications: Relieves scaling—itching—flaking of dandruff, seborrhea and psoriasis. Regular use promotes cleaner, healthier hair and scalp.

Actions: Denorex Shampoo is antiseborrheic and antipruritic. Loosens and softens scales and crusts. Coal tar helps correct abnormalities of keratinization by decreasing epidermal proliferation and dermal infiltration. Denorex also contains the antipruritic agent, menthol, which is "one of the most widely used antipruritics in dermatologic therapy of various diseases accompanied by itching". (The United States Dispensatory—26th Edition.)

Warnings: For external use only. Discontinue treatment if irritation develops. Avoid contact with eyes. Keep this and all medicines out of children's reach.

Directions: For best results, shampoo every other day. For severe scalp problems use daily. Wet hair thoroughly and briskly massage until a rich lather is obtained. Rinse thoroughly and repeat. Scalp may tingle slightly during treatment.

Professional Labeling: Same as stated under Indications.

How Supplied:
Lotion: 4 oz. and 8 oz. and 12 oz. bottles in Regular Scent, Mountain Fresh Herbal Scent, and Shampoo and Conditioner.
Gel: 2 oz. Tube and
4 oz. Tube in Regular Scent
Shown in Product Identification Section, page 434

Advanced Formula
DRISTAN®
Decongestant/Antihistamine/
Analgesic Tablets and Capsules

Active Ingredients: Each Dristan Tablet contains: Phenylephrine HCl 5 mg., Chlorpheniramine Maleate 2 mg., Acetaminophen 325 mg. Each Dristan Capsule contains: Phenylpropanolamine HCl 12.5 mg., Chlorpheniramine Maleate 2 mg., Acetaminophen 325 mg.

Product Purpose: For hours of effective multi-symptom relief of colds/flu, sinusitis, hay fever, or other upper respiratory allergies, nasal congestion, sneezing, runny nose, fever, headache and minor aches and pains.

Actions: Each ingredient in Dristan Tablets and Capsules is selected for temporary relief of symptoms of colds, sinusitis, hay fever, or other upper respiratory allergies. Each tablet/capsule contains acetaminophen as an analgesic and antipyretic, an oral nasal decongestant to reduce swollen mucosa of the upper respiratory tract, and an antihistamine as a rhinitis suppressant.
Acetaminophen is both analgesic and antipyretic. Therapeutic doses of acetaminophen will effectively reduce an elevated body temperature. Also acetaminophen is effective in reducing the discomfort of pain associated with headache.
Phenylephrine HCl and Phenylpropanolamine HCl are oral nasal decongestants (Sympathomimetic Amines), effective as vasoconstrictors to help reduce nasal/sinus congestion.
Chlorpheniramine Maleate is an antihistamine effective in the control of rhinorrhea, sneezing and lacrimation associated with elevated histamine levels in disorders of the respiratory tract.

Dosage and Administration: Adults: Two tablets or capsules every four hours, not to exceed 12 tablets or capsules in 24 hours. Children 6–12: One tablet or capsule every four hours, not to exceed six tablets or capsules in 24 hours.

Warnings: Avoid alcoholic beverages and driving a motor vehicle or operating heavy machinery while taking this product. May cause drowsiness or excitability, especially in children. Persons with asthma, glaucoma, high blood pressure, diabetes, heart or thyroid disease, difficulty in urination due to an enlarged prostate gland or taking an antidepressant drug, should use only as directed by a physician. Do not exceed recommended dosage because at higher doses nervousness, dizziness, or sleeplessness may occur. If symptoms do not improve within 7 days or are accompanied by a high fever, discontinue use and see a physician. As with any drug, if you are pregnant or nursing a baby, seek the advice of a health professional before using this product.
Do not give to children under 6. Keep this and all medication out of children's reach. In case of accidental overdose contact a physician immediately.

Professional Labeling: Same as those outlined under Indications.

How Supplied: Yellow/White uncoated tablets in tins of 12 and bottles of 24, 50 and 100. Red/white capsules (im-

Continued on next page

Whitehall—Cont.

printed "Dristan") in bottles of 20 and 40.
*Shown in Product Identification
Section, page 434*

DRISTAN®
Nasal Spray

Active Ingredients: Phenylephrine
HCl 0.5%, Pheniramine Maleate 0.2%.

Other Ingredients: Benzalkonium
Chloride 1:5000 in isotonic aqueous solution, Thimerosal preservative 0.002%
(loss is unavoidable), Alcohol 0.4%.

Indications: For temporary relief of
nasal congestion due to the common cold,
sinusitis, hay fever or other upper respiratory allergies.

Warnings: Do not exceed recommended dosage because symptoms may
occur such as burning, stinging, sneezing, or increase of nasal discharge. Do
not use this product for more than 3 days.
If symptoms persist, consult a physician.
The use of this dispenser by more than
one person may spread infection. For
adult use only. Do not give this product
to children under 12 years except under
the advice and supervision of a physician. Keep these and all medicines out of
the reach of children. In case of accidental ingestion, seek professional assistance or contact a poison control center
immediately.

Dosage and Administration: With
head upright, insert nozzle in nostril.
Spray quickly, firmly and sniff deeply.
Adults: Spray 2 or 3 times into each nostril. Repeat every 4 hours as needed.
Children under 12 years: As directed by a
physician.

Professional Labeling: Same as those
outlined under Indications.

How Supplied: 15 ml. and 30 ml. plas-
tic squeeze bottles.
*Shown in Product Identification
Section, page 434*

DRISTAN®
Long Lasting Nasal Spray

Active Ingredient: Oxymetazoline
HCl 0.05%.

Other Ingredients: Benzalkonium
Chloride 1:5000 in buffered isotonic
aqueous solution, Thimerosal preservative 0.002% (loss is unavoidable).

Indications: For temporary relief of
nasal congestion due to the common cold,
sinusitis, hay fever, or other upper respiratory allergies for up to 12 hours.

Actions: The sympathomimetic action
of Dristan Long Lasting Nasal Spray constricts the smaller arterioles of the nasal
passages, producing a prolonged, up to 12
hours, gentle and predictable decongesting effect.

Warnings: Do not exceed recommended dosage because symptoms may
occur such as burning, stinging, sneezing, or an increase of nasal discharge. Do

not use this product for more than 3 days.
If symptoms persist, consult a physician.
The use of the dispenser by more than
one person may spread infection. Keep
these and all medicines out of the reach
of children. In case of accidental ingestion, seek professional assistance or contact a poison control center immediately.

Dosage and Administration: With
head upright, insert nozzle in nostril.
Spray quickly, firmly and sniff deeply.
Adults and children 6 years of age and
over, spray 2 or 3 times into each nostril.
Repeat twice daily—morning and evening. Not recommended for children under six.

Professional Labeling: Same as those
outlined under Indications.

How Supplied: 15 ml. and 30 ml. plas-
tic squeeze bottles.
*Shown in Product Identification
Section, page 434*

FREEZONE®
Solution

Active Ingredients: Salicylic Acid
13.6% w/w in collodion vehicle. Alcohol
content 20.5% and Ether 64.8% (some
loss unavoidable).

Indications: For removal of corns and
calluses.

Actions: Freezone penetrates corns
and calluses painlessly, layer by layer,
loosening and softening the corn or callus so that the whole corn or callus can be
lifted off or peeled away in just a few
days.

Warnings: Highly Flammable. Keep
away from fire or flame. Avoid smoking
during use and until product has dried. If
product gets into the eye, flush with water to remove film and continue to flush
with water for 15 minutes. Avoid inhaling vapors. Do not use this product if you
are a diabetic or have poor blood circulation because serious complications may
result. Do not use on irritated skin or on
any area that is infected or reddened.
Care should be used to avoid contact of
product with skin surrounding corn or
callus. Do not use this product on soft
corns. If infection or inflammation occurs, see a physician immediately. Store
at room temperature away from heat.
Replace cap securely. For external use
only on the foot or toe. In case of accidental ingestion, contact a physician or call a
Poison Control Center immediately.
KEEP THIS AND ALL MEDICINES
OUT OF THE REACH OF CHILDREN.

Precautions: Apply Freezone on corn
or callus only. Avoid surrounding skin.
In applying Freezone between the toes,
hold toes apart until thoroughly dry.

Dosage and Administration: Bathe
feet with soap and warm water for several minutes. Dry thoroughly. To avoid
irritating or infecting the skin surrounding the corn or callus, confine the liquid
to the corn or callus only. Using rod in
cap, apply product one drop at a time to
sufficiently cover each hard corn or cal-

lus only; let dry. Repeat procedure daily
until the corn or callus is removed. Do
not use medication for more than 14
days.

Professional Labeling: Same as outlined under Indications.

How Supplied: Available in a .31 fl.
oz. glass bottle.

MEDICATED CLEANSING PADS
By The Makers of Preparation H®
Hemorrhoidal Remedies

Active Ingredients: Witch hazel (50%
w/v). Other ingredients: Water, Glycerin
(10% w/v), Methylparaben, Octoxynol-9,
Alcohol 7.4%.

Indications: Hemorrhoidal tissue irritation, anal cleansing wipe; everyday
hygiene of the outer vaginal area, final
cleansing step at diaper changing time.

Actions: Medicated Cleansing Pads
are scientifically developed, soft cloth
pads which are impregnated with a solution specially designed to gently soothe,
freshen and cleanse the anal or genital
area. Medicated Cleansing Pads are superior for a multitude of types of personal hygiene uses and are especially
recommended for hemorrhoid sufferers.

Warnings: In case of rectal bleeding,
consult physician promptly. In case of
continued irritation, discontinue use and
consult a physician.

Precaution: Keep this and all medicines out of the reach of children.

Dosage and Administration: As a
personal wipe—use as a final cleansing
step after regular toilet tissue or instead
of tissue, in cases of special sensitivity.
As a compress—hemorrhoid sufferers
will get additional relief by using Medicated Cleansing Pads as a compress. Fold
pad and hold in contact with inflamed
anal tissue for 10 to 15 minutes. Repeat
several times daily while inflammation
lasts.

How Supplied: Jars of 40's and 100's.

MOMENTUM®
Muscular Backache Formula

Active Ingredients: Aspirin 500 mg.,
Phenyltoloxamine Citrate 15 mg., per
tablet.

Indications: For the relief of pain due
to stiffness and tight, inflamed muscles.

Actions: The combination of aspirin
and phenyltoloxamine citrate act to relieve the pain of tense, knotted muscles.
As pain subsides, muscles loosen and become less stiff, more relaxed and mobil-
ity is increased.

Warning: Do not drive a car or operate
machinery while taking this medication
as this preparation may cause drowsiness in some persons. Keep this and all
medicines out of children's reach. In case
of accidental overdose, contact a physician immediately.

Caution: As with any drug, if you are
pregnant or nursing a baby, seek the ad-

vice of a health professional before using this product.

Dosage and Administration: Adults: Two tablets upon rising, then two tablets as needed at lunch, dinner, and bedtime. Dosage should not exceed 8 tablets in any 24-hour period. Not recommended for children.

Professional Labeling: Same as those outlined under Indications.

How Supplied: Bottles of 24 and 48 white, uncoated tablets.

OUTGRO®
Solution

Active Ingredients: Tannic Acid 25%, Chlorobutanol 5%, Isopropyl Alcohol 83% (by volume).

Indications: Provides fast, temporary relief of pain of ingrown toenails.

Actions: Outgro temporarily relieves pain, reduces swelling and eases inflammation accompanying ingrown toenails. Daily use of Outgro toughens tender skin—allowing the nail to be cut and thus preventing further pain and discomfort. Outgro does not affect the growth, shape or position of the nail.

Warnings: Flammable. Keep away from fire or flame. Avoid smoking during use and until product has dried. For external use only. Do not use Outgro solution for more than 7 days. If no improvement is seen after 7 days, discontinue use and consult a physician. If you have diabetes or circulatory impairment, do not use this product and see a physician for treatment of ingrown toenail. Do not apply this product to open sores. If toe is infected or if redness and swelling of your toe increases, or if a discharge is present around the nail, stop using this product and see your physician. In case of accidental ingestion, contact a physician or call a Poison Control Center immediately. KEEP THIS AND ALL MEDICINES OUT OF THE REACH OF CHILDREN.

Directions: Cleanse affected toes thoroughly. Using rod in cap, either apply Outgro Solution liberally in the crevice where the nail is growing into the flesh OR place a small piece of cotton into the affected nail groove and wet cotton thoroughly with Outgro solution. Let dry thoroughly. Repeat several times daily. Replace cotton in nail groove daily. Outgro will toughen tender skin allowing the nail to be cut. Do not use Outgro solution for more than 7 days. In some instances, temporary discoloration of the nail and surrounding skin may occur.

Professional Labeling: Same as outlined under Indications.

How Supplied: Available in .31 fl. oz. glass bottles.

OXIPOR VHC®
Lotion for Psoriasis

Active Ingredients: Coal Tar Solution 48.5%, Salicylic Acid 1.0%, Benzocaine 2.0%, Alcohol 81% by volume.

Indications: Clinically proven to relieve itching, redness and help dissolve and clear away the scales and crusts of psoriasis.

Actions: Coal tar solution helps control cell growth and therefore prevents formation of new scales. Salicylic acid has a keratolytic action which helps peel off and dissolve away scales. Benzocaine is a local anesthetic that gives prompt relief from pain and itching. Alcohol is the solvent vehicle.

Warnings: For external use only. Shake well before using. Avoid contact with eyes or mucous membranes. Use caution in exposing skin to sunlight after applying this product. It may increase your tendency to sunburn for up to 24 hours after application. DO NOT USE this product in or around the rectum or in the genital area or groin except on the advice of a doctor. Store at room temperature. Flammable. Keep away from fire or flame. Avoid smoking during application and until product has dried. Do not chill.
Not for prolonged use. If condition persists or if a rash or irritation develops, discontinue use and consult a physician. Keep out of reach of children.

Dosage and Administration: SKIN: Wash affected area before applying to remove loose scales. With a small wad of cotton, apply twice daily. Allow to dry before contact with clothing.
SCALP: Apply to scalp with fingertips making sure to get down to the skin itself. Leave on for as long as possible, even overnight. Shampoo. Then remove all loose scales with a fine comb. This product may temporarily discolor light-colored hair. Discoloration can be prevented by reducing the time the product is left on the scalp. Also be sure to rinse product out of hair thoroughly.

Professional Labeling: Same as those outlined under Indications.

How Supplied: Available in 1.9 oz. and 4.0 oz. glass bottles.

PREPARATION H®
Hemorrhoidal Ointment
PREPARATION H®
Hemorrhoidal Suppositories

Active Ingredients: Live Yeast Cell Derivative, supplying 2,000 units skin respiratory factor per ounce of ointment or suppository base. Shark liver oil 3.0%; in a specially prepared base with Phenylmercuric Nitrate 1:10,000 (as a preservative).

Indications: To help shrink swelling of hemorrhoidal tissues caused by inflammation, and to give prompt, temporary relief in many cases from pain and itch in tissues.

Actions: Live Yeast Cell Derivative acts to: A) Increase the oxygen utilization of dermal tissue. B) Increases collagen formation. C) Increases the rate of wound healing. Shark liver oil has been incorporated to act as a protectant which softens and soothes the tissue. Preparation H also lubricates inflamed, irritated surfaces to help make bowel movements less painful.

Precaution: In case of bleeding, or if your condition persists, a physician should be consulted.

Dosage and Administration: Ointment: Apply freely, night, morning, after each bowel movement and whenever symptoms occur. Lubricate applicator before each application and thoroughly cleanse after use.
Suppository: Remove wrapper and insert one suppository night, morning, after each bowel movement and whenever symptoms occur. Store at controlled room temperature in cool place but not over 80° F.

Professional Labeling: Same as those outlined under Indications.

How Supplied: Ointment: Net wt. 1 oz. and 2 oz.
Suppository: 12's, 24's and 48's.
Shown in Product Identification Section, page 434

PRIMATENE®
Mist
(Epinephrine)

Active Ingredients: Each spray delivers approximately 0.2 mg. Epinephrine. A 0.5% w/w (= 5.5 mg./cc.) solution of U.S.P. Epinephrine containing Absorbic Acid as a preservative in an inert propellant. Alcohol 34%.

Indications: Provides temporary relief from acute paroxysms of bronchial asthma.

Warnings: For INHALATION ONLY. Contents under pressure. Do not puncture or throw container into incinerator. Using or storing near open flame or heating above 120° F may cause bursting.
Do not use unless a diagnosis of asthma has been established by a physician. Reduce dosage if bronchial irritation, nervousness, restlessness or sleeplessness occurs. Overdose may cause nervousness and rapid heartbeat. Use only on the advice of a physician if heart disease, high blood pressure, diabetes, or thyroid disease is present. If difficulty in breathing persists, or if relief does not occur within 20 minutes of inhalation, discontinue use and seek medical assistance immediately. As with any drug, if you are pregnant or nursing a baby, seek the advice of a health professional before using this product. Children under 6 years of age should use Primatene Mist only on the advice of a physician. KEEP THIS AND ALL MEDICINES OUT OF REACH OF CHILDREN.

Continued on next page

Whitehall—Cont.

PRIMATENE®
(continued from previous — Mist with mouthpiece)

Directions:
1. Take plastic cap off mouthpiece. (For refills, use mouthpiece from previous purchase).
2. Take plastic mouthpiece off bottle.
3. Place other end of mouthpiece on bottle.
4. Turn bottle upside down. Place thumb on bottom of mouthpiece over the circular button and forefinger on top of vial. Empty the lungs as completely as possible by exhaling.
5. Place mouthpiece in mouth with lips closed around opening. Inhale deeply while squeezing mouthpiece and bottle together. Release immediately and remove unit from mouth, then complete taking the deep breath, drawing medication into your lungs, holding breath as long as comfortable.
6. Then exhale slowly keeping lips nearly closed. This distributes the medication in the lungs.

Dosage: Start with one inhalation by squeezing mouthpiece and bottle together. Release immediately and remove unit from mouth. Then wait at least one minute. If not relieved, use Primatene Mist once more; do not repeat treatment for at least 4 hours.

Professional Labeling: Same as stated under Indications.

How Supplied: ½ fl. oz. (15 cc) with mouthpiece.
½ fl. oz. (15 cc) refill
¾ fl. oz. (22.5 cc) refill

Shown in Product Identification Section, page 434

PRIMATENE®
Mist Suspension
(Epinephrine Bitartrate)

Active Ingredients: Each spray delivers 0.3 mg. Epinephrine Bitartrate equivalent to 0.16 mg. Epinephrine base. Contains Epinephrine Bitartrate 7.0 mg. per cc. in an inert propellant.

Indications: Provides temporary relief from acute paroxysms of bronchial asthma.

Warnings: For INHALATION ONLY. Contents under pressure. Do not puncture or throw container into incinerator. Using or storing near open flame or heating above 120° F may cause bursting.
Do not use unless a diagnosis of asthma has been established by a physician. Reduce dosage if bronchial irritation, nervousness, restlessness or sleeplessness occurs. Overdose may cause nervousness and rapid heartbeat. Use only on the advice of a physician if heart disease, high blood pressure, diabetes, or thyroid disease is present. If difficulty in breathing persists, or if relief does not occur within 20 minutes of inhalation, discontinue use and seek medical assistance immediately. As with any drug, if you are pregnant or nursing a baby, seek the advice of a health professional before using this product. Children under 6 years of age

should use Primatene Mist only on the advice of a physician. KEEP THIS AND ALL MEDICINES OUT OF REACH OF CHILDREN.

Administration: Directions: 1. Shake well. 2. Hold inhaler with nozzle down while using. Empty the lungs as completely as possible by exhaling. 3. Purse the lips as in saying "o" and hold the nozzle up to the lips, keeping the tongue flat. As you start to take a deep breath, squeeze nozzle and can together, releasing one full application. Complete taking deep breath, drawing medication into your lungs. 4. Hold breath for as long as comfortable. This distributes the medication in the lungs. Then exhale slowly, keeping the lips nearly closed. 5. Rinse nozzle daily with soap and hot water after removing from vial. Dry with clean cloth.

Dosage: Start with one inhalation—then wait at least one minute; if not relieved, use Primatene Mist Suspension once more; do not repeat treatment for at least 4 hours.

Professional Labeling: Same as stated under Indications.

How Supplied: ⅓ fl. oz. (10 cc.) pocket-size aerosol inhaler.

PRIMATENE®
Tablets

Available in two formulas, "M" or "P", depending on state. See details below in section on "How Supplied".

Active Ingredients: Theophylline 130 mg., Ephedrine Hydrochloride 24 mg., Phenobarbital 8 mg. (⅛ gr.) per tablet. In those states where Phenobarbital is ℞ only, Pyrilamine Maleate 16.6 mg. is substituted for the Phenobarbital.

Indications: For relief and control of attacks of bronchial asthma and associated hay fever.

Actions: Theophyilline and ephedrine both produce bronchodilation through relaxation of bronchial muscle spasm, as occurs in attacks of bronchial asthma. Because theophylline is a methylxanthine and ephedrine is a sympathomimetic, they are believed to have different mechanisms of action.

Warning: If symptoms persist, consult your physician. Some people are sensitive to ephedrine and, in such cases, temporary sleeplessness and nervousness may occur. These reactions will disappear if the use of the medication is discontinued. Do not exceed recommended dosage.
People who have heart disease, high blood pressure, diabetes or thyroid trouble should take this preparation only on the advice of a physician. "M" Formula may cause drowsiness. People taking the "M" Formula should not drive or operate machinery. "P" Formula may be habit forming.

Caution: As with any drug, if you are pregnant or nursing a baby, seek the advice of a health professional before using

this product. Keep all medicines out of reach of children.

Dosage and Administration: Adults —1 or 2 tablets initially and then one every 4 hours, as needed, not to exceed 6 tablets in 24 hours. Children (6-12): One half adult dose. For children under 6, consult a physician.

Professional Labeling: Same as stated under Indications.

How Supplied: Available in two forms coded "M" or "P". "M" formula, containing pyrilamine maleate, is available in those states where phenobarbital is ℞ only. "P" formula, containing phenobarbital, is available in all other states. Both "M" and "P" formulas are supplied in glass bottles of 24 and 60 tablets.

Shown in Product Identification Section, page 434

SEMICID®
Vaginal Contraceptive Suppositories

Description: Semicid is a safe, effective, vaginal contraceptive in suppository form.
Convenient, individually wrapped, no hormones, odorless, non-messy.

Active Ingredient: Each suppository contains nonoxynol-9, 100 mg.

Indication: For the prevention of pregnancy.

Actions: Semicid dissolves in the vagina and blends with natural vaginal secretions to provide double birth control protection: a physical barrier, plus an effective sperm killing barrier that covers the cervical opening and adjoining vaginal walls. Each Semicid suppository contains the maximum allowable amount of nonoxynol-9, the most widely used nonprescription spermicide.
Semicid requires no applicator and has no unpleasant taste or odor. Semicid is not messy and it does not drip or run like foams, creams and jellies. And it's not awkward to use like the diaphragm. As with all spermicides, some Semicid users experience irritation in using the product, but for years most women have used Semicid safely and effectively with full satisfaction. Also, Semicid does not effervesce like some suppositories, so it is not as likely to cause a burning feeling.
Semicid is approximately as effective as vaginal foam contraceptives in actual use, but is not as effective as the Pill or IUD.
Semicid provides effective contraceptive protection when used properly. However, no contraceptive method or product can provide an absolute guarantee against becoming pregnant.

Dosage and Administration: To use, just unwrap one suppository and insert it deeply into the vagina. It is essential that Semicid be inserted at least 15 minutes before intercourse, however Semicid is also effective when inserted up to 1 hour before intercourse. If intercourse is delayed for more than 1 hour after Semicid is inserted, or if intercourse is repeated, then another suppository must be inserted. Semicid can be used as frequently as needed.

Warnings: Do not insert in urethra. Do not take orally. If irritation occurs, discontinue use. If irritation persists, consult your physician. Keep this and all contraceptives out of the reach of children.

How to Store: Keep Semicid at Room Temperature (Not over 86°F or 30°C).

Precautions: If douching is desired, one should wait at least six hours after intercourse before douching. If either partner experiences irritation, discontinue use. If irritation persists, consult a physician.
If your doctor has told you that you should not become pregnant, ask your doctor if you can use Semicid.
If menstrual period is missed, a physician should be consulted.

How Supplied: Strip Packaging of 3's, 10's and 20's.
Shown in Product Identification Section, page 434

SLEEP–EZE 3™
Nighttime Sleep Aid Tablets
Diphenhydramine Hydrochloride

Description: Sleep-eze 3 is a nighttime sleep-aid that contains a widely used ingredient, clinically tested for safety and efficacy.

Active Ingredient: Diphenhydramine Hydrochloride, 25 mg. per tablet.

Indication: Helps to reduce difficulty in falling asleep.

Action: Sleep-eze 3 (diphenhydramine) is an antihistamine with anticholinergic and sedative action.

Warnings: Do not give to children under 12 years of age. Insomnia may be a symptom of serious underlying medical illness. If sleeplessness persists continuously for more than 2 weeks, consult your physician. As with any drug, if you are pregnant or nursing a baby, seek the advice of a health professional before using this product.
Do not take this product if you have asthma, glaucoma, or enlargement of the prostate gland except under the advice and supervision of a physician. In case of accidental ingestion or overdose, contact a physician or Poison Control Center immediately. Keep this and all medicines out of children's reach.

Drug Interaction: Take this product with caution if alcohol is being consumed.

Precaution: This product contains an antihistamine and will cause drowsiness. It should be used only at bedtime.

Dosage and Administration: Take 2 tablets 20 minutes before going to bed.

Professional Labeling: Same as outlined under Indications.

How Supplied: Packages of 12's, 24's, and 48's.

Winthrop-Breon Laboratories
90 PARK AVENUE
NEW YORK, NY 10016

BREONESIN®
brand of guaifenesin capsules, USP

Description: Each red, oval-shaped BREONESIN capsule contains 200 mg of guaifenesin in an easy-to-swallow, soft gelatin capsule. BREONESIN contains no sugar or alcohol.

Indications: BREONESIN is indicated for the temporary relief of coughs. BREONESIN is an expectorant which helps to loosen phlegm (sputum) and bronchial secretions, and acts to thin mucus. Coughs due to minor throat and bronchial irritation that occur with the common cold are temporarily relieved.

Warnings: Persistent cough may indicate a serious condition. Consult your physician if cough persists for more than 1 week, recurs, or is accompanied by high fever, rash, or persistent headache. Do not take this product for persistent coughs due to smoking, asthma, or emphysema, or coughs accompanied by excessive secretions, except under the advice and supervision of your physician. As with any drug, if you are pregnant or nursing a baby, seek the advice of a health professional before using this product.

Dosage: *Adults and Children 12 years of age and over:* 1 or 2 capsules every 4 hours, not to exceed 12 capsules in a 24-hour period. *Children under 12 years:* as directed by your physician.
Store at controlled room temperature, between 15°C and 30°C (59°F and 86°F).

How Supplied: Capsules of 200 mg (red), bottle of 100 (NDC 0024-1050-10)
Marketed by
Winthrop-Breon Laboratories
New York, NY 10016
Mfg. by R.P. Scherer Corp.
Clearwater, Florida 33518
Shown in Product Identification Section, page 435

BRONKOLIXIR®

Composition: Each 5 mL teaspoonful contains:
Ephedrine sulfate, USP..................12 mg
Guaifenesin, USP............................50 mg
Theophylline, USP ....15 mg
Phenobarbital, USP..........................4 mg
(Warning: May be habit forming.)
in a cherry-flavored solution containing alcohol, USP, 19% (v/v).

How Supplied: Bottle of 16 fl oz

BRONKOTABS®

Composition: Each tablet contains ephedrine sulfate, USP, 24 mg; guaifenesin, USP, 100 mg; theophylline, USP, 100 mg; phenobarbital, USP, 8 mg. (Warning: May be habit forming.)

How Supplied: Bottle of 100 (NDC 0024-1006-10)
Bottle of 1000 (NDC 0024-1006-00)

FERGON® CAPSULES
FERGON® TABLETS
brand of ferrous gluconate
FERGON® ELIXIR

Composition: FERGON (ferrous gluconate, USP) is stabilized to maintain a minimum of ferric ions. It contains not less than 11.5 percent iron. Each FERGON Capsule contains 435 mg of ferrous gluconate, yielding 50 mg of elemental iron. Each FERGON tablet contains 320 mg. FERGON Elixir 6% contains 300 mg per teaspoon.

Action and Uses: FERGON preparations produce rapid hemoglobin regeneration in patients with iron deficiency anemias. FERGON is better utilized and better tolerated than other forms of iron because of its low ionization constant and solubility in the entire pH range of the gastrointestinal tract. It does not precipitate proteins or have the astringency of more ionizable forms of iron, does not interfere with proteolytic or diastatic activities of the digestive system, and will not produce nausea, abdominal cramps, constipation or diarrhea in the great majority of patients. The pellets of ferrous gluconate contained in FERGON Capsules are coated to permit maximum availability of iron in the upper small bowel, the site of maximum absorption. FERGON preparations are indicated in anemias amenable to iron therapy (1) hypochromic anemia of infancy and childhood; (2) idiopathic hypochromic anemia; (3) hypochromic anemia of pregnancy; and (4) anemia associated with chronic blood loss.

Dosage and Administration: *Adults*—1 FERGON Capsule daily for mild to moderate iron deficiency anemia. For more severe anemia the dosage may be increased. One to two FERGON tablets or one to two teaspoons of FERGON Elixir daily. *For children and infants,* consult physician.

How Supplied: FERGON Capsules, bottle of 30 (NDC 0024-1016-03). FERGON, tablets of 320 mg (5 grains), bottle of 100 (NDC 0024-1015-10), bottle of 500 (NDC 0024-1015-50), and bottle of 1,000 (NDC 0024-1015-00). FERGON Elixir 6% (5 grains per teaspoon), bottle of 1 pint (NDC 0024-1019-16).
Shown in Product Identification Section, page 435

MEASURIN®
Timed-Released Aspirin

Description: Each tablet contains 10 grains aspirin.

How Supplied: Tablets—bottle of 60 (NDC 0024-1025-06)

Winthrop Consumer Products

Division of Sterling Drug Inc.
90 PARK AVENUE
NEW YORK, NY 10016

BRONKAID® Mist

Description: BRONKAID Mist, brand of epinephrine, USP, 0.5%, contains ascorbic acid as preservative in an inert propellant. Alcohol 33% (w/w). Each activation of the measured dose valve delivers 0.27 mg epinephrine.

Action: Epinephrine is a sympathomimetic amine which relaxes bronchial muscle spasm, as occurs in attacks of bronchial asthma.

Indication: For temporary relief of acute paroxysms of bronchial asthma

Warnings: FOR ORAL INHALATION ONLY. Do not use unless a diagnosis of asthma has been established by a doctor. Reduce dosage if nervousness, restlessness, sleeplessness, or bronchial irritation occurs. Do not use if high blood pressure, heart disease, diabetes, or thyroid disease is present, unless directed by a physician. If prompt relief is not obtained, consult your physician.
Avoid spraying in eyes. Contents under pressure. Do not break or incinerate. Do not use near open flame or store at temperature above 120°F. Keep out of reach of children.

Precaution: Children under 6 years of age should use BRONKAID Mist only on the advice of a physician. Avoid indiscriminate use of BRONKAID Mist as many people do with similar medications. Use only when actually needed for relief. Overdose may cause rapid heart beat and nervousness.

Dosage and Administration: Start with one inhalation, then wait at least one minute. If not relieved, use BRONKAID Mist once more. Do not repeat treatment for at least 4 hours. If difficulty in breathing persists, consult your physician.

Directions for Use:
1. Remove cap and mouthpiece from bottle.
2. Remove cap from mouthpiece.
3. Turn mouthpiece sideways and fit metal stem of nebulizer into hole in flattened end of mouthpiece.
4. Exhale, as completely as possible. Now, hold bottle **upside down** between thumb and forefinger and close lips loosely around end of mouthpiece.
5. Inhale deeply while pressing down firmly on bottle, once only.
6. Remove mouthpiece and hold your breath a moment to allow for maximum absorption of medication. Then exhale slowly through nearly closed lips.

After use, remove mouthpiece from bottle and replace cap. Slide mouthpiece over bottle for protection. When possible, rinse mouthpiece with tap water immediately after use. Soap and water will not hurt it. A clean mouthpiece always works better.

How Supplied: Bottles of ½ fl oz (15 mL) NDC 0024-4082-15 with actuator. Also available—refills (no mouthpiece) in 15 mL (½ fl oz) NDC 0024-4083-16 and 22.5 mL (¾ fl oz) NDC 0024-4083-22

BRONKAID® Mist Suspension

Active Ingredients: Each spray delivers 0.3 mg epinephrine bitartrate equivalent to 0.16 mg epinephrine base. Contains epinephrine bitartrate 7.0 mg per cc in an inert propellant.

Indication: Provides temporary relief from acute paroxysms of bronchial asthma.

Warnings: For INHALATION ONLY. Contents under pressure. Do not puncture or throw container into incinerator. Using or storing near open flame or heating above 120°F may cause bursting. Do not use unless a diagnosis of asthma has been established by a physician. Reduce dosage if bronchial irritation, nervousness, restlessness, or sleeplessness occurs. Overdose may cause nervousness and rapid heartbeat. Use only on the advice of a physician if heart disease, high blood pressure, diabetes, or thyroid disease is present. If difficulty in breathing persists, or if relief does not occur within 20 minutes of inhalation, discontinue use and seek medical assistance immediately. Children under 6 years of age should use BRONKAID Mist Suspension only on the advice of a physician. Keep this and all medicines out of reach of children.

Administration: (1) SHAKE WELL. (2) HOLD INHALER WITH NOZZLE DOWN WHILE USING. Empty the lungs as completely as possible by exhaling. (3) Purse the lips as in saying the letter "O" and hold the nozzle up to the lips, keeping the tongue flat. As you start to take a deep breath, squeeze nozzle and can together, releasing one full application. Complete taking deep breath, drawing medication into your lungs. (4) Hold breath for as long as comfortable. This distributes the medication in the lungs. Then exhale slowly keeping the lips nearly closed. (5) Rinse nozzle daily with soap and hot water after removing from vial. Dry with clean cloth.

Dosage: Start with one inhalation—then wait at least one minute; if not relieved, use BRONKAID Mist Suspension once more; do not repeat treatment for at least 4 hours.

Professional Labeling: Same as stated under Indication.

How Supplied: ⅓ fl oz (10 cc) pocket-size aerosol inhaler (NDC 0024-4082-10) with actuator

BRONKAID® Tablets

Description: Each tablet contains ephedrine sulfate 24 mg, guaifenesin (glyceryl guaiacolate) 100 mg, and theophylline 100 mg.

Actions: Theophylline and ephedrine both produce bronchodilation through relaxation of bronchial muscle spasm, as occurs in attacks of bronchial asthma, although they do so through different mechanisms. Guaifenesin produces an expectorant action by increasing the water content of bronchial mucus, probably by way of a vagal reflex.

Indication: For symptomatic control of bronchial asthma

Precautions: The recommended dosage of BRONKAID tablets is appropriate for home medication for the symptoms of bronchial congestion and bronchial asthma. If this dosage does not afford relief, and symptoms persist or worsen, it is an indication that the nature of your illness requires the attention of a physician. Under these conditions, or if fever is present, do not experiment with home medications. Consult your physician. Individuals with persistent coughs, high blood pressure, diabetes, heart or thyroid disease should use only as directed by a physician. If dryness of throat, nervousness, restlessness or sleeplessness occurs, discontinue the dosage and consult your physician. Occasionally, in certain individuals, this preparation may cause urinary retention and, if so, discontinue medication. Do not exceed recommended dosage unless directed by a physician.

Warning: As with any drug, if you are pregnant or nursing a baby, seek the advice of a health professional before using this product.

Dosage and Administration: *Adult Dosage:* 1 tablet every three or four hours. Do not take more than 5 tablets in a 24-hour period. Swallow tablets whole with water.
Children (6 to 12): ½ tablet every three or four hours. Do not administer more than 5 times in a 24-hour period. Do not administer to children under 6 unless directed by a physician. Swallow whole with water.
Morning Dose: An early dose of 1 tablet (for adults) can relieve the coughing and wheezing caused by the night's accumulation of mucus, and can help you start the day with better breathing capacity.
Before an Attack: Many persons feel an attack of asthma coming on. One BRONKAID tablet beforehand may stop the attack before it starts.
During the Day: The precise dose of BRONKAID tablets can be varied to meet your individual needs as you gain experience with this product. It is advisable to take 1 tablet before going to bed, for nighttime relief. However, be sure not to exceed recommended daily dosage.

How Supplied:
Boxes of 24 (NDC 0024-4081-02)
Boxes of 60 (NDC 0024-4081-06)

CAMPHO–PHENIQUE® GEL

Description: Contains phenol 4.7% (w/w) and camphor 10.8% (w/w) in an aromatic gel.

Actions: Pain-relieving antiseptic for cold sores, fever blisters, insect bites, cuts, burns, sores.

Indications: For relief of pain and to combat infection from minor injuries and skin lesions.

Warnings: Not for prolonged use. Not to be used on large areas. In case of deep or puncture wounds, serious burns, or persisting redness, swelling or pain, discontinue use and consult physician. If rash or infection develops, discontinue use and consult physician. Do not bandage if applied to fingers or toes.

Avoid using near eyes. If product gets into the eye, it should be washed out thoroughly with water and medical attention obtained. Keep this and all medicines out of the reach of children. In case of accidental ingestion, seek professional assistance or contact a poison control center immediately.

Directions for Use: For external use. Apply directly to injury or sore three or four times a day.

How Supplied: Tubes of .23 oz (6.5 g) NDC 0024-0212-01 and .50 oz (14 g) NDC 0024-0212-02

CAMPHO–PHENIQUE® Liquid

Description: Contains phenol 4.7% (w/w) and camphor 10.8% (w/w) in an aromatic oily solution.

Actions: Pain-relieving antiseptic for sores, cuts, burns, insect bites, fever blisters, and cold sores.

Indications: For relief of pain and to combat infection from minor injuries and skin lesions.

Warnings: Not for prolonged use. Not to be used on large areas or in or near the eyes. In case of deep or puncture wounds, serious burns, or persisting redness, swelling or pain, discontinue use and consult physician. If rash or infection develops, discontinue use and consult physician. Do not bandage if applied to fingers or toes.

Keep this and all medicines out of children's reach. In case of accidental ingestion, seek professional assistance or contact a poison control center immediately.

Directions for Use: For external use. Apply with cotton three or four times daily.

How Supplied:
Bottles of ¾ fl oz (NDC 0024-5150-05)
  1½ fl oz (NDC 0024-5150-06)
  4 fl oz (NDC 0024-5150-04)

HALEY'S M-O®
Laxative Lubricant

Description: An emulsion of Phillips'® Milk of Magnesia with 25 percent pure mineral oil.

Action: Laxative and lubricant preparation; the mineral oil acting as a lubricant and the Milk of Magnesia as a mild saline cathartic.

Indications: For the relief of constipation especially in patients with hemorrhoids, obstetric and cardiac patients, and in geriatric patients where straining at stool is contraindicated.

Contraindications: Abdominal pain, nausea, vomiting, or other symptoms of appendicitis.

Warnings: Not to be used when abdominal pain, nausea, vomiting, or other symptoms of appendicitis are present. Habitual use of laxatives may result in dependency upon them. When used daily or with frequent regularity, do not take within two hours of a meal because mineral oil may interfere with the absorption of pro-Vitamin A.

As with any drug, if you are pregnant or nursing a baby, seek the advice of a health professional before using this product.

Keep this and all medicines out of the reach of children. In case of accidental overdose, seek professional assistance or contact a poison control center immediately.

Dosage and Administration: *Adults,* as mild laxative, 1 to 2 tablespoons upon arising or at bedtime. For constipation, 2 tablespoons on arising and at bedtime. *Children 3 to 6 years*—1 to 2 teaspoons; 7 *to 12 years*, 2 to 4 teaspoons. *Under 3 years,* as directed by physician.

How Supplied: Haley's M-O is available as Regular and Flavored (sugar-free) in bottles of:
Regular— 8 fl oz (NDC 0024-3130-08)
  16 fl oz (NDC 0024-3130-16)
  32 fl oz (NDC 0024-3130-32)
Flavored— 8 fl oz (NDC 0024-3230-08)
  16 fl oz (NDC 0024-3230-16)
  32 fl oz (NDC 0024-3230-32)

NaSal™
Saline (buffered)
0.65% Sodium chloride
Nasal Spray
Nose Drops

Description: Both the nasal spray and nose drops contain sodium chloride 0.65% buffered with phosphates and preserved with benzalkonium chloride 0.02% and thimerosal 0.001%.

Actions: Rapid acting nasal moisturizer. Formulated to match the pH of normal nasal secretions to help prevent stinging or burning.

Indications: Provides soothing relief for clogged nasal passages—without stinging or burning. Provides prompt relief for dry, inflamed nasal membranes due to colds, low humidity, allergies, minor nose bleeds, overuse of topical nasal decongestants, and other nasal irritations. As an ideal nasal moisturizer, it can be used in conjunction with oral decongestants.

Adverse Reactions: No associated side effects. (Safe for use during pregnancy.)

Dosage and Administration: *Spray*— For adults and children six years of age

and over: with head upright, spray twice in each nostril as needed or as directed by physician. To spray, squeeze bottle quickly and firmly. *Nose Drops*—For infants and adults: 2 to 6 drops in each nostril as needed or as directed by physician.

How Supplied: Nasal Spray—plastic squeeze bottles of 15 mL (½ fl oz) NDC 0024-1316-01.
Nose Drops—MonoDrop® bottles of 15 mL (½ fl oz) NDC 0024-1315-01.

Long Acting
NEO–SYNEPHRINE® II
xylometazoline hydrochloride
Nasal Spray 0.1%
Vapor Nasal Spray 0.1%
Nose Drops 0.1%
Children's Nose Drops 0.05%

Description: *Adult Strength Nasal Spray* and *Nose Drops* contain xylometazoline hydrochloride 0.1% with benzalkonium chloride and thimerosal 0.001% as preservatives. *Adult Strength Vapor Nasal Spray* contains xylometazoline hydrochloride 0.1% with aromatics (menthol, eucalyptol, camphor, methyl salicylate) and benzalkonium chloride and thimerosal 0.001% as preservatives. *Children's Nose Drops* contain xylometazoline hydrochloride 0.05% with benzalkonium chloride and thimerosal 0.001% as preservatives.

Action: Long-acting Nasal Decongestant

Indications: Provides long-lasting, 8 to 10 hour, temporary relief of nasal congestion due to common cold, sinusitis, hay fever, or other upper respiratory allergies, makes breathing through the nose easier, reduces swelling of nasal passages, and shrinks swollen membranes.

Warnings: Nasal Spray 0.1% and Nose Drops 0.1% should be administered only to adults. Do not give this product to children under 12 years. Children's Nose Drops 0.05% should be given only to children from 2 to 12 years of age. Do not give to children under 2 years of age unless under advice and supervision of a physician. Do not exceed recommended dosage because symptoms may occur such as burning, stinging, sneezing, or increase of nasal discharge. Do not use this product for more than three days. If symptoms persist, consult a physician. The use of this dispenser by more than one person may spread infection. Keep this and all drugs out of the reach of children. In case of accidental ingestion, seek professional assistance or contact a poison control center immediately. Do not use if allergic to xylometazoline.

Continued on next page

This product information was effective as of January 1, 1985. Current detailed information may be obtained directly from Winthrop Consumer Products, Division of Sterling Drug Inc., by writing to 90 Park Avenue, New York, NY 10016.

Winthrop—Cont.

Dosage and Administration: *Spray 0.1% for adults*—Always hold head upright to spray. Insert nosepiece into nostril pointing it slightly backward. To spray, squeeze bottle quickly and firmly. Spray two or three times into each nostril every 8 to 10 hours. Do not use more than three times daily.
Solution 0.1% for adults and children over 12—two or three drops in each nostril every 8 to 10 hours. Do not use more than three times daily.
Solution 0.05% for children 2 through 12 years of age—two or three drops in each nostril every 8 to 10 hours. Do not use more than 3 times daily.

How Supplied: *Nasal Spray Adult Strength*—plastic squeeze bottles of 15 mL (½ fl oz) NDC 0024-1338-01; *Vapor Nasal Spray Adult Strength*—squeeze bottles of 15 mL (½ fl oz) NDC 0024-1339-01.
Nose Drops Adult Strength—bottles of 30 mL (1 fl oz) with dropper NDC 0024-1336-02; *Children's Strength 0.05%*—bottles of 30 mL (1 fl oz) with dropper NDC 0024-1337-02.

NEO-SYNEPHRINE®
phenylephrine hydrochloride

Action: Rapid-acting nasal decongestant.

Indications: For temporary relief of nasal congestion due to common cold, hay fever or other upper respiratory allergies, or associated with sinusitis.

Precautions: Some hypersensitive individuals may experience a mild stinging sensation. This is usually transient and often disappears after a few applications. Do not exceed recommended dosage. Follow directions for use carefully. If symptoms are not relieved after several applications, a physician should be consulted. Frequent and continued usage of the higher concentrations (especially the 1% solution) occasionally may cause a rebound congestion of the nose. Therefore, long-term or frequent use of this solution is not recommended without the advice of a physician.
Prolonged exposure to air or strong light will cause oxidation and some loss of potency. Do not use if brown in color or contains a precipitate.

Adverse Reactions: Generally very well tolerated; systemic side effects such as tremor, insomnia, or palpitation rarely occur.

Dosage and Administration: *Topical*—dropper or spray. The *0.25% solution* is adequate in most cases *(0.125% for infants)*. In resistant cases, or if more powerful decongestion is desired, the *0.5 or 1% solution* should be used. Also used as *0.5% jelly.*

How Supplied: Nasal spray 0.25%—15 mL (for children and for adults who prefer a mild nasal spray)—NDC 0024-1348-03; nasal spray 0.5%—15 mL (for

adults)—NDC 0024-1353-01 and 30 mL (1 fl oz) NDC 0024-1353-05; nasal spray 1%—15 mL (extra strength for adults)—NDC 0024-1352-02; nasal solution 0.125% (for infants and small children), 1 fl oz bottles—NDC 0024-1345-02; nasal solution 0.25% (for children and adults who prefer a mild solution), 1 fl oz bottles—NDC 0024-1347-01 and 16 fl oz bottles—NDC 0024-1347-06; nasal solution 0.5% (for adults), 1 fl oz bottles—NDC 0024-1351-01; nasal solution 1% (extra strength for adults), 1 fl oz bottles—NDC 0024-1355-01 and 16 fl oz bottles—NDC 0024-1355-06; and water soluble nasal jelly 0.5%, ⅝ oz tubes—NDC 0024-1367-01.
Also available — NEO-SYNEPHRINE Mentholated Nasal Spray 0.5% (for adults), ½ fl oz bottles—NDC 0024-1364-01.

NEO-SYNEPHRINE® 12 HOUR
oxymetazoline HCl

Nasal Spray 0.05%
Vapor Nasal Spray 0.05%
Nose Drops 0.05%
Children's Drops 0.025%

Description: *Adult Strength Nasal Spray* and *Nose Drops* contain oxymetazoline hydrochloride 0.05% with benzalkonium chloride and phenylmercuric acetate 0.002% as preservatives. *Adult Strength Vapor Nasal Spray* contains oxymetazoline hydrochloride 0.05% with aromatics (menthol, eucalyptol, camphor, methyl salicylate) with benzalkonium chloride and thimerosal as preservatives. *Children's Nose Drops* contain oxymetazoline hydrochloride 0.025% with benzalkonium chloride and phenylmercuric acetate 0.002% as preservatives.

Action: 12 HOUR Nasal Decongestant.

Indications: Provides temporary relief, for up to 12 HOURS, of nasal congestion due to colds, hay fever, sinusitis, or allergies. NEO-SYNEPHRINE 12-HOUR Nasal Sprays and Nose Drops contain oxymetazoline which provides the longest-lasting relief of nasal congestion available. It decongests nasal passages up to 12 HOURS, reduces swelling of nasal passages, and temporarily restores freer breathing through the nose.

Warnings: Do not exceed recommended dosage because symptoms may occur such as burning, stinging, sneezing, or increase of nasal discharge. (Nasal Spray 0.05%, Vapor Nasal Spray 0.05%, Nose Drops 0.05% not recommended for children under 6; Children's Drops 0.025% not recommended for children under 2.) Do not use these products for more than 3 days. If symptoms persist, consult a physician. The use of this dispenser by more than one person may spread infection.
Keep this and all medicines out of the reach of children. In case of accidental ingestion seek professional assistance or contact a poison control center immediately.

Dosage and Administration: *Adult Strength Nasal Spray*—For adults and children 6 years of age and over: With head upright, spray two or three times in each nostril twice daily—morning and evening. To spray, squeeze bottle quickly and firmly.
Adult Strength Nose Drops—For adults and children 6 years of age and over: two or three drops in each nostril twice daily—morning and evening.
Adult Strength Vapor Nasal Spray—For adults and children 6 years of age and over: With head upright, spray two or three times in each nostril twice daily—morning and evening. To spray, squeeze bottle quickly and firmly. Contains cooling menthol vapors.
Children's Nose Drops—Specially formulated for children 2 through 5 years. Children 2 to under 6 years of age: two or three drops in each nostril twice daily—morning and evening.

How Supplied: *Nasal Spray Adult Strength*—plastic squeeze bottles of 15 mL (½ fl oz) NDC 0024-1390-03 and 30 mL (1 fl oz) NDC 0024-1394-01; *Vapor Nasal Spray Adult Strength*—squeeze bottles of 15 mL (½ fl oz) NDC 0024-1391-03; *Nose Drops Adult Strength*—bottles of 15 mL (½ fl oz) with dropper (NDC 0024-1392-01); *Children's Strength 0.025%*—bottles of 15 mL (½ fl oz) with dropper (NDC 0024-1393-01)

NTZ®
Long Acting
Oxymetazoline hydrochloride
Nasal Spray 0.05%
Nose Drops 0.05%

Description: Both the nasal spray and nose drops contain oxymetazoline hydrochloride 0.05% with benzalkonium chloride and phenylmercuric acetate 0.002% as preservatives.

Actions: 12 Hour Nasal Decongestant

Indications: Provides temporary relief, for up to 12 hours, of nasal congestion due to colds, hay fever, sinusitis, or allergies. Oxymetazoline hydrochloride provides the longest-lasting relief of nasal congestion available. It decongests nasal passages up to 12 hours, reduces swelling of nasal passages, and temporarily restores freer breathing through the nose.

Warnings: Not recommended for children under six. Do not exceed recommended dosage because symptoms may occur such as burning, stinging, sneezing, or increase of nasal discharge. Do not use these products for more than 3 days. If symptoms persist, consult a physician. The use of these dispensers by more than one person may spread infection.
Keep these and all medications out of the reach of children. In case of accidental ingestion seek professional assistance or contact a poison control center immediately.

Dosage and Administration: Intranasally by spray and dropper. *Nasal*

Spray—For adults and children 6 years of age and over: With head upright, spray 2 or 3 times in each nostril twice daily—morning and evening. To spray, squeeze bottle quickly and firmly. *Nose Drops*—For adults and children 6 years of age and over: 2 or 3 drops in each nostril twice daily—morning and evening.

How Supplied: *Nasal Spray*—plastic squeeze bottles of 15 mL (½ fl oz) NDC 0024-1312-02
Nose Drops—bottles of 15 mL (½ fl oz) with dropper (NDC 0024-1311-03)

pHisoAc® BP
Acne Medication

Description: pHisoAc BP is a colorless, greaseless, and odorless cream which contains 10% benzoyl peroxide.

Actions: pHisoAc BP helps clear and prevent acne and related skin blemishes. It kills the bacteria that can cause acne.

Precautions: For external use only. Do not use this medication on very sensitive skin or if there is a sensitivity to benzoyl peroxide. This product may cause irritation, characterized by redness, burning, itching, peeling, or possibly swelling. More frequent use or higher concentration may aggravate such irritation. Mild irritation may be reduced by using the product less frequently or in a lower concentration. If irritation becomes severe, discontinue use. If irritation still continues, consult a doctor or pharmacist. Keep away from eyes, lips, mouth, and sensitive areas of the neck. This product may bleach hair or dyed fabrics. Keep this and all medicines out of reach of children. In case of accidental overdose, seek professional assistance or contact a poison control center immediately. Keep tube tightly closed. Avoid excessive heat.

Administration: Cleanse the skin thoroughly and dry well before applying medication. Test on small area for one or two days. If no excessive dryness or undue irritation occurs, cover the entire affected area with a thin layer one to three times daily. Because excessive drying of the skin may occur, start with one application daily, then gradually increase to two or three times daily if needed or as directed by a doctor.

How Supplied: Tubes of 1 oz.

pHisoDerm®
Skin Cleanser and Conditioner

Description: pHisoDerm, a nonsoap emollient skin cleanser, is a unique liquid emulsion containing Sodium Octoxynol-2 Ethane Sulfonate, White Petrolatum, Water, Petrolatum and Lanolin and Lanolin Alcohol, Sodium Benzoate, Octoxynol-1, Methylcellulose, and Lactic Acid. pHisoDerm contains no soap, perfumes, or irritating alkali. Its pH value, unlike that of soap, lies within the pH range of normal skin.

Actions: pHisoDerm is well tolerated and can be used frequently by those persons whose skin may be irritated by the use of soap or other alkaline cleansers, or by those who are sensitive to the fatty acids contained in soap. pHisoDerm contains an effective detergent for removing soil and acts as an active emulsifier of all types of oil—animal, vegetable, and mineral.

pHisoDerm produces suds when used with any kind of water—hard or soft, hot or cold (even cold sea water)—at any temperature and under acid, alkaline, or neutral conditions.

pHisoDerm deposits a fine film of lanolin cholesterols and petrolatum on the skin during the washing process and, thereby, helps protect against the dryness that soap can cause.

Indications: A sudsing emollient cleanser for use on skin of infants, children, and adults.
Useful for removal of ointments and cosmetics from the skin.

Directions: For external use only.
HANDS. Squeeze a few drops of pHisoDerm into the palm, add a little water, and work up a lather. Rinse thoroughly.
FACE. After washing your hands, squeeze a small amount of pHisoDerm into the palm or onto a small sponge or washcloth, and work up a lather by adding a little water. Massage the suds onto the face for approximately one minute. Rinse thoroughly. Avoid getting suds into the eyes.
BATHING. First wet the body. Work a small amount of pHisoDerm into a lather with hands or a soft wet sponge, gradually adding small amounts of water to make more lather. When using a washcloth use more pHisoDerm. Spread the lather over all parts of the body. Rinse thoroughly.
BABY BATHING. First wet the baby's body. Work a small amount of pHisoDerm into a lather with hands or a soft wet sponge, gradually adding small amounts of water to make more lather. Spread the lather over all parts of the baby's body, including the head. Avoid getting suds into the baby's eyes. Wash the diaper area last. Be sure to carefully cleanse all folds and creases. Rinse thoroughly. Pat the baby dry with a soft towel.

Caution: pHisoDerm suds that get into the eyes accidentally during washing should be rinsed out promptly with a sufficient amount of water.
pHisoDerm is intended for external use only. pHisoDerm should not be poured into measuring cups, medicine bottles, or similar containers since it may be mistaken for baby formula or medications. If swallowed, pHisoDerm may cause gastrointestinal irritation.
pHisoDerm should not be used on persons with sensitivity to any of its components.

How Supplied: pHisoDerm is supplied in three formulations for regular, dry, and oily skin. It is packaged in sanitary squeeze bottles of 5 and 16 ounces. The regular formula is also supplied in squeeze bottles of 9 ounces and plastic bottles of 1 gallon.

Dry Skin Formula: A high emolliency cleansing formulation that is especially suitable for people with dry skin. It can also help prevent dry skin chapping. This formula can be used for bathing babies, children, and adults to keep skin naturally soft and supple.

Oily Skin Formula: A low emolliency cleansing formulation designed for skin that is especially oily. This formulation is not recommended for use in bathing babies.
Also available—pHisoDerm–Fresh Scent for regular skin in squeeze bottles of 5, 9, and 16 ounces.

pHisoPUFF®
Nonmedicated Cleansing Sponge

Description: pHisoPUFF is a nonmedicated cleansing sponge with a special dual layer construction combining a white polyester fiber side and a green sponge side.

Actions: pHisoPUFF cleanses two ways: (1) white fiber side for extra thorough cleansing to gently remove the top layer of dead skin cells, free the dirt, debris, and oil trapped in this layer and reveal new, fresh skin cell layers and (2) green sponge side works to cleanse and rinse skin clean. Using this side will help apply your cleanser or soap more evenly. Also good for removing eye makeup.

Precautions: Do not use pHisoPUFF fiber side on skin that is irritated, sunburned, windburned, damaged, broken, or infected. Do not use on skin which is prone to rashes or itching.

Administration: For the green sponge side: Wet pHisoPUFF with warm water, apply pHisoDerm® or another skin cleanser of your choice, and develop a lather. Glide sponge over your face up and down, back and forth, or in a circle; whatever is the easiest for you. Rinse face and dry.
For the white fiber side: Wet pHisoPUFF with warm water, apply pHisoDerm or another skin cleanser of your choice, and develop a lather. Try pHisoPUFF on the back of your hand before using it on your face. Experiment by changing the pressure and speed with which you move it. Now move pHisoPUFF gently and slowly over your face. Use no more than a few seconds on each area. You can move it in any direction, whichever comes natural to you. Rinse face and dry. As you use this fiber side more often, usage and pressure may be increased to best fit your skin sensitivity. Always rinse your pHisoPUFF thoroughly each time you

Continued on next page

This product information was effective as of January 1, 1985. Current detailed information may be obtained directly from Winthrop Consumer Products, Division of Sterling Drug Inc., by writing to 90 Park Avenue, New York, NY 10016.

Winthrop—Cont.

use it. Hold under running water, let it drain, then give it a few quick shakes.

How Supplied: Box of 1 pHisoPUFF.

WinGel®
Liquid and Tablets

Description: Each teaspoon (5 ml) of liquid and each tablet contain a specially processed, short polymer, hexitol stabilized aluminum-magnesium hydroxide equivalent to 180 mg of aluminum hydroxide and 160 mg of magnesium hydroxide. Mint flavored. Smooth, easy-to-chew tablets.

Action: Antacid.

Indications: An antacid for the relief of acid indigestion, heartburn, and sour stomach.

Warnings: *Adults and children over 6*—Patients should not take more than eight teaspoonfuls or eight tablets in a 24-hour period or use the maximum dosage of the product for more than 2 weeks, except under the advice and supervision of a physician.
Absorption of other drugs may be interfered with by the aluminum in the product.

Drug Interaction Precautions: This product should not be taken if the patient is presently taking a prescription antibiotic drug containing any form of tetracycline.

Dosage and Administration: *Adults and children over 6*—1 to 2 teaspoonfuls or 1 to 2 tablets up to four times daily, or as directed by a physician.

Professional Labeling: For the symptomatic relief of hyperacidity associated with the diagnosis of peptic ulcer, gastritis, peptic esophagitis, gastric hyperacidity, and hiatal hernia.

Acid Neutralization: WINGEL Liquid 23.2 mEq/2 teaspoons; WINGEL Tablets 24.6 mEq/2 tablets.

How Supplied: Liquid—bottles of 6 fl oz (NDC 0024-2247-03) and 12 fl oz (NDC 0024-2247-05).
Tablets—boxes of 50 (NDC 0024-2249-05) and 100 (NDC 0024-2249-06).

IDENTIFICATION PROBLEM?
Consult the
Product Identifcation Section
where you'll find
products pictured
in full color.

Wyeth Laboratories
Division of American Home
Products Corporation
P.O. BOX 8299
PHILADELPHIA, PA 19101

Wyeth
Tamper-Resistant/Evident Packaging

Statements alerting consumers to the specific type of Tamper-Resistant/Evident Packaging appear on the bottle labels and cartons of all of Wyeth's over-the-counter products. This includes plastic cap seals on bottles, individually wrapped tablets or suppositories, and sealed cartons. This packaging has been developed to better protect the consumer.

ALUDROX®
Antacid
(alumina and magnesia)
ORAL SUSPENSION • TABLETS

Composition: *Suspension*—each 5 ml teaspoonful contains 307 mg aluminum hydroxide [$Al(OH)_3$] as a gel and 103 mg of magnesium hydroxide. *Tablets*—each tablet contains 233 mg aluminum hydroxide as a dried gel and 83 mg magnesium hydroxide.

Indications: For temporary relief of heartburn, upset stomach, sour stomach, and/or acid indigestion.

Directions: *Suspension*—Two teaspoonfuls (10 ml) every 4 hours or as directed by a physician. Medication may be followed by a sip of water if desired. *Tablets*—Two tablets as required for approved indications. Tablets must be chewed before swallowing.

Warnings: Do not take more than 12 teaspoonfuls (60 ml) of suspension, nor more than 16 tablets, in a twenty-four-hour period or use respective maximum dosages for more than two weeks except under the advice and supervision of a physician. As with any drug, if you are pregnant or nursing a baby, seek the advice of a health professional before using this product.

Drug Interaction Precautions: Do not take this product if you are presently taking a prescription antibiotic drug containing any form of tetracycline.
Keep at Room Temperature, Approx. 77°F (25°C)
Suspension should be kept tightly closed and shaken well before use. Avoid freezing.
Keep this and all drugs out of the reach of children.

How Supplied: *Oral Suspension*—bottles of 12 fluidounces.
Tablets—boxes of 100; each tablet is sealed in cellophane so that a day's supply can be conveniently carried.
Shown in Product Identification Section, page 435

Professional Labeling: Consult 1985 Physicians' Desk Reference.

AMPHOJEL®
Antacid
(aluminum hydroxide gel)
ORAL SUSPENSION • TABLETS

Composition: *Suspension*—Each 5 ml teaspoonful contains 320 mg aluminum hydroxide [$Al(OH)_3$] as a gel. *Tablets* are available in 0.3 and 0.6 g strengths. Each contains, respectively, the equivalent of 300 mg and 600 mg aluminum hydroxide as a dried gel. The 0.3 g (5 grain) tablet is equivalent to about 1 teaspoonful of the suspension and the 0.6 g (10 grain) tablet is equivalent to about 2 teaspoonfuls.

Indications: For temporary relief of heartburn, upset stomach, sour stomach, and/or acid indigestion.

Directions: *Suspension*—Two teaspoonfuls (10 ml) to be taken five or six times daily, between meals and on retiring or as directed by a physician. Medication may be followed by a sip of water if desired. *Tablets*—Two tablets of the 0.3 g strength, or one tablet of the 0.6 g strength, five or six times daily, between meals and on retiring or as directed by a physician. It is unnecessary to chew the 0.3 g tablet before swallowing.

Warnings: Do not take more than 12 teaspoonfuls (60 ml) of suspension, or more than twelve 0.3 g tablets, or more than six 0.6 g tablets in a 24 hour period or use this maximum dosage for more than two weeks except under the advice and supervision of a physician. May cause constipation. As with any drug, if you are pregnant or nursing a baby, seek the advice of a health professional before using this product.

Drug Interaction Precautions: Do not use this product if you are presently taking a prescription antibiotic containing any form of tetracycline.
Keep tightly closed and store at room temperature, Approx. 77°F (25°C)
Suspension should be shaken well before use. Avoid freezing.
Keep this and all drugs out of the reach of children.

How Supplied: *Suspension*—Peppermint flavored; without flavor—bottles of 12 fluidounces. *Tablets*—a convenient auxiliary dosage form—0.3 g (5 grain) bottles of 100; 0.6 g (10 grain), boxes of 100.
Shown in Product Identification Section, page 435

Professional Labeling: Consult 1985 Physicians' Desk Reference.

BASALJEL®
(basic aluminum carbonate gel)
SUSPENSION •CAPSULES
•SWALLOW
TABLETS

Composition: Suspension—each 5 ml teaspoonful contains basic aluminum carbonate gel equivalent to 400 mg aluminum hydroxide. Extra Strength Suspension—each 5 ml teaspoonful contains basic aluminum carbonate gel equivalent to 1000 mg aluminum hydroxide. Capsule contains dried basic aluminum carbonate gel equivalent to 608 mg of dried aluminum hydroxide gel or 500 mg aluminum hydroxide. Tablet contains dried basic aluminum carbonate gel equivalent to 608 mg of dried aluminum hydroxide gel or 500 mg aluminum hydroxide.

Indications: For the symptomatic relief of hyperacidity associated with the diagnosis of peptic ulcer, gastritis, peptic esophagitis, gastric hyperacidity and hiatal hernia.

Warnings: No more than 24 tablets/capsules/teaspoonfuls of BASALJEL, and no more than 12 teaspoonfuls of BASALJEL Extra Strength Suspension should be taken in a 24-hour period. Dosage should be carefully supervised since continued overdosage, in conjunction with restriction of dietary phosphorous and calcium, may produce a persistently lowered serum phosphate and a mildly elevated alkaline phosphatase. A usually transient hypercalciuria of mild degree may be associated with the early weeks of therapy.

Dosage and Administration: Suspension—two teaspoonfuls (10 ml) in water or fruit juice taken as often as every two hours up to twelve times daily. Two teaspoonfuls have the capacity to neutralize 28 mEq of acid. Extra Strength Suspension—one teaspoonful (5 ml) as often as every two hours up to twelve times daily. One teaspoonful is equivalent to two capsules or tablets and has the capacity to neutralize 22 mEq of acid. Capsules—two capsules as often as every two hours up to twelve times daily. Two capsules have the capacity to neutralize 26 mEq of acid. Swallow Tablets—two tablets as often as every two hours up to twelve times daily. Two tablets have the capacity to neutralize 28 mEq of acid. The sodium content of each dosage form is as follows: 0.1 mEq/5 ml for the suspension, 1.0 mEq/5 ml for the extra strength suspension, 0.12 mEq per capsule, and 0.09 mEq per tablet.

Precautions: May cause constipation. Adequate fluid intake should be maintained in addition to the specific medical or surgical management indicated by the patient's condition.

Drug Interaction Precautions: Alumina-containing antacids should not be used concomitantly with any form of tetracycline therapy.

How Supplied: Suspension—bottles of 12 fluidounces.
Extra Strength Suspension—bottles of 12 fluidounces.
Capsules—bottles of 100 and 500.
Swallow Tablets (scored)—bottles of 100.
Shown in Product Identification Section, page 435

COLLYRIUM
a neutral borate solution with antipyrine
SOOTHING EYE LOTION

Description: Contains 0.4% antipyrine, boric acid, borax and not more than 0.002% thimerosal (mercury derivative).

Indications: Soothes, cleanses and refreshes tired or irritated eyes resulting from long use, as in reading or close work or due to exposure to sun, strong light, irritation from dust, wind, etc.

Directions: To open, twist off and discard disposable cap. After every use, reclose by placing threaded eyecup on bottle. Rinse eyecup with clean water immediately before and after each use, and avoid contamination of rim and interior surface of cup. Apply the half-filled cup, pressing it tightly to the eye to prevent the escape of the liquid, and tilt the head well backward. Open eyelids wide and rotate eyeball to insure thorough bathing with the lotion.

Warnings: If irritation persists or increases, discontinue use and consult physician. Do not use in conjunction with a wetting solution for contact lens or other eye lotions containing polyvinyl alcohol. Keep tightly closed at Room Temperature, Approx. 77°F (25°C)

How Supplied: Bottles of 6 fl. oz. with eyecup.
Shown in Product Identification Section, page 435

COLLYRIUM $_2$™
Eye Drops with Tetrahydrozoline

Collyrium $_2$™ Eye Drops contain tetrahydrozoline hydrochloride (0.05%), zinc sulfate (0.25%), and glycerin (1.0%), with boric acid and sodium borate as buffering agents, and benzalkonium chloride (0.01%) and edetate disodium (0.1%) as preservatives.

Indications: For the relief of redness of the eyes due to minor irritations, temporary relief of burning and irritation due to dryness of the eye and/or discomfort due to minor irritations of the eye or to exposure to wind and sun.

Warnings: To avoid contamination of this product, do not touch tip of container to any other surface. Replace cap after using.
If you experience eye pain, changes in vision, continued redness or irritation of the eye, or if the condition worsens or persists for more than 72 hours, discontinue use and consult a doctor.
If you have glaucoma, do not use this product except under the advice and supervision of a doctor.
Overuse of this product may produce increased redness of the eye.
Do not use if solution changes color or becomes cloudy, or with povidone-containing contact lens wetting solutions.
Keep out of the reach of children.

Directions for using Collyrium $_2$™ Eye Drops: Tilt head back, gently pull down lower eyelid, and instill 1 to 2 drops in the affected eye(s). Then release the lower lid, close the eye, rotate the eye once or twice before opening.
Repeat this procedure up to for times daily.

How Supplied: Bottles of ½ fl. oz. with built-in eye dropper.
Shown in Product Identification Section, page 435

NURSOY®
Soy protein formula
READY–TO–FEED
CONCENTRATED LIQUID

Breast milk is preferred feeding for newborns. Nursoy® milk-free formula is intended to meet the nutritional needs of infants and children who are allergic to cow's milk protein or intolerant to lactose. It contains no corn syrup solids. Professional advice should be followed.

Ingredients: (in normal dilution supplying 20 calories per fluidounce): 87% water; 6.7% sucrose; 3.4% oleo, coconut, oleic (safflower) and soybean oils; 2.3% soy protein isolate; 0.10% potassium citrate; 0.09% monobasic sodium phosphate; 0.04% calcium carbonate; 0.04% dibasic calcium phosphate; 0.03% magnesium chloride; 0.03% calcium chloride; 0.03% soy lecithin; 0.03% calcium carrageenan; 0.03% calcium hydroxide; 0.03% l-methionine; 0.01% sodium chloride; 0.01% potassium bicarbonate; ferrous, zinc, and cupric sulfates; (68ppb) potassium iodide; ascorbic acid; choline chloride; alpha tocopheryl acetate; niacinamide; calcium pantothenate; riboflavin; vitamin A palmitate; thiamine hydrochloride; pyridoxine hydrochloride; beta-carotene; phytonadione, folic acid; biotin; activated 7-dehydrocholesterol; cyanocobalamin.

PROXIMATE ANALYSIS
at 20 calories per fluidounce
READY-TO-FEED and CONCENTRATED LIQUID:

	(W/V)
Protein	2.1%
Fat	3.6%
Carbohydrate	6.9%
Ash	0.35%
Water	87.0%
Crude fiber	not more than 0.01%
Calories/fl. oz.	20

Vitamins, Minerals: In normal dilution, each quart contains:

A	2,500	IU
D$_3$	400	IU
E	9	IU
K$_1$	0.1	mg
C (ascorbic acid)	55	mg
B$_1$ (thiamine)	0.67	mg
B$_2$ (riboflavin)	1	mg
B$_6$	0.4	mg
B$_{12}$	2	mcg
Niacin mg equivalents	9.5	
Pantothenic acid	3	mg
Folic acid	50	mcg
Choline	85	mg
Inositol	26	mg
Biotin	35	mcg
Calcium	600	mg
Phosphorus	420	mg
Sodium	190	mg
Potassium	700	mg
Chloride	355	mg
Magnesium	65	mg
Manganese	0.2	mg
Iron	12	mg
Copper	0.45	mg

Continued on next page

Wyeth—Cont.

Zinc	3.5	mg
Iodine	65	mcg

Preparation: *Ready-to-Feed* (32 fl. oz. cans of 20 calories per fluidounce formula)—shake can, open and pour into previously sterilized nursing bottle; attach nipple and feed. Cover opened can and immediately store in refrigerator. Use contents of can within 48 hours of opening.

Concentrated Liquid—For normal dilution supplying 20 calories per fluidounce, use equal amounts of Nursoy® liquid and cooled, previously boiled water. *Note: Prepared formula should be used within 24 hours.*

How Supplied: *Ready-to-Feed*—presterilized and premixed, 32 fluidounce (1 quart) cans, cases of 6; *Concentrated Liquid*—13 fluidounce cans, cases of 24.

SMA®
Iron fortified
Infant formula
READY–TO–FEED
CONCENTRATED LIQUID
POWDER

Breast milk is the preferred feeding for newborns. Infant formula is intended to replace or supplement breast milk when breast feeding is not possible or is insufficient, or when mothers elect not to breast feed.

Good maternal nutrition is important for the preparation and maintenance of breast feeding. Extensive or prolonged use of partial bottle feeding, before breast feeding has been well established, could make breast feeding difficult to maintain. A decision not to breast feed could be difficult to reverse.

Professional advice should be followed on all matters of infant feeding. Infant formula should always be prepared and used as directed. Unnecessary or improper use of infant formula could present a health hazard. Social and financial implications should be considered when selecting the method of infant feeding.

SMA® is unique among prepared formulas for its fat blend, whey-dominated protein composition, amino acid pattern and mineral content. SMA®, utilizing a hybridized safflower (oleic) oil, became the first infant formula offering fat and calcium absorption equal to that of human milk, with a physiologic level of linoleic acid. Thus, the fat blend in SMA® provides a ready source of energy, helps protect infants against neonatal tetany and produces a ratio of Vitamin E to polyunsaturated fatty acids (linoleic acid) more than adequate to prevent hemolytic anemia.

By combining reduced minerals whey with skimmed cow's milk, SMA® adjusts the protein content to within the range of human milk, reverses the whey-protein to casein ratio of cow's milk so that it is like that of human milk, and reduces the mineral content to a physiologic level.

The resultant 60:40 whey-protein to casein ratio provides protein nutrition superior to a casein-dominated formula. In addition, the essential amino acids, including cystine, are present in amounts close to those of human milk. So the protein in SMA® is of high biologic value.

The physiologic mineral content makes possible a low renal solute load which helps protect the functionally immature infant kidney, increases expendable water reserves and helps protect against dehydration.

Use of lactose as the carbohydrate results in a physiologic stool flora and a low stool pH, decreasing the incidence of perianal dermatitis.

Ingredients: SMA® Concentrated Liquid or Ready-to-Feed. Water; nonfat milk; reduced minerals whey; lactose; oleo, coconut, oleic (safflower), and soybean oils; soy lecithin; calcium carrageenan. *Minerals:* Potassium bicarbonate; calcium chloride and citrate; potassium chloride; sodium citrate; ferrous sulfate, sodium bicarbonate; zinc, cupric, and manganese sulfates. *Vitamins:* Ascorbic acid, alpha tocopheryl acetate, niacinamide, vitamin A palmitate, calcium pantothenate, thiamine hydrochloride, riboflavin, pyridoxine hydrochloride, beta-carotene, folic acid, phytonadione, activated 7-dehydrocholesterol, biotin, cyanocobalamin.

SMA® Powder. Nonfat milk; reduced minerals whey; lactose; oleo, coconut, oleic (safflower), and soybean oils; soy lecithin.
Minerals: Calcium chloride; sodium bicarbonate; calcium hydroxide; ferrous sulfate; potassium hydroxide and bicarbonate; potassium chloride; zinc, cupric, and manganese sulfates.
Vitamins: Ascorbic acid, alpha tocopheryl acetate, niacinamide, vitamin A palmitate, calcium pantothenate, thiamine hydrochloride, riboflavin, pyridoxine hydrochloride, beta-carotene, folic acid, phytonadione, activated 7-dehydrocholesterol, biotin, cyanocobalamin.

PROXIMATE ANALYSIS
at 20 calories per fluidounce
READY-TO-FEED, POWDER, and CONCENTRATED LIQUID:

	(w/v)
Fat	3.6%
Carbohydrate	7.2%
Protein	1.5%
60% Lactalbumin (whey protein)	0.9%
40% Casein	0.6%
Ash	0.25%
Crude Fiber	None
Total Solids	12.6%
Calories/fl. oz.	20

Vitamins, Minerals: In normal dilution each quart contains 2500 IU vitamin A, 400 IU vitamin D_3, 9 IU vitamin E, 55 mcg vitamin K_1, 0.67 mg vitamin B_1(thiamine), 1 mg vitamin B_2(riboflavin), 55 mg vitamin C (ascorbic acid), 0.4 mg vitamin B_6(pyridoxine hydrochloride), 1 mcg vitamin B_{12}, 9.5 mg equivalents niacin, 2 mg pantothenic acid, 50 mcg folic acid, 14 mcg biotin, 100 mg choline, 420 mg calcium, 312 mg phosphorus, 50 mg magne-

sium, 142 mg sodium, 530 mg potassium, 355 mg chloride, 12 mg iron, 0.45 mg copper, 3.5 mg zinc, 150 mcg manganese, 65 mcg iodine.

Preparation: *Ready-to-Feed* (8 and 32 fl. oz. cans of 20 calories per fluidounce formula)—shake can, open and pour into previously sterilized nursing bottle; attach nipple and feed. Cover opened can and immediately store in refrigerator. Use contents of can within 48 hours of opening.

Powder—(1 pound can)—For normal dilution supplying 20 calories per fluidounce, use 1 scoop (or 1 standard tablespoonful) of powder, packed and leveled, to 2 fluidounces of cooled, previously boiled water. For larger amount of formula, use ¼ standard measuring cup of powder, packed and leveled, to 8 fluidounces (1 cup) of water. Three of these portions make 26 fluidounces of formula.

Concentrated Liquid—For normal dilution supplying 20 calories per fluidounce, use equal amounts of SMA® liquid and cooled, previously boiled water.

Note: Prepared formula should be used within 24 hours.

How Supplied: *Ready-to-Feed*—presterilized and premixed, 32 fluidounce (1 quart) cans, cases of 6; 8 fluidounce cans, cases of 24 (4 carriers of 6 cans). *Powder*—1 pound cans with measuring scoop, cases of 6. *Concentrated Liquid*—13 fluidounce cans, cases of 24.

Also Available: SMA® lo-iron. For those who appreciate the particular advantages of SMA®, the infant formula closest in composition nutritionally to mother's milk, but who sometimes need or wish to recommend a formula that does not contain a high level of iron, now there is SMA® lo-iron with all the benefits of regular SMA® but with a reduced level of iron of 1.4 mg per quart. Infants should receive supplemental dietary iron from an outside source to meet daily requirements.

Concentrated Liquid—13 fl. oz. cans, cases of 24. *Powder*—1 pound cans with measuring scoop, cases of 6. *Ready-to-feed*—32 fl. oz. cans, cases of 6.

Preparation of the standard 20 calories per fluidounce formula of SMA® lo-iron is the same as SMA® iron fortified given above.

SIMECO®
Antacid/Anti–Gas
(aluminum hydroxide gel, magnesium hydroxide, simethicone)
ORAL SUSPENSION

Composition: Each teaspoonful (5 ml) contains aluminum hydroxide gel, equivalent to 365 mg of dried gel, USP, 300 mg of magnesium hydroxide, and 30 mg of simethicone.

Indications: For temporary relief of heartburn, upset stomach, sour stomach, and/or acid indigestion accompanied by gas.

Directions: 1 or 2 teaspoonfuls, undiluted or with a little water, to be taken

3 or 4 times daily between meals and at bedtime or as directed by a physician.

Warnings: Do not take more than 8 teaspoonfuls (40 ml) in a 24-hour period or use the maximum dosage for more than two weeks except under the advice and supervision of a physician. Do not use this product except under the advice and supervision of a physician if you have kidney disease. As with any drug, if you are pregnant or nursing a baby, seek the advice of a health professional before using this product.

Drug Interaction Precautions: Do not take this product if you are presently taking a prescription antibiotic containing any form of tetracycline.
Sodium Content: 0.3 to 0.6 mEq per teaspoonful.
Keep tightly closed at Room Temperature, Approx. 77°F (25°C).
Keep from freezing. Shake well before using.
Keep this and all drugs out of the reach of children.

How Supplied: Oral Suspension—Cool mint flavor, available in 12 fluidounce bottles.
Shown in Product Identification Section, page 435

Professional Labeling: Consult 1985 Physicians' Desk Reference.

WYANOIDS®
Hemorrhoidal Suppositories

Description: Each suppository contains 15 mg extract belladonna (0.19 mg equiv. total alkaloids), 3 mg ephedrine sulfate, zinc oxide, boric acid, bismuth oxyiodide, bismuth subcarbonate, and peruvian balsam in cocoa butter and beeswax. Wyeth Wyanoids have an unusual "torpedo" design which facilitates insertion and insures retention.

Indications: For the temporary relief of pain and itching of hemorrhoidal tissue in many cases.

Warning: Not to be used by persons having glaucoma or excessive pressure within the eye, by elderly persons (where undiagnosed glaucoma or excessive pressure within the eye occurs most frequently), or by children under 6 years of age, unless directed by a physician. Discontinue use if blurring of vision, rapid pulse, or dizziness occurs. Do not exceed recommended dosage. Not for frequent or prolonged use. If dryness of the mouth occurs, decrease dosage. If eye pain occurs, discontinue use and see your physician immediately as this may indicate undiagnosed glaucoma. In case of rectal bleeding, consult physician promptly.

Usual Dosage: One suppository twice daily for six days.

Directions: Remove wrapper of suppository and insert suppository rectally with gentle pressure, pointed end first. Use preferably upon arising and at bedtime.

How Supplied: Boxes of 12.
Shown in Product Identification Section, page 435

W. F. Young, Inc.
111 LYMAN STREET
SPRINGFIELD, MA 01103

ABSORBINE JR.

Active Ingredient: Acetone, Menthol, Wormwood, Chloroxylenol and Thymol formulated with essential oils and tinctures.

Indications: For fast relief from sore, aching muscles due to overexertion.

Actions: Absorbine Jr. rubbed on the skin dilates peripheral blood vessels to speed fresh invigorating blood flow to the point of pain.

Warnings: Keep out of the reach of children. Extremely flammable. Keep away from fire, sparks and heated surfaces. For external use only.

Symptoms and Treatment of Oral Overdosage: In case of accidental ingestion contact a physician immediately.

Dosage and Administration: Apply Absorbine Jr. full strength and massage gently 3 or 4 times daily. For severe strains see your doctor.

How Supplied: Available in 1 oz., 2 oz., 4 oz. applicator bottles. Also available in 12 oz. non-applicator bottle.
Shown in Product Identification Section, page 435

Youngs Drug Products Corp.
P.O. BOX 385
865 CENTENNIAL AVENUE
PISCATAWAY, NJ 08854

Sole Distributors for products manufactured by
HOLLAND-RANTOS COMPANY, INC.

KOROMEX®
CONTRACEPTIVE CREAM

Composition: KOROMEX CONTRACEPTIVE CREAM... Pearly-white in appearance... for those patients whose aesthetic preference is for a preparation with a lesser lubrication factor. Active ingredient is Octoxynol 3.0%—in a base of purified water, propylene glycol, stearic acid, sorbitan stearate, polysorbate 60, boric acid and fragrance. pH buffered and adjusted to 4.5.

Indications: Contraception and vaginal lubrication in conjunction with a vaginal diaphragm.

Warning: Keep this and all medication out of the reach of children.

Administration and Dosage: Approximately 2 teaspoonsful of KORO-

MEX CONTRACEPTIVE CREAM is placed on the dome surface of the diaphragm coming in direct contact with the cervix. The cream is then spread over the rubber and around the rim.

How Supplied: #225 KOROMEX C/C CREAM large refill (4.05 oz.—115 grams).

KOROMEX® CONTRACEPTIVE CRYSTAL CLEAR GEL

Description: KOROMEX CRYSTAL CLEAR GEL is colorless, unscented, non-staining, non-irritating, non-greasy, and lubricating.

Active Ingredient: Nonoxynol-9 2.0% in a base of purified water, propylene Glycol, Cellulose Gum, Boric Acid, Sorbitol and simethicone. pH 4.5

Indications: Contraceptive and vaginal lubrication in conjunction with a vaginal diaphragm.

Actions: Spermicidal

Warnings: Keep this and all medication out of the reach of children.

Side Effects: Should sensitivity to the ingredients or irritation of the vagina or penis develop, the patient should discontinue use and be instructed to consult a physician.

Dosage and Administration: Approximately 2 teaspoonfuls of KOROMEX GEL is placed on the dome surface of the diaphragm coming in direct contact with the cervix. The GEL is then spread over the rubber and around the rim.

How Supplied: #615 KOROMEX CONTRACEPTIVE CRYSTAL CLEAR GEL (4.44 oz.–126 grams).

KOROMEX® CONTRACEPTIVE FOAM

Description: KOROMEX CONTRACEPTIVE FOAM is a pure white delicately fragranced aerosol foam. It is highly spermicidal, non-staining, non-greasy.

Composition: Active ingredient is nonoxynol-9 12.5% in a base of water, propylene glycol, propellant 114, Isopropyl alcohol, Laureth-4, cetyl alcohol, propellant 12, PEG-50 stearate and fragrance.

Action: Spermicidal.

Indication: Contraception.

Side Effects: Should sensitivity to the ingredients or irritation of the vagina or penis develop, the patient should discontinue use and be instructed to consult a physician.

Warning: Contents under pressure. Do not puncture or incinerate container. Do not expose to heat or store at temperatures above 120° F. KEEP OUT OF REACH OF CHILDREN.

Continued on next page

Youngs Drug—Cont.

Dosage and Administration: One applicatorful of KOROMEX CONTRACEPTIVE FOAM should be inserted prior to each intercourse.

The patient may have intercourse any time up to one hour after the foam has been inserted. If intercourse is repeated, another applicatorful of the KOROMEX FOAM should be inserted.

When KOROMEX CONTRACEPTIVE FOAM is used, a cleansing douche is not essential. However, if a douche is recommended or desired, the patient should be instructed to wait at least 6 hours after intercourse.

How Supplied: KOROMEX CONTRACEPTIVE FOAM 40 gms. (1.41 oz.) can with applicator and purse for storage.

KOROMEX® CONTRACEPTIVE JELLY

Composition: KOROMEX CONTRACEPTIVE JELLY contains the active ingredient nonoxynol-9 3.0%—in a base of purified water, propylene glycol, cellulose gum, boric acid, sorbitol, starch, simethicone and fragrance. pH buffered and adjusted to 4.5. Pleasantly scented to meet the patient's aesthetic requirements. Homogenized to help eliminate the primary patient complaint of messiness.

Indications: Contraception and vaginal lubrication alone or in conjunction with a vaginal diaphragm.

Warning: Keep this and all medication out of the reach of children.

Administration and Dosage: Approximately 2 teaspoonsful of KOROMEX CONTRACEPTIVE JELLY is placed on the dome surface of the diaphragm coming in direct contact with the cervix. The jelly is then spread over the rubber and around the rim. When KOROMEX CONTRACEPTIVE JELLY is used alone, one applicatorful is inserted up to one hour before intercourse.

How Supplied: #115 KOROMEX C/C JELLY—large refill (4.44 oz.—126 grams).

NYLMERATE[II]® Solution Concentrate

Composition: SD alcohol 23A 50% v/v, purified water, acetic acid, boric acid, polysorbate 20, nonoxynol-9, sodium acetate, FD & C Blue #1, D & C Yellow #10.

Action and Uses: A cleansing acidified buffered vaginal irrigant. In recommended dilution pH is 4.5, thereby aiding in adjusting the vaginal pH. Helps relieve and combats offensive odors and pruritus by removing accumulated discharges.

Useful as an adjunct in specific vaginal therapy or routine vaginal cleansing.

Directions: One tablespoonful or ½ capful (filled to the top line inside of cap) to one quart of warm water. Do not add solution until the water is first added to the douche bag, then mix thoroughly.

Warning: Do not use more than twice weekly unless directed to do so by the physician. Do not use full strength. If irritation occurs, discontinue use.

How Supplied: 16 fluid oz. (473 ml) in a plastic bottle with measuring cap.

TRANSI–LUBE®
The Sexual Foaming Lubricant

Description: TRANSI-LUBE is a sexual lubricant that closely approximates the normal female transudate to enhance sexual pleasure. This medically oriented lubricant has the mild taste and aroma of strawberries. It is non-greasy, non-staining, non-irritating, maintains its lubricity for a long period of time, and is aesthetically acceptable to men and women. TRANSI-LUBE IS NOT A CONTRACEPTIVE.

Indications For Use: To enhance sexual pleasure. For improved sexual communication and response regardless of any physical or psychological disability.

Note: TRANSI-LUBE is not intended as a body lubricant. Genital play or sexual arousal is pleasantly enhanced when both partners use TRANSI-LUBE.

Contains: Purified water, isobutane propane, propylene glycol, sorbitol, PEG 14M, ceteth 10, methyl and propyl parabens, citric acid and flavor.

Side Effects: Should sensitivity to the ingredients or irritation of the vaginal area or penis develop, discontinue use. Due to the propellant, some coldness or irritation may be felt if placed directly on the penis or vagina. It is preferable to place the product on the hand, waiting 10 to 15 seconds before application.

Caution: Do not insert nozzle into the vagina or any body orifice for direct application.

Warning: FLAMMABLE—do not use near flame or while smoking. Contents under pressure. Do not puncture or incinerate. Do not store above 120° F. Keep out of reach of children. Use only as directed. Intentional misuse by deliberately concentrating and inhaling the contents can be harmful or fatal.

Packaging: Containers of 1.76 oz. (50 grams).

TRIPLE X®

Active Ingredients: Pyrethrins 0.3%, piperonyl butoxide, technical 3.00% equivalent to 2.4% (butylcarbityl) (6-propylpiperonyl) ether and to 0.6% related compounds, petroleum distillate 1.20% and benzyl alcohol 2.4%. Inert ingredients 93.1%

Indications: Triple X is indicated for the treatment of infestations of head lice, body lice and pubic (crab) lice and their eggs.

Actions: Triple X kills head lice (Pediculus humanus capitis De G.), body lice (Pediculus humanus humanus L.), and crab and pubic lice (Pediculus pubis L.), and their eggs.

Triple X is non-staining and easily removed with water. Triple X leaves no odor when it is washed out.

Precautions: This product is for external use only. Keep out of reach of children.

Causes eye irritation. Do not get in eyes. Harmful if swallowed. Do not inhale. Avoid contact with mucous membranes. In case of infection or skin irritation, discontinue use and consult a physician. Consult a physician if infestation of eyebrows and eyelashes occurs.

Should be used with caution by ragweed sensitized person.

Do not contaminate water, food or feed by storage or disposal. Do not transport or store below 32°F. Do not reuse container. Wrap container and put in trash collection.

Statement of Practical Treatment: If swallowed—Call a physician or Poison Control Center immediately. Drink one or two glasses of water and induce vomiting by touching the back of the throat with finger. Repeat until vomit fluid is clear. Do not induce vomiting or give anything by mouth to an unconscious person.

If inhaled—Remove victim to fresh air. Apply respiration if indicated.

If in eyes—Flush eyes with plenty of water. Call a physician if irritation persists.

Dosage and Administration: It is a violation of Federal Law to use this product in a manner inconsistent with its labeling. This Product Is For External Use On Humans Only.

Apply undiluted to infested areas until entirely wet. DO NOT USE ON EYELASHES OR EYEBROWS. Allow treatment to remain 10 minutes, but no longer. Then wash thoroughly with warm water and shampoo or soap. Dead lice and eggs may require removal with a fine comb. A second treatment must be made in 7 to 10 days to kill any newly hatched lice.

To avoid reinfestation with head, pubic or body lice, all clothing and bed linen should be disinfected by washing in hot water and drying, using the hot cycle for at least 20 minutes, or by dry-cleaning. Combs and brushes should be soaked in water above 135°F for 5 to 10 minutes. Sexual partners should be treated simultaneously. Rooms inhabited by infested patients should be thoroughly vacuumed.

General Information: HEAD LICE, live on the scalp, laying small white eggs (nits) on the hair shaft close to the scalp. The nits are mostly easily found on the nape of the neck or behind the ears. All personal headgear, scarves, coats, and bed linen should be disinfected by machine washing in hot water and drying, using the hot cycle of a dryer for at least

20 minutes. Personal articles of clothing or bedding that cannot be washed may be dry-cleaned or sealed in a plastic bag for a period of about 2 weeks. Personal combs and brushes may be disinfected by soaking in hot water (above 130°F) for 5 to 10 minutes. Thorough vacuuming of rooms inhabited by infested patients is recommended.

CRAB OR PUBIC LICE, generally transmitted by sexual contacts, are very small and look almost like brown or grey dots on the skin. Crab lice usually cause intense itching and lay small white eggs (nits) on the hair shaft close to the skin surface. In hairy individuals, the crab louse may be present on the short hairs of the thighs and trunk, underarms and occasionally on the beard and mustache. Sexual partners should be treated simultaneously to avoid reinfestation. All underware should be disinfected by machine washing in hot water, then drying, using the hot cycle for at least 20 minutes.

BODY LICE, and their eggs are generally found in the seams of clothing, particularly in the waistline and armpit area. They move to the skin to feed, then return to the seams of the clothing, where they lay their eggs. All clothing should be disinfected by the same procedure outlined for head lice. Clothing should be sealed for at least 30 days in a plastic bag for body lice because the nits (eggs) can remain dormant for a period of up to 30 days.

How Supplied: In 2 and 4 fl. oz. bottles. A fine-toothed comb to aid in removal of deal lice and nits and a packet of Youngs Foaming Shampoo to help rinse away Triple X are included in each package.

Products are cross-indexed by

generic and chemical names

in the

YELLOW SECTION

IDENTIFICATION PROBLEM?

Consult the

Product Identifcation Section

where you'll find

products pictured

in full color.

Memorandum

Diagnostics Devices and Medical Aids

This section is intended to present product information on Diagnostics. Devices and Medical Aids designed for home use by patients. The information concerning each product has been prepared, edited and approved by the manufacturer.

The Publisher has emphasized to manufacturers the necessity of describing products comprehensively so that all information essential for intelligent and informed use is available. In organizing and presenting the material in this edition the Publisher is providing all the information made available by manufacturers.

In presenting the following material to the medical profession. the Publisher is not necessarily advocating the use of any product.

Ames Division
Miles Laboratories, Inc.
POST OFFICE BOX 70
ELKHART, IN 46515

MICROSTIX®-Nitrite Kit
In–home dip and read test for nitrite in urine, an indicator of urinary tract infection
For in vitro diagnostic use

Active Ingredient: Reagents: P-arsanilic acid and 1,2,3,4-tetrahydrobenzo(h)quinolin-3-ol plus a buffer in solid state reagent strip format.

Indications: MICROSTIX®-Nitrite is an in-home test kit that has reagent strip tests that will detect nitrite in urine, an indicator of urinary tract infection.

Actions: The three MICROSTIX®-Nitrite test strips are to be used to test first morning urine specimens on three consecutive mornings. To achieve best results, the urine should be retained in the bladder for at least four hours, and should be tested immediately upon urinating. Ninety percent of urinary tract infections are caused by bacteria that convert nitrate in the urine to nitrite. If nitrite is present in urine, the test strip will turn a pink color. When this positive result occurs, the person should contact her/his doctor for treatment.
Shown in Product Identification Section, page 403

VISIDEX® II Reagent Strips
Visual Test for Glucose in Whole Blood

Summary and Explanation: A VISIDEX® II Reagent Strip is a disposable plastic strip with two reagent pads for determining the concentration of glucose in whole blood. A semipermeable membrane serves as a barrier to blood cell migration into the reagent area.

The reagent strip is for visual interpretation only. It is ready to use upon removal from the bottle. One large drop of whole blood sufficient to cover both reagent pads is applied to a VISIDEX II Reagent Strip. The lower range pad responds optimally to glucose concentrations of 20–110 mg/dL (1–6.0 mmol/l); the higher range pad responds optimally to glucose concentrations of 140–800 mg/dL (8–44 mmol/l). After timing and blotting, semiquantitative results are read from a color chart. The ability of users to develop skill and consistency in timing and blotting, and to interpret test results, improves with experience. It is strongly recommended, therefore, that users practice doing the procedure in order to become proficient in their technique.

Because the concentration of glucose provides an indication of the body's ability to metabolize carbohydrates, VISIDEX II Reagent Strips can be used to monitor blood glucose levels of diabetic patients on a routine basis to assist in controlling the diabetic condition. Significant hypoglycemic and hyperglycemic results are readily recognized with the test (see Limitations of Procedure for Neonatal Specimens).

Warnings and Precautions: VISIDEX II Reagent Strips are for in vitro diagnostic use.

Storage and Handling: Proper storage and handling of VISIDEX II Reagent Strips is important for accurate and dependable results.

Storage: Store unreacted VISIDEX II Reagent Strips at temperatures under 30°C (86°F) in a cool, dry place. Do not refrigerate unreacted strips. Use prior to expiration date shown on the bottle label and within 6 months after first opening. Mark the first opening date on bottle label.

Handling: Avoid exposing VISIDEX II Reagent Strips to moisture, light and heat to guard against altered reagent activity. Do not remove desiccant from bottle and keep tightly capped. Do not touch test areas of the reagent strip. Keep reagent areas away from contaminating substances often found in working areas. All unused strips must remain in the original bottle. Transfer to any other container may cause reagent strips to deteriorate and become unreactive.

Quality Control: DEXTRO-CHEK® NORMAL Control should be used any time performance is questioned. Use of the control determines reagent strip performance by identifying any VISIDEX II reagent pad deterioration or improper technique (timing, blotting, etc.) in the use of the strips. Acceptable performance is assured when the control test result falls within the range specified in the DEXTRO-CHEK NORMAL Control package insert. Discoloration or darkening of the reagent area prior to use may also be an indication of deterioration and may be identified by comparing the reagent pads with the "DRY UNREACTED REAGENT PADS" color block on the bottle label.

Specimen Collection and Preparation: Sufficient blood to perform the test may be obtained from fingertip or earlobe. If desired, a venous whole blood sample may also be used. VISIDEX II is not intended for use with serum or plasma.

Availability: From local authorized Ames distributors, Self-Testing Centers and selected retail pharmacies. VISIDEX II Reagent Strips are available in bottles of 25 strips (#2660) or 100 strips (#2661). DEXTRO-CHEK® NORMAL Control (#5591) is available in a carton containing two 5mL vials. AMES DEXTRO System® Lancet (#5574), AUTOLET®Kit (#2790) and AUTOLET® Platforms Regular Puncture (#2791) and Super Puncture (#2797) are also available.
Shown in Product Identification Section, page 403

Apothecary Products, Inc.
11531 RUPP DRIVE
BURNSVILLE, MN 55337

EZY–DOSE® MEDICINE SPOON

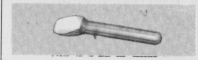

Colorful, unbreakable plastic tube spoon. Accurately calibrated with dose measurements in tsp. and ml. Special spoon design minimizes tongue contact with medication and spillage. 1, 2, and 3 tsp. sizes available in 5 assorted colors. All graduations are imprinted in white for easy reading.
Shown in Product Identification Section, page 403

EZY–DOSE®
NITRO–FRESH® NITROGLYCERINE PILL HOLDER

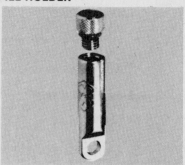

Chrome-plated, soild brass case is heat and light resistant. Diamond tooled screw cap keeps case waterproof, pill protected. Attaches to neck chain or keyring for easy access.
Shown in Product Identification Section, page 403

EZY–DOSE® ORAL SYRINGE WITH DOSAGE–KORC

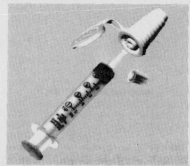

Easy, accurate dosing of liquid medication. Dosage-Korc eliminates spillage of liquid medication when withdrawing from bottle. Calibrated with tsp. and ml. Syringe tip is designed for easy medication administration. 1 and 2 tsp. sizes available.
Shown in Product Identification Section, page 403

EZY–DOSE®
7–DAY PILL REMINDER

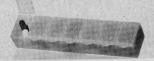

Durable plastic container with 7 compartments. Each compartment's snaplock lid is marked (also in brail) with the day of the week. Improves patient compliance, eliminates dosage errors. Small, medium, and large sizes in assorted colors.

Shown in Product Identification Section, page 403

EZY–DOSE® SPOON DROPPER

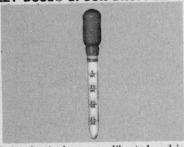

Safe, plastic dropper calibrated and imprinted in easy to read tsp. and ml measurements. Allows placement of medication onto back of tongue past taste buds. ½, 1 and 2 tsp. sizes available.

Shown in Product Identification Section, page 403

MEDI–SET™

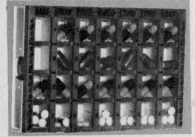

Multiple-medication control device to prevent dosage errors. Sturdy plastic, ideal for pills that must be taken up to 4 times a day, 7 times a week. Clear sliding covers lock into place. 6"L × 4"W × 1¼"D. Replacement medication trays and schedules available.

Shown in Product Identification Section, page 403

MEDTIME MINDER™

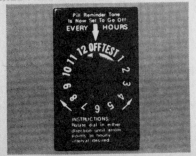

Automatic medication reminder. Compact size (1" w × 2" h). Velcro strip easily attaches device to any patients vial. Fits in a pocket. After setting only once, alarm continues to sound at regular intervals to remind patient to take medicine. Patient never forgets again.

Shown in Product Identification Section, page 403

W. A. Baum Co., Inc.
620 OAK STREET
COPIAGUE, NY 11726

HI/LO® BAUMANOMETER®
Blood Pressure Kit

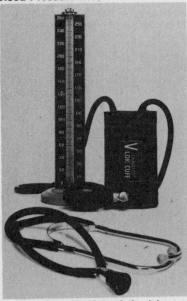

An increasing number of physicians are recommending that hypertensive patients have their blood pressure measured at home to supplement measurements made in the doctor's office. Home recordings can help reveal the true level of a patient's blood pressure and assist the physician in regulating dosage of antihypertensive drugs.

The Hi/Lo® Kit was designed for home use as directed by a physician. It includes:

Mercury-gravity Sphygmomanometer, calibrated to 260 mm/Hg—Complete CALIBRATED® V-LOK® Inflation System—Double-tube Stethoscope—Illustrated Instruction Booklet—Record Charts—Sturdy Storage Carton

Products are cross-indexed by generic and chemical names in the
YELLOW SECTION

Beecham Products
DIVISION OF BEECHAM INC.
POST OFFICE BOX 1467
PITTSBURGH, PA 15230

ACU–TEST®
In-Home Pregnancy Test

Active Ingredients: hCG on sheep red blood cells, hCG antiserum from rabbits.

Indications: An *in vitro* pregnancy test for use in the home.

Actions: Indicates the presence of human chorionic gonadotropin, a hormone of pregnancy, in the urine.

Precautions: For use on or after the 9th day following the day when the menstrual period was due. The physician should be consulted if pregnancy is indicated.

Administration: Perform test exactly according to instructions, using the first morning urine.

How Supplied: Packages of one or two tests each with test tube, dropper and buffer solution.

Boehringer Mannheim Diagnostics, Inc.
Bio-Dynamics Division
9115 HAGUE ROAD
INDIANAPOLIS, IN 46250

ACCU–CHEK™ bG
Blood Glucose Monitor

The Accu-Chek™ bG Blood Glucose Monitor (Cat. No. 790) is a portable, battery-operated device which gives rapid quantitative determinations of blood glucose levels when used in conjunction with Chemstrip bG® Reagent Strips. The Accu-Chek™ bG uses a single drop of blood on a Chemstrip bG® Test Strip to provide a reliable blood glucose result. Monitoring an individual's blood glucose level provides an immediate indication of the degree to which his diabetes is controlled, eliminating the inaccuracies of urine testing. The Accu-Chek™ bG system is designed to be accurate, economical, and easy to use.

A calibration strip for use with Accu-Chek™ bG Blood Glucose Monitor is provided with each 50-strip vial of Chemstrip bG® Reagent Strips (Cat. No. 00503). This calibration strip programs the instrument to respond to the specific reaction characteristics of the group of strips in use. The calibration strip remains in place until that particular vial of test strips is consumed. This calibration technique allows adjustment for lot-to-lot variations in test strip manufacturing, calibrates the instrument at multiple points, and ensures a high level of accuracy.

The Operator's Manual which accompanies the Accu-Chek™ bG Blood Glucose Monitor provides complete instructions for use as well as testing and operating

Continued on next page

Boehringer Mannheim—Cont.

suggestions. Bio-Dynamics Glucose Control Solution (Cat. No. 00519) is available to ensure the user of the monitor's reliability.

Accu-Chek™ bG Blood Glucose Monitor Cat. No. 790

For Ordering/Pricing/Technical Information: Call 1-800-428-4674; in Indiana, call 1-800-382-5200.

CHEMSTRIP bG®
Test for Glucose in Whole Blood

Summary and Explanation: CHEMSTRIP bG® is a test strip for the semi-quantitative visual estimation of glucose in whole blood that is used to provide information on the status of carbohydrate metabolism. The reagent test area is attached to an inert plastic strip and is made up of two distinct zones, each of different reagent concentrations, specifically designed to provide optimal sensitivity to varying glucose levels ranging from 20 mg/dl to 800 mg/dl.
CHEMSTRIP bG Reagent Strips are packaged in an aluminum vial with a tight-fitting cap containing a drying agent. Each CHEMSTRIP bG is stable and ready for use when removed from the vial.
The determination of glucose levels in whole blood CHEMSTRIP bG is based on the glucose oxidase/peroxidase reaction demonstrated by Keston[1], Comer[2] and Free, et al.[3] Bio-Dynamics has modified this procedure by substituting tetramethylbenzidine (TMB) for tolidine as an indicator in the lower (proximal) zone, and by using, in addition to o-tolidine, 3-amino-9 (γ-aminopropyl)-carbazole-dihydrochloride (APAC) in the upper (distal) zone.

Test Principle: Both zones of the reagent area contain the enzymes glucose oxidase, peroxidase and color indicators. D-glucose is oxidized to γ-D-gluconolactone with glucose oxidase acting as a catalyst. The hydrogen peroxide that results from this reaction oxidizes indicators in the presence of peroxidase. The intensities of the colors formed are proportional to the glucose concentration in the specimen.
The semi-quantitative estimation of glucose is determined by visual comparison of both zones with colors for 20, 40, 80,

120, 180, 240, 400 and 800 mg/dl on the vial label.
[See table below].
FOR IN VITRO DIAGNOSTIC USE
CHEMSTRIP bG Reagent Strips are stable in the original capped vial until the listed expiration date. In order to avoid exposure to moisture, the vial must be closed immediately after removal of a strip, using the original stopper which contains a drying agent.
Storage: Store at temperatures under 30°C (86°F); do not freeze.

Specimen Collection and Preparation: For the determination of blood glucose levels, a large drop of fresh capillary blood from the fingertip or ear lobe may be used. Venous blood may also be used; however, the test should be performed within 30 minutes of specimen collection since glucose in blood undergoes glycolysis at a rate of approximately 5% each hour at room temperature with leukocytosis and bacterial contamination accelerating the process.[4] If a refrigerated venous specimen is used, be sure all samples are brought to room temperature (20–25°C) before performing the test. Blood specimens containing common anticoagulants and preservatives, such as sodium heparin or sodium EDTA may be used; however, *fluoride must be avoided as a preservative.*

Procedure:
How Supplied: 25 Test Strips in an aluminum vial containing a drying agent Cat. No. 00501. Vial of 50 test strips with calibration strip included, may be read visually or with Accu-Chek™ bG Blood Glucose Monitor. Cat. No. 00503.
Materials Required But Not Provided: Surgical cotton and timer (i.e., stopwatch or watch with second hand).
Perform the test according to the following instructions:
1. **Carefully** place a large drop of whole blood onto the reagent area of the CHEMSTRIP bG. **DO NOT SMEAR.** Simultaneously start a timer.
   NOTE: Both zones of the reagent area must be completely covered.
2. After **exactly 60 seconds,** using moderate pressure, wipe off blood with a dry cotton ball. Lightly wipe the strip two more times using the clean side of the cotton ball.
   NOTE: All blood or cotton residues must be wiped from the test area.
3. After waiting an **additional 60 seconds** (total time elapsed: 2 minutes), match the colors on the test strip to the color scale on the vial label. If the col-

ors developed are darker than those for 240 mg/dl, wait an additional 60 seconds (total time elapsed: 3 minutes), before comparing the final reaction colors with the color scale. The color scale printed on the Chemstrip bG vial label is lot specific. Never read Chemstrip bG test strips using a scale other than that on the vial in which the strips are packaged.
NOTE: Intermediate values can be estimated when the colors of the strip zones fall between those on the vial label. For Example: If the lower zone on the strip matches the lower zone 80 on the vial, and the upper zone of the strip matches the upper zone 120 on the vial; the estimated value is 100.
4. If strip is to be saved for future reference, the following procedure is recommended:
   a. Label and date the strip for future reference.
   b. Store the reacted strip in a CHEMSTRIP bG vial, taking care to replace the cap securely.
Stability of Reacted Strips: The developed color is stable for 7 days up to 320 mg/dl or for 4 days above 320 mg/dl when stored as recommended above.[5]

Calibration: Calibration of the CHEMSTRIP bG by the user is not required. The color blocks on the vial label are calibrated by the use of precise standards during manufacturing.

Quality Control: Quality control for this procedure consists of following good laboratory techniques, ensuring that strips have been properly stored and specimens have been handled according to instructions. The analyst should be aware of the sources of error outlined under Limitations of Procedure. Each laboratory should establish its own goals for adequate standards of performance.

Results: Results are obtained by direct comparison with the color blocks printed on the vial label. Consult physician for interpretation of results. No calculations are required.

Limitations of Procedure: This procedure is free from interference if fresh capillary blood is used. Both test zones are specific for D-glucose. Other sugars which may also be present in blood do not react. Reducing substances such as uric acid, ascorbic acid, etc. (when occurring in physiological blood concentrations) do not affect the reaction. Treatment with heparin or ethylenediaminetetraacetic acid salts as well as with the usual plasma expanders does not affect the results. *Do not use preservatives that contain fluoride.*
Hematocrit values between 30–70% have no significant effect on test results. Extended exposure to air and light may result in values lower than those obtained on the initial reading. It is recommended that the reacted strips be stored under the conditions outlined in item 4 of the Procedure Section.

Reagent Composition For Chemstrip bG

Upper (Distal) Zone:		Lower (Proximal) Zone:	
o-Tolidine	21.5 μg	Tetramethylbenzidine	20.5 μg
3-Amino-9 (γ-aminopropyl)-carbozole-dihydrochloride	0.72 μg	Peroxidase (horseradish)	6.8 U
Peroxidase (horseradish)	6.0 U	Glucose oxidase (*Aspergillus niger*)	0.28 U
Glucose oxidase (*Aspergillus niger*)	0.30 U	Buffer	88.0 μg
Buffer	85.0 μg	Non-reactive ingredients	757 μg
Non-reactive ingredients	899 μg		

Expected Values (Fasting):

70–100 mg glucose/dl whole blood[4]
Hypoglycemia is manifest in children and adults at blood glucose levels below 50 mg/dl, and in neonates at levels below 30 mg/dl.[6]

Performance Characteristics: The performance characteristics of CHEMSTRIP bG Reagent Strips have been determined both in the laboratory and in clinical tests. Parameters of importance to the user are sensitivity, specificity, accuracy, precision and stability.
Generally the tests have been developed to be specific for the constituent to be measured with the exception of interferences listed previously. The stability data has been developed by testing at various temperatures and environmental conditions.
Accuracy:[7] A comparison study of the CHEMSTRIP bG test strip (y) and the Beckman Glucose Analyzer (x) yielded the following data:

$N = 200$
$y = 1.06_x - 11.6$
$r = 0.978$
$bias = 1.8$ mg/dl
at a mean value of 166.3 mg/dl
Precision is difficult to assess in a test of this type because of the variability of the human eye. It is for this reason that each user is encouraged to develop his own standards for performance.

References:

1. Keston, A., in Abstracts of Papers, 129th Meeting, Amer. Chem. Soc., Dallas, Texas; p. 31c (April, 1956).
2. Comer, J., *Anal. Chem. 28*:1748 (1956).
3. Free, A., et al., *Clin. Chem. 3*:163 (1957).
4. Schmidt, F., Handbook of Diabetes Mellitus, Pfeiffer, F., ed., Vol. 2, p. 938 (1971).
5. Kubilis, P., et al., publication in progress.
6. Forster, H., *Fortschr. Med. 94*:129 (1976).
7. Piepho, S. L., et al: Paper presented at 40th Annual Meeting of The American Diabetes Association, Washington, D.C., June 1980.

CHEMSTRIP bG®
Blood Glucose Test Kit

Chemstrip bG® Blood Glucose Test Kit (Cat. No. 00505) contains all supplies necessary for the diabetic to initiate an independent self blood glucose monitoring program.
The Test Kit contains one vial of 25 Chemstrip bG® Reagent Strips, 25 sterile lancets for finger pricking, 25 cotton balls for wiping the reacted test strip, and 25 alcohol pads for cleansing the intended puncture site. The kit also contains an illustrated, step-by-step procedure guide, and a booklet of helpful information regarding the use of Chemstrip bG® to achieve and maintain control of diabetes.
After cleansing the fingertip with an alcohol pad, in accordance with the procedure guide, the user will prick the finger to obtain a drop of blood. This drop of blood is applied to the test pads of a Chemstrip bG® Reagent Strip, and after wiping the blood from the test pads and

observing the appropriate reaction periods, the final reaction color is visually compared to the color chart on the vial label.
For Ordering/Pricing/Technical Information: Call 1-800-428-4674; in Indiana, call 1-800-382-5200.

Carter Products
Division of Carter-Wallace, Inc.
767 FIFTH AVENUE
NEW YORK, NY 10153

ANSWER®
At–Home Early Pregnancy Test Kit (Results in 1 Hour)

Active Ingredients: Each kit contains Beta-HCG antiserum (rabbit) and HCG on sheep red blood cells, dried (test tube with chemical material and a Buffer solution (plastic vial with test liquid).

Indications: A diagnostic aid for early determination of pregnancy, based on the presence of Human Chorionic Gonadotropin (HCG) in the urine. The sensitivity of ANSWER is such that pregnancy can often be determined as early as the 9th day _after_ an expected menstrual period.

Actions: ANSWER is a rapid, specific test. Based on its sensitivity, most urine specimens contain an adequate concentration of HCG to be detected nine days after the day the period was expected. In studies conducted with untrained people, 98% of the time the test was performed correctly.

Directions for Use:

A. **Urine Collection—Before you start the test.**
Collect a small amount of your first morning urine in a clean, well-rinsed glass container. The container must be washed and rinsed absolutely clean since any trace of detergent could give a false reading.
The test should be performed immediately. However, if you cannot do this, keep the urine sample covered in the refrigerator until you are ready to do the test. Sediment may form, but do _not_ shake the container of urine. Only the clear urine at the top of the container should be used. Be sure to test your urine the _same_ day it is collected. Be sure to bring urine to room temperature before testing.
Note: If urine is cloudy, pink, or red in color or has a strong odor, do not perform the test, as certain substances can cause false test results.

B. **Performance of the test.**

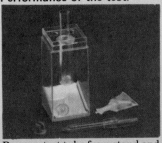

1. Remove test tube from stand and tap

it gently to make sure the chemical material is at the bottom of the test tube. Remove stopper from the test tube and replace tube in stand. Keep the stopper because you will use it later.

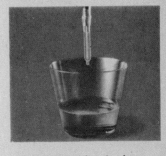

2. Fill dropper with urine by squeezing the rubber bulb.
Practice squeezing out 2 drops exactly.

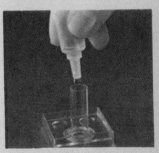

3. Empty 2 drops of urine from dropper into test tube.

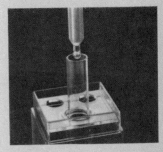

4. Remove plastic vial and hold with the tip pointing up making sure no liquid is in the neck of the vial. Snap off tip of vial, turn vial over, and carefully squeeze exactly 2 drops of the liquid from the vial into the test tube. Discard vial after use.

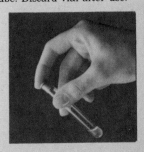

5. Replace stopper in test tube. Remove test tube from stand. DO NOT TURN

Continued on next page

Carter—Cont.

TUBE OVER. Keep tube upright and gently swirl the bottom of the tube until the chemical is completely mixed with liquid (about 10 seconds).

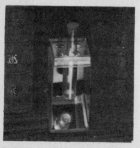

6. Replace test tube in the stand. Place the stand (with the mirror facing you) on a solid surface away from vibration, such as on a heavy chest or bookcase where it will not be hit or bumped or otherwise disturbed, and where the mirror can be easily seen. Allow to remain UNDISTURBED at room temperature for 1 hour.
Keep stand away from heat, vibration, and direct sunlight. Do not place stand on the refrigerator or on the same table or kitchen counter as a mixer or blender since these can cause vibrations when they are running. Do not place it on the stove, next to a heater, or in the window because heat or direct sunlight can disturb the test. Make sure stand is not moved during this 1-hour period.

C. **How to read the test (results).**
The test is to be read no sooner than 1 hour and no later than 2 hours after the tube is placed in the stand above the mirror.
Do not pick up or touch stand or tube.
Read results by looking at the bottom of

PREGNANCY HORMONE
NOT DETECTED

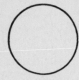

No Ring

PREGNANCY HORMONE DETECTED

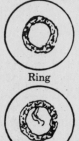

Ring

Ring

the tube in the mirror at base of stand. If the image you see in the mirror shows no ring as in illustration 1, pregnancy hormone is not detected.
If the image you see in the mirror shows a well-formed ring or doughnut-like ring, as in illustrations 2 and 3, pregnancy hormone is detected.

Important: This test is not intended to replace your doctor's diagnosis: If your test result shows pregnancy hormone detected, this should be confirmed by your doctor. If your result shows pregnancy hormone not detected, you may want to retest in one week. If you miss a second period, see your doctor.

Warnings: DO NOT REUSE, USE ONLY ONCE AND DISCARD.
Sometimes, around the time of "change of life" or in the case of certain diseases, ANSWER will show the presence of a hormone resembling the pregnancy hormone in your urine, even though you may not be pregnant. If your test result shows pregnancy hormone is detected, you should see your doctor. If you have missed a period or for any reason you think that you may be pregnant no matter what the result of the test, you should see your doctor. Don't guess; if you are not sure of your test result, consult your doctor.
ANSWER is not meant to replace an examination by your doctor. If you have been taking medication, the test may not work. In this case, you should have a test performed by your doctor or a professional laboratory. No test is perfect. Laboratory test results and a doctor's examination go hand in hand. Although the ANSWER method of detecting pregnancy is reliable, it is not 100% accurate. False results (pregnancy hormone detected when there is no pregnancy or pregnancy hormone not detected when the woman is pregnant) can occur in about 5% of women tested.

Precaution:
• Store the whole kit in a cool, dry place, not more than 30°C (86°F). Do not put in the freezer.
• ANSWER is not for internal use (it is for in vitro diagnostic use). Keep it out of the reach of children.
• Use only as directed. Do not use earlier than 9 days after the day you expected your period.
• Do not use after the expiration date stamped on the box.
• If the liquid in the plastic vial is cloudy, do not use the kit. Return to place of purchase for a new kit.

How Supplied: Available in kits of one test each. Each kit includes a test tube containing Beta-Human Chorionic Gonadotropin antiserum (rabbit) and Human Chorionic Gonadotropin on sheep red blood cells, dried with buffer and preservative (0.1% sodium azide); a plastic vial containing a buffer solution; a dropper for transferring urine; and a stand for conducting the test. The stand

includes a mirror for convenient reading without disturbing the test.
Shown in Product Identification Section, page 406

Fotomedics, Inc.
5000 CEDAR PLAZA PARKWAY
ST. LOUIS, MO 63128

CERVICOGRAPHY™
State-of-the-Art Diagnosis of Cervical Cancer

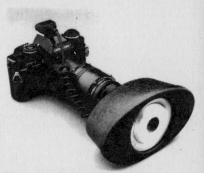

Summary and Explanations:
Cervicography™ represents the most recent advancement in cervical cancer detection. This non-invasive patented test takes an average of only 30 seconds when performed in conjunction with a gynecological examination.
The Cerviscope™ (pictured above), a specially made camera and light/lens system, is used to provide a reliable and simple method of photographing the cervix. The Cerviscope produces a special type of photographic evidence called a Cervigram™, which allows the entire cervix to be visible on one slide by providing a microscopic picture of the cervix. The Cervigram is comparable to direct colposcopic magnification and resolution. The resulting magnification (16x) makes the detection of cervical lesions and other precancerous changes more apparent in their earliest stages. Cervicography also provides an efficient method for diagnosis of Herpes and Condyloma.
Cervicography was developed to help reduce the "false-negative" rate of the pap smear (cytology) and to overcome some of colposcopy's inherent drawbacks. The reported frequency of false-negative pap smears varies among individual studies but falls in the range of 2 to 45%. It has been demonstrated that the combination of cytology and colposcopy can improve the accuracy of cervical cancer detection. However, screening by colposcopy is impractical and uneconomical. The cost of the colposcope is substantial. More importantly, there are not enough gynecologists with colposcopic expertise; and the key for success in colposcopy is determined and limited by the expertise of the examiner. The training in colposcopy is time-consuming and expensive. Furthermore, because colposcopic findings are recorded in a written description of the vascular and tissue pattern of the cervix, there is no opportunity for an objective review of the documentation of the findings.

Cervicography overcomes these problems. A physician can be trained in one hour to perform a Cervigram. In Cervicography, the cervix is illuminated and the Cerviscope is focused on the cervix by moving it back and forth. When the cervix is in focus the Cervigram is taken. The Cervigrams are processed by specially trained technicians and then sent to National Testing Laboratories for diagnosis by a specially trained physician /evaluator. All evaluators must be experienced colposcopists who have been trained and certified to evaluate Cervigrams by the Medical College of Wisconsin. The cervigram is returned to the physician with a diagnosis, providing a permanent, objective photographic record with which future changes in the cervix can be compared and used for subsequent consultations.

Dr. Adolf Stafl, M.D., of The Medical College of Wisconsin, demonstrated that the detection rate of the pap smear in combination with Cervicography increased the early detection rate and diagnostic accuracy of these two methods to 98%, thus correcting the "false-negative" rate of the pap smear while increasing the much needed early detection of cervical cancer. Because the early detection of cervical cancer is of primary importance in treating this disease, Cervicography now provides the physician with the necessary data to properly care for the patient when cervical cancer does appear.

Cervicography can be performed quickly and inexpensively by a physician or by a properly trained health care professional in conjunction with a gynecological exam. The Cervicography test is covered by most major insurance carriers.

Helena Laboratories
Home Health Care Div.
1530 LINDBERGH
P.O. BOX 752
BEAUMONT, TX 77704

COLOSCREEN SELF-TEST (CS-T)™
Fecal Occult Blood Test

Description: ColoScreen Self-Test (CS-T)™ is a simple, sanitary, one-step home test for the detection of occult blood in stool. No stool sample collection or hazardous reagents are needed. The test is based on the detection of hemoglobin released into the toilet bowl water from the stool. A special reagent impregnated in the test pad will change color if blood is present.

To use, the patient drops the pad in the toilet bowl, looks for a color change, and then flushes. Because this is a non-guaiac test, no dietary fruit and vegetable restrictions are necessary. Other fecal occult blood dietary restrictions, such as red meat and vitamin C, should be observed.

Each pad contains four test areas, plus positive and negative controls. Each kit contains three pads plus instructions.
Cat. No. 5175—Case of 12 kits.
Ordering/Pricing Information: (800) 231-5663

Consumer Information: (800) 231-4002
Shown in Product Identification Section, page 410

Lavoptik Company, Inc.
661 WESTERN AVENUE N.
ST. PAUL, MN 55103

LAVOPTIK® Eye Cups

Description: Device—Sterile disposable eyecups.

How Supplied: Individually bagged eyecups are packed 12 per box, NDC 10651-01004.

Menley & James Laboratories
a SmithKline Beckman company
ONE FRANKLIN PLAZA
P. O. BOX 8082
PHILADELPHIA, PA 19101

HEMOCCULT®HOME TEST

Description: Hemoccult®Home Test (HHT) is a guaiac-based test for fecal occult blood. It is marketed to consumers for the early detection of hidden blood in the stool.

How It Works: HHT works on the same principle as the Hemoccult II Test (SmithKline Diagnostics), detecting blood by a color-producing reaction of the peroxide in the HHT developer and peroxidase in the blood.

Interpretation: Experience with this type of test has shown that 4–5 percent of users will have a positive test result, i.e., blood present. Of this 4–5 percent, half will have blood from neoplasms, some of which may be malignant. The remainder will have a positive result from some other colorectal disease, interfering foods or drugs, or with no cause identified.

Note: Consumer labeling emphasizes that the HHT is a screen to detect occult blood, and that is **not** a test for colorectal cancer. The instructions inform users whose test results show the presence of blood in the stool to discuss the results with their physician. Under those circumstances, physicians may wish to elicit a history, including a family history, and perform a physical examination with particular attention to the GI tract. Diagnostic procedures may be indicated, as well as repeat testing for occult blood using Hemoccult II Test (SmithKline Diagnostics) with particular attention to dietary and medication limitations.

Diet Limitations: Peroxidase-rich foods may produce a positive reaction when no blood is present, and should be avoided prior to using the HHT to reduce the chance of a false-positive result. Examples of such foods are red meat (beef, lamb), turnips, broccoli, cauliflower, horseradish and melons.

Drug Limitations: Drugs known to interfere with test results are vitamin C (in excess of 250 mg), aspirin, NSAID's, iron, rectal ointments and reserpine.

Performance: Use of the test involves testing two small fecal specimens from each of three consecutive bowel movements. Directions for use of the test are written so as to be easily understood by non-health care professionals.

Copies of the HHT instructions for consumers as well as information regarding the use of the test, are available to health care professionals. Write: Hemoccult®Home Test, Menley & James Laboratories, M87, P.O. Box 8082, Philadelphia, PA 19101.

A toll-free number is available to consumers with questions concerning the test: 1-800-441-3890 (Continental US only) or 1-800-428-4323 (PA only).
Shown in Product Identification Section, page 416

Monoclonal Antibodies, Inc.
2319 CHARLESTON RD.
MOUNTAIN VIEW, CA 94043

OvuSTICK™
Self-Test

What the Test Does:
The OvuSTICK™ Self-Test is a complete personal system to help you and your doctor predict the time of ovulation.

How the Test Works:
The OvuSTICK™ Self-Test detects LH in your urine. It does this with a special plastic stick (called the OvuSTICK). When there is very little LH, the OvuSTICK stays white. When there is more, the OvuSTICK turns blue.

By regularly testing your urine, you can see the LH surge. Your OvuSTICK probably will be white or light blue during most of your cycle and darker blue during the LH surge.

Each kit includes a special test called a Surge Guide. The color of the OvuSTICK tested with the Surge Guide will help you recognize your LH surge. This will help you and your doctor predict the time of ovulation.

Do not take anything in this kit internally.

How to Collect and Store Your Urine:
Start collecting your urine on Day 10 of your cycle. Collect once a day in one of the Cups that are supplied. Use a new Cup each time. Try to collect at about the same time each day. For best results, collect between 10:00 AM and 8:00 PM. Do not collect your first urine after waking. Be sure to write down the time when you collect your urine.

You need at least one hour to perform this test. If you do not have that much time, cover your urine with a Lid. You can store it at room temperature for up to eight hours or in the refrigerator for up to 24 hours. Do not freeze it. For best

Continued on next page

Monoclonal Antibodies—Cont.

results, test your urine on the day that you collect it.

When to Start Testing:

Perform the Surge Guide on Day 9 of your menstrual cycle (Count the first day of bleeding as Day 1.) Start testing your urine on Day 10 of your cycle. Then go on testing every day until you have used all tests in the kit.

Your doctor may give you more directions if your cycle is typically shorter than 26 days or longer than 33 days.

Procedure

Prepare: Empty the liquid in Vial A into Tube B.

For Surge Guide: Partially fill the empty Vial A with water and add 10 drops to Tube B.

For Test 1 to 9: Partially fill the empty Vial A with urine and add 10 drops to Tube B.

Mix and Wait: Place the OvuSTICK in Tube B and rapidly move up and down for one minute. Set a timer and wait 30 minutes.

Rinse and Wait: Remove the OvuSTICK from Tube B and rinse each side for two to three seconds. Then place it in Tube C. Set a timer and wait 30 minutes.

Rinse and Read: Remove the OvuSTICK from Tube C and rinse each side for two to three seconds. Read the results and choose the color number that best matches the OvuSTICK.

How to Read Your Results:

You must read the result of each test right away, while the OvuSTICK is still wet. Use the drawing supplied with the Kit to find the color that best matches your OvuSTICK. If you have trouble deciding between two colors, choose the darker one.

Find the color number that is below the color you chose. Then, on the OvuSTICK Holder, write that color number under the heading for the test that you just completed. Below that, write the date and the time when you collected your urine.

Keep the used OvuSTICK, so that your doctor can see it. Put it in the correct slot of the OvuSTICK Holder, with the rounded end pointing down. Push it all the way in. You can do this while the OvuSTICK is wet. Then put the OvuSTICK Holder in the kit box. (The drawing shows you how an OvuSTICK fits in the OvuSTICK Holder.)

How to Recognize Your LH Surge:

After performing each Test, you must decide if you are having an LH surge. To do this, compare the color number of the Test to the color number of the Surge Guide. **Always compare the color numbers to decide if you are having an LH surge—never compare the OvuSTICKs to each other.** Make your decision in the following way:

- If your Test color number is **smaller** than or **equal** to your Surge Guide color number, you probably are **not** having an LH surge.
- If your Test color number is **larger** than your Surge Guide color number,

you probably **are** having a LH surge. You are likely to ovulate within one and a half days.

When you have an LH surge, follow the directions that your doctor has given you.

Be sure to contact your doctor if any of the following things happen:

- Your Test color numbers are larger than your Surge Guide color number for four days in a row or more.
- You use all of the tests in this kit, and none of the Test color numbers are larger than your Surge Guide color number.
- You have any concerns or questions about the results.

The OvuSTICK™ Self-Test must be used and interpreted under the care of your doctor.

Clinical Performance:

Forty-two (42) consumers performed the OvuSTICK Self-Test. Ninety-three percent (93%) of these consumers correctly identified the presence of the LH surge.

The kit contains:

10 OvuSTICKs (plastic sticks coated on the rounded end the mouse monoclonal antibody for LH)—enclosed individual foil pouches

10 Vial A's (contain buffered saline, surfactant, preservative, and red dye)

1 Tube B for use with the Surge Guide (contains mouse monoclonal antibody for LH linked to akaline phosphatase, human glycoprotein hormone producing color comparable to 35 ± 5 mIU/ml LH, and red dye)

9 Tube B's for use with Tests 1 to 9 (contain mouse monoclonal antibody for LH linked to akaline phosphatase

10 Tube C's (contain substrate, buffer, cofactor, a preservative)

10 Cups with Lids

1 OvuSTICK Holder

1 Pamphlet of Directions

Storage:

Store the kit below 86°F (30°C). Do not freeze it.

Orange Medical Instruments

3183-F AIRWAY AVENUE COSTA MESA, CA 92626

BETASCAN™ Reagent Strips
Blood Glucose Test Strips

Active Ingredients:

O-Tolidine	37.5 µg
Tetramethylbenzidine	22.0 µg
Diaminofluorene	15.0 µg
Glucose Oxidase	
(Aspergillus niger)	0.2 I.U.
Peroxidase (horseradish)	1.4 I.U.
Nonreactive ingredients	98% w/v

Summary and Explanation: BetaScan Reagent Strips are disposable, plastic test strips for determining the level of glucose in whole blood. At the beginning of a 60-second time period, one drop of whole blood is applied to the reagent strip area which then changes color in response to the glucose concentration in the blood.

For semiquantitative estimation of blood

glucose, a color chart on the vial label can be used. For more quantitative results and for people who have problems reading the different color concentration values, the BetaScan strip can be read in an OMI BetaScan A™ Self Blood Glucose Meter or the Ames Glucometer®.

Precaution: BetaScan Reagent Strips are intended for in vitro diagnostic use.

Dosage and Administration:

1. Patient applies a large drop of blood to the reagent pad and waits 60 seconds.
2. After 60 seconds blood is removed with special blotting paper or washed off.
3. Results are obtained one to two seconds after blotting by comparing with the color chart.

How Supplied: 50 strips per vial.

BETASCAN TRENDSTRIPS™
Blood Glucose Test Strips

Active Ingredients:

Upper Pad

O-Tolidine Dihydrochloride	26.0 µg
Peroxidase (horseradish)	0.75 I.U.
Glucose Oxidase	
(Aspergillus niger)	0.3 I.U.
Non-Reactive Ingredients	98% w/v

Lower Pad

O-Tolidine Dihydrochloride	26.0 ug
Peroxidase (horseradish)	0.75 I.U.
Glucose Oxidase	
(Aspergillus niger)	0.3 I.U.
F,D&C Yellow Dye #5	4.0 µg
Nonreactive Ingredients	98% w/v

Summary and Explanation: BetaScan TrendStrip™ is a disposable plastic test strip containing two reagent pads needed to measure the amount of glucose in whole blood. The test strip is made of two zones, each of which contains a different indicator designed to provide the optimal sensitivity for blood glucose levels ranging from 0 to 800 mg/dL. A semi-permeable membrane covers these pads to facilitate removal of blood from the surface. Strips are packaged in an aluminum can with tight fitting cap. Each strip is stable and ready to use when removed from the can. Both reagent pad reactions are based on the action of glucose oxidase, peroxidase and color indicators. Glucose oxidase catalyzes the oxidation of glucose in blood by oxygen in the atmosphere, producing gluconic acid and hydrogen peroxide. In the presence of peroxidase, indicators in the reagent strip are oxidized to produce color. The intensities of the colors formed are then proportional to the glucose concentration in the specimen.

The semi-quantitative estimation of glucose is determined by visual comparison of both zones with colors for 0, 20, 40, 80, 120, 180, 240, 400 and 800 mg/dL on the label.

Warnings: TrendStrips are for IN VITRO DIAGNOSTIC USE ONLY. In case of abnormal results, consult your physician. TrendStrips should not be used as the basis of self-diagnosis of diabetes.

Dosage and Administration:

1. Patient applies large drop of blood covering both reagent pads.
2. Wait 60 seconds and remove blood by wiping with soft tissue or cotton ball.

3. Wait an additional 60 seconds (120 seconds total elapsed time) and compare colors on test strip with the color chart on the vial.
4. For quantitative measurements, TrendStrips can be used with Trend-Meter or BetaScan B blood glucose meters.

How Supplied: Available in vials of 50 and 25 strips.

Ortho Pharmaceutical Corporation
Advanced Care Products Division
RARITAN, NJ 08869

ADVANCE®
Pregnancy Test

Active Ingredients: Human Chorionic Gonadotropin (HCG) alpha chain specific monoclonal antibody HCG, beta-chain specific antibody/enzyme conjugate, chromogenic substrate solution, and buffer solution.

Indications: An in-vitro pregnancy test for use in the home that can detect the presence of HCG in the urine as early as three (3) days past last missed period.

Actions: ADVANCE will accurately detect the presence or absence of HCG in urine in just thirty minutes. It is as accurate as pregnancy test methods used in many hospitals.

Dosage and Administration: Perform the test according to instructions. If, after thirty minutes, a blue color appears on the rounded end of the COLORSTICK, the patient can assume she is pregnant. If the rounded end of the COLORSTICK remains white, and no blue color can be seen, no pregnancy hormone has been detected and the patient is probably not pregnant. The test results may be affected by certain health conditions such as an ovarian cyst or ectopic pregnancy. For additional reassurance, a toll-free telephone number is included in each package insert. This service is staffed by Registered Nurses who can answer any questions the patient may have about her results, or how she performed the test.

How Supplied: Each ADVANCE test contains a plastic COLORSTICK, a plastic vial containing buffer solution, a glass tube containing dried test chemicals, a glass tube containing color developing solution, a test stand with urine collector, and instructions for use.

Storage: Store at room temperature (59°–86°F). Do not freeze.
Shown in Product Identification Section, page 419

DAISY 2®
Pregnancy Test

Active Ingredients: Human Chorionic Gonadotropin (HCG) on red blood cells, HCG antibodies, and diluent solution.

Indications: An in-vitro pregnancy test for use in the home that can detect the presence of HCG in the urine as early as three (3) days past last missed period.

Actions: DAISY 2® provides a double-check test method that accurately detects the presence or absence of HCG in urine in just forty-five minutes. It is the same pregnancy test method used in many hospitals.

Dosage and Administration: Perform the test according to instructions. If, after forty-five minutes, a dark brown ring is reflected in the mirror below the test tube, the patient is probably pregnant. If no ring is visible, no pregnancy hormone has been detected and the patient is probably not pregnant. All home pregnancy test kits recommend a second test if the first test indicates that the patient is not pregnant, and her period does not begin within a week. This second test may be needed because the patient may have miscalculated her period, or her body may not have accumulated enough hormone for a true reading. The test results may be affected by various other factors, such as certain medication and proteinuria, so many women like the reassurance that comes from double-checking their results. DAISY 2® makes this double-checking easy and convenient by providing two complete and identical tests in each kit. In addition, a toll-free telephone number is included in each package insert. This service is staffed by Registered Nurses who can answer any questions the patient may have about her results, or how she performed the test.

How Supplied: Each DAISY 2® Kit contains everything needed to perform two tests: Two test tubes with reagents, two vials of diluent solution, two droppers, one urine collection lid, a stand with mirror for reading test results, and complete directions.

Storage: Store at room temperature (59°–86°F). Do not freeze.
Shown in Product Identification Section, page 419

FACT™
Pregnancy Test

Active Ingredients: Human Chorionic Gonadotropin (HCG) on erythrocytes, HCG antiserum, and buffer solution.

Indications: An in-vitro pregnancy test for use in the home that can detect the presence of HCG in the urine as early as three (3) days past last missed period.

Actions: FACT will accurately detect the presence or absence of HCG in urine in just forty-five minutes. It is the same pregnancy test method used in many hospitals.

Dosage and Administration: Perform the test according to instructions. If, after forty-five minutes, a dark brown ring is reflected in the mirror below the test tube, the patient is probably pregnant. If no ring is visible, no pregnancy hormone has been detected and the patient is probably not pregnant. The test results may be affected by various other factors such as certain medication and proteinuria. For additional reassurance, a toll-free telephone number is included in each package insert. This service is staffed by Registered Nurses who can answer any questions the patient may have about her results, or how she performed the test.

How Supplied: Each FACT kit contains a glass test tube with Human Chorionic Gonadotropin (HCG) on erythrocytes and HCG antiserum, a plastic vial containing buffer solution, a dropper, a test stand with urine collector and complete instructions for use.

Storage: Store at room temperature (59–86°F). Do not freeze.
Shown in Product Identification Section, page 419

Sportmed Technology Ltd.
2180 BELGRAVE AVENUE
SUITE 495
MONTREAL, QUEBEC, CANADA
H4A2L8

THE FITNESS APPRAISAL KIT

Description: Scientifically validated fitness appraisal kit included on 3 audio cassettes. System includes:
1. MMATT—Maximal multistage aerobic Track Test
2. 20 Meter shuttle run test
3. Placed Muscular Endurance Test
4. Flexibility Evaluation
5. Lung Volume measurement
6. Body Fat Assessment
7. Nutritional Assessment Program $100.00
To order call Toll Free—1-800-361-3651

Thought Technology Ltd.
2180 BELGRAVE AVENUE
SUITE 495
MONTREAL, QUEBEC, CANADA
H4A2L8

BIOFEEDBACK 5™ RELAXATION SYSTEM

Description: Thought Technology has brought together, in one compact, convenient and economical package, a new generation of biofeedback devices that measure five psychophysiological parameters of stress, GSR, temperature, EMG, heartrate and blood volume pulse with clinical accuracy. A biofeedback system that is portable, affordable and complete. The Biofeedback 5 contains:

GSR/TEMP 2™
Monitors fluctuations in either skin resistance or temperature caused by stress-related sympathetic activity, and translates them into an audible tone or visual readout. Patients can, with practice

Continued on next page

Thought Technology Ltd—Cont.

quickly learn to lower the tone and develop relaxation skills.

HR/BVP 100T™

A dual-function meter that provides absolute heart rate and relative blood volume pressure. The latter is an extremely responsive measurement, registering changes from beat-to-beat.

EMG 100T™

Monitors EMG activities of various muscle areas for biofeedback training and muscle rehabilitation. Detects signals of less than .3 uv RMS. Output has 1% accuracy of both raw and RMS for research and biofeedback data acquisition. Unit includes 2 logarithmic meter scales (.2–20; 20–200 uv) and provides proportional tone and threshold feedback when connected to GSR 2.

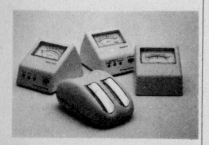

BIOFEEDBACK 5 DIGITAL™

This version includes the TEMP/SC 200T meter, which provides a precise digital readout as well as superior aural feedback through built-in speakers. Temperature response is immediate and the skin conductivity mode more accurate and applicable for clinical use. Used with the other monitors in the set, the TEMP/SC 200T provides digital readouts for all the parameter of stress, as well as two-channel monitoring.

Indications: For stress-related symptoms and conditions, either alone or as an adjunct to pharmacological treatment, these systems help patients learn stress control by themselves.

Warnings: None

Also Available:
1) Each of the systems in THE BIOFEEDBACK 5 can be purchased separately as: GSR 2, GSR/TEMP 2, EMG 100T, HR/BVP 200T, TEMP/SC 100T.
2) CALMSET 3—monitors EMG, GSR and temperature in a headset.
3) CALMTONE™ Stereo Controller.
4) CALMPUTE™ Micro-computer interface and software.
5) A complete line of clinical biofeedback software.

How Supplied: All U.S. orders are sent from Thought Technology's N.Y. warehouse, via U.P.S.
To order: Call toll free in USA: 1-800-361-3651

Warner-Lambert Company
201 TABOR ROAD
MORRIS PLAINS, NJ 07950

e·p·t® plus™
Early Pregnancy Test

- An **easy-to-read color change** tells you if you are pregnant in two hours.
- Color indicating E.P.T. PLUS is conveniently **portable** not sensitive to vibration or light.
- **Accurate** as many tests used in hospitals and labs.
- May be used as early as the ninth "late day" after a missed period.

FIRST, FAMILIARIZE YOURSELF WITH THE TEST KIT COMPONENTS:

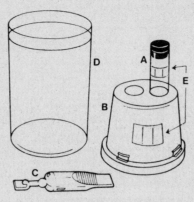

(A) **Glass test tube** with rubber stopper, containing the test reagent chemicals. Leave stopper in place until you are ready to perform the test.
(B) **Test holder.**
(C) **Plastic vial**—contains special buffer solution.
(D) **Lid,** use this to collect and hold the urine for the test.
(E) **Test results illustrations,** for convenient reading of test results.
IMPORTANT: For accurate test results, follow all instructions carefully.

What E.P.T. PLUS is

E.P.T. PLUS is a simple urine test that can be done accurately, quickly and safely at home. You can even carry E.P.T. PLUS with you in your pocket or purse. E.P.T. PLUS will tell you if you are pregnant in 2 hours from the time you start the test. The directions are easy to follow.
Nothing is taken internally.

What E.P.T. PLUS does

When you become pregnant you begin to produce a hormone called HCG—Human Chorionic Gonadotropin. This hormone appears in your urine. When the HCG level is high enough, E.P.T. PLUS will detect the presence of the HCG in the urine. This HCG level occurs at about the *ninth day* after the day on which you expected your period. It is possible to get a positive result before the ninth day (indicating you may be pregnant) although in many cases the level of HCG will not be sufficient to give an accurate, clear reading before that time. We advise that you wait until at least your ninth "late day" so that you can test with greater confidence.

When to use E.P.T. PLUS

You may use E.P.T. PLUS as early as your ninth late day. Count the day your period should have started as Day One. On Day Nine, you can use your E.P.T. PLUS test, for by that time sufficient pregnancy hormone should be present in your urine, if you are indeed pregnant. Of course you can use your E.P.T. PLUS on any day after Day Nine, as well. Do **not** use your E.P.T. PLUS test **earlier** than nine days after your missed period. If you are unsure of the date when your period should have begun, then count from the date you are most sure of. On the the ninth day after that date you can carry out the test, as well as on any day after that time.

Use only the first morning urine

If you are pregnant, the pregnancy hormone is most concentrated in the first urine specimen of the day. Collect it in the lid provided or in any other clean container. Wash the container and rinse it well with clear tap water to eliminate soap film before you use it. If you do not have enough time to do the test the first thing in the morning, you can cover and store your first morning urine specimen in the refrigerator (not in freezer)—but be sure to do the test on the same day the urine was collected. Let the urine warm to room temperature (for 15 to 20 minutes) before testing.
NOTE: If after your urine has been stored for several hours a sediment has formed at the bottom of the container, do **not** mix or shake the urine—just use the urine at the top of the container when you collect it in the plastic vial.

Performing the E.P.T. PLUS test

Before you actually start, read all the directions carefully.
COLLECTING THE FIRST MORNING URINE

Be sure that whatever you use to collect the urine—bowl or tumbler or enclosed test kit lid—is thoroughly rinsed in clear tap water before use.
You should use only first morning urine for carrying out the test. This is important because the early morning urine has the highest concentration of pregnancy hormone.
SETTING UP THE TEST

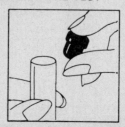

1. Remove the glass test tube (A) from the test holder (B). Remove the rubber stopper and put the tube back in the holder. Keep the stopper, you will need it again later on.

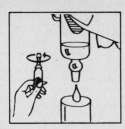

2. Remove the plastic vial (C) from the test holder (B). Do not be concerned about the amount of fluid in the vial. This is the exact amount necessary. Be sure that no liquid is in the neck of the plastic vial. Twist off the top of vial and squeeze out its entire contents into the glass test tube (A). Keep the empty plastic vial.

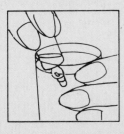

3. Now fill the empty plastic vial (C) with urine as you would with a medicine dropper.

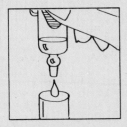

4. Carefully place 3 drops of urine into the test tube (A) by gently squeezing the plastic vial (C). Try to use just three drops, but remember that a tiny bit more or less will not hurt the test. If you have never used a dropper before, practice filling it and squeezing out drops one by one.

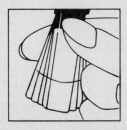

5. Take the test tube (A) and securely press back the rubber stopper. Shake the test tube gently until the contents are well mixed.

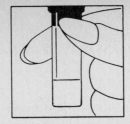

6. Now, when holding the test tube against artificial or daylight, you will observe the liquid to be an intensive red color.

WAITING TIME OF THE TEST
The test tube can be put in its holder and the holder kept anywhere convenient. Or you can take only the test tube with you in your pocket or purse. Vibration or light **does not** affect the E.P.T. PLUS test. You may read the test results 2 hours after setting up the test. Therefore, note the time you started the test. If you are pregnant, a color change may occur after one hour.

Reading the test results
Two hours after having done the test, look at the color of the liquid against day or artificial light. Compare the color you see with the following illustrations. Test result illustrations are also included on the test tube and test holder for your added convenience.
If the pregnancy hormone is present in your urine, the liquid will have become **lighter** in color. If there is **any** color change from the original intense red, you may assume that you are pregnant.

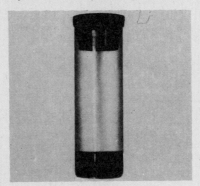

RED
NEGATIVE (−)
If the liquid **does not** change color, this means that no pregnancy hormone has been detected, and you are probably not pregnant. Your overdue period should begin soon. In the unlikely event that a week passes and you still have not menstruated, you should perform another test, using a new EPT PLUS kit; because 1) you may have miscalculated your period; 2) there may not yet have been sufficient HCG in your urine at the time of the first test; or 3) the test might have been performed incorrectly. If the second test still gives a negative result, there is little chance that you are pregnant. However, there could be other important reasons why your period has not begun and you should see your physician.

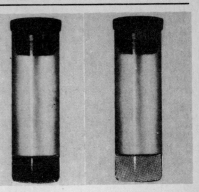

**PINK   LIGHT GREY TO
POSITIVE (+)   COLORLESS**
If the liquid **clearly does** change color, as indicated in the illustration, your urine does contain the pregnant hormone, and you can assume you are pregnant.
You should now plan to consult your physician, who is best able to advise you. (In certain rare cases HCG levels may be elevated even though you are not pregnant. Your physician can determine this.)

> **IMPORTANT: If you are pregnant a positive result may be evident at one hour. However, only the test result read within a one to two hour period after setting up the test is a reliable one. Any color-change after two hours should be disregarded.**

E.P.T. PLUS accuracy
In tests comparing E.P.T. PLUS to a laboratory test E.P.T. PLUS, when used by consumers, according to label directions, including a repeat test when indicated, was 98% accurate in diagnosing pregnant conditions and 94% accurate in diagnosing nonpregnant conditions. Laboratory tests were 98% and 96% accurate respectively in these same groups of women (Table).
HOW DOES E.P.T. PLUS COMPARE TO A LABORATORY PREGNANCY TEST?

In women who were—	E.P.T. PLUS was correct	LAB test was correct
Pregnant	98%	98%
Not Pregnant	94%	96%
Overall Accuracy	98%	97%

INGREDIENTS** FURNISHED
Each test kit contains:
1. Gold sol particles coated with monoclonal HCG antibodies.
2. Also contains special aqueous buffer solution.
** Not to be taken internally. For In Vitro Diagnostic Use.
Store below 86° Fahrenheit (30° Centigrade).
Do not freeze.

Questions about E.P.T. PLUS?
Call us toll-free 7 a.m. to 5 p.m. E.S.T.

Continued on next page

Warner-Lambert—Cont.

weekdays at 1-800-562-0266.
In New Jersey, call collect at (201) 540-2458.
Shown in Product Identification Section, page 432

EARLY DETECTOR™
In-Home Test for the Detection of Hidden Blood in the Stool

Description: Early Detector is an *in-vitro* diagnostic test to detect hidden blood in the stool.

Indications: There is uniform medical agreement that the earlier colorectal cancer is diagnosed and appropriate treatment instituted, the more favorable the disease prognosis. Among the early warning signs, rectal bleeding is considered the most sgnificant symptom. The primary at-risk groups include people over the age of 40, plus those with a family history of colorectal cancer, or the presence, or family history of familial polyposis of the colon.
In-home tests such as Early Detector are considered one of the most effective methods for large-scale screening.

Actions: Early Detector is a gum guaiac based, *in-vitro* diagnostic kit that tests for occult blood in three successive bowel movements. The procedure is simple, more acceptable to patients, and easy to perform in the privacy of the home.

Directions for Use: Complete, illustrated, easy-to-follow directions are included with each test. People who are actively bleeding from other conditions such as hemorrhoids or menstruation should not take the test. Some medications such as aspirin, iron supplements, vitamin C (over 250 mg. per day), rectal ointments, and anti-inflammatory drugs can cause an error in results. For two days before and throughout the test period, patients should avoid red or rare meat, turnips, horseradish and vitamin C supplements in their diets.

How Supplied: The Early Detector In-Home Test contains 3 specimen pads with Activity Indicator® test verification spots, developer solution, a packet containing a developer tablet and an instruction booklet.

Early Detector
The Early Detector in-home test finds hidden blood in the stool. The test is fast, painless, and simple. Blood in the stool can be a sign of a number of conditions. Some of these are ulcers, diverticulosis, hemorrhoids and cancer of the colon and rectum. Early Detector can alert you and your doctor to conditions which may require medical help. Read all the instructions before you perform the test. Follow the step-by-step guide with care to get accurate results.
Why should I use Early Detector?
Blood in the stool can be a sign of various conditions, including ulcers, diverticulosis, hemorrhoids and cancer of the colon and rectum. But you may not be aware of

this blood. Therefore, you may not seek the medical treatment you may need. Now there's Early Detector. The Early Detector Test is a fast, painless, and simple method of finding hidden blood in the stool. The Early Detector Test can be done in the privacy of your own home. There is nothing to mail in. You perform the test. You read the results.
How does Early Detector work?
Early Detector is a simple version of a standard laboratory test for hidden blood in the stool. The test is easy to do. After a bowel movement, you use a specimen pad to pat the anal area to get a stool specimen. The Early Detector Developer Solution is applied to the stool specimen. A chemical reaction will take place between the solution and stool specimen. If there is hidden blood in the stool, the area around the specimen will turn blue.
How often should I use Early Detector?
After age 40, when colo-rectal disease is most prevalent, annual screening for hidden blood in the stool with Early Detector is advisable. However, people who have a medical history of hidden blood in the stool or have a family history of gastrointestinal medical disorders should perform the test more often. The ease and convenience of Early Detector allows for more frequent and convenient screening.
What chemicals are found in Early Detector?
The final prepared Developer Solution has a stable mixture of hydrogen peroxide, gum guaiac, and denatured ethyl alcohol in water.
Each specimen pad has a positive Activity Indicator® which contains hematin, a chemical which when sprayed with Developer Solution will turn blue.
What are the precautions I should take?
The chemicals in Early Detector are not for internal use. Early Detector is made for outside the body use (**FOR IN VITRO DIAGNOSTIC USE**). Do not eat or drink this test.
Use the developer solution within two months after adding the tablet.
(Record Date on Page 13).
EARLY DETECTOR DEVELOPER SOLUTION MAY BE IRRITATING. DO NOT GET IN EYES. IF CONTACT OCCURS, FLUSH PROMPTLY WITH WATER.
Keep the Early Detector Developer Solution away from heat and light. Keep the bottle tightly capped when not in use.
CAUTION: FLAMMABLE. DO NOT USE NEAR OPEN FLAME. KEEP OUT OF REACH OF CHILDREN.
How should Early Detector be stored?
Store at room temperature (59°F–86°F)—do not refrigerate. Keep away from light and heat. Protect from direct sunlight. Keep developer solution tightly capped when not in use. Your Early Detector Test has:

3 Individually wrapped Specimen Pads with Activity Indicator®

1 Bottle Developer Solution
1 Packet Containing Developer Tablet
1 Instruction Booklet With Photographs.

How do I prepare myself to use the Early Detector Test Kit?
● Do not perform the test if you are actively bleeding from other conditions that may show up in the stool specimen. Some conditions are hemorrhoids or menstrual bleeding.

● INTERFERING SUBSTANCES
Some medicines such as aspirin, iron supplements and anti-inflammatory drugs for arthritis may cause the test to turn blue, even when blood due to a medical problem is not present in the stool (false positive result). Vitamin C (over 250 mg. daily) may prevent blood which may be present in the stool from turning the paper blue (false negative result). Such medicines should not be taken two (2) days prior to or during the test period. If your doctor has prescribed any of these medicines for you, check with him/her to see if it is permissible for you to stop taking your drugs for a few days. The use of rectal ointments should also be avoided while taking the test.

(See chart following page)

● Instructions for Special Diet. **FOR TWO DAYS BEFORE AND THROUGHOUT THE TEST PERIOD, FOLLOW THE SPECIAL DIET GUIDELINES BELOW.**

Do not eat:	Do eat foods such as:
Red or Rare Meat	Poultry
Turnips	Fish
Horseradish	Vegetables
Vitamin C Supplements	Fruit
(over 250 mg daily)	Peanuts
	Popcorn
	Bran Cereal

If you know that any of the above cause you discomfort, or if you are on a special diet or taking prescription medications check with your doctor before performing the test.

Instructions
Follow these with care to insure accurate results. Read all instructions before starting test.

NOTE: DEVELOPER SOLUTION SHOULD HAVE BEEN PREPARED AT LEAST 60 MINUTES PRIOR TO USE. To properly perform the test you will need to sample and test three successive bowel movements. It is important to do this test on all three bowel movements in a row. (If you miss one, continue test until three samples have been tested.) Gastrointestinal problems often bleed off and on. If you test three stool specimens in a row, you will have a better chance of finding hidden blood in the stool. You should do all three tests even if the first and second tests do not show hidden blood.

USE THESE INSTRUCTIONS FOR EACH TEST
STEP 1.
Wash hands thoroughly before using this

test. Have a specimen pad and developer solution bottle close to the toilet or sink.

STEP 2.

After a bowel movement, take a specimen pad and **fold the Activity Indicator spots under to keep them free of stool.**

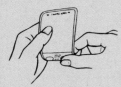

STEP 3.

Gently pat (*do not wipe*) the anal area to get a smear of stool.

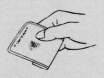

STEP 4.

Shake bottle well. Remove the clear plastic overcap from developer solution bottle. Hold bottle upright and specimen pad 1–3 inches away. Press firmly on the bottle top and spray repeatedly to wet the entire stool specimen. Be sure to spray the two Activity Indicator spots on bottom of pad. Five sprays should fully soak the pad.

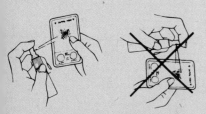

Caution: Do not spray on clothing or furniture.

STEP 5.

READ THE RESULTS IN 30–60 SECONDS. COLOR MAY FADE AFTER 60 SECONDS.

The Activity Indicator spots on the bottom of the specimen pad will show that the test is working. **The spots do not show whether there is blood in the stool.** When you spray the spots, the positive spot will turn blue and the negative spot will not change color.

NOTE: If the positive spot is blue before you spray the pad the specimen pad should not be used. If the spot does not turn blue after you have sprayed it with developer solution, do not continue test. Call toll free number for assistance.

Now look at the area on and around the stool specimen **Any trace of blue color**

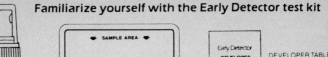
Familiarize yourself with the Early Detector test kit

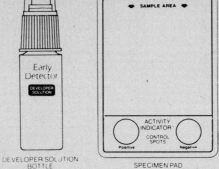

DEVELOPER SOLUTION BOTTLE   SPECIMEN PAD

Early Detector DEVELOPER TABLET   DEVELOPER TABLET

ACTIVITY INDICATOR CONTROL SPOTS   Positive   Negative

Positive Activity Indicator ® will turn blue after you spray with developer solution.

Negative Activity Indicator will not change color.

of any shade or intensity is a positive result (except in the Activity Indicator positive spot). No trace of blue color on or around the stool specimen is a negative result. See color photo for examples of positive/negative test results (Page 12 of booklet). After reading results, flush the specimen pad in the toilet.

NOTE: If you are color blind, have someone help you read the test.

STEP 6.

Record each test result in the space provided in the Record of Early Detector Test Results (last page).

IMPORTANT: If any of the three tests show a trace of blue color, you should consult with your doctor as soon as you can. Discontinue testing and consult with your doctor if your first or second test is positive.

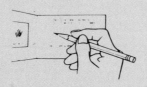

STEP 7. Wash hands thoroughly after using each test.

What do the results mean?

If a blue color (positive reading) is anywhere on the specimen pad (except in the positive circle of the Activity Indicator) this shows that there may be blood in the stool. Be sure to check edges of the smear area. If you see **ANY** blue anywhere on the specimen pad area (except in the positive circle of the Activity Indicator) within 30–60 seconds after you have sprayed the developer solution on the stool sample, the test is positive. This does not always mean that you have a serious medical problem. The blue color may be caused by the food you have eaten or the medicines you are taking or other conditions such as ulcers or hemorrhoids. As with all tests for hidden blood, the results do not give conclusive evidence of any specific disease. Early Detector is a screening tool, a diagnostic aid. It is **not** made to take the place of

routine physical examinations or other tests your doctor may wish to perform. If you have a positive result from your test, you should consult with our doctor as soon as you can. Remember **only one** specimen pad of the three tests you have done has to show a blue color for you to consult with your doctor.

If your tests showed no trace of blue color this means that at the time of taking the test there was no detectable blood in the stool. However, this does not mean you are free of disease. Not all gastrointestinal disorders bleed. You may have other symptoms which led you to use this test, such as bowel habit changes (e.g. diarrhea or constipation lasting longer than 2 weeks), unexplained weight loss lasting 2 or more weeks or visually evident blood in the stool (red or black). If so, even if your tests are negative, you should consult with your doctor.

What are the limitations of the test? As with all tests for hidden blood, results with Early Detector cannot prove the presence or absence of bleeding or illness. Early Detector is not made to replace tests that your doctor may wish to perform.

Tests to find hidden blood are being used and evaluated both in clinical practices and at leading medical centers.

Past results show that:

● In health screening surveys, the positive rate has been about 2% to 5%. Positive means any trace of blue color. However, this does not always mean that you have a serious medical problem. The blue color may be caused by the food you have eaten or the medicines you are taking.

Tests have shown that consumers can perform this test and read the results as well as a testing laboratory.

FOR ANY INFORMATION OR ASSISTANCE YOU MAY NEED CONCERNING EARLY DETECTOR YOU MAY CALL TOLL FREE 1-800-E.D. HELPS

Shown in Product Identification Section, page 432

Educational Material

Part 1 contains a listing of books, booklets, brochures and other materials that can be obtained by contacting manufacturers listed in this edition.

Part 2 provides you with the names and addresses of organizations that can be contacted if you need help for a specific health problem.

Part 1— MANUFACTURERS' SERVICE MATERIAL

ALBERTO-CULVER
Taming Your Taste For Salt   Free
A booklet containing helpful hints on reducing your sodium intake plus recipes.

ANABOLIC
Anabolism Journal of Preventive Medicine   Paid
Quarterly publication discussing current topics in nutritional science.

ARIZONA NATURAL PRODUCTS
Garlic vs Candida Albicans   Free
Arizona Natural Odorless Garlic Product Flyer
Flyer describing products available and a brief write-up on allicin.

BEECHAM
"A Personal Guide to Feminine Freshness"   Free
16-page illustrated booklet on vaginal infections, feminine hygiene and douching.
"Feminine Hygiene and You"   Free
14-minute color film explains how a woman's body works (reproductive system, menstrual cycle, and vaginal secretions) then explains douching.

BEIERSDORF
Unna Booklet   Free
The history of Dr. Paul Gerson Unna and the Unna Boot.
Wound Management   Free
A guide to bandages, dressings, and infection control.

JOHN BORNEMAN & SONS

What is Homeopathy?   Free
16-page booklet which examines the general principles of Homeopathy, Homeopathic remedies, and how to use them and some short experiments presenting scientific evidence for the activity of Homeopathic remedies.

Fine Homeopathic Remedies   Free
24-page catalogue and descriptive brochure describing some general points concerning Homeopathy, as well as some more commonly used remedies & products.

Principles of Homeopathic Prescribing   Free
4-page discussion of the basic concepts of Homeopathy and their application in practice.

The Reliability of Homeopathic Remedies   Free
18-page exposition utilizing both texts and photographs of the manufacturing and preparation of Homeopathic remedies.

Oscillococcinum®   Free
Text detailing the preparation, use, pathogenesis, and general information on Oscillococcinum®, a Homeopathic remedy used for the relief of symptoms of cold and flu.

Preparation of Mother Tinctures   Free
A four-color pamphlet detailing the process for preparation of quality Homeopathic Mother Tinctures.

Precision   Free
Brochure outlining the principles and uses of Homeopathic remedies and products. A micro-dose therapy based on the law of ''like cures like''.

Tube and Dose   Free
Brief description of a new dosage form designed for the presentation of Homeopathic remedies.

BURROUGHS WELLCOME

Pamphlets   Free
Miscellaneous patient information pamphlets on gout, herpes, eye and ear preparations, colds and allergies.

CARNATION

Calcium Booster Ideas (NRI-391/PDR)   Free
A consumer brochure with tips and recipes for increasing calcium intake.

CHATTEM CONSUMER PRODUCTS

PMS: A Review for Health Professionals
Booklet describing PMS, current theories of cause, and treatments. Written for health professionals.

PMS: Premenstrual Syndrome   Free
Brochure describing PMS, how to know if you have it and what you can do about it. Includes diary for self-monitoring of PMS symptoms. Written for consumers.

COMMERCE DRUG

Baby Ray Teething Booklet   Free
Facts parents should know about tooth development and the teething process.

Propa-PH Skin Care Booklet   Free
A guide for teenagers on proper skin care.

Everything you should know about your new braces   Free
Booklet which answers questions dental brace-wearers ask.

How to select the right medicine for relief of:
Toothache pain, denture pain, dental brace irritation,
teething pain, canker sore/cold sore pain   Free
Brochure describing various types of minor mouth pain and the specific medicine to use for each type.

GLENBROOK

What Your Doctor Wants You to Know About Aspirin   Free
Facts on the use of aspirin.

Care for Your Back   Free
Use of aspirin, ice massage and exercise in lower back pain therapy.

Reducing the Risk of Stroke   Free
Booklet

Recurrent TIA's and Stroke   Free
Booklet

Aspirin and Your Arthritis   Free
The use of aspirin for arthritis and anti-inflamation effect.

HOECHST-ROUSSEL

Changes, Cycles and Constipation   Free
Pamphlet describing constipation and its causes, with instructions on prevention and self-treatment, and when to consult a physician.

What You Should Know About Hemorrhoids and Fissures   Free
Pamphlet describing these conditions, with instructions on self-care and when to consult a physician; available in English and Spanish.

LACTAID
Digestive Disease Clearinghouse   Free
A reprint of a newsletter published by the DD Clearinghouse which provides several addresses of organizations concerned with digestive problems. Suggests several publications on lactose intolerance/digestion. It also discusses what the DD Clearinghouse is and how to contact it.
Why LactAid? The Problem and the Answer   Free
Pamphlet discussing lactose intolerance, its nutritional implications and LactAid/LactAid treated milk.

LEDERLE
Calcium Crisis in the American Woman's Diet   Free
8 page pamphlet describing why today's women need to supplement their diet with calcium.
The Myth About Athletes Foot   Free
Consumer pamphlet describing the treatment and prevention of athletes foot.

MEDICONE
Clinical Evaluation Fact Cards and Samples   Free
Medical study in usage of our rectal suppositories.

NATREN
Superdophilus   Free
Brochure on use, dosage, technical data, sources, etc.
Bifido Factor   Free
Brochure on use, dosage, technical data, sources, etc.

ORANGE MEDICAL
BetaScan Reagent Strip   Free
Brochure
TrendStrips   Free
Brochure

PADDOCK
Glutose Pamphlet   Free
Describes Glutose in greater detail with clinical studies. Also contains general management of hypoglycemia.
Emulsoil Pamphlet   Free
Describes Emulsoil in greater detail as it relates to preparing the bowel for X-ray procedures of the gastrointestinal tract.

PARTHENON
Bismuth Subgallate as an Effective Means for the Control of Ileostomy Odor:
A Double Blind Study   Free
A Study

PURDUE FREDERICK
Facts About Douching   Free
Facts on douching with visual description of methods of douching with Betadine Medicated Douche.
Fiber and Your Health   Free
Explanation of dietary fiber and its importance, with recommendation for usage and a listing of disorders associated with diets low in fiber.
Your Betadine Antiseptic Guide to First Aid   Free
Description on caring for cuts, burns, and scrapes using Betadine Antiseptics.
A Guide to the Relief of Constipation   Free
A booklet describing constipation and how the laxative Senokot-S can be used for relief.
Making Your Pregnancy Even Happier For You   Free
A booklet to aid the pregnant woman in relieving constipation, homorrhoids, morning sickness and weight control.

ROCHE
The HOW TO Book on Antibacterial Medication   Free
Booklet describing when and how to take antibacterials; how to know they are working and how to avoid problems.
The HOW TO Book on Arthritis Medication   Free
Booklet looking at types of arthritic disorders and medicines used to treat them; how to prevent common side effects.
The HOW TO Book on Diuretic Medication   Free
Book reviewing what diuretics do; how to reduce salt intake and importance of potassium levels.
The HOW TO Book on Sleep Medication   Free
Book providing information on how to use sleep medications as part of a total effort to deal with insomnia.
The HOW TO Booklet on Tranquilizer Medication   Free
Booklet giving guidelines for using tranquilizers properly; how to avoid problems and to use as a part of a total effort.
The WHAT IF Book   Free
Booklet answering questions about the medication you are taking.

SEARLE CONSUMER PRODUCTS

Constipation: What You Can Do About It   Free
Booklet

Diverticular Disease: Answers to Your Questions   Free
Booklet

Hemorrhoids: Ways to Prevent and Treat Them   Free
Booklet

The High-Fiber Diet: How It Can Aid Your Health   Free
Booklet

Irritable Bowel Syndrome: Answers to Your Questions   Free
Booklet

"The Sweet Facts" (Equal Low-Calorie Sweetener)*   Free
Folder

Understanding Arthritis   Free
Booklet

STELLAR

"First Aid Prevention for Swimmer's Ear"   Free
Patient information on cause and care of preventing swimmer's ear.

Star-Otic Patient Instruction Pads   Paid
Instructions for patients on use of Star-Otic to prevent swimmer's ear.

Part 2—HEALTH ASSOCIATIONS AND ORGANIZATIONS

**Alcohol and Drug Problems
Association of North America**
444 North Capitol St., N.W.
Washington, D.C. 20001
(202) 737-4340

**Alcoholics Anonymous World
Services, Inc.**
P.O. Box 459
Grand Central Station
New York, N.Y. 10163
(212) 686-1100

**Alzheimer's Disease and
Related Disorders Association**
360 N. Michigan Ave.
Suite 1102
Chicago, Ill. 60601
(312) 853-3060

**American Anorexia Bulimia
Association, Inc.**
133 Cedar Lane
Teaneck, N.J. 07666
(201) 836-1800

**American Association of
Poison Control Centers**
University of Maryland
20 N. Pine St.
Baltimore, MD 21201

AARP Pharmacy Service
510 King St. #420
Alexandria, VA. 22314
(703) 684-0244

American Brittle Bone Society
1256 Merrill Drive
West Chester, Pa. 19382
(215) 692-6248

American Cancer Society
777 Third Avenue
New York, N.Y. 10017
(212) 371-2900

**American Council on
Alcohol Problems**
2908 Patricia Drive
Des Moines, Iowa 50322
(515) 276-7752

American Dental Association
211 E. Chicago Avenue
Chicago, Ill. 60611

American Diabetes Association
2 Park Avenue
New York, N.Y. 10016
(212) 683-7444

American Dietetic Association
430 North Michigan Avenue
Chicago, Ill. 60611
(312) 280-5000

American Foundation for the Blind
15 W. 16th Street
New York, N.Y. 10011
(212) 620-2000

American Heart Association
7320 Greenville Avenue
Dallas, TX. 75231
(214) 750-5300

American Liver Foundation
998 Pompton Avenue
Cedar Grove, N.J. 07009
(201) 857-2626

American Lung Association
1740 Broadway
New York, N.Y. 10019

American Medical Association
535 N. Dearborn Street
Chicago, Ill. 60610
(312) 645-5000

American Osteopathic Association
212 E. Ohio Street
Chicago, Ill. 60611
(312) 280-5800

**American Physical Fitness
Research Institute**
654 No. Sepulveda Blvd.
Los Angeles, CA. 90049

**American Physical Therapy
Association**
1111 North Fairfax Street
Alexandria, VA. 22314
(703) 684-2782

**American Red Cross
Medical Operations**
National Headquarters
1730 E. St., N.W.
Washington, DC 20006
(202) 639-3011

American Society of Internal Medicine
1101 Vermont Ave., NW
Suite 500
Washington, D.C. 20005
(202) 289-1700

Arthritis Foundation
1314 Spring Street, N.W.
Atlanta, GA. 30309
(404) 872-7100

**Asthma and Allergy Foundation
of America**
1302 18th Street, N.W.
Washington, D.C. 20036
(202) 293-2950

Center for Sickle Cell Disease
2121 Georgia Ave., N.W.
Washington, D.C. 20059
(202) 636-7930

Citizens Alliance for VD Awareness
222 W. Adams Street
Chicago, Ill. 60606
(312) 236-6339

Cystic Fibrosis Foundation
6000 Executive Blvd.
Suite 510
Rockville, M.D. 20852

**Division of Sexually Transmitted
Diseases**
Centers for Disease Control
Freeway Office Park
Room 172
Atlanta, GA. 30333
(404) 329-2580

**The Epilepsy Foundation
of America**
4351 Garden City Drive
Suite 406
Landover, M.D. 20785
(301) 459-3700

**Food and Drug Administration
Press Office**
15B-42
5600 Fishers Lane
Rockville, M.D. 20857
(301) 443-4177 (301) 443-3285

**Food and Nutrition Board
National Academy of Sciences**
2101 Constitution Ave., N.W.
Washington, D.C. 20418
(202) 334-2581

**Institute of Rehabilitation Medicine
NYU Medical Center**
400 East 34th Street
New York, N.Y. 10016
(212) 340-5500

Joslin Diabetes Center
1 Joslin Place
Boston, MA. 02215
(617) 732-2415

**Juvenile Diabetes Foundation
International**
60 Madison Avenue
New York, New York 10010
(212) 889-7575

HEALTH ASSOCIATIONS AND ORGANIZATIONS

Leukemia Society of America
733 Third Avenue
New York, N.Y. 10017

**March of Dimes
Birth Defects Foundation**
1275 Mamaroneck Avenue
White Plains, N.Y. 10605
(914) 428-7100

**Medic-Alert Foundation
International**
2323 Colorado
P.O. Box 1009
Turlock, CA. 95381
(800) 344-3226

Muscular Dystrophy Association
810 7th Avenue
New York, N.Y. 10019
(212) 586-0808

**National Association of Anorexia
Nervosa & Associated Disorders**
Box 271
Highland Park, ILL. 60035
(312) 831-3438

National Association of the Deaf
814 Thayer Avenue
Silver Spring, MD. 20910
(301) 587-1788

**National Association of
Rehabilitation Facilities**
Box 17675
Washington, D.C. 20041
(703) 556-8848

**National Association for
Sickle Cell Disease**
3460 Wilshire Blvd.
Suite 1012
Los Angeles, Calif. 90010-2273
(213) 731-1166 1 (800)-421-8453

National Council on Alcoholism
12 West 21st St.
New York, N.Y. 10010
(212) 206-6770

National Federation of the Blind
1800 Johnson Street
Baltimore, MD. 21230
(301) 659-9314

**National Foundation for
Ileitis and Colitis**
444 Park Avenue South
New York, N.Y., 10016
(212) 685-3440

National Health Council
70 W. 40th Street
New York, N.Y. 10018
(212) 869-8100

National Hemophilia Foundation
19 W. 34th Street
Room 1204
New York, N.Y. 10001
(212) 563-0211

**National Institute on Alcohol Abuse
and Alcoholism
National Clearinghouse for
Alcohol Information**
P.O. Box 2345
Rockville, MD. 20852
(301) 468-2600

**National Institute on Drug Abuse
National Clearinghouse
for Drug Abuse Information**
P.O. Box 416
Kensington, MD. 20795
(301) 443-6500

National Institutes of Health
9000 Rockville Pike
Bethesda, MD. 20205
(301) 496-4000
  National Cancer Institute
  National Eye Institute
  National Heart, Lung, and Blood
  Institute
  National Institute of Allergy and
  Infectious Diseases
  National Institute of Arthritis,
    Diabetes, Digestive and Kidney
    Diseases
  National Institute of Child Health
  and Human Development
  National Institute of Dental
    Research
  National Institute of Environmental
  Health Sciences
  National Institute of General
    Medical Sciences
  National Institute of Neurological
    and Communicative Disorders
    and Strokes
  National Institute on Aging

National Kidney Foundation
2 Park Avenue
New York, N.Y. 10016
(212) 889-2210

National Mental Health Association
1021 Prince Street
Alexandria, VA. 22314
(703) 684-7722

National Multiple Sclerosis Society
205 E. 42nd Street
New York, N.Y. 10017
(212) 986-3240

National Parkinson Foundation
1501 N.W. 9th Avenue
Miami, Fla. 33136
(305) 547-6666

National Rehabilitation Association
633 S. Washington Street
Alexandria, VA. 22314
(703) 836-0850

**National Society for
Children and Adults with Autism**
1234 Massachusetts Ave., N.W.
Suite 1017
Washington, D.C. 20005
(202) 783-0125

National Society to Prevent Blindness
79 Madison Avenue
New York, N.Y. 10016-7896

**National Spinal Cord Injury
Association**
149 California Street
Newton, MA. 02158
(617) 964-0521

**Office on Smoking and Health
Technical Information Center**
5600 Fishers Lane
Park Building Room 1-16
Rockville, MD. 20857

**Planned Parenthood Federation
of America, Inc.**
810 Seventh Avenue
New York, N.Y. 10019
(212) 603-4695

Psoriasis Research Institute
(formerly the International Psoriasis
Research Foundation)
Post Office Box V
Stanford, CA. 94305
(415) 326-1848

**United Cerebral Palsy Associations,
Inc.**
66 E. 34th Street
New York, N.Y. 10016
(212) 481-6300

United Ostomy Association
2001 W. Beverly Blvd.
Los Angeles, CA. 90057
(213) 413-5510

**Wellness and Health Activation
Networks**
P.O. Box 923
Vienna, VA. 22180

Conversion Tables

Metric Doses With Approximate Apothecary Equivalents

The approximate dose equivalents represent the quantities usually prescribed by physicians using, respectively, the metric and apothecary system of weights and measures. When prepared dosage forms such as tablets, capsules, etc. are prescribed in the metric system, the pharmacist may dispense the corresponding approximate equivalent in the apothecary system and vice versa. (Note: A milliliter [mL] is the approximate equivalent of a cubic centimeter [cc]). Exact equivalents, which appear in the United States Pharmacopeia and the National Formulary, must be used to calculate quantities in pharmaceutical formulas and prescription compounding:

LIQUID MEASURE Metric	Approximate Apothecary Equivalents	**LIQUID MEASURE** Metric	Approximate Apothecary Equivalents	**LIQUID MEASURE** Metric	Approximate Apothecary Equivalents	**LIQUID MEASURE** Metric	Approximate Apothecary Equivalents
1000 mL	1 quart	3 mL	45 minims	30 mL	1 fluid ounce	0.25 mL	4 minims
750 mL	$1\frac{1}{2}$ pints	2 mL	30 minims	15 mL	4 fluid drams	0.2 mL	3 minims
500 mL	1 pint	1 mL	15 minims	10 mL	$2\frac{1}{2}$ fluid drams	0.1 mL	$1\frac{1}{2}$ minims
250 mL	8 fluid ounces	0.75 mL	12 minims	8 mL	2 fluid drams	0.06 mL	1 minim
200 mL	7 fluid ounces	0.6 mL	10 minims	5 mL	$1\frac{1}{4}$ fluid drams	0.05 mL	$\frac{3}{4}$ minim
100 mL	$3\frac{1}{2}$ fluid ounces	0.5 mL	8 minims	4 mL	1 fluid dram	0.03 mL	$\frac{1}{2}$ minim
50 mL	$1\frac{3}{4}$ fluid ounces	0.3 mL	5 minims				

WEIGHT Metric	Approximate Apothecary Equivalents	**WEIGHT** Metric	Approximate Apothecary Equivalents	**WEIGHT** Metric	Approximate Apothecary Equivalents	**WEIGHT** Metric	Approximate Apothecary Equivalents
30g	1 ounce	30mg	1/2 grain	500mg	$7\frac{1}{2}$ grains	1.2 mg	1/50 grain
15g	4 drams	25mg	3/8 grain	400mg	6 grains	1 mg	1/60 grain
10g	$2\frac{1}{2}$ drams	20mg	1/3 grain	300mg	5 grains	800 µg	1/80 grain
7.5g	2 drams	15mg	1/4 grain	250mg	4 grains	600 µg	1/100 grain
6g	90 grains	12mg	1/5 grain	200mg	3 grains	500 µg	1/120 grain
5g	75 grains	10mg	1/6 grain	150mg	$2\frac{1}{2}$ grains	400 µg	1/150 grain
4g	60 grains (1 dram)	8mg	1/8 grain	125mg	2 grains	300 µg	1/200 grain
3g	45 grains	6mg	1/10 grain	100mg	$1\frac{1}{2}$ grains	250 µg	1/250 grain
2g	30 grains ($\frac{1}{2}$ dram)	5mg	1/12 grain	75mg	$1\frac{1}{4}$ grains	200 µg	1/300 grain
1.5g	22 grains	4mg	1/15 grain	60mg	1 grain	150 µg	1/400 grain
1g	15 grains	3mg	1/20 grain	50mg	$\frac{1}{4}$ grain	120 µg	1/500 grain
750mg	12 grains	2mg	1/30 grain	40mg	$\frac{2}{3}$ grain	100 µg	1/600 grain
600mg	10 grains	1.5mg	1/40 grain				

Approximate Household Equivalents

For household purposes, an American Standard Teaspoon is defined by the American National Standards Institute as containing 4.93 ± 0.24 mL. The USP states that in view of the almost universal practice of employing teaspoons ordinarily available in the household for administration of medicine, the teaspoon may be regarded as representing 5 mL. Household units of measure often are used to inform patients of the size of a liquid dose. Because of difficulties involved in measuring liquids under normal conditions of use, household spoons are not appropriate when accurate measurement of a liquid dose is required. When accurate measurement of a liquid dose is required, the USP recommends that a calibrated oral syringe or dropper be used.

1 fluid dram = 1 teaspoonful = 5 mL
2 fluid drams = 1 dessertspoonful = 10 mL
4 fluid drams = 1 tablespoonful = 15 mL
2 fluid ounces = 1 wineglassful = 60 mL
4 fluid ounces = 1 teacupful = 120 mL
8 fluid ounces = 1 tumblerful = 240 mL

Temperature Conversion Table:

$$9 \times °C = (5 \times °F) - 160$$
Centigrade to Fahrenheit = (°C × 9/5) + 32 = °F
Fahrenheit to Centigrade = (°F − 32) × 5/9 = °C

Milliequivalents per Liter (mEq/L)

$$mEq/L = \frac{\text{weight of salt (g)} \times \text{valence of ion} \times 1000}{\text{molecular weight of salt}}$$

$$\text{weight of salt (g)} = \frac{mEq/L \times \text{molecular weight of salt}}{\text{valence of ion} \times 1000}$$

Pounds—Kilograms (kg) Conversion

1 pound = 0.453592 kg
1 kg = 2.2 pounds

Memorandum

Memorandum

Memorandum